Essential Neurology

Essential Neurology

Edited by Steven Graham

hayle
medical

New York

Hayle Medical,
750 Third Avenue, 9th Floor,
New York, NY 10017, USA

Visit us on the World Wide Web at:
www.haylemedical.com

ISBN: 978-1-63241-669-8

Cataloging-in-Publication Data

Essential neurology / edited by Steven Graham.
p. cm.
Includes bibliographical references and index.
ISBN 978-1-63241-669-8
1. Neurology. 2. Nervous system. 3. Nervous system--Diseases. I. Graham, Steven.
RC346 .E87 2019
616.8--dc23

Table of Contents

Preface... IX

Chapter 1   **Migraine-related disability and co-morbid depression among migraineurs**........................ 1
            Biniyam Alemayehu Ayele and Yared Mamushet Yifru

Chapter 2   **Comparison of the perioperative time courses of matrix
            metalloproteinase-9 (MMP-9) and its inhibitor (TIMP-1) during carotid
            artery stenting (CAS) and carotid endarterectomy (CEA)** 7
            Ákos Mérei, Bálint Nagy, Gábor Woth, János Lantos, Ferenc Kövér,
            Lajos Bogár and Diána Mühl

Chapter 3   **Do fragments and glycosylated isoforms of alpha-1-antitrypsin in CSF mirror
            spinal pathophysiological mechanisms in chronic peripheral neuropathic pain?
            An exploratory, discovery phase study** 14
            Emmanuel Bäckryd, Sofia Edström, Björn Gerdle and Bijar Ghafouri

Chapter 4   **Acute spontaneous intracerebral hemorrhage and traumatic brain injury are
            the most common causes of critical illness in the ICU and have high
            early mortality** 28
            Ye-Ting Zhou, Dao-Ming Tong, Shao-Dan Wang, Song Ye,
            Ben-Wen Xu and Chen-Xi Yang

Chapter 5   **A retrospective case series of segmental zoster paresis of limbs: clinical,
            electrophysiological and imaging characteristics** 35
            Ying Liu, Bing-Yun Wu, Zhen-Shen Ma, Juan-Juan Xu, Bing Yang,
            Heng Li and Rui-Sheng Duan

Chapter 6   **Altered levels of circulating insulin-like growth factor I (IGF-I)
            following ischemic stroke are associated with outcome** 44
            N. David Åberg, Daniel Åberg, Katarina Jood, Michael Nilsson,
            Christian Blomstrand, H. Georg Kuhn, Johan Svensson, Christina Jern and
            Jörgen Isgaard

Chapter 7   **Efficacy and safety of minimal invasive surgery treatment in hypertensive
            intracerebral hemorrhage** 56
            Yiping Tang, Fengqiong Yin, Dengli Fu, Xinhai Gao, Zhengchao Lv and
            Xuetao Li

Chapter 8   **Characterization of the symptoms of neurogenic orthostatic hypotension and
            their impact from a survey of patients and caregivers** 67
            Daniel O. Claassen, Charles H. Adler, L. Arthur Hewitt and
            Christopher Gibbons

Chapter 9   **Targeting the Notch1 oncogene by miR-139-5p inhibits glioma metastasis and epithelial-mesenchymal transition (EMT)** 76
Jianlong Li, Qingbin Li, Lin Lin, Rui Wang, Lingchao Chen, Wenzhong Du, Chuanlu Jiang and Ruiyan Li

Chapter 10   **"Recurrent multiple cerebral infarctions related to the progression of adenomyosis"** 89
Yasuhiro Aso, Ryo Chikazawa, Yuki Kimura, Noriyuki Kimura and Etsuro Matsubara

Chapter 11   **Clinical characteristics and short-term prognosis of LGI1 antibody encephalitis** 93
Weishuai Li, Si Wu, Qingping Meng, Xiaotian Zhang, Yang Guo, Lin Cong, Shuyan Cong and Dongming Zheng

Chapter 12   **Altered development of dopaminergic neurons differentiated from stem cells from human exfoliated deciduous teeth of a patient with Down syndrome** 101
Thanh Thi Mai Pham, Hiroki Kato, Haruyoshi Yamaza, Keiji Masuda, Yuta Hirofuji, Hiroshi Sato, Huong Thi Nguyen Nguyen, Xu Han, Yu Zhang, Tomoaki Taguchi and Kazuaki Nonaka

Chapter 13   **Electroclinical characteristics of seizures arising from the precuneus based on stereoelectroencephalography (SEEG)** 110
Yanfeng Yang, Haixiang Wang, Wenjing Zhou, Tianyi Qian, Wei Sun and Guoguang Zhao

Chapter 14   **Wearables for gait and balance assessment in the neurological ward - study design and first results of a prospective cross-sectional feasibility study with 384 inpatients** 121
Felix P. Bernhard, Jennifer Sartor, Kristina Bettecken, Markus A. Hobert, Carina Arnold, Yvonne G. Weber, Sven Poli, Nils G. Margraf, Christian Schlenstedt, Clint Hansen and Walter Maetzler

Chapter 15   **Intracranial pressure responsiveness to positive end-expiratory pressure is influenced by chest wall elastance: a physiological study in patients with aneurysmal subarachnoid hemorrhage** 129
Han Chen, Kai Chen, Jing-Qing Xu, Ying-Rui Zhang, Rong-Guo Yu and Jian-Xin Zhou

Chapter 16   **Planning for an uncertain future in progressive neurological disease: a qualitative study of patient and family decision-making with a focus on eating and drinking** 137
Gemma Clarke, Elizabeth Fistein, Anthony Holland, Jake Tobin, Sam Barclay and Stephen Barclay

Chapter 17   **Surgical treatment and perioperative management of intracranial aneurysms in Chinese patients with ischemic cerebrovascular diseases** 148
Yangrui Zheng and Chen Wu

Chapter 18   **The management of common recurrent headaches by chiropractors: a descriptive analysis of a nationally representative survey** 153
Craig Moore, Andrew Leaver, David Sibbritt and Jon Adams

Chapter 19   **Atypical sensory processing pattern following median or ulnar nerve injury** 162
Pernilla Vikström, Anders Björkman, Ingela K. Carlsson, Anna-Karin Olsson and Birgitta Rosén

Chapter 20   **Long-term, telephone-based follow-up after stroke and TIA improves risk factors: 36-month results from the randomized controlled NAILED stroke risk factor trial**.. 168
Joachim Ögren, Anna-Lotta Irewall, Lars Söderström and Thomas Mooe

Chapter 21   **Visual outcome is similar in optic neuritis patients treated with oral and i.v. high-dose methylprednisolone: a retrospective study on 56 patients**........................ 177
Magdalena Naumovska, Rafi Sheikh, Boel Bengtsson, Malin Malmsjö and Björn Hammar

Chapter 22   **Comorbidity of migraine with ADHD in adults**.. 184
Thomas Folkmann Hansen, Louise K. Hoeffding, Lisette Kogelman, Thilde Marie Haspang, Henrik Ullum, Erik Sørensen, Christian Erikstrup, Ole Birger Pedersen, Kaspar René Nielsen, Henrik Hjalgrim, Helene M. Paarup, Thomas Werge and Kristoffer Burgdorf

Chapter 23   **Study protocol: Care of Late-Stage Parkinsonism (CLaSP)**................................ 192
Monika Balzer-Geldsetzer, Joaquim Ferreira, Per Odin, Bastiaan R. Bloem, Wassilios G. Meissner, Stefan Lorenzl, Michael Wittenberg, Richard Dodel and Anette Schrag

Chapter 24   **Comparative effectiveness of betainterferons and glatiramer acetate for relapsing-remitting multiple sclerosis**.. 200
G. J. Melendez-Torres, Xavier Armoiry, Rachel Court, Jacoby Patterson, Alan Kan, Peter Auguste, Jason Madan, Carl Counsell, Olga Ciccarelli and Aileen Clarke

Chapter 25   **Association between medication-related adverse events and non-elective readmission in acute ischemic stroke**... 217
James A. G. Crispo, Dylan P. Thibault, Yannick Fortin, Daniel Krewski and Allison W. Willis

Chapter 26   **The psychometric properties of the Childhood Health Assessment Questionnaire (CHAQ) in children with cerebral palsy** 227
Soojung Chae, Eun-Young Park and Yoo-Im Choi

Permissions

List of Contributors

Index

Preface

The disorders of the central and peripheral nervous system are studied, diagnosed and treated under neurology. These conditions include Parkinson's disease, Alzheimer's disease, neuromuscular diseases, neuropathy, and infections and tumors of the nervous system, among others. Such disorders may affect the peripheral, central or autonomic nervous system. These are diagnosed using a range of diagnostic techniques from MRI, CAT and EEG scans to nerve conduction studies and needle electromyography. Lumbar puncture is a common procedure for assessing a patient's cerebrospinal fluid. Surgical interventions for the management of neurological disorders can be a viable option in certain cases, while in others medications and physiotherapy are recommended management strategies. An active area of research in neurology is the role of genetics in the development of neurologic diseases. This book elucidates the concepts and innovative models around prospective developments with respect to neurology. It presents researches and studies performed by experts across the globe. It is meant for students who are looking for an elaborate reference text on neurology.

The information contained in this book is the result of intensive hard work done by researchers in this field. All due efforts have been made to make this book serve as a complete guiding source for students and researchers. The topics in this book have been comprehensively explained to help readers understand the growing trends in the field.

I would like to thank the entire group of writers who made sincere efforts in this book and my family who supported me in my efforts of working on this book. I take this opportunity to thank all those who have been a guiding force throughout my life.

Editor

Migraine-related disability and co-morbid depression among migraineurs

Biniyam Alemayehu Ayele*[ORCID] and Yared Mamushet Yifru

Abstract

Background: Migraine headache is a neurologic disorder which mainly affects younger and productive segment of population. Migraine not only causes pain; but also affects quality of life in terms of low productivity and economic loss. The main aim of this study was to examine migraine-related disability, co-morbid depression, and relationship between the two.

Methods: A cross-sectional study was conducted among migraineurs who visited two neurology referral clinics. The study was conducted between June 1st 2016 to December 30th 2016. Migraine disability assessment score [MIDAS] and patient health questionnaire [PHQ-9] were used to assess disability and depression, respectively.

Results: A total of 70 patients participated in the study. Fifty-three (74.3%) of our study participants were women. Fifty one (72.9%) study participants were between age group 20–40 years. Migraine without aura was the most common subtype (70%); migraine with aura accounted for the other 28.6%. The mean (± SD) headache frequency and intensity was 23.4 ± 14.9 days and 7.4 ± 1.2 respectively. Major depressive disorder was common in this group (41.4%). The mean MIDAS and PHQ-9 scores were 46.7 ± 30 and 9.2 ± 4.4 respectively. More than two-thirds (74.3%) of our participants had severe disability. We found a statistically significant correlation between migraine-related disability and co morbid depression among our participants($r = 0.318$, p-value $= 0.007$).

Conclusion: The positive correlation observed between migraine-related disability and co-morbid depression warrant routine screening and treatment of disability and depression in migraineurs; In addition, the observed high degree of disability among our participants may indicate sub optimal treatment of these patients.

Keywords: Migraine, Depression, Disability, Co morbidity, PHQ-9, MIDAS

Background

Migraine is a disabling neurologic disorder; characterized by recurrent and often unilateral headaches. Migraine causes substantial psychological and economic impact on the individual and society at large [1]. It is three times more common in women than men. Symptoms such as: nausea, vomiting, photophobia and phonophobia are often present in most migraineurs; and a few report osmophobia [2]. Migraine is common. According to the Global Burden of Disease survey (GBD 2010), its estimated prevalence was close to 15% among the general population [3]. In patients with migraine, recurrent episodes have the potential to progress to the more frequent and severe attacks of chronic migraine (CM), which affects 2.4% of the general, population [4]. Migraine headache is classified into two broad categories; migraine with aura and migraine without aura. Migraine without aura is a clinical syndrome characterized by headache and associated autonomic features but without any warning symptoms, also known as aura. Migraine with aura is characterized by focal neurological symptoms that may precede or sometimes accompany headache [5].

Ethiopia is the second most populous country in Africa, with a population of more than 100 million. Population-based studies done in Ethiopia in the past two decades have shown the prevalence of migraine headache to be between 3 to 17.7% [6, 7]. In a recent

* Correspondence: biniyam.alemayehu@aau.edu.et; biniyam.a7@gmail.com
Department of Neurology, College of Health Science, Addis Ababa Univeristy, PO BOX: 6396, Addis Ababa, Ethiopia

Ethiopian study of migraine in relation to psychiatric co-morbidities, participants with moderate to severe depressive symptoms had a 3-fold increased odds of migraine compared with those with minimal or no depressive symptoms, and the odds of migraine increased with increasing severity of depressive symptoms [8]. Migraine is documented as a major cause of disability worldwide. According to the World Health Report, migraine is the 19th leading cause of Years of Life with Disability. In addition, the global Burden of Headache reported migraine as the leading cause of disability among neurological disorders; and globally migraine was ranked as the seventh highest cause of disability [9–11].

It has long been known that migraine is associated with a number of medical and psychiatric conditions. One of the most common psychiatric co-morbidity is depression; which is reported in up to 80% of patients, especially in chronic migraine [12]. Patients with migraine are two to four times more likely to develop lifetime major depression as compared to those without migraine [13]. Different Studies suggest that the presence of depression in migraine patients significantly increase the level of disability that these patients experience in their daily life. As such, depression is associated with a greater incidence of severe disability. Patients with severe disability are six times more prone to have depression compared to those with lower disability [13, 14].

The Presence of clinical depression in a migraineurs is not only associated with more frequent and severe headaches, it also has the risk of transforming episodic migraine to chronic migraine. Chronic migraine is more disabling and often refractory to treatment [15]. The co-existence of depression can also adversely affect the quality of life by increasing the burden of the disease [15, 16]. We did this study with the main objective, to determine the relationship between migraine-related disability co-morbid depression among migraineurs having a follow-up at two neurology referral clinics in Addis Ababa, Ethiopia.

Even though multiple studies done elsewhere confirm the positive correlation between migraine-related disability and co-morbid depression, to the authors' best knowledge, this is the first study of its kind to assess disability and depressive symptoms and their association among migraineurs in Ethiopia. As a result, we believe this study will be a baseline study for Ethiopia and other sub-Saharan countries.

Methods

This is an observational, cross-sectional, hospital based study conducted between June 1st 2016 to December 30th 2016. Demographic variables included in this study were age, sex, marital status, educational status, occupation and religion. The study was conducted at Tikur Anbessa Specialized Hospital (TASH), a university teaching hospital and the only tertiary level referral hospital in Ethiopia; located at the heart of Addis Ababa and Zewditu Memorial Hospital (ZMH), a government referral hospital also located in Addis Ababa having affiliation to Addis Ababa University.

Data collection was started after obtaining formal approval letter from Institutional Review Board (IRB) of College of Health Sciences, Addis Ababa University. Inclusion criteria was all migraine patients attending both neurology referral clinics during the study period in which a diagnosis of migraine (both migraine with aura and migraine without aura) was made by a neurologist based on the International Classification of Headache Disorders (ICHD-3) and having age greater than 13 years (by tradition patients with age > 13 years are seen at adult outpatients clinic in our hospital) [5]. An exclusion criterion was migraine patients having additional diagnosis of other primary headache disorders like tension type headache (Tables 1 and 2).

A total of 72 patients with confirmed diagnosis of migraine were interviewed. Two patients were excluded because of the co-occurrence of tension type headache with migraine headache. The demographic and clinical data were collected from structured survey questionnaire. Disability was assessed by Migraine Disability Assessment Score [MIDAS], well validated disability screening tool. MIDAS is simple to administer, easily interpreted and has been validated in population-based samples [17]. MIDAS is graded in to four grades; Grade I (little or no disability, scores range 0–5), grade II (mild disability, scores range 6–10), grade III (moderate disability, scores range 11–20), and grade IV (severe disability, 21 or greater).

The Patient Health Questionnaire [PHQ-9] was used to screen depression. PHQ-9 is a nine-question screening instrument for depressive symptoms based on Diagnostic and Statistical Manual of Mental Disorders (DSM) IV criteria to diagnose depression and also a validated tool in African population [18, 19]. PHQ-9 has also been validated in

Table 1 Diagnostic criteria for migraine without aura

A. At least five attacks fulfilling criteria B–D

B. Headache attacks lasting 4–72 h (untreated or unsuccessfully treated)

C. Headache has at least two of the following four characteristics:
  1. Unilateral location
  2. Pulsating quality
  3. Moderate or severe pain intensity
  4. Aggravation by or causing avoidance of routine physical activity (walking or climbing stairs)

D. During headache at least one of the following
  1. Nausea and/or vomiting
  2. Photophobia and Phonophobia

E. Not better accounted for by another ICHD-3 diagnosis.

Note. ICDH. The International Classification of Headache Disorders: 3rd edition. Cephalalgia. 2013; 33:9; 629–808

Table 2 Diagnostic criteria for migraine aura:-

A. At least two attacks fulfilling criteria B–C

B. One or more of the following fully reversible aura symptoms:

   1. visual

   2. sensory

   3. speech and/or language

   4. motor

   5. brainstem

   6. retinal

C. At least two of the following four characteristics:

   1. At least one aura symptom spreads gradually over 5 min, and/or two or more symptoms occur in succession

   2. Each individual aura symptom lasts 5–60 min1

   3. At least one aura symptom is unilateral2

   4. The aura is accompanied, or followed within 60 min, by headache

D. Not better accounted for by another ICHD-3 diagnosis, and transient ischemic attack has been excluded.

Note. ICDH. The International Classification of Headache Disorders: 3rd edition. Cephalalgia. 2013; 33:9; 629–808

Table 3 Frequency distribution of socio-demographic characteristics of migraine patients. $N = 70$

Variables	Number	Percent
Gender		
Male	18	25.7
Female	52	74.3
Age groups		
14–20	4	5.7
20–30	28	40
30–40	25	35.7
40–65	13	18.6
Marital status		
Single	23	32.9
Married	33	47.1
In a relationship	5	7.1
Divorced	8	11.4
Widowed	1	1.5
Occupational status		
Government employee	34	48.6
Student	9	12.9
Private business	13	18.6
House wife	7	10.0
Farmer	2	2.9
Jobless	2	2.9
Other	3	4.3
Educational status		
Illiterate	2	2.9
Read and write only	3	4.3
Primary education (1–8)	8	11.4
Secondary education (8–12)	20	28.6
Diploma	18	25.7
Degree and above	19	27.1

Ethiopia [20]. All the interviews were conducted by the two investigators; both neurologists. The statistical analysis was performed using SPSS version 20.0 computer program. Chi square test with p values and crude odds ratio (OR) with a 95% confidence interval (CI) were used to determine to statistical associations of selected variables.

A p-value < 0.05 was considered significant. Descriptive summaries were employed for socio-demographic and other clinical variables. Analytical statistics including bivariate analysis with Spearman's correlation were performed to determine the correlation between; disability and depression.

Results

Of the seventy migraine patients interviewed at the two Neurology clinics in Addis Ababa, three-fourths (74.3%) were female. More than two third (72.9%) of our study participants were between age group 20–40 years, 5.7% were < 20 years and 18.6% of them were > 40 years (Table 3). Thirty-three (47.1%) were married and 8 (11.4%) of them were divorced. Thirty four (48.6%) patients were government employees, 9 (12.9%) were students and only 2(2.9%) were unemployed. One-third (28.6%) of the study participants had a secondary school education and 27.1% had a Bachelor's degree or above educational level (Table 3).

Among women migraineurs, 31.5% experienced worsening or occurrence of their migraine headache during menses. The majority of our study participants (70%) had migraine without aura, while 28.6% of our participants reported auras of different type prior to their migraine attack. Whether patients with aura did have at times headache episodes without accompanying aura was not specifically queried. One patient found to have diagnosis of ophthalmoplegic migraine (1.4%).

The majority of participants had a diagnosis of migraine by a physician less than five years ago (54.3%), while24.3% had it for 5–10 years. The rest of our participants (21.4%) had migraine for more than 10 years (Table 4). Among our study participants 31.5% of them are on medications for migraine prophylaxis; including 25.1% on Amitriptyline, 5.9% on propranolol and 0.5% on Imipramine (Table 4).

The mean PHQ-9 score in our study was 9.2 ± 4.4. Severe depressive symptoms were present in 14.3% of study participants, while 45.7% had a PHQ-9 score between 5 and 9, indicative of mild depressive disorder. Many (41.4%) of our

Table 4 Frequency distribution of headache-related characteristics of migraine patients. $N = 70$

Migraine headache worsening/ occurring during Menses		%
	Yes	31.5
	No	68.5
	Total	100
Subtype of Migraine	Migraine without aura	70.0
	Migraine with aura	28.6
	Ophtalmopelgic migraine	1.4
	Total	100
Duration of Migraine headache	< 05 years	54.3
	5–10 years	24.3
	> 10 years	21.4
	Total	100
Migraine prophylaxis	Amitriptyline	25.1
	Propranolol	5.9
	Imipramine	0.5
	Total	31.5

participants fulfilled criteria for major depressive disorder (Table 5). The mean MIDAS score was 46.7 ± 30. Over two-third of our patients (74.3%) had severe disability, defined as MIDAS score ≥ 21, while 15.7%, had moderate and 8.6% mild disability. Only 1.4% of our study participants had little or no disability (Table 6).

Spearman's correlation was used to examine associations between co-morbid depression and disability. There was a significant ($p = 0.007$) correlation between severe disability (Grade IV) and depression (PHQ-9, Grade II-IV) for both minor and major depressive disorders, compared to non-depressed patients (PHQ-9, Grade I). Spearman's coefficient of this correlation is $r = 0.318$, indicating positive correlation between depression and severe disability (Table 7). Depression was associated with occurrence of severe disability; severe disability was found to be 8 times more common in patients with depression in comparison to those having no depression. Depressed migraine patients were five times more likely to have severe disability ($p = 0.007$) compared to non-depressed patients. In our study; we also found a statistically significant ($p = 0.002$)

Table 5 Patient Health Questioners (PHQ-9) score of migraine patients. $N = 70$

PHQ-9	Mean(SD)	9.2 ± 4.4
Minimal (0–4)	%	12.9
Mild (5–9)	%	45.7
Moderate(10–14)	%	27.1
Severe(> = 15)	%	14.3

Table 6 Migraine Disability Assessment Scale (MIDAS) score of migraine patients. $N = 70$

MIDAS Scoring	Mean(SD)	46.7 ± 30
Little or no disability (0–5)	%	1.4
Mild disability (6–10)	%	8.6
Moderate disability (11–20)	%	15.7
Severe disability (> = 21)	%	74.3

association between migraine-related disability and migraine occuring during menses (Table 8).

Discussion

Most of our participants were females, and two-thirds of them had migraine without aura. Significant proportion of the study participants fulfilled the criteria for major depressive disorders, and many of them had severe disability scores. We also found a strong correlation between disability and co- morbid depression among migraineurs. Most of the migraine- related clinical characteristics, like female preponderance, high proportion of migraine without aura observed in our study, are comparable to prior published studies on migraine from both developing and developed countries [21].

We observed one patient with diagnosis of ophthalmoplegic migraine in our study; which we also saw in other reported cases from Ethiopia in the past few years [22, 23]. When we compare our findings with the study done by Pavlović 2015 and his colleagues, in which 60% of women with migraine reported an association between migraine attack and menses [24], our finding show much lower than this, only one third of our participants reported an association between migraine attack and menses; which could be attributable to lack of awareness among our patients about the possible association between menses and migraine and not using the headache diary, which often is helpful in tracking such precipitating causes.

Close to half of our participants are government employees (Table 3) and their diagnosis of migraine was made in less than five years (Table 4). This might be due to the fact that the study was done in the capital city, Addis Ababa, where better neurologic service was started only recently.

Table 7 Correlation between degree of disability and depression among migraine patients. $N = 70$

	MIDAS score		P-value	Spearman coefficient
	MIDAS Grade < IV	MIDAS Grade IV		
PHQ-9 Grade II-IV	47	14	0.007	0.318
PHQ-9 Grade I	5	4		
Total	52	18		70

Spearman coefficient = 0.318; indicative of positive correlation. Statistically significant P-value < 0.001, 95% CI

Table 8 Association between disability and migraine during menses among migraine patients. $N = 70$

	MIDAS score		Total	P-value
	MIDAS Grade < IV	MIDAS Grade IV		0.02
Headache During menses				
Yes	7	12	19	
No	34	17	51	
Total	41	29	70	

Statistically Significant P-value < 0.05, 95% CI

Two factors may explain the higher prevalence of migraine-related disability among our study participants. First, the fact that this is a hospital based study and most likely many of our patients had prolonged treatment by general practitioners in other facilities then referred for better assessment and treatment by a neurologist. Secondly, the suboptimal treatment and lack of screening for management of disability and co -morbid events like depression may also contribute to the higher level of morbidity.

An interesting finding in this study is high proportion of our study participants were on amitriptyline for migraine prophylaxis, yet significant proportion had persistent major depressive disorder (MDD). This may be due to use of low doses of amitriptyline, which is inadequate to treat depression as well as lack of psychotherapy.

Regarding co-morbid depression based on PHQ-9 score; the mean PHQ-9 (Table 5) of our study is comparable to the finding from Canadian study, in which the mean PHQ-9 score was 8 [25]. Among our study participants, significant proportion of them fulfilled the criteria for Major depressive disorder with PHQ-9 ≥ 10 (Table 5), which is comparable to one meta-analysis which reported the incidence of depression in migraineurs to be between 8.6 to 47.9% [26].

Our mean MIDAS score (Table 6) with higher than those reported from studies done in Turkey (19.3 ± 12.3) and Italy (12 ± 8.2) [27, 28]. More than two third of our study participants had severe disability with a MIDAS score ≥ 21 (Table 6), which is much higher than the result from a similar study from Turkey, in which severe disability was noted in 40%. One study done in South Korea reported a much higher MIDAS score of 54.1 ± 49.9, mainly among chronic migraine patients in their study [29].

In our study, depression was associated with greater incidence of severe disability. Our finding is comparable to those results reported from South Korea [29] and another study reported by JL Brandes et al. [30] which showed patients with MDD had significant association with severe disability [MIDAS Grade IV], compared to non-depressed migraineurs. We also found a statistically significant (p 0.02) association between migraine-related disabilities in migraine occurring during menses; this

finding highlights the need to routinely look for aggravation of migraine during menses, so that we may be able to optimize both abortive and preventive migraine treatment in such situation.

Limitations of our study include a small sample size and the fact that this is hospital-based study with likelihood of over representation of more severe cases. As a result we acknowledge the limited generalizability of these findings to the whole population. In addition, for both the screening tools we were dependent on patient's ability to remember symptoms in the past two weeks for depression screening and three months for disability, which could have introduced recall bias.

Conclusion

We conclude from our analysis that there is a higher proportion of severe disability and co-morbid depression with positive correlation between the two in migraine. Our findings show the importance of screening for disability and depression in migraine patients, as this might guide our management approach and impact their overall therapeutic outcome.

Finally, this study points to the need for large scale longitudinal, observational study in Ethiopia to evaluate the relationship between migraine-related disability and co-morbid depression.

Abbreviations

MIDAS: Migraine Disability Assessment Score; PHQ-9: Patient Health Questioner 9; TASH: Tikur Anbessa Specialized Hospital; ZMH: Zewditu Memorial Hospital; MDD: Major Depressive Disorder

Acknowledgements

– I would like to extend my heartfelt gratitude all the nursing staffs at both neurology referral clinics were the survey was conducted, above all my heartfelt gratitude goes to all participants of this study.
– We would like to extend our greatest appreciation to prof. Douglas Dulli who spends his valuable time in correcting the typo and language errors of our manuscript.

Funding

– No funding was received from any organization or individuals.

Authors' contributions

BAA and YMY participated in data acquisition, data analysis, data interpretation and manuscript editing and preparation. Both authors read and approved the final manuscript.

Authors' information

1. Biniyam Alemayehu Ayele, MD, Assistant professor of neurology
   – Staff at department of neurology, College of Health Science, Addis Ababa Univeristy
   – Teach clinical neurology to both undergraduate medical students and graduate students including neurology residents.
   – Work as consultant neurologist at Tikur Anbessa Specialized University Hospital and Zewditu Memorial Hospital.
   – Involved in different research projects in field of neuroscience in Ethiopia.
   – Have special interest in Headache disorders, Clinical neurophysiology and movement disorders.
   – Member of International Headache society(IHS)
   – Email: biniyam.alemayehu.aau.edu.et/biniyam.a7@gmail.com
2. Yared Mamushet Yifru, MD, MSc, Headache specialist
   – Assistant professor of Neurology at department of neurology, College of Health Science Addis Ababa Univeristy, Ethiopia.
   – Teach clinical neurology to both undergraduate medical students and graduate students including neurology residents.
   – Work as consultant neurologist at Tikur Anbessa Specialized University Hospital and Zewditu Memorial Hospital.
   – Involved in different research projects in field of neuroscience in Ethiopia.
   – Have special interest in Headache disorders, strokes and movement disorders.
   – Email: yared_mty@yahoo.com

Ethics approval and consent to participate

– Ethical approval letter was obtained from Institutional Review Board of the College of Health Sciences, Addis Ababa University, with protocol number: 017/16/Neuro on meeting No: 005/16, on May25, 2016.
– All participants/their guardians gave informed written consent before taking part in the study.
– The research was performed in accordance with the Declaration of Helsinki.
– Written informed consent was obtained from patients and for those under the age of 18 years from their legal guardians before proceeding to interview.

Competing interests

– The authors declare that they have no competing interests.

References

1. L. M. Bloudek, M. Stokes, D., C. Buse,T. K. Wilcox, R. B. Lipton, P. J. Goadsby,S. F. Varon, A. M. Blumenfeld, Z. KatsaravaJ. Pascual, M. Lanteri-Minet, P. Cortelli, P. Martelletti et al. cost of healthcare for patients with migraine in five European countries- results from the international burden of migraine study (IBMS). J Headache Pain.2012; 13:361–378.
2. Robert BD, Joseph J, John CM, Scott LP. Headache and other craniofacial pain. In: Ivan G, Todd JS, Carrie ER, Jonathan HS, editors. Bradely, Neurology in clinical practice. 7th ed. China: Elsevier; 2016. p. 1695–706.
3. Vos T, Flaxman AD, Naghavi M, Lozano R, Michaud C, Ezzati M, Shibuya K, Salomon JA, Abdalla S, Aboyans V, Abraham J, Ackerman I, Aggarwal R, Ahn SY, Ali MK, Alvarado M, Anderson HR, Anderson LM, Andrews KG, Atkinson C, Baddour LM, Bahalim AN, Barker-Collo S, Barrero LH, Bartels DH, Basáñez MG, Baxter A, Bell ML, Benjamin EJ, Bennett D, et al. Years lived with disability (YLDs) for 1160 sequelae of 289 diseases and injuries 1990–2010: a systematic analysis for the global burden of disease study 2010. Lancet. 2012;380:2163–96.
4. Castillo J, Munoz P, Guitera V, et al. Epidemiology of chronic daily headache in the general population. Headache. 1998;39:190–6.
5. ICDH. The International Classification of Headache Disorders: 3rd edition. Cephalalgia. 2013;33(9):629–808.
6. Tekle Haimanot R, Seraw B, Forsgren L, Ekbom K, Ekstedt J. Migraine, chronic tension-type headache, and cluster headache in an Ethiopian rural community. Cephalalgia. 1995; https://doi.org/10.1046/j.1468-2982.1995.1506482.x.
7. Mihila Z, Tekle-Haimanot R, Dawit DK, Thomas H, Steiner TJ. The prevalence of primary headache disorders in Ethiopia. J Headache Pain. 2016; https://doi.org/10.1186/s10194-016-0704-z.
8. Bizu G, Lee BP, Seblewongel L, Markos T. Migraine and psychiatric comorbidities among sub-Saharan African adults. Headache. 2013; https://doi.org/10.1111/j.1526-4610.2012.02259.x.
9. Leonardi M, Steiner TJ, Scher AT, Lipton RB, et al. The global burden of migraine-measuring disability in headache disorders with WHO's classification of functioning, disability and health (ICF). J Headache Pain. 2005;6:429–40.
10. World Health Organization. Atlas of Headache Disorders and Resources in the World. Geneva: World Health Organization; 2011. www.who.int. ISBN 978 924 15642 12.
11. Steiner TJ, Stovner LJ, Birbeck GL, et al. Migraine - the seventh disabler. J Headache Pain. 2013;14:1.
12. Mercante JP, Peres MF, Vera G, Eliova Z, Marcio AB, et al. DEPRESSION IN CHRONIC MIGRAINE. ArqNeuropsiquiatr. 2005;63(2):217–20.
13. Breslau N, Lipton RB, et al. Co morbidity of migraine and depression. Neurology. 2003;60:1308–12.
14. Breslau N, Davis GC, et al. Migraine and major depression – a longitudinal study. HEADACHE J HEAD AND FACE PAIN. 1994;34:387–93.
15. Jette N., et al. Comorbidity of migraine and psychiatric disorders - a national population-based study. Headache 2008;48; 4: 501–16.
16. Shehbaz N, Ali S, et al. MIGRAINE - COMORBIDITY WITH DEPRESSION. Pak J Med Sci. 2007;23(1):95–9.
17. Stewart WF, et al. Reliability of the migraine disability assessment score in a population based sample of headache sufferers. Cephalalgia. 1999;19(2):107–14.
18. Monahan PO, Shacham E, Reece M, et al. Validity/reliability of PHQ-9 and PHQ-2 depression scales among adults living with HIV/AIDS in western Kenya. J Gen Intern Med. 2009;24:189–97.
19. Omoro SA, Fann JR, Weymuller EA, Macharia IM, Yueh B, et al. Swahili translation and validation of the patient health Questionnaire-9 depression scale in the Kenyan head and neck cancer patient population. Int J Psychiatry Med. 2006;36:367–81.
20. Charlotte H, Girmay M, Medhin S, et al. Validity of brief screening questionnaires to detect depression in primary care in Ethiopia. J Affect Disord. 2015;186:32–9.
21. Gobel H, Petersen-Braun M, Soyka D, et al. The epidemiology of headache in Germany - a nationwide survey of a representative sample on the basis of the headache classification of the international headache society. Cephalalgia. 1994;14:97–106.
22. Ayele BA, Mengistu G, Wako AA, et al. Adult variant of ophthalmologic migraine with recurrent 6th cranial nerve palsy in 25yrs old Ethiopian patient - case report. J Neurol Stroke. 2016; https://doi.org/10.15406/jnsk.2016.04.00158.
23. Arasho BD, et al. Ophthalmoplegic migraine in a 15-year-old Ethiopian - case report and literature review. J Headache Pain. 2009;10(1):45–9.
24. Jelena MP, Walter FS, Christa AB, Jennifer AG, Haiyan S, Dawn CB, Richard BL, et al. Burden of migraine related to menses - results from the AMPP study. J Headache Pain. 2015; https://doi.org/10.1186/s10194-015-0503-y.
25. Amoozegar F, et al. The prevalence of depression and the accuracy of depression screening tools in migraine patients. Report. Univeristy of Calgary. Alberta APRIL. 2014.
26. Antonaci F, et al. Migraine and psychiatric comorbidity -a review of clinical findings. J Headache Pain. 2011;12(2):115–25.
27. Eraslan D, Dikmen PY, et al. The relation of sexual function to migraine-related disability, depression and anxiety in patients with migraine. J Headache Pain. 2014;15:32.
28. CORALLO F COLAMC, et al. Assessment of anxiety, depressive disorders and pain intensity in migraine and tension headache patients. ActaMedicaMediterranea. 2015;31:615.
29. Kim SY, Park SP, et al. The role of headache chronicity among predictors contributing to quality of life in patients with migraine - a hospital-based study. J Headache Pain. 2014;15:68.
30. J I B, Roberson SC, et al. The relationship between co-morbid depression and migraine disability. Advanced studies in medicine. 2002;2:16.

Comparison of the perioperative time courses of matrix metalloproteinase-9 (MMP-9) and its inhibitor (TIMP-1) during carotid artery stenting (CAS) and carotid endarterectomy (CEA)

Ákos Mérei[1,3]* , Bálint Nagy[1,3,4], Gábor Woth[1,3,4], János Lantos[2], Ferenc Kövér[5], Lajos Bogár[1,4] and Diána Mühl[1]

Abstract

Background: Our aim was to compare the perioperative time courses of matrix metalloproteinase-9 (MMP-9) and its inhibitor (TIMP-1) in during carotid endarterectomy (CEA) and carotid artery stenting (CAS).

Methods: In our prospective study, twenty-five patients who were scheduled to undergo CAS were enrolled. We used a matched, historical CEA group as controls. Blood samples were collected at four time points: T1: preoperative; T2: 60 min after stent insertion; T3: first postoperative morning; and T4: third postoperative morning. Plasma MMP-9 and TIMP-1 levels were measured by ELISA.

Results: In the CEA group, the plasma levels of MMP-9 were significantly elevated at T3 compared to T1. In the CAS group, there was no significant difference in MMP-9 levels in the perioperative period. MMP-9 levels were significantly higher in the T3 samples of the CEA group compared to the CAS group. Significantly lower TIMP-1 levels were measured in both groups at T2 than at T1 in both groups. MMP-9/TIMP-1 at T3 was significantly higher than that at T1 in the CEA group compared to both T1 and the CAS group.

Conclusions: CAS triggers smaller changes in the MMP-9-TIMP-1 system during the perioperative period, which may correlate with a lower incidence of central nervous system complications. Additional studies as well as cognitive and functional surveys are warranted to determine the clinical relevance of our findings.

Keywords: Carotid stenting, Carotid endarterectomy, Matrix metalloproteinase, MMP-9, TIMP-1

Background

Ischaemic stroke is one of the leading causes of death, dementia and disability in the developed world [1, 2]. Among stroke survivors, the risk of recurrent attacks remains high. Significant stenosis of the internal carotid artery is a well-known risk factor of ischaemic stroke [3].

Intervention of the stenotic carotid artery can decrease the risk of stroke. The gold standard intervention is carotid endarterectomy (CEA), but carotid artery stenting (CAS) is a less invasive therapeutic method with increasing popularity [4–6]. Although both methods have well-known complications, clinical trials have found that the risk of death or recurrent stroke within 30 days of surgery in symptomatic patients was higher among the CAS patients than among the CEA patients [7–12]. According to the 2014 AHA/ASA stroke prevention guideline for low- or average-risk symptomatic patients, CAS is an alternative to CEA when the internal carotid

* Correspondence: merei.akos@gmail.com
[1]Department of Anaesthesiology and Intensive Therapy, Medical School, University of Pécs, Ifjúság Str. 13, Pécs HU-7624, Hungary
[3]Medical Skills Lab, Medical School, University of Pécs, Szigeti Str. 12, Pécs HU-7624, Hungary
Full list of author information is available at the end of the article

artery stenosis is greater than 70% by non-invasive imaging or greater than 50% by catheter-based imaging and if the anticipated rate of periprocedural stroke or death is less than 6% [13]. For patients younger than 70 years old, the risk of periprocedural complications (stroke, myocardial infarction or death) and the long-term risk of ipsilateral stroke is equal whether they undergo CAS or CEA [13]. CAS is also a reasonable treatment modality among patients with symptomatic severe stenosis (> 70%) and concurrent anatomic or medical conditions that increase the risks of surgery or in cases with specific circumstances such as radiation-induced stenosis or restenosis after CEA [13].

The gold standards of periprocedural stroke diagnosis are clinical parameters and neuroimaging. In recent years, various biomarkers of neural damage have been tested and validated; however, a single biomarker that is capable of identifying neural damage is not yet available [14]. Matrix metalloproteinases (MMPs) and their tissue inhibitors (TIMPs) have already been examined in CEA- and CEA-associated periprocedural stroke [15, 16]. MMPs play a crucial role in extracellular matrix turnover, degradation and remodelling. In addition, the effects of MMPs in signalling pathways have been confirmed and evaluated in various physiological and pathophysiological conditions [17–19]. Matrix metalloproteinase-9 (MMP-9) is a gelatinase enzyme and a marker of inflammation. Although it lacks specificity in the monitoring of neuronal damage, increased perivascular tissue levels and microglial production of MMP-9 were observed in acute stroke patients. Higher MMP-9 levels have been found to be associated with increased oxidative stress, apoptosis, blood-brain-barrier (BBB) dysfunction and development of cerebral oedema [20]. According to in vitro results, TIMP-1 can play a protective role in neuronal apoptosis and neurotrophic action, but in vivo data are controversial, as the possibility of secondary TIMP-1 increases as a result of BBB injury [21]. The interaction between MMPs and TIMPs is stoichiometric, and therefore, MMP/TIMP ratios can be used to reflect MMP-TIMP activity.

In one of our earlier studies, we examined the time course of CEA-related changes in MMP-9 and TIMP-1 [22]. Although Giuliani et al. investigated the levels of MMP-9 (and other biomarkers) in CEA patients versus CAS patients, the perioperative changes in the plasma levels of MMP-9 and TIMP-1 have not yet been evaluated [23]. The aim of our study was to compare the perioperative changes of the plasma levels of MMP-9 and TIMP-1 in CEA and CAS.

Methods

Our study was carried out in accordance with the ethical guidelines of the 2008 Declaration of Helsinki at the Clinical Centre of University of Pécs in Hungary between October 2013 and November 2015. The study protocol was approved by the Institutional Scientific and Human Research Ethics Committee of the University of Pécs in Hungary. Following verbal and written information about the study, all enrolled patients provide their written informed consent to participate in our study. In total, twenty-five elective CAS patients were enrolled. The exclusion criteria were a diagnosis of malignant diseases, inflammatory and systemic autoimmune disorders, psychiatric disorders and previous debilitating stroke. For all patients, a preoperative anaesthetic assessment was routinely performed prior to the elective procedures. During this assessment, signs of ongoing infections or trauma were excluded.

In a study recently published by our workgroup, a group of 54 patients undergoing CEA was evaluated [22]. In the present study, a matched subgroup of 30 patients from the previously obtained data served as a historical control.

Surgical procedures

A detailed description of the CEA procedure and blood sampling schedule is available in our prior publication [22]. The CEA group samples were collected at the following four time points (T1–4): T1, at the time of the insertion of the arterial line; T2, 60 min after cross-clamp release; T3, the first postoperative morning; and T4, the third postoperative morning.

CAS operation

CAS was performed under regional anaesthesia with lidocaine. Pre- or intraoperative sedation was not performed on our CAS patients. After catheterising the right femoral artery, diagnostic angiography was performed in all cases. After the precise localisation of the stenosis, a guide catheter was inserted with the help of a hydrophilic guide wire. Then, through this guide catheter, a microwire was inserted through the stenotic area. Once the appropriate position was achieved, the lumen was opened with the gradual dilatation of the stent. During the dilatation, 0.5 mg of intravenous atropine was administered to prevent bradycardia. CAS patients were admitted to the neurosurgery ward after the procedure for postoperative monitoring. Blood samples from CAS patients were collected via an arterial cannula. Sampling was performed at three time points (T1–3): T1, at the time of the insertion of the arterial line; T2, 60 min after stent insertion; and T3: the first postoperative morning. The fourth sampling (on the third postoperative morning) was not performed because the patients were discharged from the hospital on the second postoperative day.

Plasma was isolated from heparin-anticoagulated blood samples by low speed centrifugation at 4 °C and stored at − 80 °C until they were analysed in a single batch at the end of the study. MMP-9 and TIMP-1 levels were measured with quantitative sandwich enzyme-linked immunosorbent assay (ELISA) techniques according to the manufacturer's instructions (R&D Systems Inc., Minneapolis, MN, USA). Then, spectrophotometric (Multiskan Ascent microplate photometer, Type: 354, Thermo Electron Corporation, Waltham, MA, USA) reading of the absorbance at 450 nm was compared to standard curves. Plasma concentrations of MMP-9 and TIMP-1 were expressed as ng/ml.

Statistical analysis

Non-parametric tests were used since the data distribution was found to be not normal by the Kolmogorov-Smirnov and Shapiro-Wilk tests. CEA patients and CAS patients were compared with the Mann-Whitney U test. Kruskal-Wallis one-way ANOVA with post hoc Dunn test was used to compare data of the different time points in both patient groups. The analyses were conducted by the Statistical Package for the Social Sciences (SPSS) Statistics software, version 21.0 (IBM Corporation, USA). Values of $p < 0.05$ were considered statistically significant.

Results

Table 1 shows the demographic data, comorbidities, major complications and pre-existing medical conditions and treatments of the two analysed groups. There was no significant difference between the CAS group and the control CEA group in the number of patients enrolled, age, gender, medications, comorbidities and major complications. Age, gender, procedure laterality, previous stroke, presence of contralateral stenosis, prior ipsi- or contralateral surgery, smoking, pre-existing hypertension and diabetes treated with oral antidiabetic medication did not influence the plasma levels of MMP-9 and TIMP-1 at any time points. The plasma levels of MMP-9 among diabetic patients treated with insulin analogues were significantly higher in the T2 samples (Table 2). Lipid lowering agents and aspirin did not influence the plasma levels of MMP-9 and TIMP-1 at any time point. Baseline (T1) plasma MMP-9 levels of the patients treated with adenosine diphosphate (ADP) receptor antagonists were significantly lower (Table 3). Intraoperative hypo- or hypertension had no effect on plasma MMP-9 or TIMP-1 levels in the present study.

In the CEA group, significantly higher plasma MMP-9 levels were measured at T3 compared to baseline (T1). There were no differences in the plasma MMP-9 levels in the CAS group at any time point ($p > 0.05$). In the T3 samples, plasma MMP-9 levels were significantly higher

Table 1 Demographic and characteristic data of patients

Parameters	CEA	CAS
Patient number	30	25
Age (year)	65 ± 8	60 ± 7
Gender (male/female)	20/10	16/9
Laterality (right/left)	15/15	13/12
Degree of stenosis	83 ± 7.8%	79 ± 7.5%
Contralateral stenosis > 50% n (%)	8 (26.7)	9 (36)
Symptomatic ICA stenosis n (%)	16 (53.3)	17 (68)
Previous stroke n (%)	6 (20)	5 (20)
Time since stroke (months)	28 ± 10	27 ± 18
Previous transient ischaemic attack n (%)	10 (33.3)	12 (48)
Time since transient ischaemic attack (months)	6 ± 4	6 ± 3
Previous ipsilateral ICA procedure n (%)	4 (13.3)	7 (28)
Coexisting diseases		
Hypertension n (%)	29 (96.7)	23 (92)
Non-insulin-dependent diabetes mellitus n (%)	9 (30)	3 (12)
Insulin-dependent diabetes mellitus n (%)	3 (10)	2 (8)
Hyperlipidaemia n (%)	20 (66.7)	14 (56)
History of smoking n (%)	10 (33.3)	8 (32)
Medications		
Acetyl salicylic acid n (%)	16 (53.3)	20 (80)
ADP receptor antagonists n (%)	13 (43.3)	8 (32)
Lipid lowering agents n (%)	20 (66.7)	15 (60)
Intraoperative complications		
Hypertension n (%)	9 (30)	1 (4)
Hypotension n (%)	8 (26.7)	1 (4)
Transient shunt n (%)	3 (10)	0 (0)
Bleeding (> 100 ml) n (%)	2 (6.7)	0 (0)
Transient ischaemia n (%)	4 (13.3)	0 (0)
Stroke n (%)	0 (0)	0 (0)
Postoperative complications		
Bleeding (> 100 ml) n (%)	2 (6.7)	1 (4)
Transient ischaemia n (%)	2 (6.7)	0 (0)
Stroke n (%)	0 (0)	0 (0)

Data are presented as the mean ± standard error of mean
ICA internal carotid artery, *ADP* adenosine diphosphate

Table 2 Effect of insulin analogue on plasma MMP-9 levels

		T1	T2	T3	T4
MMP-9 (ng/ml)	IA	327.5±33.5	585.3±170.6*	414.6±138.9	509.4±202.1
	Non-IA	273.7±26.8	238.3±31.8	359.0±42.9	336.2± 54.3

Data are presented as the mean ± standard error of mean
IA patients who were treated with insulin analogue, *non-IA* patients who were not treated with insulin analogue, *T1* preoperative values, *T2* 60 min after cross-clamp release/stent insertion, *T3* postoperative day 1, *T4* postoperative day 3; and
*$p < 0.05$ compared to non-IA patients

Table 3 Effect of ADP receptor antagonists on plasma MMP-9 levels

		T1	T2	T3	T4
MMP-9 (ng/ml)	ADP antag.	233.1 ± 20.7*	299.4 ± 66.6	382.0 ± 70.2	456.6 ± 101.4
	Non-ADP antag.	346.9 ± 49.3	246.7 ± 37.4	380.7 ± 53.0	320.6 ± 66.7

Data are presented as the mean ± standard error of mean

ADP antag patients who were treated with ADP receptor antagonists, *non-ADP antag* patients who were not treated with ADP receptor antagonists, *T1* preoperative values, *T2* 60 min after cross-clamp release/stent insertion, *T3* postoperative day 1, *T4* postoperative day 3; and

* $p < 0.05$ compared to non-ADP antag

in the CEA group compared to the CAS group (Table 4 and Fig. 1).

Significantly lower plasma TIMP-1 levels were measured in both groups at T2 compared to baseline (Table 4 and Fig. 2).

MMP-9/TIMP-1 ratios at T3 were significantly higher than baseline in the CEA group and the CAS group ($p < 0.05$) (Table 4 and Fig. 3).

Discussion

Interventions on the extracranial carotid artery are relatively common vascular procedures worldwide. The gold standard intervention is still CEA; however, according to the 2014 AHA/ASA stroke prevention guideline, CAS can be equally effective and less invasive in selected cases [13]. Careful preoperative assessment and management are essential to identify the patients who may benefit from the less invasive nature of an endovascular operation compared to an open surgery.

Most studies on the MMP-9-TIMP-1 system in CEA and CAS have assessed changes at only a single time point [16, 23, 24]. Thus, our primary aim was to describe the time course of changes in MMP-9 and TIMP-1 levels during the perioperative period of CAS, compare the results to CEA and identify factors influencing these changes.

Muzahir et al. provided information regarding the correlation of MMP/TIMP levels with age, gender and diurnal activity [25]. There were no significant differences in the demographic data of the patients between the study groups, and all surgeries started in the morning;

therefore, we could not ascribe the identified differences to population bias. Although hypo- and hypertension were more prevalent in the CEA group, these complications were promptly addressed.

The role of MMP-9 and TIMP-1 in cardiovascular remodelling is being intensively investigated [26, 27]. In paediatric hypertension, Niemirska et al. found sex-related elevations in the plasma concentrations of MMP-9 and TIMP-1 [28]. In our recent study, age, gender and pre-existing hypertension did not influence the plasma levels of MMP-9 and TIMP-1 at any time point.

The plasma level of MMP-9 has been found to be an independent risk factor for atherothrombotic events [29]. Among patients with coronary artery disease, concurrent type 2 diabetes mellitus is associated with higher plasma levels of MMP-9 [30]. This highlights the role of MMP-9 in diabetes-associated atherothrombosis. In our study, diabetes treated with oral antidiabetic medication did not influence the plasma levels of MMP-9 and TIMP-1 at any time point. Noticeably, the plasma levels of MMP-9 among diabetic patients treated with insulin analogues were significantly higher 60 min after reperfusion, but the difference was no longer detectable in the T3 or T4 samples. In contrast with our results, in vitro and animal studies have found that insulin treatment specifically inhibits MMP-9 expression [31]. Additional investigation of increased case numbers is necessary to resolve this contradistinction.

The mechanism by which ADP receptor antagonists influence plasma MMP-9 levels is not clear; however, the adenosine triphosphate (ATP) induced expression of

Table 4 Plasma MMP-9, TIMP-1 and MMP-9/TIMP-1 levels in the study groups

	Group	T1	T2	T3	T4
MMP-9 (ng/ml)	CEA	290.9 ± 112.1	284.7 ± 247.5	488.6 ± 249.8*#	382.9 ± 285.4
	CAS	259.8 ± 244.9	239.1 ± 221.3	180.9 ± 159.7	–
TIMP-1 (ng/ml)	CEA	117.3 ± 43.2	81.7 ± 73.9*	88.5 ± 41.6	117.2 ± 52.3
	CAS	93.5 ± 30.9	61.7 ± 28.8*	70.7 ± 30.2	–
MMP-9/TIMP1	CEA	2.73 ± 1.37	4.39 ± 2.69	6.41 ± 3.86*#	3.40 ± 2.50
	CAS	2.78 ± 1.88	4.33 ± 3.05	2.26 ± 1.79	–

Data are presented as the mean ± standard error of mean

CEA carotid endarterectomy control group, *CAS* carotid angioplasty and stenting group, *T1* preoperative values, *T2* 60 min after cross-clamp release/stent insertion, *T3* postoperative day 1, *T4* postoperative day 3

* $p < 0.05$ compared to T1

# $p < 0.05$ compared to CAS

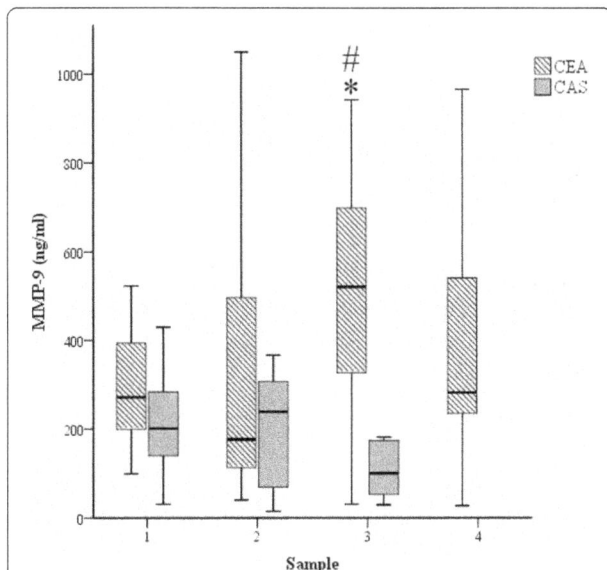

Fig. 1 Changes in plasma MMP-9 concentrations in the two patient groups. CEA: carotid endarterectomy group (striated); and CAS: carotid artery stenting group (grey). Samples: 1, preoperative values; 2, 60 min after cross-clamp release/stent insertion; 3, postoperative day 1; and 4, postoperative day 3. *: $p < 0.05$ compared to sample 1; and #: $p < 0.05$ compared to CAS

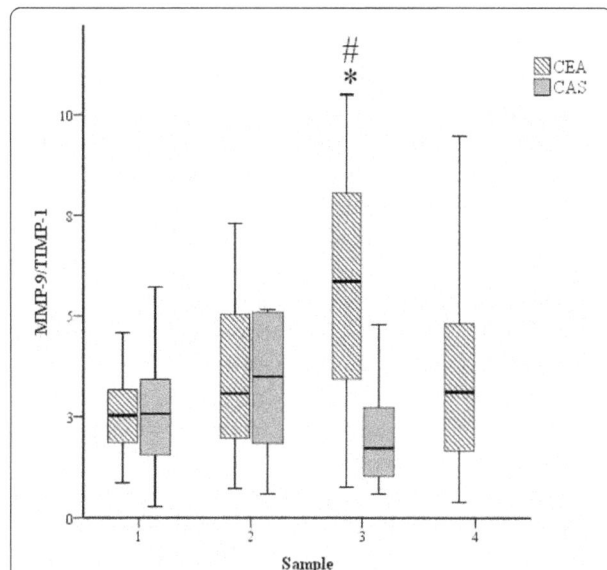

Fig. 3 Changes in plasma MMP-9/TIMP-1 ratios in the two patient groups. CEA: carotid endarterectomy control group (striated); and CAS: carotid artery stenting group (grey). Samples: 1, preoperative values; 2, 60 min after cross-clamp release/stent insertion; 3, postoperative day 1; and 4, postoperative day 3. *: $p < 0.05$ compared to sample 1; and #: $p < 0.05$ compared to CAS

MMP-9 has been investigated in different cell types [32, 33]. Choi et al. found that ATP induced microglial activation through the non-transcriptional activation of MMP-9, which can be inhibited by a P2Y receptor antagonist (including clopidogrel) in cell culture [34].

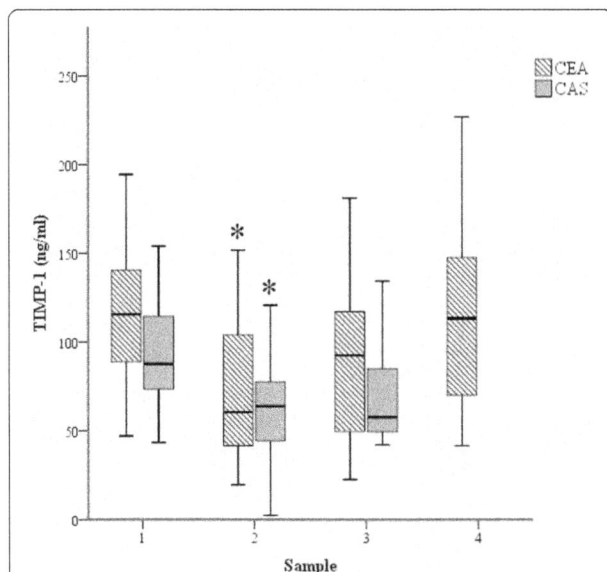

Fig. 2 Changes in plasma TIMP-1 concentrations in the two patient groups. CEA: carotid endarterectomy control group (striated); and CAS: carotid artery stenting group (grey). Samples: 1, preoperative values; 2, 60 min after cross-clamp release/stent insertion; 3, postoperative day 1; and 4, postoperative day 3. *: $p < 0.05$ compared to sample 1

Sternberg et al. observed a reduction in MMP-9 plasma levels after clopidogrel administration in acute ischaemic stroke [35]. TIMPs can inhibit MMP-dependent platelet adhesion and aggregation. The effect of TIMPs on platelet aggregation can be enhanced by aspirin and ADP receptor antagonists. Reduced platelet aggregation caused by ADP receptor antagonist treatment may retroactively influence the expression of TIMPs [36].

After a transient ischaemic attack or ischaemic stroke, both the increase of MMP and decrease of TIMP levels can occur as a result of ischaemic damage and, later, as a result central nervous system repair [37, 38]. The significant increase of MMP-9 levels in the CEA group on the first postoperative day may indicate subclinical BBB dysfunction and/or microembolisation [16]. Using diffusion-weighted magnetic resonance imaging, Tedesco et al. observed a higher incidence of postprocedural microembolisation after CAS than after CEA [39], but Montorsi et al. found that the risk of microembolisation could be decreased with a proximal endovascular occlusion approach [40]. Another cause of the higher MMP-9 in the CEA group on the first postoperative day could be the longer carotid flow restriction compared to the endovascular procedure (CAS). The significant decrease of TIMP-1 in both groups during the study may be an indicator of increased extracellular matrix turnover following reperfusion [37, 38]. The higher MMP-9/TIMP-1 ratio on the first postoperative day in the CEA group originated from the higher plasma MMP-9 levels but seems to have been not significantly influenced by the TIMP-1 levels.

Limitations of our study: The extent of the resulting tissue damage from the two surgical procedures (CEA and CAS) are different. MMP-9 and TIMP-1 are commonly viewed as biomarkers of different pathophysiological conditions, but they also have biological properties and thus could potentially affect outcomes. As previously described by Agren et al., elevated MMP-9 levels are present in healing wounds, which may contribute to the elevated MMP-9 levels on the day after CEA surgery [41]. Another limitation of our study is that preoperative MRI was not routinely performed to determine the size of the previous ischaemic lesion; however, previous debilitating stroke was one of our exclusion criteria. Although the presence of contralateral carotid artery stenosis did not influence the plasma levels of MMP-9 and TIMP-1 at any time point, an examination of the effects of atherosclerosis in other arteries was not part of our study.

Conclusions

According to our study, there were no significant differences in the incidence of neurological complications between the two groups during the perioperative period. However, the endovascular procedure triggers smaller changes in the MMP-9-TIMP-1 system, which may suggest a lower incidence of central nervous system damage. This finding may originate from a lower incidence of BBB dysfunction and/or microembolisation and a shorter carotid flow restriction time; however, the exact mechanism is not completely clear. Postoperative neuroimaging (such as MRI) may help identify subclinical changes; however, postoperative neuroimaging in a complication-free group was not performed. Additional studies in a larger group of patients, including a cognitive and functional survey at 1 and 6 months, are necessary to identify subtle differences in the functional outcome between the two procedures.

Abbreviations
ADP: Adenosine diphosphate; ATP: Adenosine triphosphate; BBB: Blood-brain-barrier; CAS: Carotid artery stenting; CEA: Carotid endarterectomy; ELISA: Enzyme-linked immunosorbent assay; IA: Insulin analogue; ICA: Internal carotid artery; MMP-9: Matrix metalloproteinase-9; MMPs: Matrix metalloproteinases; TIMP-1: Tissue inhibitor of matrix metalloproteinase-1; TIMPs: Tissue inhibitor of matrix metalloproteinases

Acknowledgements
The authors are grateful for all the help and support from their technical co-workers and nurses in the Department of Anaesthesia and Intensive Therapy and the Department of Neurosurgery at the University of Pécs as well as Csilla Fajtik from the Department of Surgical Research and Techniques for providing the supportive help in completing the present study.

Funding
This study was supported by the Higher Education Institutional Excellence Program of the Ministry of Human Capacities in the framework of the research project 20765–3/2018/FEKUTSTRAT at University of Pécs and was supported by PTE ÁOK-KA-2017-07.

Authors' contributions
ÁM participated in the design of the study, data acquisition, performed the statistical analysis and drafted the manuscript. BN participated in the design of the study, data acquisition, statistical analysis and drafted the manuscript. GW participated in the data interpretation, statistical analysis and drafted the manuscript. JL participated in the design of the study, data interpretation and performed blood sample analysis. FK participated in the design of the study and performed endovascular surgery. LB participated in data interpretation and revised the manuscript. DM participated in design of the study and revised the manuscript. All authors read and approved the final manuscript.

Competing interests
The authors declare that they have no competing interests.

Author details
Department of Anaesthesiology and Intensive Therapy, Medical School, University of Pécs, Ifjúság Str. 13, Pécs HU-7624, Hungary. [2]Department of Surgical Research and Techniques, Medical School, University of Pécs, Szigeti Str. 12, Pécs HU-7624, Hungary. [3]Medical Skills Lab, Medical School, University of Pécs, Szigeti Str. 12, Pécs HU-7624, Hungary. [4]Department of Operational Medicine, Medical School, University of Pécs, Szigeti Str. 12, Pécs HU-7624, Hungary. [5]Department of Neurosurgery, Medical School, University of Pécs, Rét Str. 2, Pécs HU-7623, Hungary.

References
1. Zorowitz RD, Chen E, Bianchini Tong K, Laouri M. Costs and rehabilitation use of stroke survivors: a retrospective study of Medicare beneficiaries. Top Stroke Rehabil. 2009;16:309–20.
2. Soler EP, Ruiz VC. Epidemiology and risk factors of cerebral ischemia and ischemic heart diseases: similarities and differences. Curr Cardiol Rev. 2010;6:138–49.
3. Dickerson LM, Carek PJ, Quattlebaum RG. Prevention of recurrent ischemic stroke. Am Fam Physician. 2007;76:382–8.
4. Liapis CD, Bell PRF, Mikhailidis D, Sivenius J, Nicolaides A, Fernandes e Fernandes J, et al. ESVS guidelines. Invasive treatment for carotid stenosis: indications, techniques. Eur J Vasc Endovasc Surg. 2009;37:1–19.
5. Yip H-K, Sung P-H, Wu C-J, Yu C-M. Carotid stenting and endarterectomy. Int J Cardiol. 2016;214:166–74.
6. Featherstone RL, Dobson J, Ederle J, Doig D, Bonati LH, Morris S, et al. Carotid artery stenting compared with endarterectomy in patients with symptomatic carotid stenosis (international carotid stenting study): a randomised controlled trial with cost-effectiveness analysis. Health Technol Assess. 2016;20:1–94.
7. Meier P, Knapp G, Tamhane U, Chaturvedi S, Gurm HS. Short term and intermediate term comparison of endarterectomy versus stenting for carotid artery stenosis: systematic review and meta-analysis of randomised controlled clinical trials. BMJ. 2010;340:c467.
8. Meller SM, Salim Al-Damluji M, Gutierrez A, Stilp E, Mena-Hurtado C. Carotid stenting versus endarterectomy for the treatment of carotid artery stenosis: contemporary results from a large single center study. Catheter Cardiovasc Interv. 2016;88(5):822–30.
9. Bonati LH, Ederle J, McCabe DJH, Dobson J, Featherstone RL, Gaines PA, et al. Long-term risk of carotid restenosis in patients randomly assigned to endovascular treatment or endarterectomy in the carotid and vertebral artery transluminal angioplasty study (CAVATAS): long-term follow-up of a randomised trial. Lancet Neurol. 2009;8:908–17.
10. SPACE Collaborative Group, Ringleb PA, Allenberg J, Brückmann H, Eckstein H-H, Fraedrich G, et al. Thirty day results from the SPACE trial of stent-protected angioplasty versus carotid endarterectomy in symptomatic patients: a randomised non-inferiority trial. Lancet. 2006;368:1239–47.
11. Bonati LH, Ederle J, Dobson J, Engelter S, Featherstone RL, Gaines PA, et al. Length of carotid stenosis predicts peri-procedural stroke or death and restenosis in patients randomized to endovascular treatment or endarterectomy. Int J Stroke. 2014;9:297–305.
12. Choi JC, Johnston SC, Kim AS. Early outcomes after carotid artery stenting compared with endarterectomy for asymptomatic carotid stenosis. Stroke. 2015;46:120–5.
13. Kernan WN, Ovbiagele B, Black HR, Bravata DM, Chimowitz MI, Ezekowitz MD, et al. Guidelines for the prevention of stroke in patients with stroke and transient ischemic attack: a guideline for healthcare professionals from the american heart association/american stroke association. Stroke. 2014;45:2160–236.

14. Li J, Wang Y. Blood biomarkers in minor stroke and transient ischemic attack. Neurosci Bull. 2016:1–6.

15. Ramos-Fernandez M, Bellolio MF, Stead LG. Matrix Metalloproteinase-9 as a marker for acute ischemic stroke: a systematic review. J Stroke Cerebrovasc Dis. 2011;20:47–54.

16. Molloy K, Thompson M, Schwalbe E, Bell PR, Naylor A, Loftus I. Elevation in plasma MMP-9 following carotid endarterectomy is associated with particulate cerebral embolisation. Eur J Vasc Endovasc Surg. 2004;27:409–13.

17. Lorente L, Martín MM, Labarta L, Díaz C, Solé-Violán J, Blanquer J, et al. Matrix metalloproteinase-9, –10, and tissue inhibitor of matrix metalloproteinases-1 blood levels as biomarkers of severity and mortality in sepsis. Crit Care. 2009;13:R158.

18. Mühl D, Nagy B, Woth G, Falusi B, Bogár L, Weber G, et al. Dynamic changes of matrix metalloproteinases and their tissue inhibitors in severe sepsis. J Crit Care. 2011;26:550–5.

19. Mühl D, Ghosh S, Uzuelli JA, Lantos J, Tanus-Santos JE. Increases in circulating matrix metalloproteinase-9 levels following fibrinolysis for acute pulmonary embolism. Thromb Res. 2010;125:549–53.

20. Chaturvedi M, Kaczmarek L. Mmp-9 inhibition: a therapeutic strategy in ischemic stroke. Mol Neurobiol. 2014;49:563–73.

21. Crocker SJ, Pagenstecher A, Campbell IL. The TIMPs tango with MMPs and more in the central nervous system. J Neurosci Res. 2004;75:1–11.

22. Nagy B, Woth G, Mérei Á, Nagy L, Lantos J, Menyhei G, et al. Perioperative time course of matrix metalloproteinase-9 (MMP-9), its tissue inhibitor TIMP-1 & S100B protein in carotid surgery. Indian J Med Res. 2016;143:220–6.

23. Giuliani E, Genedani S, Moratto R, Veronesi J, Carone C, Bonvecchio C, et al. Neural damage biomarkers during open carotid surgery versus endovascular approach. Ann Vasc Surg. 2014;28:1671–9.

24. Gaudet JG, Yocum GT, Lee SS, Granat A, Mikami M, Connolly ES, et al. MMP-9 levels in elderly patients with cognitive dysfunction after carotid surgery. J Clin Neurosci. 2010;17:436–40.

25. Tayebjee MH, Lip GYH, Blann AD, MacFadyen RJ. Effects of age, gender, ethnicity, diurnal variation and exercise on circulating levels of matrix metalloproteinases (MMP)-2 and –9, and their inhibitors, tissue inhibitors of matrix metalloproteinases (TIMP)-1 and –2. Thromb Res. 2005;115:205–10.

26. Marchesi C, Dentali F, Nicolini E, Maresca AM, Tayebjee MH, Franz M, et al. Plasma levels of matrix metalloproteinases and their inhibitors in hypertension. J Hypertens. 2012;30:3–16.

27. Galis ZS, Khatri JJ. Matrix metalloproteinases in vascular remodeling and Atherogenesis. Circ Res. 2002;90(3):251–62.

28. Niemirska A, Litwin M, Trojanek J, Gackowska L, Kubiszewska I, Wierzbicka A, et al. Altered matrix metalloproteinase 9 and tissue inhibitor of metalloproteinases 1 levels in children with primary hypertension. J Hypertens. 2016;34:1815–22.

29. Blankenberg S, Rupprecht HJ, Poirier O, Bickel C, Smieja M, Hafner G, et al. Plasma concentrations and genetic variation of matrix metalloproteinase 9 and prognosis of patients with cardiovascular disease. Circulation. 2003;107(12):1579–85.

30. Marx N, Froehlich J, Siam L, Ittner J, Wierse G, Schmidt A, et al. Antidiabetic PPARγ-activator rosiglitazone reduces MMP-9 serum levels in type 2 diabetic patients with coronary artery disease. Arterioscler Thromb Vasc Biol. 2003;23(2):283–8.

31. Schuyler CA, Ta NN, Li Y, Lopes-Virella MF, Huang Y. Insulin treatment attenuates diabetes-increased atherosclerotic intimal lesions and matrix metalloproteinase 9 expression in apolipoprotein E-deficient mice. J Endocrinol. 2011;210:37–46.

32. Wesley UV, Bove PF, Hristova M, McCarthy S, van der Vliet A. Airway epithelial cell migration and wound repair by ATP-mediated activation of dual oxidase 1. J Biol Chem. 2007;282:3213–20.

33. Huwiler A, Akool e-S, Aschrafi A, Hamada FMA, Pfeilschifter J, Eberhardt W. ATP potentiates interleukin-1 beta-induced MMP-9 expression in mesangial cells via recruitment of the ELAV protein HuR. J Biol Chem. 2003;278(51):51758–69.

34. Choi MS, Cho KS, Shin SM, Ko HM, Kwon KJ, Shin CY, et al. ATP induced microglial cell migration through non-transcriptional activation of matrix Metalloproteinase-9. Arch Pharm Res. 2010;33:257–65.

35. Sternberg Z, Chichelli T, Sternberg D, Sawyer R, Ching M, Janicke D, et al. Relationship between inflammation and aspirin and Clopidogrel antiplatelet responses in acute ischemic stroke. J Stroke Cerebrovasc Dis. 2016;25:327 34.

36. Santos-Martínez MJ, Medina C, Jurasz P, Radomski MW. Role of metalloproteinases in platelet function. Thromb Res. 2008;121:535–42.

37. Montaner J, Alvarez-Sabín J, Molina C, Anglés A, Abilleira S, Arenillas J, et al. Matrix metalloproteinase expression after human Cardioembolic stroke. Stroke. 2001;32(8):1759–66.

38. Zhao B-Q, Wang S, Kim H-Y, Storrie H, Rosen BR, Mooney DJ, et al. Role of matrix metalloproteinases in delayed cortical responses after stroke. Nat Med. 2006;12:441–5.

39. Tedesco MM, Lee JT, Dalman RL, Lane B, Loh C, Haukoos JS, et al. Postprocedural microembolic events following carotid surgery and carotid angioplasty and stenting. J Vasc Surg. 2007;46:244–50.

40. Montorsi P, Caputi L, Galli S, Ciceri E, Ballerini G, Agrifoglio M, et al. Microembolization during carotid artery stenting in patients with high-risk, lipid-rich plaque: a randomized trial of proximal versus distal cerebral protection. J Am Coll Cardiol. 2011;58:1656–63.

41. Agren MS, Jorgensen IN, Andersen M, Viljanto J, Gottrup P. Matrix metalloproteinase 9 level predicts optimal collagen deposition during early wound repair in humans. Br J Surg. 1998;85:68–71.

Do fragments and glycosylated isoforms of alpha-1-antitrypsin in CSF mirror spinal pathophysiological mechanisms in chronic peripheral neuropathic pain? An exploratory, discovery phase study

Emmanuel Bäckryd[*] iD, Sofia Edström, Björn Gerdle and Bijar Ghafouri

Abstract

Background: Post-translational modifications (PTMs) generate a tremendous protein diversity from the ~ 20,000 protein-coding genes of the human genome. In chronic pain conditions, exposure to pathological processes in the central nervous system could lead to disease-specific PTMs detectable in the cerebrospinal fluid (CSF). In a previous hypothesis-generating study, we reported that seven out of 260 CSF proteins highly discriminated between neuropathic pain patients and healthy controls: one isoform of angiotensinogen (AG), two isoforms of alpha-1-antitrypsin (AT), three isoforms of haptoglobin (HG), and one isoform of pigment epithelium-derived factor (PEDF). The present study had three aims: (1) To examine the multivariate inter-correlations between all identified isoforms of these seven proteins; (2) Based on the results of the first aim, to characterize PTMs in a subset of interesting proteins; (3) To regress clinical pain data using the 260 proteins as predictors, thereby testing the hypothesis that the above-mentioned seven discriminating proteins and/or the characterized isoforms/fragments of aim (2) would be among the proteins having the highest predictive power for clinical pain data.

Methods: CSF samples from 11 neuropathic pain patients and 11 healthy controls were used for biochemical analysis of protein isoforms. PTM characterization was performed using enzymatic reaction assay and mass spectrometry. Multivariate data analysis (principal component analysis and orthogonal partial least square regression) was applied on the quantified protein isoforms.

Results: We identified 5 isoforms of AG, 18 isoforms of AT, 5 isoforms of HG, and 5 isoforms of PEDF. Fragments and glycosylated isoforms of AT were studied in depth. When regressing the pain intensity data of patients, three isoforms of AT, two isoforms of PEDF, and one isoform of angiotensinogen "reappeared" as major results, i.e., they were major findings both when comparing patients with healthy controls and when regressing pain intensity in patients.

Conclusions: Altered levels of fragments and/or glycosylated isoforms of alpha-1-antitrypsin might mirror pathophysiological processes in the spinal cord of neuropathic pain patients. In particular, we suggest that a putative disease-specific combination of the levels of two different N-truncated fragments of alpha-1-antitrypsin might be interesting for future CSF and/or plasma biomarker investigations in chronic neuropathic pain.

Keywords: Alpha-1-antitrypsin, Cerebrospinal fluid, Neuropathic, Pain, Pathophysiology

* Correspondence: emmanuel.backryd@regionostergotland.se
Pain and Rehabilitation Center, and Department of Medical and Health Sciences, Linköping University, Linköping, Sweden

Background

A substantial part of our knowledge about the pathophysiology of pain has been acquired through animal experiments. Although there are obvious similarities between species, there are also differences, and translating evidence from animals to humans in this field is far from trivial [1]. The quest for *human* biomarkers, which would mirror the pathophysiology of different chronic pain conditions, must be understood against this background. Biomarkers would be useful for diagnosis and prognosis of different pain conditions, for the evaluation of treatment response, and for the development of drugs; they could also serve as surrogate endpoints (i.e., as substitutes for clinical endpoints) [2].

Post-translational modifications (PTMs) generate a tremendous protein diversity from the ~ 20,000 protein-coding genes of the human genome, the complexity of the proteome being several orders of magnitude greater than the coding capacity of the genome [3–5]. After the genome, mapping the proteome is next in turn [6]. Whereas the genome is constant, the proteome is continuously modulated by genome-environment interactions [7, 8]. PTMs modulate enzyme activity, protein turnover and localization, protein-protein interactions, various signaling cascades, DNA repair, and cell division [5].

Glycosylation, i.e. when a carbohydrate is attached to a protein, is one type of PTM [5]. The glycosylation form of a protein can be altered significantly because of changes in cellular pathways and processes resulting from inflammatory conditions, neurodegeneration, or cancer [9]. These potentially detectable protein modifications may lead to the discovery of specific and sensitive biomarkers [10]. Protein fragments, i.e. proteins that have been truncated either at the N- or C-terminal end of the amino acid sequence, are also potential specific biomarkers [11]. Indeed, in the context of dementia, the term "protein fragmentology" has been used [12], as has the term "degradome research" [13]. In the pain field, such a well-known neuropeptide as Substance P has biologically active and detectable fragments [14].

In chronic pain conditions, exposure to pathological processes in the central nervous system (CNS) could perhaps lead to a disease-specific fragmentation process detectable in the cerebrospinal fluid (CSF). Protein fragments are also interesting because their smaller size would enable them to cross the blood-brain barrier (BBB) easier than full-length proteins, and hence fragments would probably be easier to detect in blood [12].

Neuropathic pain is defined as pain caused by a lesion or disease in the somatosensory nervous system [15]. In a previous comparative two-dimensional gel electrophoresis study [16], we described seven CSF proteins highly discriminating between neuropathic pain patients and healthy controls. These seven proteins were one isoform of angiotensinogen (AG), two isoforms of alpha-1-antitrypsin (AT), three isoforms of haptoglobin (HG), and one isoform of pigment epithelium-derived factor (PEDF). The three aims of the present exploratory, discovery phase study [17] were:

1. To examine the multivariate inter-correlations between all identified isoforms of these seven proteins, using multivariate data analysis by projection (MVDA) [18, 19]. The focus here was not on discriminant analysis but rather on the internal correlation structure between these isoforms in health vs. neuropathic pain. Our hypothesis was that neuropathic pain is associated with an altered correlation structure between the different isoforms of a particular protein, compared to healthy controls.
2. Based on the results of the first aim above, to characterize PTMs in a subset of interesting proteins. Because protein fragments seem especially promising as biomarkers (their generation by disease-specific processes could reduce the overlap between diagnostic groups) [12], special attention was given to fragmented proteins [11].
3. Returning to MVDA and focusing on the patients, to regress clinical pain parameters (pain intensity and pain duration), using all the proteomic data (260 proteins) of our previous study as predictor variables [16]. We wanted to test the hypothesis that the above-mentioned seven discriminating proteins and/or the characterized isoforms/fragments of aim (2) above would be among the proteins having the highest predictive power for either pain intensity or pain duration.

Hence, the purpose of the study was not to conduct clinical biomarker research at the validation stage; instead, this was a pre-clinical exploratory study in the early discovery stage [17, 20].

Methods
Patients
The patients have been described extensively in a previous paper [16]. All pain patients included in this study were participating in a clinical trial of intrathecal bolus injections of the analgesic ziconotide [21]. Inclusion criteria were: 1) patient, at least 18 years of age, suffering from chronic (≥6 months) neuropathic pain due to trauma or surgery, who had failed on conventional pharmacological treatment; 2) average Visual Analogue Scale chronic Pain Intensity (VASPI) last week ≥40 mm [22]; 3) patient capable of judgment, i.e. able to understand information regarding the drug, the mode of administration and evaluation of efficacy and side effects; 4) signed informed consent.

After informed consent, the following data were registered: basic demographic data; pain diagnosis; pain duration; present and past medical history; concomitant medication. A medical examination was performed. All patients had at least probable post-traumatic/post-surgical neuropathic pain according to the criteria published by Treede et al. [23], and all were or had been candidates for Spinal Cord Stimulation. Detailed patient characteristics have been published elsewhere [16, 21]. After CSF sampling, the patient received an intrathecal bolus injection of ziconotide according to the protocol of the clinical trial.

For an overview of patients vs healthy controls, see Table 1.

Healthy controls

Healthy controls were recruited by local advertisement at the Faculty of Health Sciences, Linköping University, Sweden, and by contacting healthy subjects from earlier studies. After informed consent, a structured interview was conducted to ensure the absence of any significant medical condition. The following areas were specifically assessed in the interview: earlier major trauma; back, joints, muscles or skeletal disease; heart or vascular disease; lung or bronchial disease; psychiatric symptoms; neurological, ear or eye disease; digestive tract disease; kidney, urinary or genital disease; skin disease; tumor or cancer; endocrine disease; hematological disease; birth defects; other disease, disability or allergy. Moreover, the presence of a known bleeding disorder was specifically inquired for.

The absence of a chronic pain condition was ensured by a structured questionnaire covering sociodemographic data,

presence of pain now, location of pain now, generalization of pain, presence of intermittent pain, duration of persistent pain. The questionnaire also covered anxiety and depressive symptomatology using Hospital Anxiety and Depression Scale [24], coping aspects (i.e., catastrophizing) using Pain Catastrophizing Scale [25], and health-related quality of life aspects using Short Form-36 (SF-36) [26], in order to ensure that the controls were healthy. Subjects were also given the possibility to make a pain drawing about Pain Now, Pain at worst and Pain at best. Musculoskeletal pain was more deeply assessed by VASPI last month for 9 specific anatomical locations: neck; shoulders; arms; hands; upper back; lower back; hips; knees; feet. Concomitant medicines were registered. A medical examination was performed, including assessment for fibromyalgia tender points.

Procedures

For every subject in this study, intrathecal access was obtained by lumbar puncture with a 27 GA pencil-point Whitacre needle (BD Medical, Franklin Lakes, New Jersey, USA) and a 10 ml sample of CSF was drawn in five numbered syringes of 2 ml each. Each sample was immediately cooled on ice and transported to the Painomics® laboratory, Linköping University Hospital, centrifuged and divided in aliquots and stored at − 70°C until analysis.

Biochemical analyses

The comparative proteomic study between patients and healthy controls was performed as described in our previously study [16]. Briefly, 100 μg of depleted CSF proteins from each subject (11 patients and 11 healthy

Table 1 Overview of patients and healthy controls

Variables	Patients (n = 11)	Healthy controls (n = 11)	Statistics p-value
Age (years)	58 (35–75)	23 (20–28)	< 0.001*
Sex (% female)	55%	55%	1.0
Body Mass Index (kg/m²)	24.7 (20.2–30.0)	22.6 (20.8–26.5)	0.065
Pain duration (months)	65 (30–180)	0	< 0.001*
Pain intensity (0–100 mm)[a]	72 (40–87)	0	< 0.001*
Opioid dose[b] (mg/day)	0 (0–480)	0	0.076
On opioids (%)	45%	0%	0.035*
On tricyclics or duloxetine (%)	36%	0%	0.090
On gabapentinoids (%)	36%	0%	0.090
On paracetamol[c] (%)	45%	0%	0.035*
On NSAID[c] (%)	18%	0%	0.476

Data are presented as median (range) or percentages. Furthest to the right is the result of the statistical comparisons between patients and healthy controls. * denotes significant group difference

Notes:

[a]: At inclusion, patients were asked to grade their average pain intensity for last week on a Visual Analogue Scale 0–100 mm, whereas the pain status of healthy controls was investigated by an extensive structured interview. All controls were free of pain

[b]: In oral morphine equivalents

[c]: Excluding treatment "as needed". NSAID: Non-Steroidal Anti-Inflammatory Drug

controls) were separated by 2-DE, visualized by silver staining and the protein patterns were digitalized and quantified using CCD camera (VersaDoc™ Imaging system 4000 MP, Bio-Rad) in combination with a computerized imaging 12-bit system designed for evaluations of 2-DE patterns (PDQuest 8.0.1 Bio-Rad). The different gel images were evaluated and protein spots were quantified according to spot optical densities (SOD). The generated SODs were evaluated for significant differences between the groups.

For the characterization of the different protein isoforms, a pooled CSF sample from patients and a pooled sample from healthy subjects were used. The samples were desalted, lyophilized and dissolved in urea sample buffer solution, as has been described in detail elsewhere [16]. Protein concentration was determined before and after desalting step using Bradford assay [16]. To examine N-glycosylation, 300 μg of CSF proteins were incubated in presence or absence of an *N*-glycosidase PNGase F (Sigma Aldrich) at 37 °C overnight using conditions recommended by the supplier and as has been described in detail elsewhere [27]. The proteins were then analyzed by 2-DE.

The interesting protein spots were excised from the gels, trypsinated and identified by liquid chromatography tandem mass spectrometry (LC-MS/MS) using Linear Trap Quadropole (LTQ) Orbitrap Velos Pro hybrid (Thermo Fisher Scientific) in conjunction with nano flow HPLC system (EASY-Nlc II, Thermo Fisher Scientific). Data processing of the spectra was performed using MaxQuant software, and the generated mass list was searched against SwissProt human protein sequence database as previously described [16]. When identifying fragments of proteins, the position of the matched peptides within the theoretical sequence of the protein were computed using the proteomic tool Compute *pI/MW* (http://www.expasy.org/proteomics). The calculated pI/*MW* of the fragment was controlled to be in agreement with the apparent mass and *pI* on the 2D-gel.

Statistics

Traditional univariate statistical methods can quantify level changes of individual substances but disregard interrelationships between them and thereby ignore system-wide aspects. Therefore, we used SIMCA version 13.0 (Umetrics AB, Umeå, Sweden) for MVDA computations. Conceptually, imagine a multidimensional space where each protein is a dimension ("k" dimensions). Each subject (patient or control) will be a point in this k-dimensional space. Due to a combination of technological development (rendering high "k") and practical/economic constraints (leading to a low number of subjects "n"), todays data tables in the omics field often have a low subjects-to-variables ratio (n < <<k). Classical regression

techniques like multiple linear regression (MLR) or logistic regression (LR), which were developed in the early days of the twentieth century, are not suited for such high-dimensional and multi-collinear data. Hence, todays data table often break one of the underlying assumption behind MLR and LR, namely that the predictor (X) variables are fairly independent. MLR and LR also assume that a high subject-to-variables ratio is present (e.g., > 5), and they have difficulties coping with missing data. Due to the above-mentioned drawbacks of classical regression techniques (with regression coefficients becoming unstable and their interpretability breaking down), the modern MVDA methods of Principal Component Analysis (PCA) and Orthogonal Partial Least Squares (OPLS) regression were used instead. PCA and OPLS can handle subject-to-variables ratios < 1, and they cope well with both multi-collinearity and missing data. OPLS is a recent, easier-to-interpret modification of Partial Least Squares (PLS). The MVDA workflow and the reporting of parameters necessary for evaluating model quality were in accordance with the paper published by Wheelock & Wheelock [19]. For all MVDA analyses, data were log-transformed when needed (using the SIMCA function "auto transform selected variables as appropriate") and scaling to unit variance was applied [18, 19].

For Aim 1 we used PCA, which is the foundation of all latent variable projection methods, separately for patients ($n = 11$) and healthy controls ($n = 11$), focusing on all the isoforms of the seven proteins mentioned in the introduction. Each isoform had previously been quantified by SOD [16]. In a multivariate data set, important information can be found in the correlation structure of the whole data set, i.e. in the inter-correlations between all the variables taken together as a whole. PCA entails the definition of a few latent variables that describe the underlying structure in the data. The latent variables (called principal components, PC) are uncorrelated to each other, and they summarize and simplify the data, separating information from noise and enabling to find relevant patterns in the data. Optimal model dimensionality (i.e. number of PCs) is determined by cross-validation, which is a practical and reliable way to test the significance of a PCA model. This is default in SIMCA. Hence, PCA can be viewed as a form of multivariate correlation analysis. PCA also enables the identification of multivariate outliers and deviant subgroup, as assessed by Hotelling's T2 statistic (T^2 Critical 95%) and by distance to model in X-space (DModX). The R^2 value indicates how well the model explains the dataset, and cross-validated Q^2 is a measure of the predictive power of the model. If R^2 is substantially greater than Q^2 (a difference > 0.3 is mentioned in the literature) [18], the robustness of the model is poor, suggesting overfitting [19].

A PC relates to each original variable by a loading, which has a value between − 1 and + 1. Variables with high loadings (ignoring the sign) are considered to be of large or moderate importance for the PC under consideration. Hence, PCA is a data visualization technique that models the correlation structure of a dataset, presenting the relationship between variables in a loading plot. On a loading plot, variables close to each other are positively correlated, and variables that are unimportant for the model are found around the origin of the plot (i.e., variables with loadings near zero do not contribute to the model) [18].

For Aim 3, OPLS was used to regress (predict) two clinical variables in patients: VASPI last week and pain duration. Hence, the outcome variable (Y) was one of these two clinical variables, whereas the predictor variables (X:s) where the relative quantification of 260 proteins by SOD in accordance with our previous study [16]. Concerning optimal model dimensionality (i.e. the number of latent variables) and R2/Q2, see above.

In OPLS, the importance of each variable for the model can be measured as a Variable Influence on Projection (VIP) value. This indicates the relevance of each X-variable pooled over all dimensions and Y-variables – the group of variables that best explain Y. Variables with VIP ≥ 1.0 and having a 95% confidence interval not including zero are usually considered significant, but in this study VIP≥ 1.5 was used. The direction of the relationship (positive or negative) was determined by sign of the corresponding loading.

For traditional univariate statistics, all computations were made using IBM® SPSS® Statistics version 23. Spearman's rho correlation coefficient was used for bivariate correlation analysis, and Mann-Whitney U test or Fisher's exact test were used for comparing groups (for continuous and categorical data, respectively). A two-sided significance level of 0.05 was chosen.

Results

Correlation structure in patients vs. controls (aim 1)

We identified 5 isoforms of AG, 18 isoforms of AT, 5 isoforms of HG, and 5 isoforms of PEDF – amounting to a total of 33 proteins. Hence, we generated a SIMCA data table consisting of 22 individuals (rows) and spot optical densities from 33 proteins (columns). To enable quick identification when looking at loading plots (see below), AG, AT, HG, or PEDF was added to the original spot number. Moreover, on basis of their location on the gels, five groups of AT were identified, which were referred to by Roman numeral I-V; AT5106 did not belong to any group (Fig. 1). Because of the large number of missing values in AT group V (3 isoforms with missing values in 68%, 68% and 63% of cases, respectively), proteins from that group were not included in the analysis

of Aim 1. Hence, the statistical models described below were based on 30 protein variables.

First, an unsupervised PCA model for healthy controls ($n = 11$) was computed. The model had one PC ($R^2 = 0.31$, $Q^2 = 0.12$). No multivariate outliers were found. The loadings column plot of the model is depicted in Fig. 2a. Then, an unsupervised PCA model for patients was computed ($n = 11$). The model had one PC ($R^2 = 0.29$, $Q^2 = 0.02$). No multivariate outliers were found. The loadings column plot of the model is depicted in Fig. 2b. Then, the two loadings column plots were compared (Fig. 2a and b), focusing on the seven proteins with the highest discriminatory power between patients and healthy controls according to our previous study [16], namely AG3409, AT5106, IV_AT1505, HG1211, HG1203, HG2205, and PEDF3308:

- **AG3409:** In healthy controls, AG3409 is separated from the four other isoforms of AG, and these four isoforms inter-correlated positively, ie the loading values (p [1]) were similar. This correlation structure is disrupted in patients in the sense that, in patients, it is AG4404 that is separated from the four other isoforms of AG.
- **AT5106:** In Fig. 2b, the p [1] value of I_AT111 (black column) is almost the same as that of AT5106 (white column), i.e. these two proteins inter-correlated positively in patients. In healthy controls (Fig. 2a), this was not the case. We have previously shown that AT5106 was downregulated in patients, whereas I_AT111 (although not being one of the seven highest discriminating proteins) was upregulated [16]. Hence, in patients, a down-regulated isoform of AT correlated by PCA to an up-regulated isoform of AT. However, looking at these two proteins with traditional bivariate correlation (i.e., not multivariate PCA), there was no statistically significant association between them, neither in patients nor in healthy controls.
- **IV_AT1505:** In both patients and healthy controls, IV_AT1505 is close to zero, meaning that this isoform does not contribute much to the two PCA models. IV_AT1505 also remains fairly isolated from the other isoforms of group IV. The remaining isoforms of group IV of AT positively inter-correlate in a similar way in both health and disease.
- **HG1211, HG1203, HG2205**: No clear correlation structure was discernable for these three isoforms. The same was true for the two other isoforms of HG.
- **PEDF3308:** It was difficult to discern a clear pattern concerning PEDF3308 and its isoforms.

Post-translational modifications (aim 2)

Based on the above-mentioned correlation between AT5106 and I_AT111 (albeit by PCA, not traditional bivariate

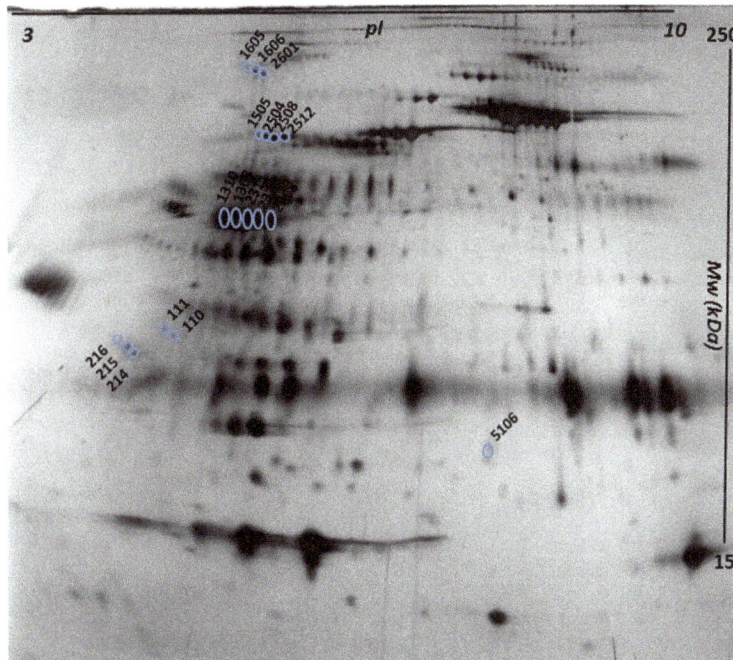

Fig. 1 Typical cerebrospinal fluid two-dimensional electrophoresis gel, highlighting the 18 isoforms alpha-1-antitrypsin with their spot number. Proteins separate according to pI (range 3–10) and according to Mw (range 15–250 kDa)

correlation), we decided to focus the biochemical part of the present paper on characterizing some of the post-translational modifications and fragments of AT. The 18 isoforms of AT are highlighted in Fig. 1, and the analyzed isoforms are shown in Table 2. As can be seen in Table 2, we found six truncated forms of AT, and we were able to show that seven isoforms were N-glycosylated. Three of the N-glycosylated isoforms (spots 1605, 1606, and 2601) belonged to AT group V which, as described above, had a large proportion of missing values. However, at least one AT group V isoform was present in seven out of 11 patients compared to two out of 11 healthy controls ($p = 0.04$, Fisher's exact test).

AT5106 and I_AT111, which were positively inter-correlated in patients by PCA, were both confirmed to be N-terminal truncated fragments. IV_AT1505 was N-glycosylated.

Regression of clinical pain parameters (aim 3)

First, pain intensity data in patients ("VASPI last week") was regressed, using the 260 proteins from our earlier study as predictor variables (X-variables). The OPLS model on 11 patients with "VASPI last week" as outcome variable (Y-variable) rendered three components ($R^2 = 0.99$, $Q^2 = 0.43$), and the results are summarized in Table 3. Notably, the protein having the highest VASPI-VIP (as well as a high and significant Spearman's rho) was a

previously not identified isoform of alpha-1-antitrypsin (spot 2515, Table 3).

Of the proteins described in Aim 1 (including Table 2), the following four proteins had a high VIP (i.e. VIP≥ 1.5) *and* a significant Spearman's rho correlation coefficient:

- PEDF3308 had VIP = 2.38, which was the second-highest VIP of the model (rank 2 out of 260 proteins). The bivariate correlation between "VASPI last week" and PEDF3308 was positive (rho = 0.75, $p = 0.008$), Fig. 3.
- I_AT110 had VIP = 1.83 (rank 13 out of 260 proteins). The bivariate correlation between "VASPI last week" and I_AT110 was negative (rho = − 0.676, $p = 0.022$). Going back to Fig. 2b, it can be seen that I_AT110 positively inter-correlated with I_AT111 (and hence with AT5106) in patients, and this was confirmed by classical bivariate correlation (rho = 0.664, $p = 0.026$); in healthy controls, no such correlation existed between I_AT110 and I_AT111 (rho = 0.191, $p = 0.574$).
- I_AT111 had VIP = 1.75 (rank 19 out of 260 proteins). The bivariate correlation between "VASPI last week" and I_AT111 was negative (rho = − 0.781, $p = 0.005$), Fig. 4.
- AG3409 had VIP = 1.73 (rank 20 out of 260 proteins). The bivariate correlation between "VASPI

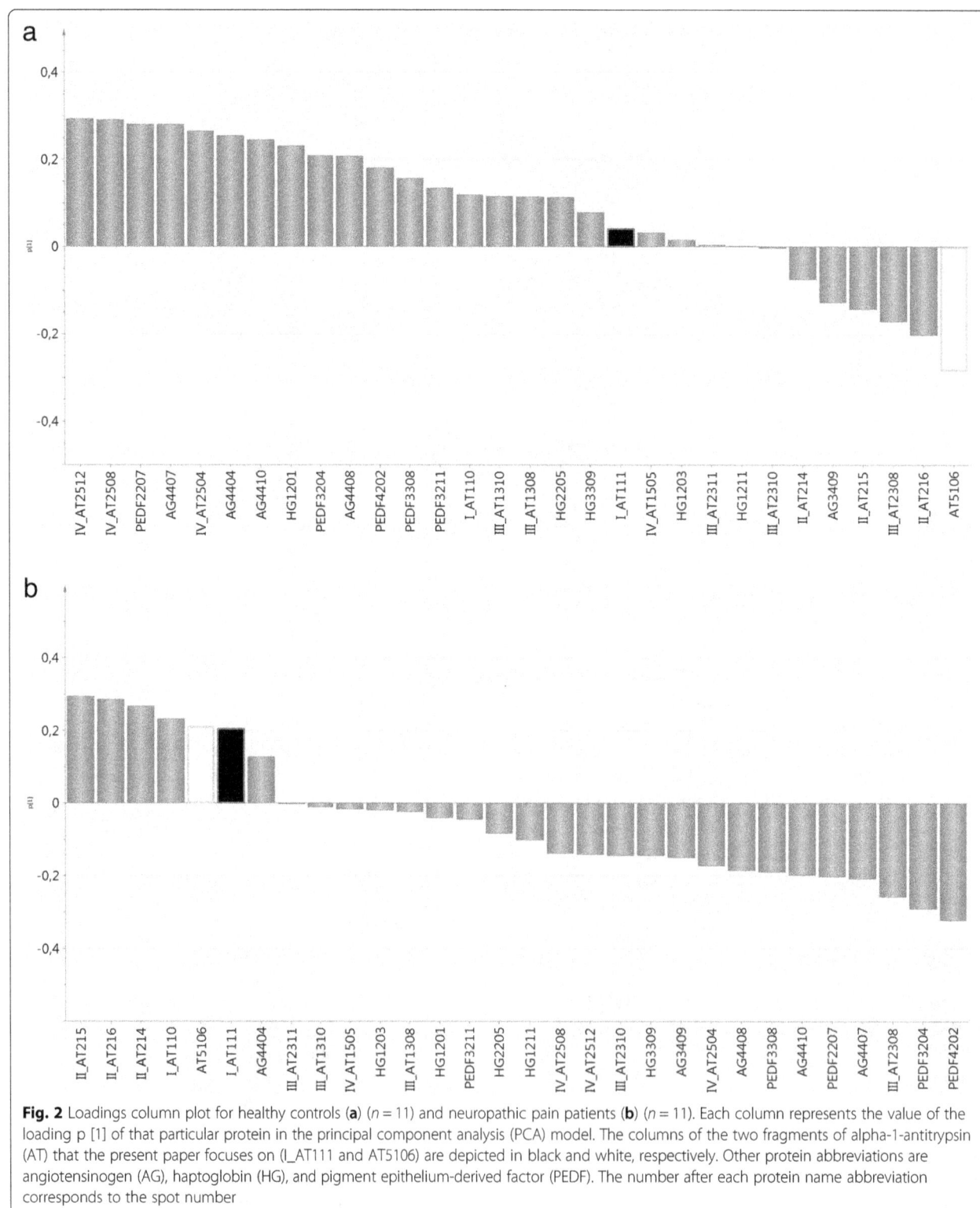

Fig. 2 Loadings column plot for healthy controls (**a**) (*n* = 11) and neuropathic pain patients (**b**) (*n* = 11). Each column represents the value of the loading p [1] of that particular protein in the principal component analysis (PCA) model. The columns of the two fragments of alpha-1-antitrypsin (AT) that the present paper focuses on (I_AT111 and AT5106) are depicted in black and white, respectively. Other protein abbreviations are angiotensinogen (AG), haptoglobin (HG), and pigment epithelium-derived factor (PEDF). The number after each protein name abbreviation corresponds to the spot number

last week" and AG3409 was positive (rho = 0.81, *p* = 0.003), Fig. 5.

Moreover, PEDF3211, which was one of the five iso-forms of PEDF in Aim 1 above, also had a very high

VASPI-VIP (VIP = 2.14, rank 4 out of 260 proteins), albeit with a non-significant Spearman's rho (rho = 0.58, *p* = 0.064).

Hence, three isoforms of AT, two isoforms of PEDF, and one isoform of angiotensinogen "reappeared" as

Table 2 Post-translational modifications (PTMs) of 18 isoforms of cerebrospinal fluid alpha-1-antitrypsin

SPOT NUMBER	Mw (kDa)	pI	Unique peptides	Peptides position START-END	PTM
1605	153.0	5.50	18	35–418	N-glycosylation
1606	153.0	5.52	18	35–418	N-glycosylation
2601	153.0	5.54	18	35–418	N-glycosylation
1310	70.9	5.25	14	35–418	–
1308	69.5	5.35	20	35–418	–
2311	69.5	5.39	25	35–418	–
2310	68.2	5.44	25	35–418	–
2308	68.2	5.50	31	35–418	–
216	36.7	4.78	6	180–411	N-terminal truncation
215	35.4	4.80	16	126–418	N-terminal truncation
214	33.4	4.90	6	35–241	C-terminal truncation
111	38.9	5.10	10	126–418	N-terminal truncation
110	37.4	5.15	16	154–418	N-terminal truncation
5106	19.4	6.50	7	299–418	N-terminal truncation
1505	57.6	5.3	12	35–418	N-glycosylation
2504	60.9	5.5	12	35–418	N-glycosylation
2508	68.3	5.5	12	35–418	N-glycosylation
2512	68.2	5.4	12	35–418	N-glycosylation

major results when regressing VASPI, i.e., they were major findings both in the present study and in our previous study [16].

Then, pain duration in patients was regressed using the 260 proteins from our earlier study as predictor variables (X-variables). The OPLS model on 11 patients with "pain duration" as outcome variable (Y-variable) had 3 components ($R^2 = 0.99$, $Q^2 = 0.54$), and the results are summarized in Table 4. Of the proteins described above in Aim 1 (including Table 2), seven proteins had a high VIP for pain duration (i.e. VIP≥1.5), but none of these proteins had a significant Spearman's rho correlation coefficient for pain duration. Among these seven proteins, however, the presence of AG3409 was noted, as it was rather highly ranked among the 260 proteins (VIP = 1.95, rank 12 and rho = − 0.39, $p = 0.233$).

Discussion

The results presented in this paper suggest that fragments of AT might be considered as potential biomarkers for pathophysiological processes in the spinal cord of patients suffering from chronic peripheral neuropathic pain. AT in CSF is considered to be plasma-derived [28], but exposure to pathological processes in the central nervous system during diffusion from plasma to CSF could potentially lead to a disease-specific fragmentation process detectable in the CSF. However, local CNS production of AT in pathological conditions is also a possibility [29, 30].

The results presented here should be viewed as hypothesis-generating [31], and the low number of subjects

in the study is of course a strong limitation, as is the age difference between the groups. Another limitation is the fact that the patients were using analgesics, introducing a potential confounding effect; moreover, concerning paracetamol and Non-Steroidal Anti-Inflammatory Drugs (NSAID), the percentages reported in Table 1 might perhaps somewhat underestimate the size of this problem because treatment "as needed" was not recorded. The difficulties inherent in CSF sampling (not least in pain patients) should however be remembered, and the usefulness of the CSF for CNS biomarker studies should be emphasized [13, 32]. Human pain proteomic CSF studies that actually report biomarker candidates are rare, and those that have been published typically report about 10 subjects per group [33, 34].

Protein fragments are emerging as important potential biomarkers in medicine in general [11]. Indeed, in the context of dementia research, the term "protein fragmentology" has been used [12]. What makes protein fragments so interesting in a CNS context is that their small size could enable them to cross the BBB easier than full-length proteins, and they would theoretically therefore be easier to detect in plasma [12]. As taking a blood sample is much easier than doing a lumbar puncture for CSF analysis, this is a very important practical aspect to take into consideration when searching for useable biomarkers.

Three fragments of AT stand out as especially interesting: AT5106, I_AT111, and I_AT110. AT5106 is a very small fragment (Table 2 and Fig. 1), and in our previous study it had the second-highest discriminatory power between

Table 3 Proteins associated with Visual Analogue Pain Intensity last week (VASPI) in patients with peripheral neuropathic pain

SPOT NB	VASPI-VIP	Protein name	Bivariate correlation with VASPI	
			Spearman's rho	p-value
2515	2.41	Alpha-1-antitrypsin	0.77	0.005*
3308	2.38	Pigment epithelium-derived factor	0.75	0.008*
4204	2.31	Fibrinogen gamma chain	0.72	0.012*
3211	2.14	Pigment epithelium-derived factor	0.58	0.064
7001	2.11	Prostaglandin-H2 D-isomerase	0.63	0.040*
6105	2.01	Kallikrein-6	0.62	0.041*
6104	2.00	Prostaglandin-H2 D-isomerase	−0.54	0.084
1111	1.97	Apolipoprotein E	0.66	0.028*
2405	1.89	Antithrombin	0.65	0.031*
2514	1.87	Beta-Ala-His dipeptidase	0.46	0.163
6613	1.84	Serotransferrin	0.70	0.016*
110	1.83	Alpha-1-antitrypsin	−0.68	0.022*
6206	1.79	Serotransferrin	0.52	0.104
1506	1.78	Beta-Ala-His dipeptidase	0.14	0.678
8004	1.77	Prostaglandin-H2 D-isomerase	−0.26	0.440
7202	1.76	Procollagen C-endopeptidase enhancer 1	0.38	0.244
111	1.75	Alpha-1-antitrypsin	−0.78	0.005*
3409	1.73	Angiotensinogen	0.81	0.003*
6205	1.72	Serotransferrin	−0.45	0.163
8108	1.67	Prostaglandin-H2 D-isomerase	−0.40	0.226
4611	1.66	Hemopexin	0.48	0.140
1205	1.64	Complement factor B	−0.62	0.041*
2205	1.64	Haptoglobin	0.30	0.375
2522	1.63	prothrombin	0.40	0.226
7713	1.62	plasminogen	−0.73	0.103
3302	1.61	Antithrombin	0.55	0.081
2504	1.61	Alpha-1-antitrypsin	0.37	0.257
8414	1.60	IgG heavy chain	−0.44	0.177
6304	1.58	Beta-2-glycoprotein 1	−0.21	0.535
8204	1.57	Prostaglandin-H2 D-isomerase	0.24	0.473
9507	1.56	Complement C4-A	−0.28	0.399
5620	1.55	Serum Albumin	0.42	0.204
3204	1.53	Pigment epithelium-derived factor	0.56	0.075
8413	1.52	IgG heavy chain	−0.23	0.491
7407	1.50	IgG heavy chain	−0.26	0.440

Note: Proteins are listed in decreasing order of importance according to Variable Influence on Projection (VIP) of the OPLS model. Only protein isoforms with VIP ≥ 1.5 are reported (see Methods section). Spot NB refers to the marked protein spot in Additional file 1: Figure S1

groups, being down-regulated in patients [16]. The correlation of AT5106 with I_AT111 in patients (as revealed by comparing the PCA column loading plots, Fig. 2a and b), lead to a particular interest also in the latter fragment. Indeed, I_AT111 turned out to be an important predictor of VASPI by MVDA, and it correlated negatively with VASPI by traditional bivariate statistics (Fig. 4). In our previous study, I_AT111 was shown to be up-regulated in patients [16]. We therefore speculate that the combination of down-regulated N-truncated AT5106 and up-regulated N-truncated I_AT111 could mirror disease-specific processes in the spinal cord. The negative correlation with

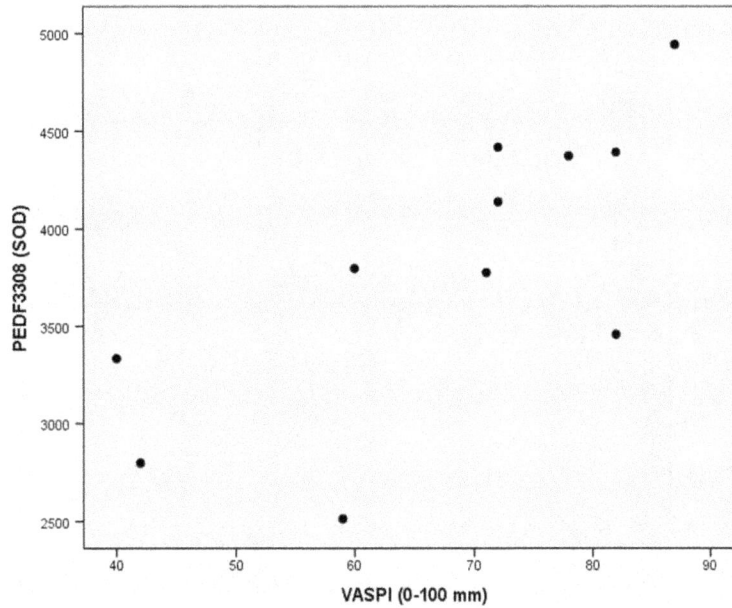

Fig. 3 Pain intensity vs PEDF spot 3308. Scatter plot of Visual Analogue Scale Pain Intensity (0–100 mm) last week (VASPI) vs. spot optical density (SOD) of pigment epithelium-derived factor (PEDF) spot 3308 in the cerebrospinal fluid of patients with peripheral neuropathic pain ($n = 11$). Spearman's rho $= 0.75$, $p = 0.008$

VASPI could perhaps indicate that I_AT111 indirectly mirrors the efficacy of anti-nociceptive mechanisms, i.e. it would be up-regulated in patients, and those who have more of it would have less activity in the nociceptive pathways. Does I_AT111 hence indirectly mirror an anti-inflammatory compensating mechanism in the spinal cord? The speculative nature of this line of reasoning must be emphasized. By PCA as well as by traditional bivariate correlation, it is also notable that I_AT111 and I_AT110 positively inter-correlated in patients but not in healthy controls. All in all, we speculate that the interactions of these three fragments of AT

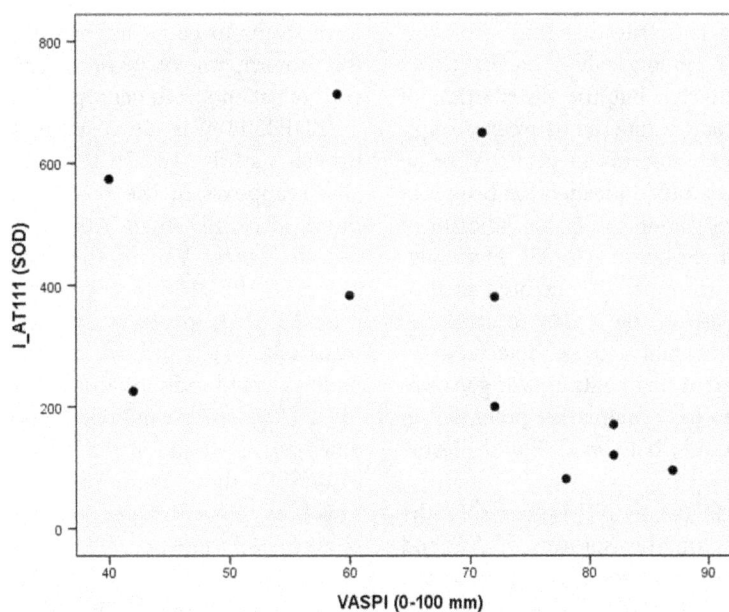

Fig. 4 Pain intensity vs AT spot 111. Scatter plot of Visual Analogue Scale Pain Intensity (0–100 mm) last week (VASPI) vs. spot optical density (SOD) of alpha-1-antitrypsin (AT) spot 111 in the cerebrospinal fluid of patients with peripheral neuropathic pain ($n = 11$). Spearman's rho $= -0.781$, $p = 0.005$

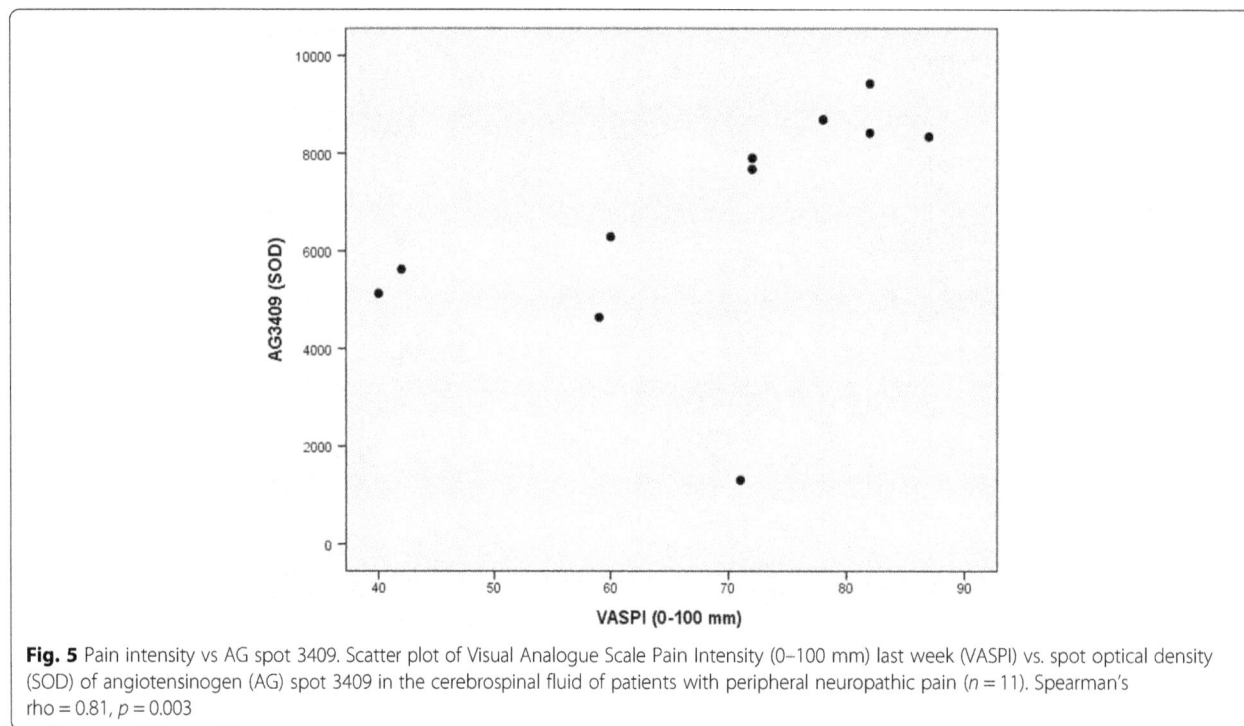

Fig. 5 Pain intensity vs AG spot 3409. Scatter plot of Visual Analogue Scale Pain Intensity (0–100 mm) last week (VASPI) vs. spot optical density (SOD) of angiotensinogen (AG) spot 3409 in the cerebrospinal fluid of patients with peripheral neuropathic pain (n = 11). Spearman's rho = 0.81, p = 0.003

might mirror disease-specific processes in the spinal cord.

Isoform IV_AT1505, which was one of the seven most discriminating proteins in our earlier study [16], did not contribute to the PCA models of Aim 1 and did not appear as a result of Aim 3.

Turning to glycosylated isoforms of AT, subgroup V (consisting of V_AT1605, V_AT1606, and V_AT2601, Fig. 1) appears interesting. It is true that these isoforms have a high percentage of missing values (in 68%, 68% and 63% of cases, respectively), but the distribution of glycosylated isoforms of group V differed between groups, the presence of glycosylated isoforms in group V being associated with the patients group. Indeed, it has been said that the pattern of AT glycosylation can be an indicator of the immune modulatory properties of AT [35]. The drawback of "big" glycosylated isoforms, as compared to protein fragments, is their relatively low ability to cross the BBB and hence lower probability to be detectable in plasma. All in all, we think that fragments and/or glycosylated isoforms of AT seem to have "biomarker potential" in pain medicine. Further studies, both in CSF and plasma [35], seem warranted.

Although we chose to focus on AT isoforms in the present study, future work on the isoforms of AG and PEDF would be interesting. Concerning AG3409, which had the highest discriminative power between groups in our previous study [16], it is notable that it reappears in the results of Aim 3 in the present paper (Fig. 5). Although this of course might be a false positive finding, it

is nonetheless interesting that the same protein reappears when regressing clinical parameters in the patients group. Hence, AG3409 discriminated between patients and healthy controls [16], but was *also* positively correlated to VASPI (and had a high VIP when regressing pain duration). The renin-angiotensin system seems to be involved in nociception processing [36, 37], and is a potential pain therapeutic target [38–40]; investigating this particular isoform seems to be an important line of future work. Does this isoform mirror pro-nociceptive activity in the spinal cord of patients with neuropathic pain?

PEDF3308 was down-regulated in patients in our previous study [16]. In the present study, this isoform also reappears in the results of Aim 3, and this even more forcefully than AG3409 as PEDF3308 had the *second-highest* VIP of the model (rank 2 out of 260 proteins). PEDF3308 correlated positively with VASPI (Fig. 3). PEDF protects against glutamate-caused excitotoxicity [41], and we therefore speculate that our findings could indicate a direct anti-nociceptive activity of PEDF3308, which would be "consumed" in patients (hence down-regulated and at the same time positively correlated to VASPI – those "consuming" more of it having less pain). This is of course extremely speculative, but seems to make physiological sense.

Going back to AT, one might wonder why such a well-known protein would be a specific biomarker for a pathological pain condition. In this context, it is important to remember that PTMs are very important physiologically. PTMs modulate enzyme activity, protein turnover and

Table 4 Proteins associated with pain duration in patients with peripheral neuropathic pain

SPOT NB	Pain duration-VIP	Protein name	Bivariate correlation with pain duration	
			Spearman's rho	p-value
2312	2.31	Zinc-Alpha-2-glycoprotein	0.50	0.120
7712	2.27	Plasminogen	0.82	0.023*
1205	2.26	Complement factor B	0.78	0.005*
7711	2.23	Plasminogen	0.61	0.148
3502	2.16	Hemopexin	0.55	0.082
3309	2.15	Haptoglobin	0.29	0.392
4309	2.14	Haptoglobin	0.71	0.071
2106	2.09	Apolipoprotein E	0.55	0.079
206	2.07	Haptoglobin	0.77	0.072
2601	2.05	Alpha-1-antitrypsin	0.89	0.019*
3106	2.03	Clusterin	−0.67	0.024*
3409	1.95	Angiotensinogen	−0.39	0.233
409	1.93	Alpha-2-HS-glycoprotein	0.46	0.159
1203	1.86	Haptoglobin	0.52	0.105
7713	1.86	Plasminogen	0.77	0.072
6001	1.82	Alpha-1-antitrypsin	−0.54	0.091
2311	1.82	Alpha-1-antitrypsin	0.38	0.245
6611	1.75	Serotransferrin	−0.57	0.067
6614	1.73	Serotransferrin	−0.58	0.062
6610	1.72	Serotransferrin	−0.67	0.023*
3111	1.71	Prostaglandin-H2 D-isomerase	−0.54	0.085
412	1.69	Alpha-2-HS-glycoprotein	0.44	0.179
6609	1.67	Serotransferrin	−0.72	0.013*
1211	1.67	Haptoglobin	0.30	0.377
3210	1.66	Haptoglobin	0.52	0.098
3010	1.66	Tetranectin	−0.21	0.527
2310	1.63	Alpha-1-antitrypsin	0.25	0.466
7403	1.61	Complement C3	0.59	0.055
4105	1.61	Prostaglandin-H2 D-isomerase	−0.51	0.113
5306	1.59	Pigment epithelium-derived factor	−0.60	0.050
2108	1.57	Apolipoprotein E	−0.56	0.073
208	1.56	Haptoglobin	0.35	0.290
8001	1.55	Phosphatidylethanolamine binding protein	−0.46	0.154
1111	1.53	Apolipoprotein E	−0.55	0.082

Note: Proteins are listed in decreasing order of importance according to Variable Influence on Projection (VIP) of the OPLS model. Only protein isoforms with VIP ≥ 1.5 are reported (see Methods section). Spot NB refers to the marked protein spot in Additional file 1: Figure S1

localization, protein-protein interactions, various signaling cascades, DNA repair, and cell division [5]. It is becoming increasingly clear that PTMs are important in both health and disease. For instance, posttranslational glycosylation patterns are said to be an extremely sensitive indicator of intracellular conditions, and the fields of glycoproteomics is emerging as an important contributor in the search for biomarkers in different medical conditions [42]. Hence, PTM-patterns are probably important when trying to identify the molecular "fingerprints" of different pain conditions. Other important forms of PTMs include acetylation, deamidation, hydroxylation, nitration, palmitoylation, phosphorylation, sulfation and ubiquitination [5, 43]. Therefore, looking only at *total* levels of a particular protein is probably often too simplistic, and an "old" and well-known protein like AT might very well, due to PTMs, mirror disease-specific processes. The familiarity of AT should not make one a priori consider it uninteresting as a biomarker.

In the words of Pavlou et al., we have studied "a small number of samples from diseased and nondiseased groups" in order to "identify molecules exhibiting discriminating potential" [17]. To correctly evaluate our findings, it is important to understand that the present study was not intended to generate clinical biomarker candidates. If that had been our purpose, dozens or perhaps hundreds of samples would have been necessary. Instead, using the terminology proposed by Pavlou et al., this was an early discovery phase, pre-clinical exploratory study [17]. For such studies, in which the aim is to strive towards a better understanding of molecular pathology in humans, the study design requirements are different from clinical biomarker studies [20].

Conclusions

On the basis of the findings reported in the present paper, we present the hypothesis that fragments and/or glycosylated isoforms of alpha-1-antitrypsin might be considered as potential biomarkers of the pathophysiological processes in the spinal cord of neuropathic pain patients. The biomarker potential of protein fragments should be taken into account by pain researchers. Biomarkers with high specificity and sensitivity are difficult to find, and the combinatorial power of a panel of different biomarkers has been suggested as a solution this problem [44]. This is in line with modern systems biology [45], the focus lying not on a particular "magic bullet" protein but on networks of mutually interacting proteins. In such a context, the above-mentioned combination of down-regulated N-truncated AT5106 and up-regulated N-truncated I_AT111 could perhaps be of value. More research is needed, both in CSF and plasma, in order to perhaps confirm this hypothesis.

Abbreviations

AG: Angiotensinogen; AT: Alpha-1-antitrypsin; BBB: Blood-brain barrier; CNS: Central nervous system; CSF: Cerebrospinal fluid; HG: Haptoglobin; MVDA: Multivariate data analysis by projection; OPLS: Orthogonal partial least squares projection to latent structures; PC: Principal component; PCA: Principal component analysis; PEDF: Pigment epithelium-derived factor; PTM: Post-translational modification; SOD: Spot optical density; VASPI: Visual analogue scale pain intensity; VIP: Variable influence on projection

Acknowledgements

This paper is dedicated to the memory of our dear co-worker Patrik Olausson, who passed away while this paper was being peer-reviewed. Patrik took part in the biochemical analyses and in the critical revision of the original manuscript.

Funding

This study was supported by the Swedish Research Council (K2015-99x-21874-05-4), Region Östergötland and AFA Insurance (140341). The funders had no role in study design, data collection and analysis, decision to publish, or preparation of the manuscript.

Authors' contributions

EB, BGe, and BGh designed the study. EB collected the CSF samples. Biochemical analyses were made by SE and BGh. Statistical analyses were made by EB. EB, BGe, and BGh interpreted the data. EB and BGh drafted the article, and all authors revised it critically. All authors approved the final version.

Competing interests

The authors declare that they have no competing interests.

References

1. Mao J. Translational pain research: achievements and challenges. J Pain. 2009;10:1001–11.
2. Borsook D, Becerra L, Hargreaves R. Biomarkers for chronic pain and analgesia. Part 1: the need, reality, challenges, and solutions. Discov Med. 2011;11:197–207.
3. Internat. Human Genome Sequencing Consortium. Finishing the euchromatic sequence of the human genome. Nature. 2004;431:931–45.
4. Jensen ON. Modification-specific proteomics: characterization of post-translational modifications by mass spectrometry. Curr Opin Chem Biol. 2004;8:33–41.
5. Karve TM, Cheema AK. Small changes huge impact: the role of protein posttranslational modifications in cellular homeostasis and disease. J Amino Acids. 2011;2011:207691.
6. Kim MS, Pinto SM, Getnet D, Nirujogi RS, Manda SS, Chaerkady R, Madugundu AK, Kelkar DS, Isserlin R, Jain S, et al. A draft map of the human proteome. Nature. 2014;509:575–81.
7. Niederberger E, Geisslinger G. Proteomics in neuropathic pain research. Anesthesiology. 2008;108:314–23.
8. Niederberger E, Kuhlein H, Geisslinger G. Update on the pathobiology of neuropathic pain. Expert Rev Proteomics. 2008;5:799–818.
9. Pan S, Chen R, Aebersold R, Brentnall TA. Mass spectrometry based glycoproteomics--from a proteomics perspective. Mol Cell Proteomics. 2011;10:R110 003251.
10. Drake PM, Cho W, Li B, Prakobphol A, Johansen E, Anderson NL, Regnier FE, Gibson BW, Fisher SJ. Sweetening the pot: adding glycosylation to the biomarker discovery equation. Clin Chem. 2010;56:223–36.
11. Genovese F, Karsdal MA. Protein degradation fragments as diagnostic and prognostic biomarkers of connective tissue diseases: understanding the extracellular matrix message and implication for current and future serological biomarkers. Expert Rev Proteomics. 2015;13:213–25.
12. Inekci D, Jonesco DS, Kennard S, Karsdal MA, Henriksen K. The potential of pathological protein fragmentation in blood-based biomarker development for dementia - with emphasis on Alzheimer's disease. Front Neurol. 2015;6:90.
13. Lai ZW, Petrera A, Schilling O. The emerging role of the peptidome in biomarker discovery and degradome profiling. Biol Chem. 2015;396:185–92.
14. Carlsson-Jonsson A, Gao T, Hao JX, Fransson R, Sandstrom A, Nyberg F, Wiesenfeld-Hallin Z, Xu XJ. N-terminal truncations of substance P 1–7 amide affect its action on spinal cord injury-induced mechanical allodynia in rats. Eur J Pharmacol. 2014;738:319–25.
15. Jensen TS, Baron R, Haanpaa M, Kalso E, Loeser JD, Rice AS, Treede RD. A new definition of neuropathic pain. Pain. 2011;152:2204–5.
16. Bäckryd E, Ghafouri B, Carlsson AK, Olausson P, Gerdle B. Multivariate proteomic analysis of the cerebrospinal fluid of patients with peripheral neuropathic pain and healthy controls - a hypothesis-generating pilot study. J Pain Res. 2015;8:321–33.
17. Pavlou MP, Diamandis EP, Blasutig IM. The long journey of cancer biomarkers from the bench to the clinic. Clin Chem. 2013;59:147–57.
18. Eriksson L, Byrne T, Johansson E, Trygg J, Vikström C. Multi- and Megavariate data analysis: basic principles and applications. 3rd ed. MKS Umetrics AB: Malmö; 2013.

19. Wheelock AM, Wheelock CE. Trials and tribulations of 'omics data analysis: assessing quality of SIMCA-based multivariate models using examples from pulmonary medicine. Mol BioSyst. 2013;9:2589–96.

20. Mischak H, Vlahou A, Righetti PG, Calvete JJ. Putting value in biomarker research and reporting. J Proteome. 2014;96:A1–3.

21. Bäckryd E, Sorensen J, Gerdle B. Ziconotide trialing by Intrathecal bolus injections: an open-label non-randomized clinical trial in postoperative/posttraumatic neuropathic pain patients refractory to conventional treatment. Neuromodulation. 2015;18:404–13.

22. Dworkin RH, Turk DC, Farrar JT, Haythornthwaite JA, Jensen MP, Katz NP, Kerns RD, Stucki G, Allen RR, Bellamy N, et al. Core outcome measures for chronic pain clinical trials: IMMPACT recommendations. Pain. 2005;113:9–19.

23. Treede RD, Jensen TS, Campbell JN, Cruccu G, Dostrovsky JO, Griffin JW, Hansson P, Hughes R, Nurmikko T, Serra J. Neuropathic pain: redefinition and a grading system for clinical and research purposes. Neurology. 2008; 70:1630–5.

24. Zigmond AS, Snaith RP. The hospital anxiety and depression scale. Acta Psychiatr Scand. 1983;67:361–70.

25. Sullivan MJ, Bishop SR, Pivik J. The pain catastrophizing scale: development and validation. Psychol Assess. 1995;7:524–32.

26. Sullivan M, Karlsson J, Ware JE Jr. The Swedish SF-36 health survey—I. Evaluation of data quality, scaling assumptions, reliability and construct validity across general populations in Sweden. Soc Sci Med. 1995;41:1349–58.

27. Ghafouri B, Irander K, Lindbom J, Tagesson C, Lindahl M. Comparative proteomics of nasal fluid in seasonal allergic rhinitis. J Proteome Res. 2006;5:330–8.

28. Irani DN. Properties and Composition of Normal Cerebrospinal Fluid. In: Irani DN, editor. Cerebrospinal Fluid in Clinical Practice. Philadelphia, PA: Saunders; 2009. p. 67–89.

29. Jesse S, Lehnert S, Jahn O, Parnetti L, Soininen H, Herukka SK, Steinacker P, Tawfik S, Tumani H, von Arnim CA, et al. Differential sialylation of serpin A1 in the early diagnosis of Parkinson's disease dementia. PLoS One. 2012;7:e48783.

30. Gollin PA, Kalaria RN, Eikelenboom P, Rozemuller A, Perry G. Alpha 1-antitrypsin and alpha 1-antichymotrypsin are in the lesions of Alzheimer's disease. Neuroreport. 1992;3:201–3.

31. Biesecker LG. Hypothesis-generating research and predictive medicine. Genome Res. 2013;23:1051–3.

32. Roche S, Gabelle A, Lehmann S. Clinical proteomics of the cerebrospinal fluid: towards the discovery of new biomarkers. Proteomics Clin Appl. 2008;2:428–36.

33. Conti A, Ricchiuto P, Iannaccone S, Sferrazza B, Cattaneo A, Bachi A, Reggiani A, Beltramo M, Alessio M. Pigment epithelium-derived factor is differentially expressed in peripheral neuropathies. Proteomics. 2005;5:4558–67.

34. Liu XD, Zeng BF, Xu JG, Zhu HB, Xia QC. Proteomic analysis of the cerebrospinal fluid of patients with lumbar disk herniation. Proteomics. 2006;6:1019–28.

35. McCarthy C, Saldova R, Wormald MR, Rudd PM, McElvaney NG, Reeves EP. The role and importance of glycosylation of acute phase proteins with focus on alpha-1 antitrypsin in acute and chronic inflammatory conditions. J Proteome Res. 2014;13:3131–43.

36. Nemoto W, Nakagawasai O, Yaoita F, Kanno S, Yomogida S, Ishikawa M, Tadano T, Tan-No K. Angiotensin II produces nociceptive behavior through spinal AT1 receptor-mediated p38 mitogen-activated protein kinase activation in mice. Mol Pain. 2013;9:38.

37. Smith MT, Lau T, Wallace VC, Wyse BD, Rice AS. Analgesic efficacy of small-molecule angiotensin II type 2 receptor antagonists in a rat model of antiretroviral toxic polyneuropathy. Behav Pharmacol. 2014;25:137–46.

38. Finnerup NB, Baastrup C. Angiotensin II: from blood pressure to pain control. Lancet. 2014;383:1613–4.

39. Rice AS, Dworkin RH, McCarthy TD, Anand P, Bountra C, McCloud PI, Hill J, Cutter G, Kitson G, Desem N, et al. EMA401, an orally administered highly selective angiotensin II type 2 receptor antagonist, as a novel treatment for postherpetic neuralgia: a randomised, double-blind, placebo-controlled phase 2 clinical trial. Lancet. 2014;383:1637–47

40. Smith MT, Muralidharan A. Targeting angiotensin II type 2 receptor pathways to treat neuropathic pain and inflammatory pain. Expert Opin Ther Targets. 2015;19:25–35.

41. Craword SE, Fitchev P, Veliceasa D, Volpert OV. The many facets of PEDF in drug discovery and disease: a diamond in the rough or split personality disorder? Expert Opin Drug Discov. 2013;8:769–92.

42. Hua S, An HJ. Glycoscience aids in biomarker discovery. BMB Rep. 2012;45:323–30.

43. Rogowska-Wrzesinska A, Le Bihan MC, Thaysen-Andersen M, Roepstorff P. 2D gels still have a niche in proteomics. J Proteome. 2013;88:4–13.

44. Drucker E, Krapfenbauer K. Pitfalls and limitations in translation from biomarker discovery to clinical utility in predictive and personalised medicine. EPMA J. 2013;4:7.

45. Antunes-Martins A, Perkins JR, Lees J, Hildebrandt T, Orengo C, Bennett DL. Systems biology approaches to finding novel pain mediators. Wiley Interdiscip Rev Syst Biol Med. 2013;5:11–35.

Acute spontaneous intracerebral hemorrhage and traumatic brain injury are the most common causes of critical illness in the ICU and have high early mortality

Ye-Ting Zhou[1†], Dao-Ming Tong[2*†], Shao-Dan Wang[3], Song Ye[1], Ben-Wen Xu[1] and Chen-Xi Yang[1]

Abstract

Background: Critical care covers multiple disciplines. However, the causes of critical illness in the ICU, particularly the most common causes, remain unclear. We aimed to investigate the incidence and the most common causes of critical illness and the corresponding early mortality rates in ICU patients.

Methods: A retrospective cohort study was performed to examine critically ill patients (aged over 15 years) in the general ICU in Shuyang County in northern China (1/2014–12/2015). The incidences and causes of critical illnesses and their corresponding early mortality rates in the ICU were determined by an expert panel.

Results: During the 2-year study period, 1,211,138 person-years (PY) and 1645 critically ill patients (mean age, 61.8 years) were documented. The median Glasgow Coma Scale (GCS) score was 6 (range, 3–15). The mean acute physiology and chronic health evaluation II (APACHE II) score was 21.2 ± 6.8. The median length of the ICU stay was 4 days (range, 1–29 days). The most common causes of critical illness in the ICU were spontaneous intracerebral hemorrhage (SICH) (26%, 17.6/100,000 PY) and traumatic brain injury (TBI) (16.8%, 11.4/100,000 PY). During the first 7 days in the ICU, SICH was the most common cause of death (42.2%, 7.4/10,000 PY), followed by TBI (36.6%, 4.2/100,000 PY). Based on a logistic analysis, older patients had a significantly higher risk of death from TBI (risk ratio [RR], 1.7; 95% CI, 1.034–2.635), heart failure/cardiovascular crisis (RR, 0.2; 95% CI, 0.083–0.484), cerebral infarction (RR, 0.15; 95% CI, 0.050–0.486), or respiratory failure (RR, 0.35; 95% CI, 0.185–0.784) than younger patients. However, the risk of death from SICH in the two groups was similar.

Conclusions: The most common causes of critical illness in the ICU were SICH and TBI, and both critical illnesses showed a higher risk of death during the first 7 days in the ICU.

Keywords: Critical illness, Causes, Incidence, Mortality, Epidemiology, Intracerebral hemorrhage, Head injury

Background

Twenty years ago, patients with organ failure accounted for most intensive care unit (ICU) cases [1], and a high mortality rate was observed in patients who refused ICU care [2, 3]. Today, with improvements in living standards and the aging of the general population, management of critically ill patients using intensive nursing care is more common [4–6]. Multiple epidemiological studies on pre-hospital emergency medical services have been conducted [7, 8]; however, the causes of critical illnesses in the ICU, especially the most common causes, remain unclear. Moreover, it is important to determine the most common illnesses that require management in an ICU and to understand the early mortality rates associated with these illnesses during the ICU stay. The aim of this study was to investigate the incidences and causes of critical illnesses and the corresponding early mortality rates among patients admitted to the ICU from the general population of Shuyang County in northern China.

* Correspondence: dmtong@xzhmu.edu.cn
†Ye-Ting Zhou and Dao-Ming Tong contributed equally to this work.
[2]Department of Neurology, Affiliated Shuyang Hospital, Xuzhou Medical University, Xuzhou, Jiangsu, China
Full list of author information is available at the end of the article

Methods

Study design and participants

We retrospectively analyzed data that were collected from January 2014 to December 2015 for critically ill patients who were admitted to a general ICU (17 beds) in a tertiary teaching hospital—the unique three-general hospital. The hospital has a referral center (with 10 ambulances) and was responsible for all critical or emergency work within Shuyang County in northern China (38 county townships and a county town). Thus, 24 h a day, almost all critically ill patients were sent directly to the ICU. Therefore, this hospital was a strong source of critically ill patients, which ensured sufficient data availability. The study sample was compiled from the 2014 and 2015 data registries. During the study period, 1,211,138 people aged 15 years or older, including 697,615 women and 115,355 people aged 65 years or older, lived in the county [9]. The study was approved by the Ethical Committee on Clinical Research of the Shuyang People's Hospital in China. Because the study involved care for critical illness, written informed consent was obtained from the nearest relative or a person who had been designated to provide consent by the patient.

Procedures

To date, there are no compulsory diagnostic criteria for critical illness. Moreover, the codes for critical illnesses per the International Classification of Diseases, 10th Revision (ICD-10), are not well established. The relevant code changes according to the condition of the critically ill patient, and these conditions include coma (R40.2), cardiac arrest (I46.9), heart failure (I50), shock (R57.9), respiratory failure (J96), cardiovascular crisis and other critical events. We also identified those patients who had acute spontaneous intracerebral hemorrhage (SICH) by the code I61.9, but in this study, SICH was only limited to those with acutely non-traumatic coma. Similarly, traumatic brain injury (TBI) indicated a severe TBI (including traumatic subdural and epidural hematoma, or with intracerebral hematoma or subarachnoid hemorrhage) with sudden traumatic coma. Coma refers to a state of unconsciousness from which the patient cannot be aroused and is typified by the absence of language and motor function with a Glasgow Coma Scale (GCS) score of 3 to 8 (on a scale of 3 to 15, with lower scores indicating a lower level of consciousness). Cardiovascular crisis includes cardiogenic shock, cardiac arrest, sudden chest pain, and hypertensive crisis. Here, our retrospective study of ICU patients used the following inclusion criteria: (1) the patient (age > 15 years) exhibited an emergency- onset condition with unstable life signs or acute organ dysfunction and required transfer by emergency services to the ICU, and (2) the patient was hospitalized due to the onset a life-threatening organ dysfunction

and required monitoring in the ICU. We used the following exclusion criteria: (1) age < 15 years, (2) an additional visit to the ICU within 2 weeks, and (3) residence in the county for < 6 months. We collected the critically ill patient data from the prospective registration of their primary diagnosis in the ICU patient out-of-hospital registry. Registration was the responsibility of the physician in charge of the ICU. The data registry annual volumes included sex, age, address, the date of admission, the sole primary diagnosis, the ICU stay length, the outcome of the main processing, and a contact telephone number for the ICU patient. All patients with craniocerebral disease were verified using their electronic medical records (an emergency cranial CT scan upon admission) and were assigned an initial GCS score and an acute physiology and chronic health evaluation II (APACHE II) score.

The time window of the ICU stay for most patients was between 3 and 7 days. Early mortality was assessed during the first 7 days of the critical illness. The World Health Organization (WHO) defines a person who is over 65 years old as geriatric. Therefore, patients were divided into a geriatric group and a non-geriatric group to compare the risks of critical illness between age groups.

Death events in the ICU and their causes were identified through medical record notes and from follow-up information. Follow-up information was from our physician who was conducted inquiries by phone to the patient's closest living relative on day 7 of discharge from the ICU. Intensive care and neurology experts conducted a retrospective statistical analysis of the data of the study population during the 2-year period.

Statistical analysis

All numeric variables are expressed as the mean ± SD or median (interquartile range [IQR]) and N (%). The overall incidence and causes were analyzed. The incidence rate per year in the population of critically ill patients was documented. Incidence rates for risk during 1 year were also calculated by dividing the baseline population by the number of annual cases. We used a logistic regression analysis to determine the risk ratio (RR) for a death event comparing the geriatric patients with the non-geriatric patients. All p-values were 2-sided, and significance was set at $p < 0.05$. Data were analyzed using SPSS version 17.0 (SPSS Inc., Chicago, IL, USA).

Results

Overall analysis

During the 2-year study period, 1791 critically ill cases were registered in the ICU following hospital discharge. We excluded cases that did not meet the inclusion criteria, including patients aged < 15 years ($n = 126$), patients who had another visitation to the ICU within

2 weeks ($n = 21$), and patients who had lived in the area for < 6 months ($n = 4$). Ultimately, 1645 patients who met the criteria were designated as critically ill patients and were enrolled into the study. The survey included 1015 men (61.7%) and 630 women (38.3%), which resulted in a male-to-female ratio of 1.7:1. The ages of the patients ranged from 15 to 98 years, and the average age was 61.8 ± 0.49 years. The median initial GCS score was 6 (range, 3–15). The mean initial APACHE II score (mean ± SD) was 21.2 ± 6.8. The median length of the ICU stay was 4 days (up to 29 days).

Incidence of critical illness

During the 2-year study period, 1645 patients with an acute critical illness were documented among the total county population. The total incidence of critical illness was 67.9/100,000 person-years (PY) (Table 1). The most common acute critical illness types were strokes and neurological critical illnesses (632/2 years, 38.4%, 26.1/100,000 PY, including 577 cases of stroke/2 years, 35.1%, 23.8/100,000 PY), followed by trauma and traumatic brain injury (TBI) (397/2 years, 24.1%, 16.4/100,000 PY), cardiovascular critical diseases (140/2 years, 5.8/100,000 PY), and respiratory critical diseases (96/2 years, 4.0/100,000 PY).

The incidence of acute SICH tended to increase with increasing age, with the incidence peaking between 55 and 64 years. The incidence of TBI tended to decrease with decreasing age, with the incidence peaking between 65 and 74 years. The types and outcome of SICH and TBI during the first 7 days in the ICU are shown in Table 2.

Table 1 Incidence and ranking of emergency critical events

Critically ill events ranking	Number of cases in 2 years	Percentage (%)	Per100000 population members per year
Stroke and neurological critical ill	632	38.4	26.1
TBI and Trauma	397	24.1	16.4
Cardiovascular Critical ill	140	8.5	5.8
Respiratory Critical ill	96	5.8	4.0
After surgery or intervention	89	5.4	3.7
Gastrointestinal critical ill	74	4.5	3.1
Pesticides / drug poisoning	72	4.4	3.0
Sepsis / septic shock	48	2.9	2.0
Any cancer	32	1.9	1.3
Others	65	4.0	2.7
All	1645	100	67.9

TBI traumatic brain injury

Table 2 The types and outcome of SICH and TBI observed during the first 7 days in the ICU

Types	Number of cases in 2 years	Death (%)
SICH	427	180(42.2)
Striato-capsula,n(%)	178(41.7)	75(42.1)
Lobar,n(%)	81(10.0)	30(37.0)
Thalamus,n(%)	72(16.7)	23(31.9)
Brainstem, n(%)	61(14..3)	40(65.6)
Cerebellar, n(%)	26(6.1)	10(38.5)
Others (%),n(%)	9(2.1)	2(22.0)
TBI	276	101(36.6)
Subdural hematoma, n(%)	181(65.6)	89(49.2)
Intracerebral hemorrhage, n(%)	58(21.o)	9(15.5)
Epideural hematoma, n(%)	37(13.4)	3(8.1)
With subarachnoid hemorrhage, n(%)	201((72.8))	N/A
With contusions, n(%)	189(68.5)	N/A
With fractures, n(%)	182(65.9)	N/A

ICU intensive care unit, *SICH* spontaneous intracerebral hemorrhage, *TBI* traumatic brain injury

Causes of critical illness

Of the 1645 cases of critical illness, the most common cause of critical illness was SICH with coma (26%, 17.6/100,000 PY), followed by acute TBI with coma (16.8%, 11.4/100,000 PY), heart failure/cardiovascular crisis (8.5%, 5.8/100,000 PY), trauma (7.4%, 5.0/100,000 PY), cerebral infarction with coma (7.3%, 5.0/100,000 PY), respiratory failure (5.8%, 4.0/100,000 PY), post-surgery complication or intervention (5.4%, 3.7/100,000 PY), pesticide/drug poisoning (4.4%, 3.0/100,000 PY), metabolic dysfunction (3.7%, 2.5/100,000 PY), and gastrointestinal bleeding with shock (3.4%, 2.3/100,000 PY). Other causes of critical illness were less frequent (Fig. 1).

Incidence of death from critical illness

Four hundred eighty-nine deaths were reported in the ICU within the first 7 days of admission, with a rate of 20.2/100,000 PY. Males were at higher risk for this outcome than females (313/1015, 13.0/100,000 PY vs. 176/630, 7.4/100,000 PY, respectively; $p < 0.005$), and older patients (> 65 y old) were at higher risk than younger patents (15 y to 65 y old) (243/701, 10/100,000 PY vs. 246/944, 1/100,000 PY, respectively; $p < 0.0001$). (Table 3).

Causes of death from critical illness in the ICU

The causes of death from critical illness within the first 7 days of admission to the ICU were determined. The most common cause of death for ICU patients was SICH (180 patients, 7.4/100,000 PY), followed by acute TBI (4.2/100,000 PY), heart failure/cardiovascular crisis (2.5/100,000 PY), respiratory failure (1.2/100,000 PY), cerebral

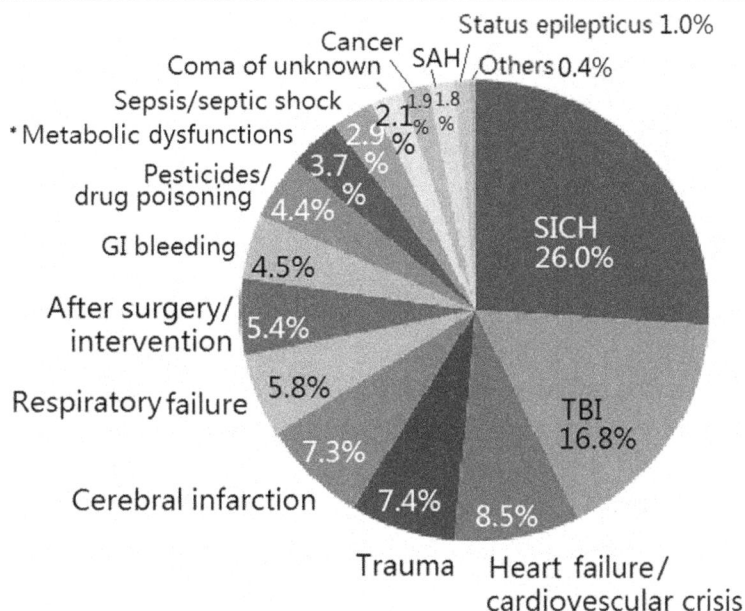

Fig. 1 The causes of critical illness in a northern China ICU. *Metabolic dysfunctions: including hypoglycemia, diabetic ketoacidosis, hyperglycemic nonketotic hyperosmolar states, kedney failure or uremia, hepatic encephalopathy, heat stroke, anoxia, and electrolyte dysfunction, etc.

infarction (0.9/100,000 PY), gastrointestinal bleeding (0.9/100,000 PY), sepsis/septic shock (0.9/100,000 PY), coma of unknown origin (0.4/100,000 PY), pesticide poisoning (0.5/100,000 PY), other traumas (0.3/100,000 PY), cancer (0.3/100,000 PY), SAH (0.3/100,000 PY), metabolic dysfunction (0.1/100,000 PY), and status epilepticus (0.04/100,000 PY) (Table 3).

Risk of death within 7 days of admission for the geriatric group vs. the non-geriatric group

Using a logistic regression analysis of the same study population, we compared the risk of death within 7 days of admission between the geriatric group and the non-geriatric group (Table 4). The risks of death from TBI (RR, 1.7; 95% CI, 1.034–2.635; $p < 0.05$), cerebral infarction (RR, 0.15; 95% CI, 0.050–0.486; $p < 0.0005$), heart failure/cardiovascular crisis (RR, 0.2; 95% CI, 0.083–0.484; $p < 0.0005$), and respiratory failure (RR, 0.35; 95% CI, 0.185–0.784; $p < 0.005$) were higher in the geriatric group than in the non-geriatric group. The risks of death from SICH, cardiac arrest with resuscitation, gastrointestinal bleeding, sepsis/septic shock, pesticide poisoning, and coma of unknown origin were not significantly different between the two age groups.

Discussion

In previous epidemiological surveys of prehospital emergency care, altered mental status [7] and trauma [8] have been reported to have the highest incidence rates. However, this study found that the incidences of these

ailments among critically ill patients in the ICU were different from those observed in previous prehospital emergency care studies. We found that stroke (35.1%, 23.8/100,000 PY) had the highest incidence rate, followed by trauma and TBI (24.1%,16.4/100,000 PY). The latter incidence may be due to the number of mild condition patients with prehospital trauma and TBI that may have been managed outside the ICU. This has been confirmed by a recent study that reported that only 20% of TBI cases account for admission to the ICU [10]. Conversely, epidemiological studies have confirmed that the incidence [11] and mortality rate for stroke are very high in China [12]. Therefore, it is likely that the care of patients with stroke has become a primary objective of ICU management.

The incidence of SICH varies in countries around the world [13], but recent studies have confirmed that the SICH incidence rate is highest in Asians (40.8–51.8/100,000 PY) [13, 14]. According to our study, SICH is a main cause of critical illness among patients admitted to the ICU, which suggests that more than 1/3 of patients with SICH need ICU care. Moreover, the fatality rate for patients with SICH within the first 7 days of admission was very high (42.2%) and similar to the fatality rate after 1 month (43–52%) that has been reported by other studies [15, 16].

TBI is the primary cause of injury-related death and disability [17], although its exact incidence is unclear. Our current study showed that TBI (16.8%, 11.4/100,000 PY) was the second most common cause of ICU

Table 3 Incidence of death due to critical illness during the first 7 days in the ICU

Charateristics	Number of cases in ICU/2 years	Death during the first 7 days in the ICU/2 years	Percentage (%)	Mortality during the first 7 days/per100000 population members per year
Overall	1645	489	29.7	20.2
Sex				
Male	1015	313	30.8§	12.9
Female	630	176	27.9§	7.3
Age				
> 65 years	701	243	34.7△	10.0
15 to 65 years	994	246	24.7△	1.0
Types of critical illness				
SICH	427	180	42.2	7.4
TBI	276	101	36.6	4.2
Heart failure/cardiovescular	140	61	43.6	2.5
Respiratory failure crisis	96	28	29.2	1.2
After surgery or intervention	89	10	11.2	0.4
GI bleedingwith shock	74	22	29.7	0.9
Cerebral infarction	120	21	17.5	0.9
Sepsis / septic shock	48	21	43.8	0.9
Pesticides/ drug poisoning	73	11	15.1	0.5
Coma of unknown origin	35	9	25.7	0.4
Trauma	121	8	6.6	0.3
Any cancer	32	7	21.9	0.3
SAH	30	7	23.3	0.3
Metabolic dysfunction	61	2	3.3	0.1
Status epilepticus	16	1	6.2	0.04
Other	7	0	0	0.0

§$p < 0.005$; △$p < 0.0001$

ICU intensive care unit, *SICH* spontaneous intracerebral hemorrhage, *TBI* traumatic brain injury

admission. TBI has a mortality rate of approximately 40.0% [18] and a disability rate of 57.4% [19]. Moreover, our data showed that the fatality rate within the first 7 days of admission was also high in cases of TBI (36.6%). However, the risks of death from TBI, heart failure/myocardial infarction, severe cerebral infarction, and respiratory failure were significantly higher

Table 4 Logistic regression analysis of the risk of death comparing the geriatric group and non-geriatric group during the first 7 days in the ICU

Critical illness	RR	95%CI	p Value
TBI	1.7	1.034–2.635	0.034
Heart failure/cardiovascular crisis	0.2	0.082–0.483	0.000
Cerebral infarction	0.15	0.049–0.460	0.001
Respiratory failure	0.35	0.159–0.790	0.011

ICU intensive care unit, *RR* risk ratio, *CI* confidence intervals, *TBI* traumatic brain injury

in the geriatric group than in the non-geriatric group. This finding indicates that older age is an important risk factor for death from most critical illnesses in the general ICU, which is consistent with a previous study [20] and may be related to that the older patients is more likely to develop an acutely fatal multiple organ failure [21]. On the contrary, the risk of death from SICH in the two groups was similar, and the SICH incidence results suggested a trend toward an increase in the younger population. This has been confirmed by one recent study [22].

Prior studies have shown that sepsis and septic shock account for 10% of ICU cases [23], whereas this study identified only 48 such cases (2.9%). Because most sepsis or septic shock diagnoses are secondary to another disease, our result may be related to our study criteria, which examined only the first diagnosis (primary disease). These patients had been transferred to specialist wards or information on sepsis/septic shock had not been included in the diagnosis.

Surprisingly, the combined incidence of SICH and TBI was almost equal to the sum of the general ICU admissions for other critical patients. This strongly suggests that addressing these two critical diseases should be a public health priority and is deserving of further attention.

Although this study was conducted in one ICU, this ICU was the county's only ICU with a referral center. Therefore, we believe that our data are informative because the results of this study are more likely to represent the true epidemic spectrum of critical illness. However, certain limitations should be acknowledged. First, although this was a prospective registration, a small number of critically ill patients may be underrepresented due to a lack of standardized criteria for defining critical illness in this population. Second, because our registration only selected a sole primary diagnosis in the ICU, some patients with sequential liver or renal failure were not documented. This may have been the cause of the low frequencies of liver and renal failures that we observed. Additionally, the causes of coma were difficult to identify because numerous comatose patients had been intubated and could not consent to brain magnetic resonance examination. However, patients with unexplained comas were rare, so this was unlikely to produce a bias in the population of critically ill patients with neurological conditions.

In conclusion, the rate of critical illness was high in Shuyang County in northern China. The most common illnesses that required care in the ICU were SICH and TBI, and both of these critical illnesses carried a higher risk of death than other illnesses. This strongly suggests that addressing these two conditions should be a public health priority and is deserving of further attention.

Abbreviations
APACHE II: Acute physiology and chronic health evaluation II; GCS: Glasgow coma scale; ICU: Intensive care unit; SICH: Spontaneous intracerebral hemorrhage; TBI: Traumatic brain injury

Funding
This work is supported by a grant from the Medical Research Council, affiliated Shuyang People's Hospital, Xuzhou Medical University (Clinical Key Specialty Construction Project of Jiangsu Provence,20160017).

Authors' contributions
ZYT and TDM were responsible for the study concept and design. ZYT, TDM, WSD, YS, XBW, and YCX were responsible for data acquisition and analysis. ZYT, TDM, WSD, YS, and YCX. were responsible for drafting the manuscript. All authors read and approved the final manuscript.

Competing interests
The authors declare that they have no competing interests.

Author details
[1]Department of Surgery, Affiliated Shuyang Hospital, Xuzhou Medical University, Xuzhou, Jiangsu, China. [2]Department of Neurology, Affiliated Shuyang Hospital, Xuzhou Medical University, Xuzhou, Jiangsu, China. [3]Department of Intensive Care Medicine, Affiliated Shuyang Hospital, Xuzhou Medical University, Xuzhou, Jiangsu, China.

References
1. Bral AL, Cerra FB. Multiple organ failure syndrome in 1990, systemic inflammatory response and organ dysfunction. JAMA. 1994;271:226–33.
2. Joynt GM, Gomersall CD, Tan P, Lee A, Cheng CA, Wong EL. Prospective evaluation of patients refused admission to an intensive care unit: triage, futility and outcome. Intensive Care Med. 2001;27(9):1459–65. pmid: 11685338. https://doi.org/10.1007/s001340101041.
3. Sinuff T, Kahnamoui K, Cook DJ, et al. Rationing critical care beds: a systematic review. Crit Care Med. 2004;32(7):1588–97. pmid:15241106. https://doi.org/10.1097/01.ccm.0000130175.38521.9f.
4. Adhikari NK, Fowler RA, Bhagwanjee S, et al. Critical care and the global burden of critical illness in adults. Lancet. 2010;376(9749):1339–46. https://doi.org/10.1016/S0140-6736(10)60446-1.
5. Cerro G, Checkley W. Global analysis of critical care burden. Lancet Respir Med. 2014;2(5):343–4. https://doi.org/10.1016/S2213-2600(14)70042-6.
6. Gomes B, Higginson IJ. Where people die (1974--2030): past trends, future projections and implications for care. Palliat Med. 2008;22(1):33–41. https://doi.org/10.1177/0269216307084606.
7. Rosamond WD, Evenson KR, Schroeder EB, et al. Calling emergency medical services for acute stroke: a study of 9–1-1 tapes[J]. Prehospital emergency care. 2005;9(1):19–23. PMID: 16036823[PubMed - indexed for MEDLINE]
8. Román MI, de Miguel AG, Garrido PC, et al. Epidemiologic intervention framework of a prehospital emergency medical service. Prehosp Emerg Care. 2005;9(3):344–54.
9. Statistical Yearbook of Jiangsu Province in 2013. Jiangsu: Population Statistics office press; 2013. p. 1–56.
10. Hefny AF, Idris K, Eid HO, et al. Factors affecting mortality of critical care trauma patients. Afr Health Sci. 2013;13(3):731–5. https://doi.org/10.4314/ahs.v13i3.30.
11. Sun YH, Zhang GH, Hu R, Wang C. Epidemiological survey of cerebrovascular disease among population in Inner Mongolia autonomous region. Chin J Epidemiol. 2015;36:925–8.
12. Chen Z. The third cause of death among netionwide reprospective sample survey report. Beijing: Chinese Peking Union Medical College press; 2008. p. 8–14.
13. van Asch CJ, Luitse MJ, Rinkel GJ, van der Tweel I, Algra A, Klijn CJ. Incidence, case fatality, and functional outcome of intracerebral haemorrhage over time, according to age, sex, and ethnic origin: a systematic review and meta-analysis. The Lancet Neurology. 2010;9(2):167–76.
14. Chan CL, Ting HW, Huang HT. The incidence, hospital expenditure, and, 30 day and 1 year mortality rates of spontaneous intracerebral hemorrhage in Taiwan. J Clin Neurosci. 2014;21(1):91–4.
15. Fogelholm R, Avikainen S, Murros K. Prognostic value and determinants of first-day mean arterial pressure in spontaneous supratentorial intracerebral hemorrhage. Stroke. 1997;28:1396–400.
16. Broderick J, Connolly S, Feldmann E, et al. Guidelines for the management of spontaneous intracerebral hemorrhage in adults: 2007 update: a
   guideline from the American Heart Association /American Stroke Association stroke council, high blood pressure research council, and the quality of care and outcomes in research interdisciplinary working group. Circulation. 2007;116(16):e391–413.
17. Coronado VG, Xu L, Basavaraju SV, et al. Surveillance for traumatic brain injury-related deaths--United States, 1997-2007. MMWR Surveill Summ. 2011;60(5):1–32.

18. Iwashyna TJ, Deane AM. Individualizing endpoints in randomized clinical trials to better inform individual patient care: the TARGET proposal. Critical Care. 2016;20:1.

19. Harrison DA, Griggs KA, Prabhu G, et al. External validation and Reca libration of risk prediction models for acute traumatic brain injury among critically ill adult patients in the United Kingdom. J Neurotrauma. 2015;32(1):1522–37.

20. Taylor MD, Tracy JK, Meyer W, et al. Trauma in the elderly: intensive care unit resource use and outcome. J Trauma. 2002;53(3):407–14.

21. Broos PL, D'Hoore A, Vanderschot P, et al. Multiple trauma in patients of 65 and over. Injury patterns. Factors influencing outcome. The importance of an aggressive care. Acta Chir Belg. 1993;93(3):126–30.

22. Wang J, Bai L, Shi M,et al. Trends in age of first-ever stroke following increased incidence and life expectancy in a low-income chinese population. Stroke.2016 11. pii: STROKEAHA.115.012466. [Epub ahead of print].

23. Angus DC, Linde-Zwirble WT, Lidicker J, Clermont G, Carcillo J, Pinsky MR. Epidemiology of severe sepsis in the United States: analysis of incidence, outcome, and associated costs of care. Crit Care Med. 2001;29:1303–131.

A retrospective case series of segmental zoster paresis of limbs: clinical, electrophysiological and imaging characteristics

Ying Liu[1], Bing-Yun Wu[1], Zhen-Shen Ma[2], Juan-Juan Xu[1], Bing Yang[3], Heng Li[3] and Rui-Sheng Duan[3*]

Abstract

Background: Segmental zoster paresis (SZP) of limbs, characterized by focal weakness of extremity, is recognized as a rare complication of herpes zoster (HZ). The following study analyzes the clinical characteristics and data from electromyography and MRI scans in patients with motor weakness after zoster infection.

Methods: One thousand three hundred ninety-three patients from our database (Shandong Provincial Qianfoshan Hospital) suffering from HZ were retrospectively reviewed from June 2015 to July 2017. Patients who fulfilled the diagnostic criteria for SZP were included in the analysis. The clinical characteristics, as well as electromyography findings and MRI scans were analyzed.

Results: SZP was present in 0.57% of patients with HZ (8/1393). The average age of symptom onset in 8 SZP patients was 69 years old (SD: 13, range 47–87). The severity of muscle weakness ranged from mild to severe. The electrophysiological testing revealed the characteristics of axonopathy. Radiculopathy (2/8), plexopathy (2/8), radiculoplexopathy (3/8) and combined radiculopathy and mononeuropathy (1/8) were also identified. MRI revealed hyperintensity of the affected spinal dorsal horns, nerve roots or peripheral nerves.

Conclusions: SZP is associated with obvious limb weakness, nerve axons lesions and localization to nerve roots, plexus or peripheral nerves.

Keywords: Herpes zoster, Segmental zoster paresis, Infectious neuropathy, Nerve conduction, Electromyography, Nerve MRI

Background

Herpes zoster (HZ) is caused by varicella-zoster virus (VZV) which is latent in the dorsal root ganglia and reactivates when the immune system is not functioning properly. The incidence of HZ is about 4–4.5 per 1000 person-years [1], which is characterized by vesicular rash and burning pain. Postherpetic neuralgia is the most common neurologic syndrome of HZ, whereas segmental zoster paresis (SZP) of limbs is a relatively rare complication, characterized by focal weakness of upper or lower extremity. The motor involvement can be observed in 0.5–5% patients with HZ [2, 3].

The exact mechanism of SZP is not clear, although the spread of virus along the nerve is presumed [4–6]. The existing literature mainly includes case reports [7–18]. Comparatively, only few studies have described case series of SZP based on electrophysiological, imaging characteristics and prognosis data. In addition, antiviral medications and corticosteroids are the most commonly applied drugs for treating SZP. The prognosis for patients with SZP is generally favorable; however, in some extreme cases it can lead to permanent disability [2].

Here, we investigated clinical, electrophysiological and imaging evidence in a case series of 8 patients with SZP, as well as possible factors influencing prognosis.

* Correspondence: ruisheng_duan@yahoo.com
[3]Department of Neurology, Shandong Provincial Qianfoshan Hospital, Shandong University, Jinan 250014, People's Republic of China
Full list of author information is available at the end of the article

Methods

Patients

The patient database in Shandong Provincial Qianfoshan Hospital was reviewed for coded diagnoses of HZ from June 2015 to July 2017. Patients with HZ were diagnosed as SZP based on the following criteria [4]: 1) Infection of HZ preceding or following limb paresis established based on historical or physical examination evidence of a cutaneous vesicular eruption; 2) geographical (same limb) and temporal (no more than 30 days) evidence of associated limb weakness which was confirmed by a neurologist; 3) the lesions of nerve roots and plexus or mononeuropathy associated with HZ which were verified using electrophysiological testing.

Weakness was identified in each affected muscle as mild (corresponding to MRC 4 or 4+), moderate (corresponding to MRC 3), severe (corresponding to MRC 2 or 1) and complete (corresponding to MRC 0).

According to the Medical Research Council scale, the muscle recovery was based on the following criteria: 1) complete recovery, if muscle strength was evaluated as grade 5 and the sensory symptom disappeared in the last follow-up visit; 2) no recovery, if no improvement in muscle strength was observed; 3) partial recovery, case between the complete and no recovery. In addition, all patients were followed up for approx. 0.5–2.0 years; the follow-up evaluation was based on sensorimotor symptom and muscle strength.

This retrospective study was approved by the medical ethics committee at our hospital.

Electrophysiology

Nihon Kohden MEB-9400 electromyograph was used to evaluate nerve injury. Surface electrodes were used to perform nerve conduction studies (NCS), including motor and sensory nerve conduction velocity (NCV), distal motor latency (DML), amplitudes of compound muscle action potentials ($CMAP_S$) and sensory nerve action potentials ($SNAP_S$).

Median motor study was performed with distal stimulation site over the median nerve at the wrist and proximal stimulation site at the antecubital fossa, recording the abductor pollicis brevis muscle. Ulnar motor study was performed with distal stimulation site over the ulnar nerve at the wrist and proximal stimulation site above the elbow, recording the abductor digiti minimi muscle. Radial motor study was performed with distal stimulation site in the forearm and proximal stimulation site in the arm, below the spiral groove, recording the extensor indicis proprius muscle.

Tibial motor study was performed with distal stimulation site slightly proximal and posterior to the medial malleolus and proximal stimulation site in the middle of the popliteal fossa, recording the abductor hallucis brevis muscle. Peroneal motor study was performed with distal stimulation site over the anterior ankle and proximal stimulation site below the fibular head, recording the extensor digitorum brevis muscle.

Axillary, suprascapular, musculocutaneous motor conduction studies were performed, recording the deltoid, supraspinatus and biceps brachii with surface electrodes repectively, and stimulation site was at Erb's point.

Antidromic and orthodromic sensory studies were performed in upper extremity or lower extremity respectively. Index finger and little finger were respectively stimulated to record SNAPs of the median and ulnar nerve.

A comparison with contralateral (asymptomatic) sides or normal values helped to determine the degree of damage. If NCV was slower than 75% of the lower limit of normal, and DML was longer than 130% of the upper limit of normal, it was regarded as demyelination. If the side-to-side amplitudes difference was greater than 50%, it was regarded as abnormal and axonal lesion.

The needle electromyography (EMG) was performed by a concentric needle electrode, which was used to find spontaneous potentials such as positive sharp waves and fibrillation potentials conventionally graded from 0 to 4+ as follows: 0 for none present; + 1 for persistent single trains of potentials (> 2–3 s) in at least two areas; + 2 for moderate number of potentials in three or more areas; + 3 for many potentials in all areas; + 4 for full interference pattern of potentials. The firing pattern (activation, recruitment and interference pattern) was assessed.

According to SNAP and spontaneous activities in paraspinal muscles, associated limb was characterized as preganglionic, postganglionic lesions or combined pre- and postganglionic lesions, and then further identified as radiculopathy, plexopathy, radiculoplexopathy and peripheral nerves [4] .

Imaging

The MRI results were reviewed by an experienced radiologist. All studies included both T1- and T2- weighted images in coronal planes, without gadolinium-enhanced T1-weighted images. All T2-weighted sequences had fat saturation or a short tau inversion recovery sequence. Nerve root, plexus, or peripheral nerve images were identified as abnormal if prolonged nerve T2 or nerve enlargement was shown based on comparison with contralateral neural structures within the imaging field.

Results

Patient demographics and clinical characteristics

Eight out of 1393 inpatients with HZ fulfilled the diagnostic criteria for SZP, accounting for 0.57%, which was confirmed by neurologic examination and electrodiagnostic evaluation. Clinical characteristics are listed in Table 1.

Table 1 Demographics and clinical characteristics in patients with segmental zoster paresis

Features	
Mean age (years)	69 (range 47–87)
Men	3 of 8
Affected myotomes	
Left upper limb	1 of 8
Right upper limb	5 of 8
Left lower limb	0 of 8
Right lower limb	2 of 8
Rash after weakness (within 30 days)	0 of 8
Mean interval between rash and weakness (days)	11.9
Diabetes mellitus	4 of 8
Immunocompromise	1 of 8
Post-herpetic neuralgia 4 months after onset	5 of 8
Myotomes corresponding to dermatomes	8 of 8
Disseminated zoster	1 of 8

Detailed information of 8 patients are described in Table 2. Three descriptive cases are described in detail in the following paragraphs.

Rash distribution in all patients corresponded to weakness distribution (Fig. 1). Although the severity of muscle weakness ranged from mild to severe, most were at least moderate. All patients had paresthesia, such as tingling and numbness, corresponding to the distribution of affected myotomes. The deep tendon reflexes were diminished or absent in distribution of affected limbs. In addition, most patients had a certain degree of post-herpetic neuralgia 4 months after onset (5/8).

Four patients had diabetes (case 2, 3, 4 and 5), while 1 patient had a 20-year history of rheumatoid arthritis and use of immunosuppressive medications (case 5). Antiviral drugs, such as acyclovir, were administered to 5 patients (case 1, 2, 5, 6, 7) orally or intravenously within 72 h after the rash appeared, 3 patients after 72 h. In addition, 4 patients received short term use of oral corticosteroids (case 2, 3, 5, 8); nevertheless, no patient experienced immediate pain or weakness relief after treatment.

The prognosis was quite different (Fig. 2). Patient 1 recovered completely 3 months after symptoms onset; this patient was placed on oral antiviral medication for 1 week. Patient 6 and 8 recovered partially through 1 or 0.5 year respectively. However, the remaining 5 patients did not recover until 0.5–2.0 years of follow-up. Their muscle strength showed no improvements and one patient's muscles seemed atrophied (case 7).

Electrophysiological characteristics

All electrophysiological examinations were performed no more than 2 weeks after weakness onset. Briefly, nerve conduction studies showed markedly decreased or absent $CMAP_S$ and $SNAP_S$ amplitudes of affected nerves, compared with the contralateral sides (Table 3). Nerve conduction velocities of affected nerves were normal or mildly decreased, which means they were faster than 75% of the lower limit of normal and above 35 m/s. Distal motor latencies were shorter than 130% of the upper limit of normal. All of these showed axonal lesions, not demyelinating lesions (Fig. 3).

All the patients showed different grades of spontaneous potentials in affected muscles. The average grade was 2+. There was a pattern of decreased recruitment of motor unit action potentials (MUAPs) in weak muscles. The positive sharp waves and fibrillation potentials in affected myotomes and the decreased recruitment of MUAPs suggested ongoing axonal lesions.

According to spontaneous activities in paraspinal muscles and $SNAP_S$ amplitudes, 2 among 8 were diagnosed with preganglionic lesions (case 1: C5-C6 radiculopathy; case 8: C5 radiculopathy), 2/8 were characterized as having postganglionic locations (case 2: upper and middle trunk lesions; case 4: lower trunk lesions) and 4 out of 8 were recognized as combined pre- and postganglionic lesions (case 3: L5-S1 radiculoplexopathy; case 5: C6-C8 radiculoplexopathy; case 6: L5 radiculoplexopathy; case 7: C7 radiculopathy and median, radial nerve lesions).

Imaging characteristics

The MRI examination was performed in 4 out of 8 patients no more than 1 week after electrophysiological testing (Fig. 4). Scans of affected brachial plexus nerves and corresponding spine segments, showed nerve enlargement and enhanced T2 signal intensity, and were in accordance with symptoms (case 5, 7 and 8). In patient 7, median and radial nerve enlargement and T2 hyperintensity were observed, although abnormality of nerve root was not identified. One patient underwent an MRI scanning on cervical spine, not the affected nerves (case 2), and axial T2-weighted image showed hyperintensity in the dorsal horns of C5–6 spinal cord levels, corresponding to her sensory symptoms.

Descriptive cases

Case 1

A 47-year-old man developed severe burning pain and a vesicular eruption in the right shoulder and anterolateral arm. Two days later after the rash, he was not able to elevate his right arm to the shoulder level or bend the forearm at the elbow joint. Additionally, he also presented with numbness in the back of the thumb. Muscle weakness was present in the right deltoid (1/5), infraspinatus (1/5), supraspinatus (1/5) and biceps (2/5), according to the MRC scale. Distal muscle strength was normal. The right biceps reflex was absent. The electrophysiological

Table 2 Characteristics of 8 patients with segmental zoster paresis

Case	Gender	Age	Interval between rash and weakness	Rash distribution	Weak distribution	Electrodiagnostic localization	Imaging findings	Prognosis	Factors
1	M	47y	2d	Right shoulder and anterolateral arm	Right C5-6 myotomes	a right incomplete C5-6 radiculopathy	–	A fast recovery (3 months)	–
2	F	70y	20d	Right lateral arm and forearm	Right C5-7 myotomes	a right incomplete brachial plexopathy (upper and middle trunk)	Hyperintensity in spinal dorsal horns at C4–5 vertebral levels	No recovery (2.0 years)	Diabetes 5y
3	M	63y	3d	Dorsum and planta of the right foot	Right L5-S1 myotomes	a right L5-S1 radiculoplexopathy	–	No recovery (1.8 years)	Diabetes 3y
4	a	80-90y a	22d	Neck first, all body then	Right C8 myotome	a right brachial plexopathy (lower trunk)	–	No recovery (1.9 years)	Diabetes 30y
5	F	87y	14d	Right lateral arm and forearm	Right C6-8 myotomes	a right incomplete C6–8 radiculoplexopathy	increased signal in the C6–8 nerve roots	No recovery (1.0 year)	Diabetes 20y
6	a	60-70y a	12d	Right buttocks and lateral calf	Right L5 myotome	a right L5 radiculoplexopathy	–	Partial recovery (1.0 year)	–
7	M	61y	15d	Left thumb, index finger and forearm	Left C6-8 myotomes	a left C7 radiculopathy and median, radial nerves	increased signal in mdian and radial nerves	No recovery (0.5 year)	–
8	F	80y	7d	Right shoulder, anterolateral arm and thumb	Right C5 myotomes	a right C5 radiculopathy	increased signal in the C5 nerve roots	Partial recovery (0.5 year)	–

To protect patient privacy, a was used

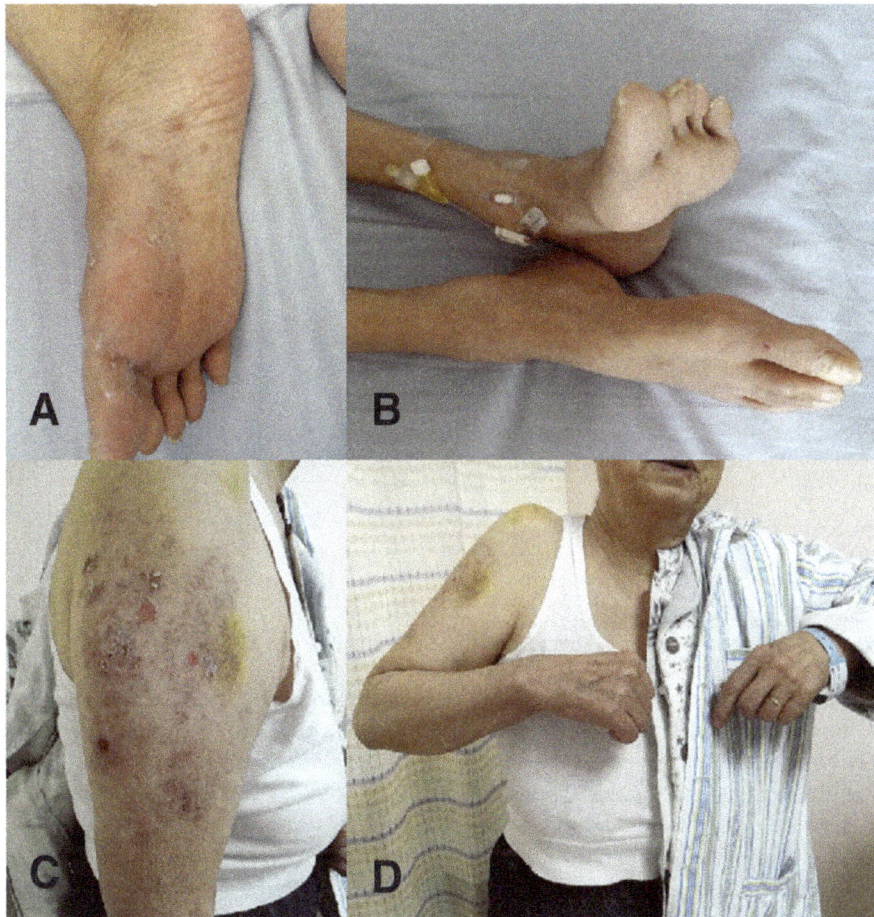

Fig. 1 Rash distribution in all patents corresponds to weakness distribution. Scars of a prior herpetic eruption and pigmentation over the dorsum and planta of the right foot were seen in patient 3, who had a foot drop (**a** and **b**). Scars from prior herpetic eruption and pigmentation over the right shoulder and anterolateral arm were seen in patient 8, who could not elevate her shoulder (**c** and **d**)

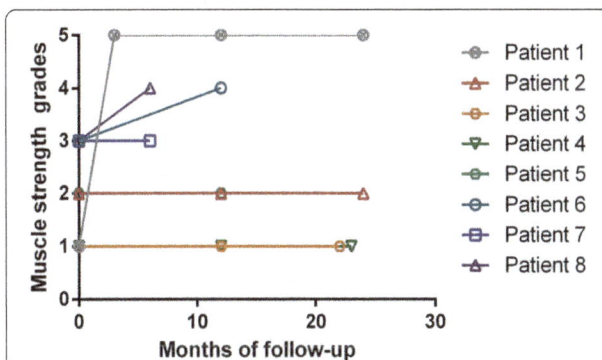

Fig. 2 Eight patients had a different prognosis. Patient 1 recovered completely 3 months after symptoms onset. Patient 6 and 8 recovered partially through 1 or 0.5 year respectively. However, the remaining five patients did not recover until 0.5–2.0 years of follow-up

examination revealed lower amplitude axillary and musculocutaneous CMAPs (12.1 and 7.3 mV, respectively) compared to contralateral sides (25.7 and 18.9 mV, respectively). The sensory nerve conduction studies were normal. Abnormal spontaneous potentials and decreased recruitments of MUAPs were present in the right deltoid, infraspinatus, biceps and C5–6 paraspinal muscles. In conclusion, the electrophysiologic findings were consistent with the incomplete lesions of C5 and C6 nerve roots.

Within 3 months follow-up period, he regained the full arm strength without any treatments. Electrophysiologically, the amplitude axillary and musculocutaneous CMAPs (21.1 and 16.6 mV, respectively) were normal. Abnormal spontaneous activities in muscles innervated by C5 and C6 nerve roots disappeared and many polyphasic MUAPs were observed.

Case 5

An 87-year-old woman developed burning pain and vesicular rash over the right lateral arm and forearm. Two

Table 3 Nerve conduction studies of patients with segmental zoster paresis

	P1	P2	P3	P4	P5	P6	P7	P8
CMAP of nerves (mV)								
Axillary	12.1(53%↓)	3.5(77%↓)		normal	4.4(51%↓)		normal	6.4(66%↓)
Suprascapular		1.7(84%↓)						3.3(76%↓)
Musculocutaneous	7.3(61%↓)	4.5(52%↓)		normal	3.6(62%↓)		normal	normal
Median	normal	normal		6.2(51%↓)	1.4(83%↓)		normal	normal
Ulnar	normal	normal		5.3(53%↓)	normal		normal	normal
Radial	normal	normal		5.2(55%↓)	normal		4.1(63%↓)	normal
Peroneal			NR			0.7(75%↓)		
Tibial			3.0(79%↓)			normal		
SNAP of nerves (μV)								
Median	normal	NR		normal	NR		2.3(77%↓)	normal
Ulnar	normal	normal		2.8(60%↓)	normal		normal	normal
Radial	normal	normal		normal	NR		4.5(64%↓)	normal
Superficial peroneal			NR			NR		
Sural			NR			normal		

The amplitudes of CMAPs and SNAPs were compared with contralateral side
CMAP compound muscle action potential, *SNAP* sensory nerve action potential, *μV* microvolt, *mV* millivolt, *NR* no response

weeks after rash, she was not able to elevate her right arm to the shoulder level, bend the forearm at the elbow joint or grip tightly. Moderate to severe weakness of C6–8 myotomes was observed, as well as the hypoesthesia over the C6–7 dermatomes. The biceps reflex was absent. The electrophysiological examination revealed decreased motor amplitudes of axillary, musculocutaneous and median nerve (4.4, 3.6 and 1.4 mV, respectively) and the absence of median and radial nerve SNAPs. The needle EMG revealed many positive sharp waves in the right deltoid, biceps, extensor digitorum communis, abductor pollicis brevis and C6 paraspinal muscles. These findings were consistent with a right incomplete C6–8 radiculoplexopathy. Brachial plexus MRI showed hyperintensity of right brachial plexus especially at the C6–8 nerve roots level. Consequently, clinical one-year follow-up revealed that the patient was still not

able to elevate her right arm to the shoulder level. Also, she presented with numbness of the thumb and post-herpetic neuralgia.

Case 7

A 61-year old man developed burning pain and vesicular rash over left thumb, index finger and forearm. Fifteen days after his rash, he noted weakness in his left hand dorsal stretch and grip. There was moderate weakness of muscles in left C6–8 myotomes and hypoesthesia over the thumb. The triceps muscle stretch reflex was absent. The electrophysiological examination revealed decreased amplitude radial CMAPs (4.1 mV) as compared to the contralateral side (11.1 mV) and decreased amplitudes median and radial nerve SNAPs. The needle EMG revealed many positive sharp waves in the left extensor digitorum communis, brachioradialis, abductor pollicis

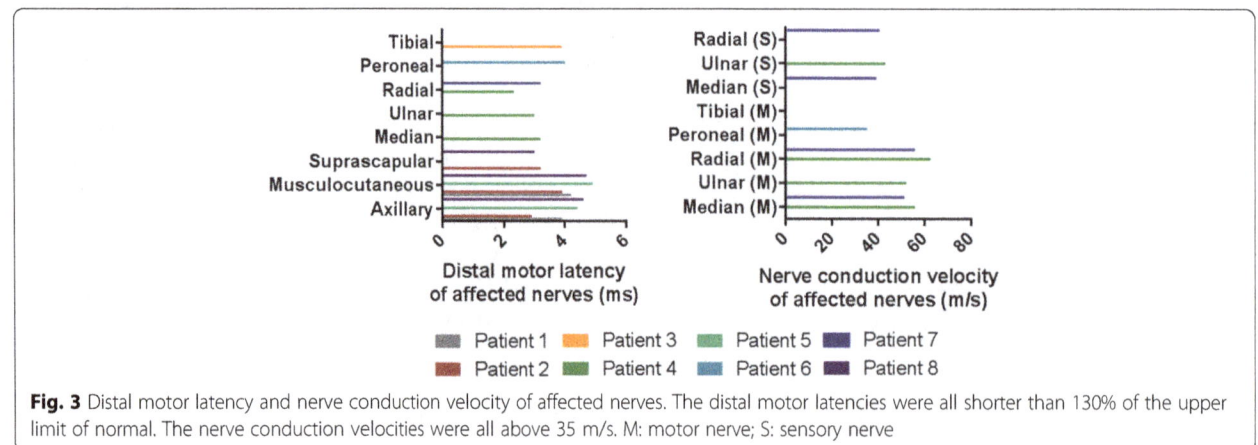

Fig. 3 Distal motor latency and nerve conduction velocity of affected nerves. The distal motor latencies were all shorter than 130% of the upper limit of normal. The nerve conduction velocities were all above 35 m/s. M: motor nerve; S: sensory nerve

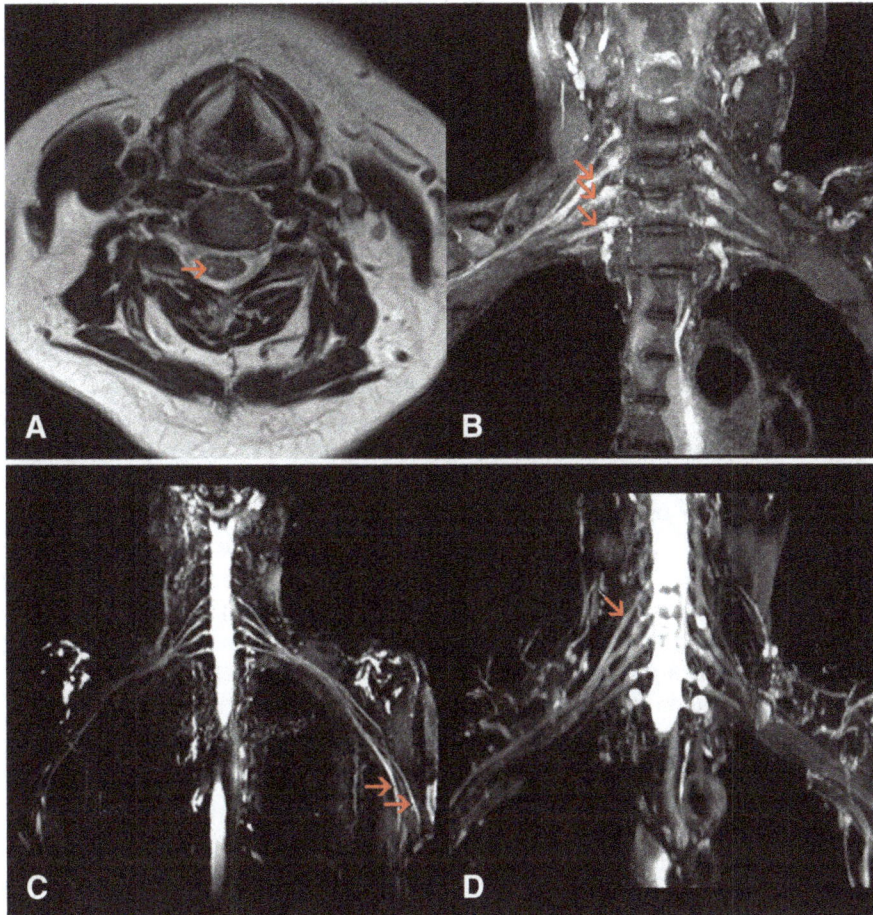

Fig. 4 Imaging characteristics of patients with SZP. Axial T2-weighted image showed the unilateral hyperintensity in the dorsal horn of C5 spinal cord in patient 2 (**a**). Brachial plexus magnetic resonance imaging showed hyperintensity of C6–8 nerve roots in patient 5 (**b**), left median and radial nerves in patient 7 (**c**) and C5 nerve roots in patient 8 (**d**)

brevis and C7 paraspinal muscles. These findings were consistent with a left median and radial nerve lesions and nerve root lesion. Moreover, brachial plexus MRI showed hyperintensity of distal median and radial nerve. Though, there was no nerve enlargement or T2 hyperintensity of nerve roots. A half-year follow-up revealed that his muscle strength did not recover, and his muscles seemed atrophied. Also, he developed post-herpetic neuralgia.

Discussion

In the present study, we confirmed that varicella-zoster virus can lead to SZP which is an uncommon complication of a common ailment, including nerve roots, brachial or lumbar plexus, and peripheral nerves lesions. The electrophysiologic and imageological findings can help demonstrate the extent and severity of affected nerves or nerve roots.

The elderly and immunocompromised patients are most susceptible to VZV [1, 9, 19]. Due to the immunosenescence in aged people, HZ infection frequently occurs [1]. It is a high incidence of disease over the age of 40; the highest incidence is found in the age group from 60 to 70. [2]. The average age in our sample was 69 years old.

Yoleri et al. have suggested that zoster paresis preferentially strikes the upper limbs and then the lower limbs [8], while according to other studies, the upper and lower extremities are equally affected [3, 20]. In the present study, upper limbs were involved in 6 out of 8 patients; which was in line with the former results. The weakness in upper limbs most commonly occurs in C5–7 segments, while the weakness in lower extremities most frequently occurs in L1–4 segments [5]. The involvement of C8 myotome is relatively rare [10]. In other words, the distribution of muscle weakness is common in the proximal muscles of the limbs and limb-girdles. In most of our cases, the upper extremities were involved, which was in accordance with this pattern; although in 3 patients the distal muscles were also involved. In 2 cases of affected lower limbs, weakness did not fit this pattern and indicated the distal weakness. Interestingly, right limbs were involved in 7 out of 8 patients, which was in accordance with previous literatures [5–18, 21–27].

Our electrophysiological study manifested low amplitudes of CMAPs or SNAPs together with many spontaneous activities in all patients, thus suggesting motor and sensory axonopathy. In axonal loss lesions, NCS and DML were normal or mildly slow. Generally, NCV was above 35 m/s and DML was shorter than 130% of the upper normal limit in axonal loss lesions. All our results from 8 patients met the criteria. Consequently, peripheral neuropathy caused by HZ with predominant axonopathy could be seen through our cases electrophysiologically. Sachs et al. have reported an electrophysiological study of zoster paresis for 22 months of follow-up, which appeared to be axonopathy and reinnervation [28].

The dorsal root ganglion is the seat of VZV previous to the HZ eruption; therefore, it is no wonder that amplitudes of SNAPs were low, showing sensory neurons or axons damage. According to existing pathologic studies, demyelination, axon degeneration and lymphocyte infiltration can be found in affected nerves, dorsal root ganglions and dorsal horns [29]. These findings were observed in the postmortem examinations long time after HZ infections. Thus, it's possible that the demyelination found in autopsy is secondary to the axon degeneration induced by HZ infection. Meanwhile, our electrophysiological examinations were performed no more than 2 weeks from the onset of weakness. Axonal degeneration may be the early presentation.

Brachial or lumbosacral plexus was affected in 5 out of 8 patients, suggesting the dorsal root ganglion (the seat of virus prior to its eruption) and ventral roots lesions. Although the precise mechanism of SZP remains unclear, it is easy to understand that the spread of VZV along nerve fibers to ventral root, ventral horn, and distal nerves can lead to corresponding lesions.

Four of our patients underwent MRI examination. MRI is a useful tool for diagnosing SZP. The imaging abnormalities included nerve enlargement and T2 signal hyperintensity of dorsal horn and brachial plexus or peripheral nerves, which were consistent with clinical symptoms and electrophysiological findings, although these imaging manifestations are not specific and could be found in peripheral nerve inflammation caused by other diseases such as neurobrucellosis [30]. The imaging abnormalities were not found in 100% of patients, while nerve T2 hyperintensity or nerve enlargement was found in 70% of patients [31]. Our patent 7 did not show imaging abnormalities at roots.

In the literature, the prognosis for SZP is generally favorable, but the return of motor function can be incomplete, while recovery time can significantly vary [10, 32]. Two-thirds of their patients had completely or almost fully recovered within a year while the other one-sixth of patients suffered from permanent weakness of extremities, which usually occurred in muscles like diaphragm, anterior tibial and the hand intrinsic muscles [2]. In our study, anterior tibial was involved in 1 patient (case 3), and hand intrinsic muscles were involved in 3 patients (case 4, 5 and 7). Nevertheless, C5–7 myotome muscles were mainly observed, even though not mentioned previously, in patient 2 who still had a poor recovery over 2.0-year follow-up. These patients had a longer recovery time than the 47-year old man. The other reason may be probably due to the older age (patient 2–7) and diabetes mellitus (patient 2–5) [14, 33].

Our study is limited by a small sample size of this rare complication of HZ and retrospective design. Some patients without clinical zoster paresis were not examined with EMG, so there might be electrophysiological abnormalities in these patients. In addition, some patients were likely to have a longer follow-up for prognostic estimation.

Conclusions

In summary, the present study highlights clinical, electrophysiological and imaging characteristics of this rare motor involvements of HZ. It is associated with significant limb weakness, obvious nerve axons lesion, and it is localized in nerve roots, plexus or peripheral nerves. The information is crucial for neurologists in order to avoid unnecessary misdiagnosis. Also, SZP should be considered in the differential diagnosis of acute painful motor weakness of limbs. The electrophysiological testing and MRI scan can be useful for confirming the diagnosis of SZP.

Abbreviations

CMAPs: Compound muscle action potentials; DML: Distal motor latency; EMG: Electromyography; HZ: Herpes zoster; MRI: Magnetic resonance imaging; MUAPs: Motor unit action potentials; NCS: Nerve conduction studies; NCV: Nerve conduction velocity; SNAPs: Sensory nerve action potentials; SZP: Segmental zoster paresis; VZV: Varicella-zoster virus

Acknowledgments

The authors thank Chun-Lin Yang and Min Zhang at Department of Neurology, Shandong Provincial Qianfoshan Hospital, Shandong University, for assistance with the preparation of this manuscript.

Funding

This work was partially supported by Taishan Scholars Construction Engineering of Shandong Province (NO. ts20130914), Medicine and Health Science Technology Development Programme of Shandong Province (NO. 2015WS0226) and Key Research and Development Plan of Shandong Province (NO. GG201709190225).

Authors' contributions

YL and RSD participated in the conception and the design of the study. YL drafted the manuscript. BYW, JJX, BY and HL participated in the acquisition of raw data and the analysis of the clinical data. ZSM performed and interpreted the imaging data. RSD provided the major funding for the study. All authors read and approved the final manuscript.

Competing interests

The authors declare that they have no competing interests.

Author details

[1]Department of Electromyography, Shandong Provincial Qianfoshan Hospital, Shandong University, Jinan 250014, People's Republic of China. [2]Department of radiology, Shandong Provincial Qianfoshan Hospital, Shandong University, Jinan 250014, People's Republic of China. [3]Department of Neurology, Shandong Provincial Qianfoshan Hospital, Shandong University, Jinan 250014, People's Republic of China.

References

1. Yawn BP, Gilden D. The global epidemiology of herpes zoster. Neurology. 2013;81(10):928–30.
2. Gupta SK, Helal BH, Kiely P. The prognosis in zoster paralysis. J Bone Joint Surg Br. 1969;51(4):593–603.
3. Thomas JE, Howard FM Jr. Segmental zoster paresis--a disease profile. Neurology. 1972;22(5):459–66.
4. Jones LK Jr, Reda H, Watson JC. Clinical, electrophysiologic, and imaging features of zoster-associated limb paresis. Muscle Nerve. 2014;50(2):177–85.
5. Kawajiri S, Tani M, Noda K, Fujishima K, Hattori N, Okuma Y. Segmental zoster paresis of limbs: report of three cases and review of literature. Neurologist. 2007;13(5):313–7.
6. Reda H, Watson JC, Jones LK Jr. Zoster-associated mononeuropathies (ZAMs): a retrospective series. Muscle Nerve. 2012;45(5):734–9.
7. Kim JG, Chung SG. Herpetic brachial plexopathy: application of brachial plexus magnetic resonance imaging and ultrasound-guided corticosteroid injection. Am J Phys Med Rehabil. 2016;95(5):e67–71.
8. Yoleri O, Olmez N, Oztura I, Sengul I, Gunaydin R, Memis A. Segmental zoster paresis of the upper extremity: a case report. Arch Phys Med Rehabil. 2005;86(7):1492–4.
9. Rastegar S, Mahdavi SB, Mahmoudi F, Basiri K. Herpes zoster segmental paresis in an immunocompromised breast cancer woman. Adv Biomed Res. 2015;4:170.
10. Kreps CE, Rynders SD, Chhabra AB, Jenkins JG. C8 myotome herpes zoster paresis. Am J Orthop. 2012;41(5):220–2.
11. Teo HK, Chawla M, Kaushik M. A rare complication of herpes zoster: segmental zoster paresis. Case Rep Med. 2016;2016:7827140.
12. Park SE, Ganji P, Ji JH, Park SH. Transient motor paresis caused by herpes zoster. J Shoulder Elb Surg. 2016;25(10):e309–12.
13. Martic V. Recurrent herpes zoster with segmental paresis and postherpetic neuralgia. Vojnosanit Pregl. 2014;71(2):214–7.
14. Namekawa M, Kameda T, Kumabe A, Mise J. Segmental zoster paresis of the right shoulder. Intern Med. 2013;52(24):2839.
15. Kang SH, Song HK, Jang Y. Zoster-associated segmental paresis in a patient with cervical spinal stenosis. J Int Med Res. 2013;41(3):907–13.
16. Yoshioka M, Kurita Y, Hashimoto M, Murakami M, Suzuki M. A case of segmental zoster paresis with enhanced anterior and posterior spinal roots on MRI. J Neurol. 2012;259(3):574–5.
17. Khan A, Camilleri J. Motor radiculopathy. BMJ Case Rep. 2012;2012:bcr2012006246.
18. Umehara T, Sengoku R, Mitsumura H, Mochio S. Neurological picture. Findings of segmental zoster paresis on MRI. J Neurol Neurosurg Psychiatry. 2011;82(6):694.
19. Andrei G, Snoeck R. Advances in the treatment of varicella-zoster virus infections. Adv Pharmacol. 2013;67:107–68.
20. Cruz-Velarde JA, Munoz-Blanco JL, Traba A, Nevado C, Ezpeleta D. Segmental motor paralysis caused by the varicella zoster virus. Clinical study and functional prognosis. Rev Neurol. 2001;32(1):15–8.
21. Chabot RH, Wirtz PW. Teaching NeuroImages: MRI findings in varicella zoster brachial plexus neuritis. Neurology. 2011;76(15):e76.
22. Alshekhlee A, Tay E, Buczek M, Shakir ZA, Katirji B. Herpes zoster with motor involvement: discordance between the distribution of skin rash and localization of peripheral nervous system dysfunction. J Clin Neuromuscul Dis. 2011;12(3):153–7.
23. Samuraki M, Yoshita M, Yamada M. MRI of segmental zoster paresis. Neurology. 2005;64(7):1138.
24. Yaszay B, Jablecki CK, Safran MR. Zoster paresis of the shoulder. Case report and review of the literature. Clin Orthop Relat Res. 2000;377:112–8.
25. Hanakawa T, Hashimoto S, Kawamura J, Nakamura M, Suenaga T, Matsuo M. Magnetic resonance imaging in a patient with segmental zoster paresis. Neurology. 1997;49(2):631–2.
26. Fabian VA, Wood B, Crowley P, Kakulas BA. Herpes zoster brachial plexus neuritis. Clin Neuropathol. 1997;16(2):61–4.
27. Braverman DL, Ku A, Nagler W. Herpes zoster polyradiculopathy. Arch Phys Med Rehabil. 1997;78(8):880–2.
28. Sachs GM. Segmental zoster paresis: an electrophysiological study. Muscle Nerve. 1996;19(6):784–6.
29. Watson CP, Deck JH, Morshead C, Van der Kooy D, Evans RJ. Post-herpetic neuralgia: further post-mortem studies of cases with and without pain. Pain. 1991;44(2):105–17.
30. Al-Sous MW, Bohlega SA, Al-Kawi MZ, McLean DR, Ghaus SN. Polyradiculopathy. A rare complication of neurobrucellosis. Neurosciences (Riyadh). 2003;8(1):46–9.
31. Zubair AS, Hunt C, Watson J, Nelson A, Jones LK Jr. Imaging findings in patients with zoster-associated plexopathy. AJNR Am J Neuroradiol. 2017; 38(6):1248–51.
32. Merchut MP, Gruener G. Segmental zoster paresis of limbs. Electromyogr Clin Neurophysiol. 1996;36(6):369–75.
33. Mondelli M, Romano C, Rossi S, Cioni R. Herpes zoster of the head and limbs: electroneuromyographic and clinical findings in 158 consecutive cases. Arch Phys Med Rehabil. 2002;83(9):1215–21.

Altered levels of circulating insulin-like growth factor I (IGF-I) following ischemic stroke are associated with outcome

N. David Åberg[1]*, Daniel Åberg[1], Katarina Jood[2], Michael Nilsson[2,3], Christian Blomstrand[2], H. Georg Kuhn[2,4], Johan Svensson[1], Christina Jern[5,6] and Jörgen Isgaard[1]

Abstract

Background: Insulin-like growth factor I (IGF-I) has neuroprotective effects in experimental ischemic stroke (IS). However, in patients who have suffered IS, various associations between the levels of serum IGF-I (s-IGF-I) and clinical outcome have been reported, probably reflecting differences in sampling time-points and follow-up periods. Since changes in the levels of post-stroke s-IGF-I have not been extensively explored, we investigated whether decreases in the levels of s-IGF-I between the acute time-point (median, 4 days) and 3 months (ΔIGF-I, further transformed into ΔIGF-I-quintiles, ΔIGF-I-q) are associated with IS severity and outcome.

Methods: In the Sahlgrenska Academy Study on Ischemic Stroke (SAHLSIS) conducted in Gothenburg, Sweden, patients with IS who had s-IGF-I measurements available were included ($N = 354$; 65% males; mean age, 55 years). Baseline stroke severity was evaluated using the National Institutes of Health Stroke Scale (NIHSS) and converted into NIHSS-quintiles (NIHSS-q). Outcomes were assessed using the modified Rankin Scale (mRS) at 3 months and 2 years.

Results: In general, the levels of s-IGF-I decreased (positive ΔIGF-I), except for those patients with the most severe NIHSS-q. After correction for sex and age, the 3rd ΔIGF-I-q showed the strongest association to mRS 0–2 [Odds Ratio (OR) 5.11, 95% confidence interval (CI) 2.18–11.9], and after 2 years, the 5th ΔIGF-I-q (OR 3.63, 95% CI 1.40–9.38) showed the strongest association to mRS 0–2. The associations remained significant after multivariate correction for diabetes, smoking, hypertension, and hyperlipidemia after 3 months, but were not significant ($p = 0.057$) after 2 years. The 3-month associations withstood additional correction for baseline stroke severity ($p = 0.035$), whereas the 2-year associations were further attenuated ($p = 0.31$).

Conclusions: Changes in the levels of s-IGF-I are associated primarily with temporally near 3-month outcomes, while associations with long-term 2-year outcomes are weakened and attenuated by other factors. The significance of the change in post-stroke s-IGF-I is compatible with a positive role for IGF-I in IS recovery. However, the exact mechanisms are unknown and probably reflects combinations of multiple peripheral and central actions.

Keywords: Insulin-like growth factor I, Ischemic stroke, Outcome

* Correspondence: david.aberg@medic.gu.se
[1]Department of Internal Medicine, Institute of Medicine, The Sahlgrenska Academy at University of Gothenburg, Gröna Stråket 8, SE-413 45 Gothenburg, Sweden

Background

Extensive studies conducted in experimental animals have demonstrated that insulin-like growth factor-I (IGF-I) exerts neuroprotective and plasticity-promoting effects [1, 2]. For humans who have suffered an ischemic stroke (IS), a few observational studies have evaluated the role of endogenous levels of serum IGF-I (s-IGF-I). In the first two studies on this topic ($N = 85$ and $N = 42$, respectively), s-IGF-I was associated with measures of improved functional outcome [3, 4]. However, s-IGF-I was analyzed at only one time-point, either within 24 h of IS onset [3] or at 19–209 days after the IS [4], and functional follow-up was performed approximately 3–6 months post-stroke [3, 4]. In addition, a previous study from our group ($N = 407$) has shown a positive association between the 3-month level of s-IGF-I and improvements in the mRS score from 3 months to 2 years, whereas there was a negative association with the 3-month mRS score [5]. Thus, although endogenous s-IGF-I has been associated with favorable IS outcome, there remain unresolved issues in terms of the importance of the: post-stroke sampling time-point; age of the patient; severity of IS; timing of the follow-up; and temporal changes in s-IGF-I level after IS.

The association between change in post-stroke s-IGF-I and IS outcome has been investigated in one small study, in which the average level of s-IGF-I increased by 8.5% from < 72 h to 7 days after the stroke ($N = 15$) [6]. However, in that study, there was relatively large inter-individual variability, and interestingly, a decrease in post-stroke s-IGF-I correlated with a better 1-month mRS score ($N = 10$) [6]. Furthermore, the local expression of IGF-I in the brain may increase after IS [7, 8], and in analogy with the increased brain uptake of IGF-I after experimental exercise [9], the transport of IGF-I from the serum into the brain may be increased after IS. In our previous study, the level of s-IGF-I was increased during the first days after the stroke (+ 11.2% on Days 0–2, as compared to healthy controls), followed by a leveling off of the s-IGF-I level on Days 3–5. Thereafter, there was an average decrease of 14.8% from Day 9 to Day 19, resulting in 3-month s-IGF-I levels that were approximately similar to those seen in healthy, age-matched controls [5]. However, we did not analyze the associations between the individual changes in s-IGF-I and IS outcome [5]. The hypothesis underlying the present study is that not only the absolute levels of s-IGF-I, but also the temporal pattern of s-IGF-I levels (as estimated by changes in the s-IGF-I levels), are of importance for IS outcome. Thus, our primary objective was to investigate whether intra-individual changes in post-stroke s-IGF-I (ΔIGF-I), from the acute phase to 3 months post-IS, are associated with functional independence 3 months after the IS, and if so, whether ΔIGF-I is also associated with functional outcome 2 years after IS. As ΔIGF-I has not been investigated extensively to date,

we explored descriptively the effects of the following parameters: first day of sampling; age; IS severity; stroke subtype; and stroke etiology. We also performed multivariate regression analyses with the inclusion of potential confounders, such as cardiovascular risk factors and IS severity.

Methods
Subjects and methods

The design of SAHLSIS has been reported elsewhere [10]. Briefly, patients (< 70 years of age) with first-ever or recurrent acute IS were recruited consecutively at four Stroke Units in western Sweden between 1998 and 2003 (see Fig. 1 for flow chart of inclusions). The final inclusion cohort with regard to ΔIGF-I had 354 subjects (Table 1). S-IGF-I was analyzed on one occasion in 2008 with a methodological intra-assay coefficient of variation (CV) of 5.1% and the biological variation showed a CV of 38% [5]. Blood sampling was performed between 08:30 and 10:30 after overnight fasting, and s-IGF-I was assayed using an IGF-binding protein (IGFBP)-blocked RIA kit (Mediagnost, Reutlingen, Germany). The acute serum samples were taken 0–19 days after the IS, with a median sampling time of 4 days [5]. The frequencies of previous hypertension, diabetes mellitus, and smoking were recorded and, the levels of low-density lipoprotein (LDL) were evaluated as previously described [10]. The ΔIGF-I values were transformed into quintiles (ΔIGF-I-q), owing to the values being skewed towards the left, as well as for convenience of presentation. The ΔIGF-I-q were defined according to ΔIGF-I: q1 = − 279.6--10, q2 = − 9.999–10, q3 = 10.001–30.7, q4 = 30.701–55.6, q5 = 55.601–178.9 ng/ml, with higher quintiles representing a decrease in s-IGF-I from the acute time-point to the 3-month time-point. Blood glucose or plasma glucose was analyzed using standardized methods at the Department of Clinical Chemistry at the Sahlgrenska University Hospital. In cases with the presence of blood glucose, these values were transformed to plasma glucose according to the formula: plasma glucose = blood glucose × 1.11. Initial stroke severity was assessed by scoring using the Scandinavian Stroke Scale (SSS), with the values being recalculated into the now more commonly used National Institutes of Health Stroke Scale (NIHSS). The algorithm used was: NIHSS = 25.68−0.43 × SSS [11], and due to a markedly skewed appearance, these scores were further transformed into quintiles: q1 = 0–0.74 (mild); q2 = 0.7401–2.03 (minor); q3 = 2.0301–3.75 (moderate); q4 = 3.75–10.2 (major); and q5 = 10.201–42 (severe). Due to many cases having minimal NIHSS scores, the first quintile was somewhat overbalanced (see Fig. 2). Stroke subtype and etiology were classified according to the Oxfordshire Community Stroke Project (OCSP) [12] and the Trial of Org 10,172 in Acute Stroke Treatment (TOAST) [13] criteria (see Table 2 for groups and abbreviations).

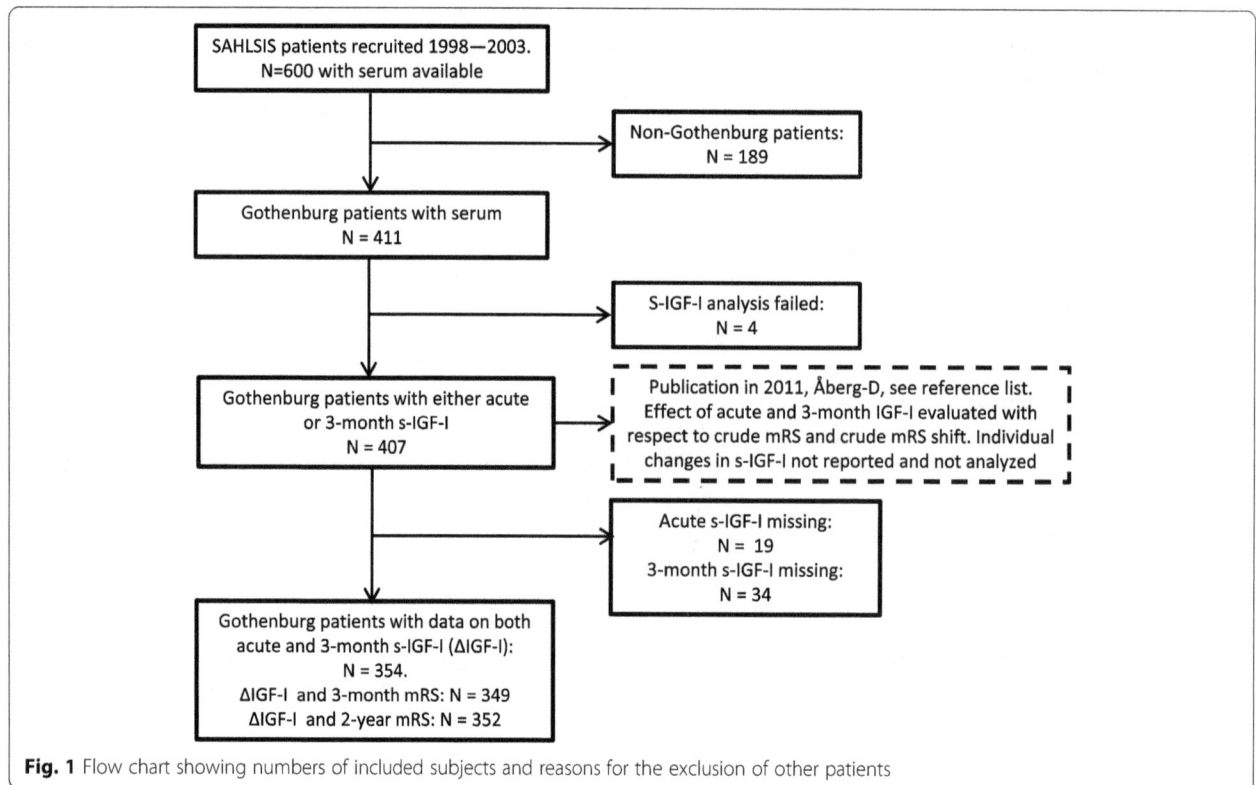

Fig. 1 Flow chart showing numbers of included subjects and reasons for the exclusion of other patients

Outcomes were assessed functionally and classified according to the modified Rankin Scale (mRS), where the levels of functional independence was classified by scores in the range of 0–2 (considered as favorable) and scores in the range of 3–6 (considered as unfavorable) [14]. Further details of the study design, patient examination, scoring scales, and protein measurements are given in the Additional file 1. A part of this report was presented as an abstract (with a modified title) at the European Stroke Conference in May 2018 [15] .

Statistical analysis

Statistical evaluation was performed using the SPSS ver. 21.0 software (SPSS Inc., Chicago, IL). In the descriptive section, comparisons between groups (stroke severity, day-of-sampling, age, stroke subtype, and etiology) were performed using analysis of variance (ANOVA), and with Dunnett's (for comparison with one reference) or Tukey's (for crosswise comparison of all groups) post hoc tests, as indicated. Comparisons between distributions were made with the Chi-square test. Crude correlations using the method of Pearson are presented.

The aim of the project was to evaluate the effect of ΔIGF-I on functional outcome (mRS) 3 months and 2 years after IS. Towards this goal, we assessed whether the crude correlations withstood subsequent binary logistic regression analysis, in which the data on functional outcome were dichotomized (favorable outcome, mRS 0–2 versus unfavorable outcome, mRS 3–6). The Odds Ratios (ORs) and 95% confidence intervals (CIs) for favorable outcome (mRS 0–2) were age- and sex-adjusted (model 1) and were relative to the lowest quintile of ΔIGF-I (ΔIGF-I-q1, i.e., an increase in ΔIGF-I). Adjustments were also made for the vascular risk factors of smoking, hypertension, diabetes, and LDL levels (model 2), initial stroke severity quintile (model 3), and finally, also for the different days of first sample (model 4). As suggested by Peduzzi and coworkers [16], the number of events per variable (EPV) needed to reduce statistical bias should exceed the included number of covariates by a factor of 10. With the eight covariates given above, and an event rate of mRS 3–6 ($N = 82$ and $N = 74$ for the 3-month and 2-year outcomes, respectively), we refrained from adding 'stroke etiology' and 'stroke subtype' as covariates. The statistical significance level was set at $p < 0.05$.

Results

Descriptive data for s-IGF-I and stroke severity and subtype

The baseline characteristics of the 354 patients from SAHLSIS (Fig. 1) with ΔIGF-I values are summarized in Table 1. ΔIGF-I, which represents the intra-individual decrease in s-IGF-I from the acute phase to 3 months post-IS, averaged 20.2 ng/mL for the entire group. ΔIGF-I only weakly correlated with age ($r = -0.12$, $p = 0.025$, $N = 354$), as compared to the acute s-IGF-I and age ($r = -0.331$, $p < 0.001$, $N = 354$) and the 3-month s-IGF-I and age

Table 1 Baseline data for patients and s-IGF-I in each of the quintiles of changing s-IGF-I (ΔIGF-I-q1–5)

Parameter	Unit		Value
n			354
Age at index ischemic stroke	Years (SD)		55.4 (11)
Sex	Missing (N)		229/125
	Male/female (fraction)		0.65
Diabetes	Yes (N/fraction)		67 (0.19)
	Missing (N)		0
Hypertension	Yes (N/fraction)		188 (0.53)
	Missing (N)		0
Current smoking	Yes (N/fraction)		136 (0.38)
	Missing (N)		0
LDL level (ng/nL)	Mean (SD)		3.3 (1.0)
	Missing (N)		27
P-glucose (acute)	Mean (SD)		6.5 (2.64)
	Missing (N)		8
P-glucose (3 m)	Mean (SD)		6.03 (2.29)
	Missing (N)		8
Stroke severity (NIHSS)	Mean (20, 80%)		5.3 (0.7, 10.2)
	Missing (N)		0
Stroke outcome (mRS) 3 m	Mean(SD)		1.85 (1.06)
	Missing (N)		5
Stroke outcome (mRS) 2 yr	mRS (SD)		1.77 (1.32)
	Missing (N)		2
Dead (3-24 m)	Yes (n/fraction)		9 (0.025)
	Missing (N)		0
s-IGF-I (acute)	ng/mL (SD)		172.8 (62.9)
	Missing (N)		0
s-IGF-I (3 m)	ng/mL (SD)		152.7 (55.7)
	Missing (N)		0
ΔIGF-I (ng/mL), all data	ng/mL (SD)		20.2 (51.0)
	Missing (N)		0
Quintile of ΔIGF-I:	ΔIGF-I (ng/mL)	s-IGF-I acute (ng/mL)	Change (%)
ΔIGF-I-q1 (SD)	− 48.3 (48.0)	146.5 (53.7)	incr. 33.0
(N)	71	71	71
ΔIGF-I-q2 (SD)	1.6 (5.8)	145.4 (44.6)	decr. 1.10
(N)	72	72	72
ΔIGF-I-q3 (SD)	20.8 (5.7)	152.5 (56.0)	decr 13.5
(N)	71	71	71
ΔIGF-I-q4 (SD)	42.5 (7.2)	178.9 (45.9)	decr 23.6
(N)	70	70	70
ΔIGF-I-q5 (SD)	85.9 (28.0)	240.5 (57.6)	decr 35.7
(N)	70	70	70

Absolute ΔIGF-I (ng/mL) represents a subtraction of acute s-IGF-I by 3-month s-IGF-I. A negative numerical value represents an increase from the acute to 3-month time point, and a positive numerical value represents a decrease. Modified Rankin scale (mRS), low density lipoprotein (LDL), National Institutes of Health Stroke Scale (NIHSS). An extended version of the table with a comparison to data presented in 2011 is found in Additional file 2: Table S1

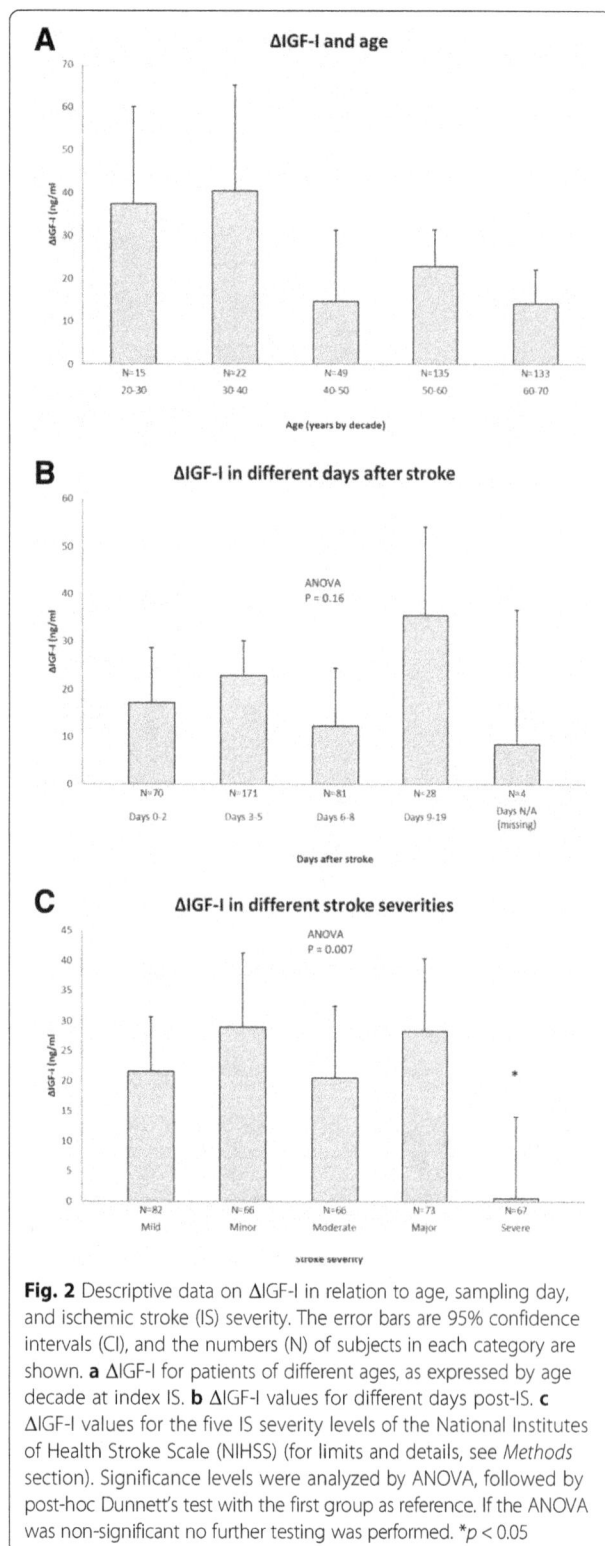

Fig. 2 Descriptive data on ΔIGF-I in relation to age, sampling day, and ischemic stroke (IS) severity. The error bars are 95% confidence intervals (CI), and the numbers (N) of subjects in each category are shown. **a** ΔIGF-I for patients of different ages, as expressed by age decade at index IS. **b** ΔIGF-I values for different days post-IS. **c** ΔIGF-I values for the five IS severity levels of the National Institutes of Health Stroke Scale (NIHSS) (for limits and details, see *Methods* section). Significance levels were analyzed by ANOVA, followed by post-hoc Dunnett's test with the first group as reference. If the ANOVA was non-significant no further testing was performed. *$p < 0.05$

ΔIGF-I regardless of the post-stroke sampling day of the first "acute" serum sample (Fig. 2b). However, ΔIGF-I was found to be related to initial stroke severity (Table 2, Fig. 2c). Specifically, there was no decrease in ΔIGF-I in the most severe IS, whereas the value of ΔIGF-I (20–29 ng/mL) was similar for all the other severities of IS. The low ΔIGF-I values noted for the patients with severe or large IS were further supported by the observed tendency towards a correlation between the ΔIGF-I quintiles and NIHSS quintiles ($r = -0.092$, $p = 0.084$, $N = 354$), and the fact that the subtype with the largest IS, total anterior cerebral infarctions (TACI), had a lower ΔIGF-I than the other subtypes (Table 2, OCSP). Moreover, the ΔIGF-I value was higher in the group of patients with IS with etiology of arterial dissection, which might be attributable in part to the younger age of these patients (Table 2, TOAST classification). These subgroups were not used in the subsequent regressions, since the numbers of subjects and events in each of the groups were relatively low. As the absolute levels of s-IGF-I are inversely related to P-glucose levels and metabolic syndrome [17–19], ΔIGF-I could potentially relate to the P-glucose levels. However, there were no correlations (acute P-glucose and ΔIGF-I; $r = -0.065$, $p = 0.23$, $N = 346$; 3-month P-glucose and ΔIGF-I, $r = -0.012$, $p = 0.83$, $N = 346$), and this parameter was not used in the subsequent regression analyses.

Multivariate regression analysis of changes in the levels of s-IGF-I and the clinical outcomes 3 months and 2 years after the IS

We investigated whether ΔIGF-I was related to IS outcome after 3 months and 2 years, using univariate (correlations) and multivariate regression analyses. Although ΔIGF-I correlated with the crude 3-month mRS score (Fig. 3a), outliers and the skewing of ΔIGF-I indicated that the ΔIGF-I quintiles were better suited to analysis of association, and the application of the widely accepted dichotomized mRS. Accordingly, the crude ΔIGF-I quintiles correlated with favorable outcome (i.e., mRS 0–2) 3 months after IS ($r = 0.21$, $p = 0.01$, $N = 349$) and 2 years after IS ($r = 0.14$, $p = 0.007$, $N = 352$). This is evidenced by the significantly different distributions of ΔIGF-I quintiles at both 3 months and 2 years for the patients with favorable outcome (mRS 0–2) and those with unfavorable outcome (mRS 3–6) of IS (Fig. 2b).

For the significant crude associations with mRS outcome 3 months and 2 years after the IS, we performed further analyses using binary logistic regression with adjustment for multiple covariates. Higher ΔIGF-I quintiles (representing decreased levels of s-IGF-I) adjusted for sex and age were indeed associated with favorable outcome in terms of mRS score after 3 months (model 1, for ΔIGF-I-q5, OR 4.63, 95% CI 2.01–10.7; Fig. 3c). This was not due to the higher level of acute s-IGF-I found in

($r = -0.264$, $p < 0.001$, $N = 354$). Furthermore, the weak negative correlation between ΔIGF-I and age was not reflected in any difference of ΔIGF-I with respect to decade of age (Fig. 2a). We found no significant difference in

Table 2 S-IGF-I for patients included by etiology, stroke subtype and severity, respectively

	Mean		Mean		Mean			
	ΔIGF-I (SD)	P	Acute IGF-I (SD)	P	3-month IGF-I (SD)	P	Age	P
Stroke severity (NIHSS†)		Dunnett, q1 vs. q2-q5						
q1 (mild)	21.6 (42.0)	N/A	162.4 (59.5)	N/A	140.8 (50.0)	N/A	53.1 (12.5)	N/A
N	82		82		82		82	
q2 (minor)	29.0 (51.0)	ns	181.9 (67.0)	ns	152.9 (53.1)	ns	55.7 (9.9)	ns
N	66		66		66		66	
q3 (moderate)	20.6 (49.5)	ns	168.1 (63.5)	ns	147.6 (56.0)	ns	54.4 (11.1)	ns
N	66		66		66		66	
q4 (major)	28.3 (72.7)	ns	181.6 (61.8)	ns	153.4 (53.6)	ns	58.4 (9.5)	0.01
N	73		73		73		73	
q5 (severe)	0.58 (58.5)	0.04	171.7 (62.5)	ns	171.2 (63.2)	0.003	54.0 (10.7)	ns
N	67		67		67		67	
Missing (n)	0		0		0		0	
Subtype (OCSP)		Tukey's crosswise						
Lacunar cerebral infarction (LACI)	21.1 (37.0)	0.09-TACI	163.9 (57.4)	ns	142.8 (48.5)	**TACI	56.6 (9.6)	0.05-POCI
N	113		113		113		113	
Partial anterior cerebral infarction (PACI)	18.1 (47.3)	ns	172.8 (67.9)	ns	154.7 (59.5)	ns	55.0 (11.3)	ns
N	104		104		104		104	
Posterior cerebral infarction (POCI)	30.7 (59.4)	**TACI	181.6 (65.4)	ns	150.9 (57.1)	ns	52.7 (12.2)	0.11-TACI
N	94		94		94		94	0.05-LACI
Total anterior cerebral infarction (TACI)	−1.5 (68.1)	**POCI	171.7 (58.4)	ns	173.3 (57.1)	**LACI	52.7 (9.3)	0.11-POCI
N	37	0.09-LACI	37		37		37	
Missing (N)	6		6		6		6	
Etiology (TOAST)		Tukey's crosswise						
Large vessel disease (LVD)	20.4 (53.7)	ns	181.1 (57.0)	*D	160.8 (57.9)	ns	59.0 (7.8)	***D, **Cr
N	51		51	0.08-CE	51		51	
Small vessel disease (SVD)	19.1 (39.6)	ns	161.4 (60.6)	***D	142.3 (53.4)	**D	58.4 (7.2)	***D, **Cr
N	69		69		69		69	
Cardioembolic (CE)	6.1 (46.2)	ns	151.2 (53.3)	***D, 0.08-LVD	145.1 (51.1)	*D	55.5)11.6	*D
N	52		52	0.15-Cr	52		52	
Cryptogenic (Cr)	20.1 (43.3)	ns	174.1 (60.7)	***D	154.0 (53.9)	0.09 vs. D	53.1 (11.9)	**LVD/SVD
N	112		112	0.15-CE	112		112	

Table 2 S-IGF-I for patients included by etiology, stroke subtype and severity, respectively (Continued)

	Mean ΔIGF-I (SD)	P	Mean Acute IGF-I (SD)	P	Mean 3-month IGF-I (SD)	P	Age	P
Arterial dissection (D)	40.1 (95.7)	*CE	223.7 (63.0)	***SVD/CE/Cr	183.6 (66.7)	**-SVD	48.1 (9.4)	***LVD/SVD
N	27		27		27		27	
Other/undetermined	26.2 (45.7)	N/A	172.2 (71.9)	*LVD	146.0 (53.7)	*CE, 0.09-Cr	54.2 (13.5)	**Cr, 0.14-D
n	43		43		43		43	
Missing (N)	0		0		0		0	

P-values less than 0.3 are specified although they are considered being not signicant (ns). * < 0.05, ** < 0.01, *** < 0.001 for Dunnett's or Tukey's post-hoc tests as indicated. As we have a slightly different number of included patients, and using NIHSS instead of SSS as it was presented in 2011, we present s-IGF-I (acute, 3-month) for comparison with the present inclusion (n = 354). TOAST = Trial of Org 10,172 in Acute Stroke Treatment [1], OCSP = Oxfordshire Community Stroke Project [4]. All variation shown is given in standard deviations (SD). N/A designates not applicable. †Scoring of neurological function is taken from the original SSS scores and converted to NIHSS (methods)

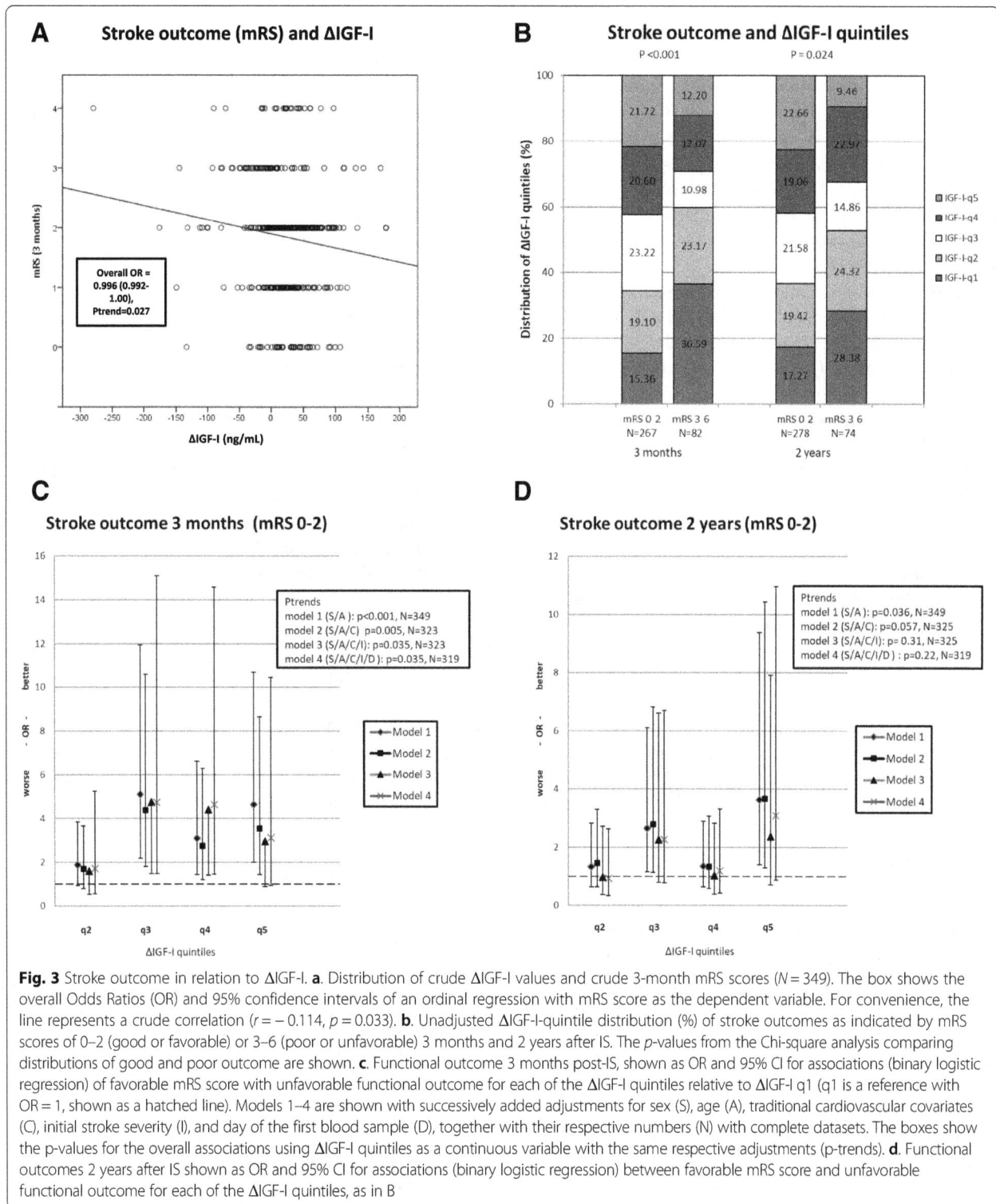

Fig. 3 Stroke outcome in relation to ΔIGF-I. **a.** Distribution of crude ΔIGF-I values and crude 3-month mRS scores (N = 349). The box shows the overall Odds Ratios (OR) and 95% confidence intervals of an ordinal regression with mRS score as the dependent variable. For convenience, the line represents a crude correlation (r = − 0.114, p = 0.033). **b.** Unadjusted ΔIGF-I-quintile distribution (%) of stroke outcomes as indicated by mRS scores of 0–2 (good or favorable) or 3–6 (poor or unfavorable) 3 months and 2 years after IS. The p-values from the Chi-square analysis comparing distributions of good and poor outcome are shown. **c.** Functional outcome 3 months post-IS, shown as OR and 95% CI for associations (binary logistic regression) of favorable mRS score with unfavorable functional outcome for each of the ΔIGF-I quintiles relative to ΔIGF-I q1 (q1 is a reference with OR = 1, shown as a hatched line). Models 1–4 are shown with successively added adjustments for sex (S), age (A), traditional cardiovascular covariates (C), initial stroke severity (I), and day of the first blood sample (D), together with their respective numbers (N) with complete datasets. The boxes show the p-values for the overall associations using ΔIGF-I quintiles as a continuous variable with the same respective adjustments (p-trends). **d.** Functional outcomes 2 years after IS shown as OR and 95% CI for associations (binary logistic regression) between favorable mRS score and unfavorable functional outcome for each of the ΔIGF-I quintiles, as in B

ΔIGF-I-q4–5 (model 1 with acute s-IGF-I as an additional covariate; data not shown). We did not explore the impact of acute s-IGF-I on outcome any further, as acute s-IGF-I has been previously demonstrated to be negatively correlated with outcome [5]. Furthermore, the 3-month associations withstood adjustment for traditional cardiovascular risk factors and adjustment for initial stroke severity (Fig. 3c, model 3). However, the associations were marginally more robust for ΔIGF-I-q3 than for ΔIGF-I-q5 (model 1, ΔIGF-I-q3: OR 5.11, 95% CI

2.18–11.9). Although 'day of first sample' did not crudely relate with ΔIGF-I (Fig. 3b), there was a biological rationale for including this parameter as a covariate (due to the initial increase in s-IGF-I; see *Introduction*), which marginally amplified the associations (Fig. 3, c and d, model 4). This was also reflected in the regression analysis in which samples collected on Days 0–2 ($N = 70$) were excluded, generating an inclusion cohort of $N = 275$. This regression analysis generated marginally higher ORs for favorable outcome ($N = 275$, model 1, ΔIGF-I-q3: OR 5.59, 95% CI 2.03–14.4).

In general, the associations were somewhat weaker for the 2-year outcome (model 1, ΔIGF-I-q5: OR 3.63, 95% CI 1.40–9.38). The association with favorable 2-year outcome persisted as a trend ($p = 0.057$) after adjustment for cardiovascular risk factors but was significant for specific ΔIGF-I-quintiles (model 2, ΔIGF-I-q5: OR 3.66, 95% CI 1.29–10.4). However, additional adjustment for initial stroke severity reduced associations to non-significant levels ($p = 0.31$). For the 2-year outcome, the association was most robust for ΔIGF-I-q5.

Discussion

Decreased level of IGF-I is associated with favorable outcome after ischemic stroke

This study investigated individual s-IGF-I changes (ΔIGF-I) from the subacute phase after IS to 3-month follow-up. In addition, we related the ΔIGF-I to outcome for up to 2 years after IS. The ΔIGF-I did not differ with respect to stroke severity, except that in the most severe stroke cases, there was only a minimal change in the levels of s-IGF-I. In general, the individual ΔIGF-I values showed that s-IGF-I decreased from the subacute phase to 3 months post-IS. There were more prominent decreases in the levels of s-IGF-I in patients with favorable outcome than in those with unfavorable outcome. A subsequent regression analysis of ΔIGF-I-q revealed robust associations with favorable outcome at 3 months and somewhat less-pronounced associations at 2 years after IS. These associations withstood adjustments for cardiovascular covariates in the 3-month and 2-year follow-ups. However, the associations withstood additional adjustment for initial stroke severity only in terms of the 3-month follow-up. Taken together, our data show that a dynamic decrease in the level of s-IGF-I from the subacute phase to 3 months post-stroke is strongly associated with better stroke outcome at 3 months, whereas the association with outcome at 2 years is weaker.

Decreasing the level of IGF-I is associated with favorable outcome, also after correction for confounders

The effect of the decrease in the level of IGF-I might be confounded by various factors, such as stroke volume, initial stroke severity, higher initial s-IGF-I, and cardiovascular factors. While the exact stroke volume was not available, the TOAST classification gave some indication of the stroke volume [13]. Accordingly, large IS (TACI) and severe IS, as opposed to other groups, exhibited a minimal ΔIGF-I (i.e., unchanged s-IGF-I). Therefore, it could be argued that the worst IS scenario, with low ΔIGF-I, could explain the statistical associations. However, even within the group of most severe IS, similar ORs for favorable outcome were noted (data not shown). Furthermore, when adding 'initial stroke severity' as a covariate in the statistical analyses, the association between ΔIGF-I and favorable 3-month outcome remained, whereas the association between ΔIGF-I and favorable 2-year outcome was weakened to statistically non-significant levels. Thus, even after correction for initial stroke severity, the association between ΔIGF-I and favorable 3-month functional outcome persisted.

In the multivariate regression analyses, the association between ΔIGF-I and IS outcome was not confounded by the level of acute s-IGF-I. This suggests that the association between ΔIGF-I and favorable outcome is independent of the acute level of IGF-I. Given the previous report on the absolute levels of IGF-I [5], we did not explore further the effects of the acute or 3-month levels of IGF-I.

The beneficial effect of ΔIGF-I was essentially unchanged by the applied adjustments for cardiovascular covariates (Fig. 3b and c). This is of importance, as the absolute levels of s-IGF-I are lower in cases of metabolic syndrome and diabetes [17–19]. In summary, the change in s-IGF-I level appears to be an independent predictor of favorable outcome 3 months after IS, as this association withstands corrections for cardiovascular covariates, absolute levels of acute IGF-I, and initial stroke severity.

Possible underlying mechanisms

In the present study, it was not possible to determine whether the changes in s-IGF-I reflect similar changes in the local availability of IGF-I in the brain. However, in experimental IS, IGF-I was upregulated early after IS, both locally [7, 8, 20] and in the serum [8], allowing for a subsequent decrease in the level of IGF-I. In our previous study, the levels of s-IGF-I increased during the first days after the stroke. The levels of s-IGF-I reached a plateau on Days 3–5, and thereafter, an average decrease of 14.8% was seen on Days 9–19, resulting in 3-month s-IGF-I levels that were approximately similar to those in healthy, age-matched controls [5]. It can be speculated that the higher levels of IGF-I around the brain injuries result in better recovery, and that after 3 months, the expression of IGF-I decreases if the injury exhibits recovery (implying that IGF-I is no longer needed). In line with this, brain injuries with little recovery would continue to have unchanged or even increased levels of IGF-I in the brain, and possibly also in the serum, after 3 months. If so, local IGF-I in the brain would not be an exacerbating agent, but instead a substance that could improve the clinical outcome of IS. From experimental studies, there is evidence that local astrocyte IGF-I expression mediates neuroprotection [21] and that locally delivered astrocyte IGF-I improves experimental stroke outcomes [22]. While the exact mechanisms are not known, they probably involve neuroprotection, as well as angiogenesis, neurogenesis, and neuronal sprouting (for reviews, see [1, 2]). Another possible explanation is that the patients with IS who exhibit a substantial recovery and favorable outcome are those with the greatest potential for transporting IGF-I from the serum into the brain [9]. Such a mechanism would give results similar to ours, although this notion is partly contradicted by our previous report that large infarctions have relatively higher absolute levels of both acute and 3-month s-IGF-I [5]. It should be pointed out that interactions between local brain IGF-I synthesis, circulating s-IGF-I (including peripheral sources and regulation from liver and bone [23]), and uptake of s-IGF-I through the blood-brain barrier are biologically plausible but very complicated to study and poorly understood in humans. A more stringent time series of IGF-I measurements in the serum and cerebrospinal fluid (CSF) in relation to IS might give some indication of the relative importance of the different sources of IGF-I.

Changes in s-IGF-I levels in relation to previous studies and significance of favorable clinical outcome

Our main finding is that ΔIGF-I is associated with favorable outcome both 3 months and 2 years post-IS, although the association with functional outcome after 2 years loses significance after adjustment for initial stroke severity. In a previous smaller study ($N = 15$), a decrease in IGF-I level during the first week of stroke was associated with shorter length of stay, greater independence at 1 month (mRS), and discharging to home vs. remaining as an inpatient [6]. As compared to the study of Mattlage and coworkers, our study has a wider range of first days of sampling and a considerably later time-point for the second sample (3 months). While the variation of the first day of sampling is a weakness in the present study, we have partly addressed this problem by correcting for this parameter in the multivariate regression analysis (Fig. 3, c and d, model 4) and by excluding Days 0–2, resulting in somewhat stronger associations between ΔIGF-I and favorable functional outcome (mRS 0–2). Thus, the combined results of the present and the previous studies clearly suggest that a post-stroke decrease in the level of s-IGF-I is associated with improved clinical outcome after IS.

In the present study, the largest beneficial effects (ORs) observed for ΔIGF-I were in ΔIGF-I-q3 (for 3-month outcomes) and in ΔIGF-I-q5 (for 2-year outcomes), which correspond to decreases in s-IGF-I of 13.5 and 35.7%, respectively (Table 1). These relatively substantial changes in s-IGF-I support the notion that s-IGF-I plays a role in stroke pathophysiology and rehabilitation. In terms of the crude unadjusted data, 42.3% of the patients who showed an increase in s-IGF-I (ΔIGF-I-q1) had an unfavorable 3-month functional outcome, as compared to 12.7–20.3% of those patients who showed a decrease in s-IGF-I (q3 - q5 of ΔIGF-I). These are rather large differences, as an unfavorable outcome (mRS 3–6) means that the patient is requires assistance with daily living activities. Furthermore, the differences in associations noted between q3 and q5 for ΔIGF-I- and mRS 0–2 are overall rather small. Our most important finding is that decreases in s-IGF-I levels contrast with no change or an increase in the post-stroke level of s-IGF-I with respect to outcome. However, this needs to be evaluated in greater detail in larger clinical studies.

Strengths and limitations

The methodological strengths of this study include consecutive recruitment of well-characterized patients with IS. Another advantage is the high hospitalization rate (84–95%) for stroke patients in Sweden [24], which has among the highest rates in Europe [25]. The relatively young age of the participants in the present study (mean age, 55 years), as compared to the mean age of all patients with IS in Sweden (approximately 76 years [26]), facilitated follow-up, with very few drop-outs and few cases of fatality, although it somewhat disfavored the inclusion of the bulk of cases of IS etiology, i.e., IS due to cardiovascular causes. In addition, the inclusion of patients of young age favored the inclusion of less-severe cases of IS. The fact that few patients were lost to follow-up makes other selection biases unlikely. The fact that the patients were recruited between 1998 and 2003 means that very few patients received thrombolysis (local arterial, $N = 4$, intravenous, $N = 0$) and that more of the patients received previous treatment with warfarin ($N = 41$) than is currently the case. Another drawback of this study is that there is no analysis of exact stroke volumes, although baseline stroke severity can be used as a marker of stroke lesion volumes with correlation coefficients of 0.62–0.64 [27, 28]. In addition, we chose to include only those patients for whom there was a complete dataset for both the subacute and 3-month s-IGF-I, giving 354 subjects, as compared to the 407 subjects in our previous report [5]. We do not believe that this introduced any systematic bias, given that the cardiovascular covariates, acute and 3-month s-IGF-I levels, and the 3-month and 2-year mRS scores were comparable to those previously reported [5] (see also the Additional file 2: Table S1). Other weaknesses include the relatively small sample size and the lack of replication in a different geographic area.

Conclusions

Decreasing levels of s-IGF-I show clear associations with favorable outcome at 3 months and 2 years after IS, suggesting that the dynamics of IGF-I regulation is of importance, independent of the actual s-IGF-I levels. After adjustment for initial stroke severity, the 3-month association remained statistically significant, whereas the 2-year association lost significance. Thus, the changes in s-IGF-I levels are associated primarily with the temporally close (3-month) outcomes, while the associations with long-term (2-year) outcomes are weakened and attenuated by other factors. The post-stroke changes in the levels of s-IGF-I are compatible with a positive role for IGF-I in IS recovery, although the exact mechanisms are uncertain and probably reflect certain combinations of different factors. Exploration of the causality warrants further studies involving intra-individual serial analyses of IGF-I levels in the serum and CSF of patients who have suffered an IS.

Abbreviations

CI: 95% confidence interval; IGF-I: Insulin-like growth factor I; IS: Ischemic stroke; mRS: Modified Rankin Scale; NIHSS: National Institutes of Health Stroke Scale; OCSP: Oxfordshire Community Stroke Project; SD: Standard deviation; SSS: Scandinavian Stroke Scale; TOAST: Trial of Org 10,172 in Acute Stroke Treatment

Acknowledgments

The authors wish to thank Dr. Vincent Collins for careful correction of the English language of the manuscript.

Funding

This study was supported by grants from the Swedish Government (ALFGBG-751111, ALFGBG-719761, the Swedish Research Council (K2015-63X-20117-10-4), the Swedish Heart Lung Foundation (20100256), the Swedish Stroke Association, the Göteborg Foundation for Neurological Research, and the Yngve Land, Rune and Ulla Amlöv, Edit Jacobson, Magnus Bergvall, Emelle, Lars Hierta, and John and Brit Wennerström foundations.

Authors contributions

NDÅ planned, designed, performed, analyzed, and wrote the paper. DÅ, MN, CB and HGK planned and wrote the paper. KJ planned, analyzed and wrote the paper. JS wrote the paper. JI and CJ planned, designed and wrote the paper. All authors contributed to and have approved the final manuscript.

Competing interests

The authors declare that they have no competing interests.

Author details

[1]Department of Internal Medicine, Institute of Medicine, The Sahlgrenska Academy at University of Gothenburg, Gröna Stråket 8, SE-413 45 Gothenburg, Sweden. [2]Department of Clinical Neuroscience, Institute of Neuroscience and Physiology, The Sahlgrenska Academy at University of Gothenburg, Gothenburg, Sweden. [3]Hunter Medical Research Institute, University of Newcastle, Newcastle, Australia. [4]Center for Stroke Research Berlin, Charité – Universitätsmedizin Berlin, Berlin, Germany. [5]Institute of Biomedicine, The Sahlgrenska Academy at University of Gothenburg, Gothenburg, Sweden. [6]Department of Clinical Genetics, The Sahlgrenska Academy at University of Gothenburg, Gothenburg, Sweden.

References

1. Åberg ND, Brywe KG, Isgaard J. Aspects of growth hormone and insulin-like growth factor-I related to neuroprotection, regeneration, and functional plasticity in the adult brain. TheScientificWorldJournal. 2006;6:53–80.
2. Sohrabji F, Williams M. Stroke neuroprotection: oestrogen and insulin-like growth factor-1 interactions and the role of microglia. J Neuroendocrinol. 2013;25(11):1173–81.
3. Denti L, Annoni V, Cattadori E, Salvagnini MA, Visioli S, Merli MF, Corradi F, Ceresini G, Valenti G, Hoffman AR, et al. Insulin-like growth factor 1 as a predictor of ischemic stroke outcome in the elderly. Am J Med. 2004;117(5):312–7.
4. Bondanelli M, Ambrosio MR, Onofri A, Bergonzoni A, Lavezzi S, Zatelli MC, Valle D, Basaglia N, Degli Uberti EC. Predictive value of circulating insulin-like growth factor I levels in ischemic stroke outcome. J Clin Endocrinol Metab. 2006;91(10):3928–34.
5. Åberg D, Jood K, Blomstrand C, Jern C, Nilsson M, Isgaard J, Åberg ND. Serum IGF-I levels correlate to improvement of functional outcome after ischemic stroke. J Clin Endocrinol Metab. 2011;96(7):E1055–64.
6. Mattlage AE, Rippee MA, Sandt J, Billinger SA. Decrease in insulin-like growth Factor-1 and insulin-like growth Factor-1 ratio in the first week of stroke is related to positive outcomes. J Stroke Cerebrovasc Dis. 2016;25(7):1800–6.
7. Beilharz EJ, Russo VC, Butler G, Baker NL, Connor B, Sirimanne ES, Dragunow M, Werther GA, Gluckman PD, Williams CE, et al. Co-ordinated and cellular specific induction of the components of the IGF/IGFBP axis in the rat brain following hypoxic-ischemic injury. Brain Res Mol Brain Res. 1998;59(2):119–34.
8. Wang J, Tang Y, Zhang W, Zhao H, Wang R, Yan Y, Xu L, Li P. Insulin-like growth factor-1 secreted by brain microvascular endothelial cells attenuates neuron injury upon ischemia. FEBS J. 2013;280(15):3658–68.
9. Carro E, Nunez A, Busiguina S, Torres-Aleman I. Circulating insulin-like growth factor I mediates effects of exercise on the brain. J Neurosci. 2000;20(8):2926–33.
10. Jood K, Ladenvall C, Rosengren A, Blomstrand C, Jern C: Family history in ischemic stroke before 70 years of age: the Sahlgrenska Academy study on ischemic stroke. Stroke 2005, 36(7):1383–1387.
11. Ali K, Cheek E, Sills S, Crome P, Roffe C. Development of a conversion factor to facilitate comparison of National Institute of Health Stroke Scale scores with Scandinavian Stroke Scale scores. Cerebrovasc Dis. 2007;24(6):509–15.
12. Bamford J, Sandercock P, Dennis M, Burn J, Warlow C. Classification and natural history of clinically identifiable subtypes of cerebral infarction. Lancet. 1991;337(8756):1521–6.
13. Adams HP Jr, Bendixen BH, Kappelle LJ, Biller J, Love BB, Gordon DL, Marsh EE 3rd. Classification of subtype of acute ischemic stroke. Definitions for use in a multicenter clinical trial. TOAST. Trial of org 10172 in acute stroke treatment. Stroke. 1993;24(1):35–41.
14. Banks JL, Marotta CA. Outcomes validity and reliability of the modified Rankin scale: implications for stroke clinical trials: a literature review and synthesis. Stroke. 2007;38(3):1091–6.
15. Åberg ND, Åberg D, Jood K, Nilsson M, Blomstrand C, Kuhn HG, Svensson J, Jern C, Isgaard J. The change in circulating insulin-like growth factor I (IGF-I) after ischemic stroke is independently associated with outcome. In: European Stroke Organisation Conference: 2018. Gothenburg: European Stroke Journal; 2018. p. 342–3. AS316–018.
16. Peduzzi P, Concato J, Kemper E, Holford TR, Feinstein AR. A simulation study of the number of events per variable in logistic regression analysis. J Clin Epidemiol. 1996;49(12):1373–9.
17. Landin-Wilhelmsen K, Wilhelmsen L, Lappas G, Rosen T, Lindstedt G, Lundberg PA, Bengtsson BA. Serum insulin-like growth factor I in a random population sample of men and women: relation to age, sex, smoking habits, coffee consumption and physical activity, blood pressure and concentrations of plasma lipids, fibrinogen, parathyroid hormone and osteocalcin. Clin Endocrinol. 1994;41(3):351–7.
18. Parekh N, Roberts CB, Vadiveloo M, Puvananayagam T, Albu JB, Lu-Yao GL. Lifestyle, anthropometric, and obesity-related physiologic determinants of insulin-like growth factor-1 in the third National Health and nutrition examination survey (1988-1994). Ann Epidemiol. 2010;20(3):182–93.
19. Spartano NL, Stevenson MD, Xanthakis V, Larson MG, Murabito JM, Vasan RS. Associations of objective physical activity with insulin sensitivity and circulating adipokine profile: the Framingham heart study. Clinical obesity. 2017;7(2):59–69.

20. Gustafson K, Hagberg H, Bengtsson BÅ, Brantsing C, Isgaard J. Possible protective role of growth hormone in hypoxia-ischemia in neonatal rats. Pediatr Res. 1999;45(3):318–23.
21. Genis L, Davila D, Fernandez S, Pozo-Rodrigalvarez A, Martinez-Murillo R, Torres-Aleman I. Astrocytes require insulin-like growth factor I to protect neurons against oxidative injury. F1000Research. 2014;3:28.
22. Okoreeh AK, Bake S, Sohrabji F. Astrocyte-specific insulin-like growth factor-1 gene transfer in aging female rats improves stroke outcomes. Glia. 2017; 65(7):1043–58.
23. Sjögren K, Liu JL, Blad K, Skrtic S, Vidal O, Wallenius V, LeRoith D, Törnell J, Isaksson OG, Jansson JO, et al. Liver-derived insulin-like growth factor I (IGF-I) is the principal source of IGF-I in blood but is not required for postnatal body growth in mice. Proc Natl Acad Sci U S A. 1999;96(12):7088–92.
24. Hallström B, Jonsson AC, Nerbrand C, Petersen B, Norrving B, Lindgren A. Lund stroke register: hospitalization pattern and yield of different screening methods for first-ever stroke. Acta Neurol Scand. 2007;115(1):49–54.
25. Malmivaara A, Meretoja A, Peltola M, Numerato D, Heijink R, Engelfriet P, Wild SH, Belicza E, Bereczki D, Medin E, et al. Comparing ischaemic stroke in six European countries. The EuroHOPE register study. Eur J Neurol. 2015; 22(2):284–91. e225-286
26. Asplund K, Hulter Asberg K, Appelros P, Bjarne D, Eriksson M, Johansson A, Jonsson F, Norrving B, Stegmayr B, Terent A, et al. The Riks-stroke story: building a sustainable national register for quality assessment of stroke care. Int J Stroke. 2011;6(2):99–108.
27. Effect of intravenous recombinant tissue plasminogen activator on ischemic stroke lesion size measured by computed tomography. NINDS; the National Institute of Neurological Disorders and Stroke (NINDS) rt-PA stroke study group. Stroke 2000, 31(12):2912–2919.
28. Menezes NM, Ay H, Wang Zhu M, Lopez CJ, Singhal AB, Karonen JO, Aronen HJ, Liu Y, Nuutinen J, Koroshetz WJ, et al. The real estate factor: quantifying the impact of infarct location on stroke severity. Stroke. 2007;38(1):194–7.

Efficacy and safety of minimal invasive surgery treatment in hypertensive intracerebral hemorrhage

Yiping Tang[1], Fengqiong Yin[2*], Dengli Fu[1], Xinhai Gao[1], Zhengchao Lv[1] and Xuetao Li[1]

Abstract

Background: Recently, minimal invasive surgery (MIS) has been applied as a common therapeutic approach for treatment of hypertensive intracerebral hemorrhage (HICH). However, the efficacy and safety of MIS is still controversial compared with conservative medical treatment or conventional craniotomy. This meta-analysis aimed to systematically assess the safety and efficacy of MIS compared with conservative method and craniotomy in treating HICH patients.

Methods: PubMed, Embase, Web of Science, and Cochrane Controlled Trials Register were used to identify relevant studies on MIS treatment of HICH up to November 2017. This study evaluated Glasgow Outcome Scale (GOS) score, Activities of Daily Living (ADL) score, pulmonary infection rate, mortality rate, and rebleeding rate for patients who underwent MIS, or conservative method, or craniotomy. Subgroup analyses were performed to compare randomization versus non-randomization and large hematoma versus small or mild hematoma. Begg's test and Egger's test were used to determine the potential presence of publication bias.

Results: Sixteen studies consisting of 1912 patients were included in this study to compare the efficacy and safety of MIS to conservative method or craniotomy. MIS contributed to a significant improvement on the prognosis of the patients comparing with conservative group or craniotomy group. Patients undergoing MIS had a lower mortality rate when compared to those receiving conservative method. Also, MIS led to a notable reduction of rebleeding rate and an effective improvement of the patient's quality of life by contrast with craniotomy. No obvious difference was found in terms of the pulmonary infection rate among the comparisons of three treatment methods. Randomization is not the potential source of heterogeneity, but hematoma volume may be a risk factor for post-operative mortality rate. No statistical evidence of publication bias among studies was found under most of comparison models.

Conclusion: This meta-analysis suggests that minimal invasive surgery is an efficient and safe method for the treatment of hypertensive intracerebral hemorrhage, which is associated with a low mortality rate and rebleeding rate, as well as a significant improvement of the prognosis and the quality life of patients when compared with conservative medical treatment or craniotomy.

Keywords: Minimal invasive surgery (MIS), Hypertensive intracerebral hemorrhage (HICH), Conservative method, Craniotomy, Meta-analysis

* Correspondence: 3536133175@qq.com
[2]Priority Ward, The Second Affiliated Hospital of Kunming Medical University, No. 374 Dianmian Avenue, Kunming 650101, Yunnan Province, China
Full list of author information is available at the end of the article

Background

Hypertensive intracerebral hemorrhage (HICH), a common neurosurgery disease, seriously endangers lives of elderly patients and produces heavy economic burden for families and society [1]. HICH generally results from hypertension-induced intracranial arterial, venous, and capillary ruptures, of which, the mechanical stress of hematoma on brain tissue is the most common reason [2]. HICH has been reported to account for 50–70% of all spontaneous intracranial hemorrhage (ICH), its morbidity and mortality both occupy the top among all types of strokes, more than 30% survivors suffer from varying degrees of disability [3, 4]. Worse, the incidence of HICH continues to rise with aged tendency of population [5]. A study reported that the HICH patients with a hematoma volume > 50 ml are of a greater probability of mortality and disability [6]. Based on the risks and harmfulness of HICH, it is urgently necessary to seek out an effective therapeutic strategy for curing the patients with hypertensive cerebral hemorrhage (HCH).

Although the renowned deleterious influences of HICH, there have been no significant breakthrough in therapeutic schedules hitherto [7]. Currently, conservative medical treatment and surgical evacuation are the main options for HICH treatment [7]. Surgical treatment can be roughly divided into conventional craniotomy and minimally invasive surgery. Conventional conservative method has been used to treat of HICH for a long time, however, which has not made great progress in recent years, and was related with high fatality rate and mortality rate [8]. Craniotomy is the major surgical treatment for HICH, which can eliminate hematoma relatively thoroughly since it is applied, however, several disadvantages should also be noted, including large trauma, general anesthesia, obvious impairment on brain tissues, high blood loss, long operation time, severe edema reaction, various complications, poor prognosis and curative effect [9, 10].

Therefore, conservative treatment and craniotomy of hematoma could not achieve a desired therapeutic effect for HICH treatment.

With the development of imaging technique, minimal invasive surgery (MIS) has been widely applied in the treatment of HICH patients recently, which can reach to the designated position accurately and establish a work channel for clearing hematoma. MIS has been proved to be superior to conservative treatment or craniotomy in some respects [11]: 1) reducing the damage to cerebral tissues and surgical trauma; 2) relieving hematoma compression by targeting hematoma region directly; 3) treating patients with intracranial deep hematoma; 4) accelerating removal of hematoma;5) lowering the mortality and side-effects, as well as improving surgical prognosis. However, some studies [9, 12, 13] showed that MIS did not decrease the mortality rate or improve the long-term outcomes comparing with conservative treatment or craniotomy. Therefore, until now, it is unable to draw an exact conclusion about the impacts of MIS on the curative effect of HICH patients. Due to above controversial conclusions, we performed a comprehensive systematic review and meta-analysis in this study to evaluate the safety and efficacy of MIS for treating HCH.

Methods

This systematic review and meta-analysis was performed to assess the safety and efficacy of minimally invasive surgery treatment for hypertensive intracerebral hemorrhage in accordance with PRISMA statement [14]. No ethical review was required in this study.

Literature search

Four international databases including PubMed, Embase, Web of Science, and Cochrane Controlled Trials Register (CCTR) were searched from the earliest date to November 2017. The following search terms were used in different combination: 'hypertensive', 'hypertension', 'cerebral hemorrhage', 'putamen hemorrhage', 'intracerebral hemorrhage', 'intracranial haemorrhage', 'cerebral bleeding', 'minimally', 'endoscopic surgery', 'keyhole', 'small bone window', and 'stereotactic drilling'. All terms were searched as subject headings and keywords. Meanwhile, Back Tracking Method was performed to ensure the integration of the included literatures.

Inclusion and exclusion criteria
Inclusion criteria

Inclusion criteria in this meta-analysis were as follows: 1. Research subjects: computed tomography (CT)-confirmed diagnosis of HICH; 2. Intervention and comparison: MIS comparing with other treatment methods, including craniotomy or conservative medical treatment; 3. Primary outcome: mortality rate, rebleeding rate, lung infection rate, and the difference in the score of therapeutic efficiency.

Exclusion criteria

Exclusion criteria were as follows: 1. Publication language: not in Chinese or English; 2. Publication type: in the form of abstracts, statements, proceedings, comments, and other unpublished grey literatures, or reviews, pathology reports, project designs, cell experiments, and animal studies. 3. Data requirement: unable to provide required data or with less data in duplicated literatures.

Data screening and quality evaluation

Two reviewers independently identified all studies according to inclusion and exclusion criteria, and assessed the quality of eligible articles. In the event of any disagreements, consensus was reached by discussion with a third reviewer. Two reviewers independently extracted the following data from each study: name of first author, publication year, country, range of eligible cases, study design (random), the type of patients, hematoma volume, number of cases, gender, age, the type of minimally invasive surgery, guideline, outcome index. All data in the charts are converted into numeric data. The third researcher was responsible for checking the extracted data.

Statistical analysis

The primary outcomes across study were calculated by the dichotomous variables, and the data of each trial were showed as a relative risk (RR) ratio with a 95% confidence interval (CI). RR > 1 and $p < 0.05$ indicated that the long-term prognosis, side effects, and mortality in minimally invasive group were higher than those in other two groups. For the significant efficiency, we used Glasgow Outcome Scale (GOS) score, and Activities of Daily Living (ADL) score. Good outcome was defined as GOS score > 4, and ADL score > 3. For all outcomes, heterogeneity was quantified via Cochran'Q statistics and I-squared (I^2) statistics [15]. A probability value of $p < 0.05$ or $I^2 < 50\%$ was judged as statistical heterogeneity, then a random-effect model was performed to analyze the pooled data; on the other hand, a fixed-effect model was used. In case of a study with uncertain methodological quality, a sensitivity analysis was conducted by eliminating the peculiar study. If all the results were reversed, the pooled result would be considered as with low sensitivity and high stability. Subgroup analyses were performed to compare randomization versus non-randomization and large hematoma versus small or mild hematoma. Begg's test and Egger's test were used to assess the potential presence of publication bias, and $p > 0.05$ was considered a low publication bias. All statistical analyses were performed using Statistical Analysis System (Version 9.0; SAS Institute, Cary, NC) and RevMan5 software (Cochrane Information Management System).

Results

Literature research

Initial comprehensive literature search identified 260 potentially relevant articles from PubMed ($n = 44$), Web of science ($n = 40$), EmBase ($n = 162$), and CCTR ($n = 14$). 81 studies were excluded as duplicates, 179 studies were remained. According to the inclusion and exclusion criteria, 160 articles were removed due to the following reasons: systematic reviews ($n = 82$),

unrelated studies ($n = 57$), other reasons causing HCH ($n = 17$), case reports ($n = 3$), and animal assay ($n = 1$). Next, we reviewed the full-text of the remaining 22 studies, and 6 studies were eliminated based on other reasons: not exactly HICH ($n = 4$) and without available data ($n = 2$). Finally, 16 studies [5, 9, 16–29] were included in this meta-analysis.

Characteristics of the included studies

A total of 16 studies, consisting of 1912 patients, were included in the meta-analysis. Six of the studies were published between 2003 and 2010 [18, 19, 24–26, 28]. Most of the patients were Chinese except for 69 Japanese. Cranial computed tomography (CT) scan was used as the puncture positioning method in all the included studies. All patients were diagnosed with one type of hypertensive intracerebral hemorrhage diseases, and had been undergone a minimally invasive surgery. Eight of the included studies were randomized controlled trials [5, 16, 19, 20, 23, 25, 26, 29]. Most of the studies provided the detailed information of cases, including the proportion of male, age, the level of high voltage in addition to T. Nakano's report [24]. 388 patients in 5 studies were treated with MIS vs. conservative method [17, 19, 20, 23, 25], whereas 1085 patients in 8 studies were treated with MIS vs. craniotomy [5, 9, 16, 18, 21, 22, 27, 29], and 439 patients in 3 studies were treated with MIS vs. craniotomy or conservative method [24, 26, 28]. The protocol of the studies was approved by the 4th Cerebrovascular Disease Conference ($n = 5$), Ethics Committee of General Hospital of Beijing Military Region ($n = 1$), and intracranial hematoma minimally invasive puncture removal techniques standardized treatment guidelines ($n = 1$), while 9 studies were not mentioned guideline. The outcomes reported in the articles were mainly based on GOS score ($n = 9$), ADL score ($n = 5$), and NIHSS ($n = 4$). The detailed data are summarized in Table 1.

Effects of interventions

Comparison of GOS score

Data from 4 studies containing 258 patients were pooled to evaluate GOS score between MIS and conservative groups; meanwhile, 5 studies with data on 352 patients were available for the comparison between MIS and craniotomy groups. Heterogeneity ($I^2 = 62.1\%$, $p = 0.032$) existed in the GOS Score comparison between MIS and craniotomy groups, therefore, the random-effects model was used. The following results showed that MIS would lead to a statistical significance comparing with conservative group ($n = 258$; RR: 1.546; 95% CI: 1.121 ~ 1.972; $p < 0.001$; Fig. 1a) or craniotomy group ($n = 352$; RR: 1.678; 95% CI: 1.099 ~ 2.590; $p = 0.017$; Fig. 1b),

Table 1 Characteristics of the included studies

First author (year)	Country	Duration	Random trail	Type of patients	Hematoma volume (ml)	Comparison of treatment methods Number (Male, Age (year), Hematoma volume (ml))			Information of minimally invasive			Outcome
						Conservative group	Craniotomy group	Minimally invasive group	Method	Puncture positioning method	Guideline	
Bo Huang (2003) [28]	China	1998–2001	No	HICH	> 30	38 (57.9%, 62.1 ± 5.8, 35–128)	38 (68.4%, 56.7 ± 5.3, 38–120)	36 (72.2%, 60.3 ± 5.1, 32–139)	Minimally invasive evacuation	Cranial CT scan	The 4th Cerebrovascular Disease Conference	NIHSS
Gang Yang (2016) [5]	China	2012–2014	Yes	HCH	> 30	–	78 (55.1%, 59.77 ± 5.06, 30–180)	78 (66.67%, 60.18 ± 5.51, 35–180)	Minimally invasive intracranial hematoma	Cranial CT scan	The 4th Cerebrovascular Disease Conference	BI
Guodong Wang (2017) [23]	China	2015–2016	Yes	Hypertensive spontaneous ICH (basal ganglia)	> 30	60 (66.67%, 55.2 ± 5.6, 31–87)	–	60 (61.67%, 60.2 ± 7.3, 33–85)	Minimally invasive intracranial hematoma	Cranial CT scan	The 4th Cerebrovascular Disease Conference	NIHSS
Guoqiang Wang (2014) [22]	China	2009–2012	No	Hypertensive spontaneous ICH	> 30	–	114 (71.9%, 55.3 ± 11.1, 30–128)	84 (73.8%, 59.4 ± 14.5, 30–144)	Minimally invasive puncture and drainage	Cranial CT scan	Ethics Committee of General Hospital of Beijing Military Region	GOS
Huili Kang (2016) [27]	China	2012–2014	No	HCH (basal ganglia)	20–40	–	30 (46.67%, 48 ± 12, 20–40)	30 (50%, 50 ± 10, 20–40)	Minimally invasive removal	Cranial CT scan	–	GOS
Jinbiao Luo (2008) [25]	China	2004–2008	Yes	Hypertensive mild hemorrhage (basal ganglia)	10–30	39 (58.97%, 54.3 ± 10.1, 10–30)	–	36 (58.33%, 56.3 ± 9.2, 10–30)	Minimally invasive directional soft tube placement	Cranial CT scan	–	GOS, ADL
Pingbo Wei (2010) [19]	China	2007–2010	Yes	HICH	20–40	39 (56.4%, 40–77, 39 ± 8)	–	31 (54.8%, 39–76, 31 ± 8) 36(52.7%, 41–80, 31 ± 9)	Minimally invasive surgery	Cranial CT scan	Intracranial hematoma minimally invasive puncture removal techniques standardized treatment guidelines	GOS
Shuwu Lin (2004) [26]	China	1995–2003	Yes	HICH		134 (52.2%, 60.9 ± 10.6, 33.5 ± 23.1)	10 (20%, 62.1 ± 11.2, 32.3 ± 22.5)	134 (48.5%, 60.1 ± 10.8, 35.0 ± 23.5)	Minimally invasive puncture and drainage	Cranial CT scan	–	ADL
T. Yamamoto (2006) [18]	Japan	2002–2006	No	HCH		–	10 (80%, 54–82, 15.9)	10 (80%, 53–86, 22.3)	Endoscopic surgery	Cranial CT scan	–	GOS
T. Nakano (2003) [24]	Japan	2000–2001	No	HICH		32	11	6	Endoscopic surgery	Cranial CT scan	–	GOS
Wenjun Wang (2017) [21]	China	2012–2016	No	HICH	> 50	–	34 (82.35%, 56.0 ± 12.37, 35.3 ± 18.28)	70 (82.35%, 61.10 ± 12.10, 68.8 ± 13.42)	Minimally invasive puncture and drainage	Cranial CT scan	–	GOS
Xinghua Xu (2017) [9]	China	2009–2014	No	Supratentorial HICH	55.2 ± 28.4/ 55.9 ± 27.6	–	69 (66.7%, 53.8 ± 13.5, 55.9 ± 27.6)	82 (7.07, 52.9 ± 12.3, 55.2 ± 28.4)	Endoscopic surgery	Cranial CT scan	–	MRS score, GOS

Table 1 Characteristics of the included studies (*Continued*)

First author (year)	Country	Duration	Random trail	Type of patients	Hematoma volume (ml)	Comparison of treatment methods Number (Male, Age (year), Hematoma volume (ml))			Information of minimally invasive			Outcome
						Conservative group	Craniotomy group	Minimally invasive group	Method	Puncture positioning method	Guideline	
Xueyuan Wang (2011) [20]	China	2004–2009	Yes	Hypertensive basal ganglia hemorrhage	20–35	30 (53.33%, 45.73 ± 11.64, 20–35)	–	32 (56.25%, 46.75 ± 10.55, 20–35)	Minimally invasive puncture and drainage	Cranial CT scan	The 4th Cerebrovascular Disease Conference	ADL
YF Yan (2015) [17]	China	2010–2013	No	Hypertensive basal ganglia hemorrhage	15–30	12 (58.33%, 47.75 ± 9.16, 22.42 ± 4.70)	–	13 (76.92%, 55.31 ± 9.97, 25.18 ± 4.15)	Neuronavigation-assisted minimally invasive	Cranial CT scan	–	GOS, NIHSS
Yi Feng (2016) [29]	China	2006–2013	Yes	HCH	< 60	–	91 (63.73%, 69.10 ± 10.26)	93 (60.21%, 66.35 ± 12.23)	Endoscope-assisted keyhole technique	Cranial CT scan	–	ADL
Zaiyu Li (2012) [16]	China	2007–2010	Yes	HICH	> 30	–	110 (74.55%, 45–79, 30)	102 (71.57%, 37–75, 30)	Minimally invasive puncture suction drainage	Cranial CT scan	The 4th Cerebrovascular Disease Conference	ADL, NIHSS

HICH Hypertensive intracerebral hemorrhage, *HCH* hypertensive cerebral hemorrhage, *ICH* intracranial hemorrhage, *CT* computed tomography, *ADL* Activities of Daily Living, *GOS* Glasgow Outcome Scale

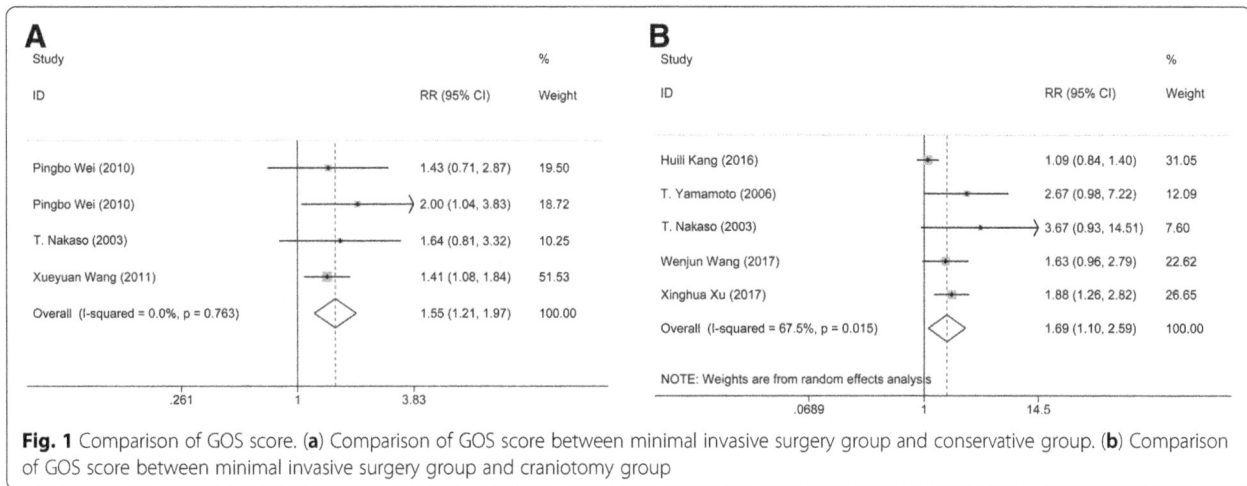

Fig. 1 Comparison of GOS score. (**a**) Comparison of GOS score between minimal invasive surgery group and conservative group. (**b**) Comparison of GOS score between minimal invasive surgery group and craniotomy group

suggesting that MIS shows a positive effect on the prognosis of the patients.

Comparison of pulmonary infection rate

Four studies containing data on 282 patients pooled pulmonary infection rate for MIS and conservative groups; meanwhile, 3 studies consisting of 486 subjects were available for the comparison between MIS and craniotomy groups. Heterogeneity ($I^2 = 77.8\%$, $p = 0.011$) was found in the pulmonary infection rate between MIS and craniotomy, assessed using a random-effect model. Clearly, no significant difference was found between the MIS and conservative group ($n = 282$; RR: 0.610; 95% CI: $0.342 \sim 1.086$; $p = 0.038$; Fig. 2a) nor craniotomy group ($n = 486$; RR: 0.700; 95% CI: $0.430 \sim 1.141$; $p = 0.449$; Fig. 2b), suggesting that MIS treatment has no positive influence on the pulmonary infection rate of patients.

Comparison of mortality rate

Data from 6 studies with 600 patients were pooled to evaluate the mortality rate between MIS and conservative group; meanwhile, 8 studies consisting of 1127 subjects were available for the comparison between MIS and craniotomy groups. No heterogeneity occurred in either the comparison between MIS and conservative method ($I^2 = 14.5\%$, $p = 0.321$) nor craniotomy ($I^2 = 44.9\%$, $p = 0.080$). Obviously, apparent statistical significance was appeared in the pooled data between the MIS and conservative group ($n = 600$; RR: 0.265; 95% CI: $0.173 \sim 0.404$; $p < 0.001$; Fig. 3a), but not craniotomy group ($n = 1127$; RR: 0.839; 95% CI: $0.649 \sim 1.086$; $p = 0.182$; Fig. 3b), suggesting that MIS treatment could yield a lower mortality rate than conservative method.

Comparison of ADL score

Four studies consisting of 696 subjects were available for the comparison between MIS and craniotomy groups.

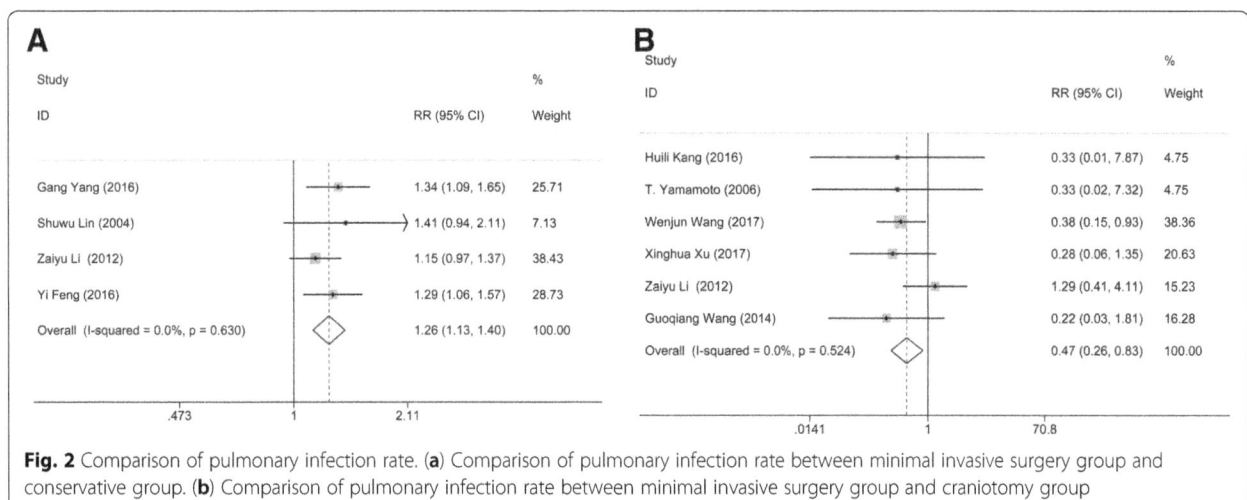

Fig. 2 Comparison of pulmonary infection rate. (**a**) Comparison of pulmonary infection rate between minimal invasive surgery group and conservative group. (**b**) Comparison of pulmonary infection rate between minimal invasive surgery group and craniotomy group

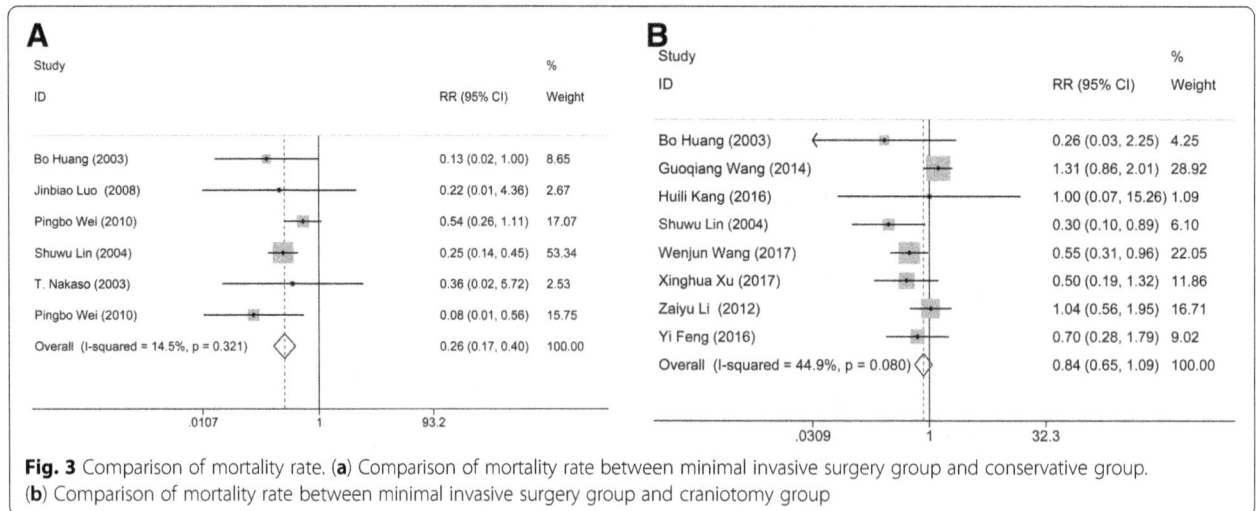

Fig. 3 Comparison of mortality rate. (**a**) Comparison of mortality rate between minimal invasive surgery group and conservative group. (**b**) Comparison of mortality rate between minimal invasive surgery group and craniotomy group

There was no heterogeneity ($I^2 = 0.0\%$, $p = 0.630$) in the comparison of ADL score between MIS and conservative method. The following results showed that MIS had a statistical significance comparing with craniotomy group ($n = 696$; RR: 1.259; 95% CI: 1.133 ~ 1.400; $p <$ 0.001; Fig. 4a), indicating that MIS treatment can effectively improve the patient's quality of life.

Comparison of rebleeding rate

Six studies containing 745 subjects pooled the data of rebleeding rate for MIS and craniotomy groups. No significant heterogeneity ($I^2 = 0.0\%$, $p = 0.524$) was found between these articles. The results showed that the rebleeding rate of the patients in MIS had a statistical significance comparing with that in craniotomy group ($n = 745$; RR: 0.468; 95% CI: 0.263 ~ 0.832; $p = 0.001$; Fig. 4b), suggesting that MIS treatment can effectively reduce the postoperative rebleeding rate.

Subgroup analysis

The data of heterogeneity analysis suggested that significant heterogeneity existed in the comparisons of GOS score between MIS and conservative method, and pulmonary infection rate between MIS and craniotomy. Based on the results of Table 2, we supposed that the sources of heterogeneity included the randomization of experiment design and the hematoma volume of HICH patients. Therefore, subgroup analyses were performed by stratified the status of randomization, and hematoma volume. The result of subgroup analysis based on the randomization of experiment design suggested that randomization would not change the pooled outcome: randomization (RR: 0.80; 95% CI: 0.50 ~ 1.28; $p = 0.358$) and no-randomization (RR: 0.86; 95% CI: 0.63 ~ 1.17; $p = 0.322$), which implied that randomization is not the potential source of heterogeneity (Fig. 5a). Also, the subgroup analysis of hematoma was conducted according to the volume of hematoma (large hematoma:

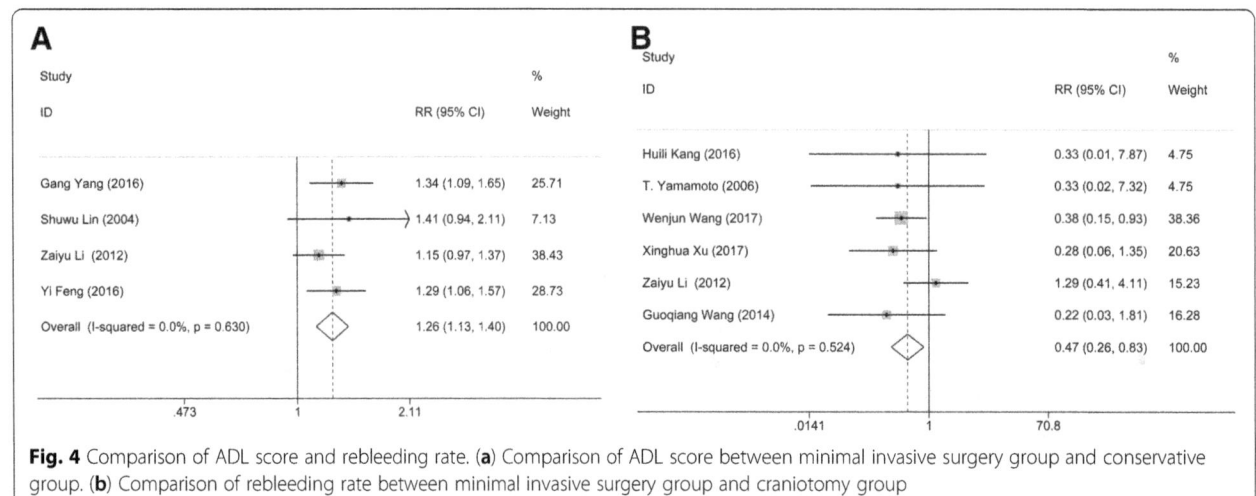

Fig. 4 Comparison of ADL score and rebleeding rate. (**a**) Comparison of ADL score between minimal invasive surgery group and conservative group. (**b**) Comparison of rebleeding rate between minimal invasive surgery group and craniotomy group

Table 2 The pooled data

		RR (95% CI)	p of RR	I^2	p of Heterogeneity	p of Begg's test	p of Egger's test
Minimally invasive group vs. conservative group	Rate of patients with a GOS score > 4 points	1.546 (1.121, 1.972)	< 0.001	0.0%	0.763	0.734	0.093
	Pulmonary infection rate	0.610 (0.342, 1.086)	0.038	0.0%	0.489	1.000	0.917
	Mortality rate	0.265 (0.173, 0.404)	< 0.001	14.5%	0.321	0.707	0.425
Minimally invasive group vs. craniotomy group	Rate of patients with a GOS score > 4 points	1.678 (1.099, 2.590)	0.017	67.5%	0.015	0.221	0.178
	Rate of patients with a ADL score > 3 points	1.259 (1.133, 1.400)	< 0.001	0.0%	0.630	0.308	0.336
	Pulmonary infection rate	0.700 (0.430, 1.141)	0.449	77.8%	0.011	0.296	0.08
	Rebleeding rate	0.468 (0.263, 0.832)	0.001	0.0%	0.524	1.000	0.656
	Mortality rate	0.839 (0.649, 1.086)	0.182	44.9%	0.080	0.386	0.132

RR relative risk, *GOS* Glasgow Outcome Scale, *ADL* activities of daily living

volume > 30 ml; small or mild hematoma: volume < 30 ml). No significant difference of the mortality rate was found between MIS and craniotomy groups when the included cases with the hematoma volume > 30 ml (RR: 0.95; 95% CI: 0.71 ~ 1.28; $p = 0.755$). Whereas, MIS would decrease the mortality rate of the HICH patients when the hematoma volume is less than a certain value (RR: 0.54; 95% CI: 0.31 ~ 0.96; $p = 0.035$) (Fig. 5b). Above demonstrated that hematoma volume may be a risk factor for post-operative mortality rate. Nonetheless, more randomized controlled trial should be included to verify whether the above conclusion was correct or not because there was no clear record about the scope of hematoma volume in the included literatures.

Publication bias
Begg's and Egger's test were conducted to assess the publication bias of this meta-analysis, and the result was shown in Table 2. Obviously, there was no statistical evidence of publication bias among studies under most of comparisons, which suggested that our pooled data is of high authenticity and reliability.

Discussion
Hypertensive intracerebral hemorrhage is one of the most common complications of hypertension. Currently, the minimally invasive surgery applied on the treatment of HICH has increased. The advantages of MIS include the well impermeability, less infection, low cost, low mortality and disability rates, better survival quality, and

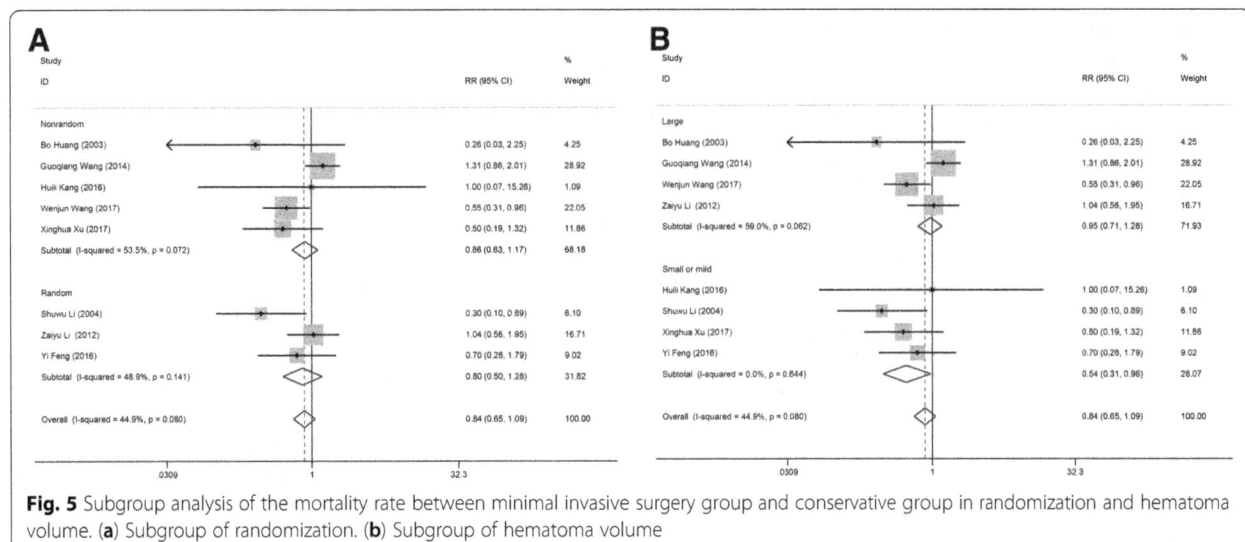

Fig. 5 Subgroup analysis of the mortality rate between minimal invasive surgery group and conservative group in randomization and hematoma volume. (**a**) Subgroup of randomization. (**b**) Subgroup of hematoma volume

fast recovery time [11]. Although most reports about the curative effect of MIS are positive, some low level of recognition also existed, and the safety and efficacy of MIS remains unproven until now. Thus, it is great value to research application of minimally invasive surgery in hypertensive intracerebral hemorrhage. This systematic review with meta-analysis pooled the data from the included 16 studies concerning the effects of MIS, conservative method, and craniotomy on HICH to confirm the safety and efficacy of MIS. The main results suggested that MIS was associated with better prognosis outcomes and quality of daily living compared with conservative method or craniotomy. Moreover, this treatment modality could significantly decrease the mortality rate and rebleeding rate of patients. However, the incidence of pulmonary infection rate showed no significant difference between three groups. Overall, these findings demonstrated that MIS could be a safe and effective strategy in treating patients with HICH.

Rebleeding and pulmonary infection are two major complications related with the outcomes during treatments. Previous study [30] has suggested that MIS could decrease the risk of complications of patients comparing with traditional craniotomy for the following reasons: 1) MIS is associated with the smaller skin incision and shorter operation time; 2) craniotomy needs more space to operate, thus contribute to brain retraction, while MIS could reduce the risk of brain edema by affording preferable visualizing to the bleeding site due to without brain retraction. In our study, the patients underwent MIS exert low re-bleeding rate than those underwent craniotomy despite hemostasis cannot be easily performed under the direct vision during MIS. The reason for this possibly due to that hematoma is removed thoroughly in craniotomy approach, then result in a drastic pressure reduce in the hematoma cavity. The originally high pressure might cause the potential rebleeding in ruptured vessels. Although there is a gradual pressure reduction during the MIS treatment with continued hematoma drainage, it can in turn keep a steady pressure in the ruptured vessels and hematoma cavity, then promote the compression of hemostasis and stop the occurrence of rebleeding. An epidemiological study reported that pulmonary infection is one of the most common complications in HICH patients after treatment [31]. Conventional craniotomy is generally associated with significant blood loss, long-time anesthesia, and large trauma in elderly patients, which easily results in some complications, such as pulmonary infection. However, no significant difference was observed in the complication of pulmonary infection between the three groups, the result was in part agree with previously reported results [32]. Moreover, MIS was more effective in preventing death compared with conservative method

but not craniotomy, which indicated that MIS was feasible in patients with HICH and its surgical efficacy was superior to that of conservative method can be achieved. In addition, we found a well-marked improvement of the prognosis and the life quality of the patients receiving MIS than those received craniotomy or conservative method, which verifies the long-term effect of MIS. The reason for these may be related with rapid and effective hematoma clearance of MIS. Puncture suction during MIS can remove hematoma rapidly, the hematoma-induced neurological damage could be relieved quickly, which lay a crucial foundation for improving the prognosis effect and living capability of patients in the future. Based on the above points, the advantages of MIS are prominent.

To further confirm whether the randomization status and the hematoma volume are the sources of heterogeneity, we performed the subgroup analysis. Subgroup analysis of randomization status found no difference in clinical outcomes in the treatment of HICH, suggesting that MIS treatment of hypertensive intracerebral hemorrhage is a safe and effective irrespective of the randomization status. Some researchers believed that the hematoma volume is an important factor for the patients received surgical treatments including MIS and craniotomy. For example, Zhou et al. [33] reported that MIS is suited to the hematomas with a volume of 25~40 ml, while, other forms of treatments like craniotomy should be performed when the volume hematomas >40 ml. Meanwhile, the research of Yamashiro et al. [14] showed that MIS was associated with lower mortality rate when the mean hematoma volume of involved patients was at the range of 99 ~ 130 ml. In this subgroup analysis, no significant difference of the mortality rate was found between MIS and craniotomy groups when the included cases with the hematoma volume > 30 ml. Whereas, MIS of hematoma volume that is less than a certain value would contribute to a lower rate of death than other treatment options, demonstrating that hematoma volume may be a risk factor for post-operative mortality rate. However, due to a lack of sufficient evidence from the included literatures of the scope of hematoma volume, this underlying benefit of hematoma volume for HICH treatment requires more relevant studies to affirm. It is failed to perform to a subgroup analysis of the ethnic because most of the involved patients were Asians and the lack of related information from other races. Previous studies have confirmed that the incidence of HICH was varying in different races [3], which is mainly responsible for the differential gene expression [33]. As we known, minimally invasive surgery treatment is not belonged to the gene therapy. Thus, we believe that there is no significant difference in the therapeutic effect of MIS on HICH patients who have different ethnic backgrounds. Also, we did not conduct a subgroup analysis of the age. In this review, most of the included trials limited the age ≥ 30 and ≤ 80 years, thus the issue of MIS applying to the patients aged < 30 or > 80 years was ignored. Generally, the older patients are associated with a higher rate of mortality and the poorer prognoses [34]. However, no final verdict was achieved in terms of whether the older series undergoing MIS show worse outcomes than the young people. Zhou et al. [33] reported that the patients aged ≥30 years treated with MIS showed a significantly favourable outcome comparing with other treatment approaches, while no statistical difference was found in the patients aged ≥18 years. On the contrary, the study of Wang et al. [20] revealed that the older the patients received MIPD (minimally invasive puncture and drainage) is accompanied with the higher risk of death and the poor short- or long-term outcome. Here, we suspect that the older series may have better outcomes than the youngsters, reasons are as follows: elderly patients with an atrophic brain have a lower intracranial pressure when compared with the younger patients with same hematoma size, and they have more time to wait until the bleeding stop. Therefore, MIS will contribute to less brain retraction and brain tissue damage, with shorter anesthesia time and less blood loss in the elderly [29].

The main advantages of our study are as follows: First, this meta-analysis is based on the comprehensive literature search of several databases to confirm all associated comparative studies, and the research process was conducted by independent reviewers according to PRISMA statement. Second, most of identified literatures were published in more famous publications in recent years, which are of high-quality and contain more comprehensive content. Third, our study does not suffer from any publication bias, suggesting the high-reliability of our pooled data. Fourth, the large sample size provides some valuable data, which enables us to compare the outcomes by minimally invasive method, conservative method, and craniotomy, then summarizes some important conclusions. Fifth, this meta-analysis refers to all available clinically related outcomes, instead of selectively reporting only a few outcomes.

Also, several limitations in our meta-analysis should be taken into consideration: First, most of the involved studies were derived from the People's Republic of China, which may restrict the applicability of our findings to some extent. Second, a few studies in our meta-analysis failed to provide the scope of hematoma volume, hence, we can't be quite sure that the hematoma volume is a risk factor for post-operative mortality rate. Third, a lot of the included studies [1, 9, 17, 18, 21, 22, 24, 27, 28] on minimally invasive approaches to HICH were retrospective

studies rather than RCTs. However, it also should be taken into account that it is very hard to carry out a prospective randomized study within a reasonable timeframe. Fourth, no studies provide the outcomes data of the side effects and the patient's discharge from hospital, which are necessary to evaluate the safety of the MIS. Despite above, the findings in all studies generated unified results, as well as the similar surgical experience and postoperative outcomes, which reassures us that these disadvantages do not deny the validity of the meta-analysis.

Conclusion

Collectively, based on the preliminary statistics and evaluation of the included 16 studies, it can be concluded that minimal invasive surgery is an efficient and safe alternative in the treatment of patients with hypertensive intracerebral hemorrhage, which has superior outcomes than conservative medical treatment or craniotomy. Although there is no improvement in pulmonary infection rate, MIS treatment is associated with the better prognosis and quality of daily living, as well as the lower mortality rate and rebleeding rate, when compared with conservative method or craniotomy. Hematoma volume may be a risk factor for post-operative mortality rate. However, more high-quality trials should be included before any claims can be putted forward.

Abbreviations
ADL: Activities of Daily Living; CI: Confidence interval; CT: Computed tomography; GOS: Glasgow Outcome Scale; HCH: Hypertensive cerebral hemorrhage; HICH: Hypertensive intracerebral hemorrhage; ICH: Intracranial hemorrhage; MIS: Minimal invasive surgery; RR: Relative risk

Authors' contribution
FQY conceived and designed the entire study; YPT and DLF analyzed the data; XHG, ZCL and XTL performed literature research and statistical analysis; YPT and XHG drafted the paper. FQY supervised the entire study and revised the manuscript before submission. All authors have read and agreed with the final version of this manuscript.

Competing interests
The authors declare that they have no competing interests.

Author details
[1]Department of Neurosurgery, The Second Affiliated Hospital of Kunming Medical University, Kunming 650101, Yunnan Province, China. [2]Priority Ward, The Second Affiliated Hospital of Kunming Medical University, No. 374 Dianmian Avenue, Kunming 650101, Yunnan Province, China.

References

1. Zhang WT, Zhao X, Jin XY. Curative effect of minimally invasive hematoma removal combining with heparin-saline continuous irrigation in 48 cases with hypertensive cerebral hemorrhage. Chin J Pract Nerv Dis. 2014;17(15):119–20.
2. Wang Y, Geng Y. Analysis of postoperative pulmonary infection and its influencing factors of patients with hypertensive intracerebral hemorrhage. Chin J Pract Nerv Dis. 2014; (13): 5–7.
3. van Asch CJ, Luitse MJ, Rinkel GJ, Van dTI, Algra A, Klijn CJ. Incidence, case fatality, and functional outcome of intracerebral haemorrhage over time, according to age, sex, and ethnic origin: a systematic review and meta-analysis. Lancet Neurol. 2010;9(2):167–76.
4. Muengtaweepongsa S, Seamhan B. Predicting mortality rate with ICH score in Thai intracerebral hemorrhage patients. Neurol Asia. 2013;18(18):131–5.
5. Yang G, Shao G. Clinical effect of minimally invasive intracranial hematoma in treating hypertensive cerebral hemorrhage. Pak J Med Sci. 2016;32(3):677–81.
6. Fiorella D, Arthur A, Bain M, Mocco J. Minimally invasive surgery for intracerebral hemorrhage: rationale, review of existing data and emerging technologies. Stroke. 2016;47(5):1399–406.
7. Morgenstern LB, Hemphill JC, Anderson C, Becker K, Broderick JP, Connolly ES Jr, Greenberg SM, Huang JN, MacDonald RL, Messé SR, Mitchell PH, Selim M, Tamargo RJ; American Heart Association Stroke Council and Council on Cardiovascular Nursing. Guidelines for the Management of Spontaneous Intracerebral Hemorrhage a Guideline for healthcare professionals from the American Heart Association/American Stroke Association. Stroke. 2010;41(9): 2108–29.
8. Chen J. The efficacy comparison of minimally invasive and conservative treatment for hypertensive cerebral hemorrhage. Clini Med Eng. 2012.
9. Xu X, Chen X, Li F, Zheng X, Wang Q, Sun G, Zhang J, Xu B. Effectiveness of endoscopic surgery for supratentorial hypertensive intracerebral hemorrhage: a comparison with craniotomy. J Neurosurg. 2018;128(2):553–9.
10. Huang JX, Ye M, Zhang WB, Lai X, Qiu QZ. Comparison of minimally invasive treatment with craniotomy in the treatment of hypertensive cerebral hemorrhage. Hainan Med J. 2012;23(2):13–5.
11. Broderick J, Connolly S, Feldmann E, Hanley D, Kase C, Krieger D, Mayberg M, Morgenstern L, Ogilvy CS, Vespa P, Zuccarello M; American Heart Association; American Stroke Association Stroke Council; High Blood Pressure Research Council; Quality of Care and Outcomes in Research Interdisciplinary Working Group. Guidelines for the management of spontaneous intracerebral hemorrhage in adults: 2007 update: a guideline from the American Heart Association/American Stroke Association stroke council, high blood pressure research council, and the quality of care and Outc. Stroke. 2008;38(6):2001–3.
12. Yamashiro S, Hitoshi Y, Yoshida A, Kuratsu J. Effectiveness of endoscopic surgery for comatose patients with large Supratentorial intracerebral hemorrhages. Neurol Med Chir. 2015;55(11):819–23.
13. Auer LM, Deinsberger W, Niederkorn K, Gell G, Kleinert R, Schneider G, Holzer P, Bone G, Mokry M, Körner E, Kleinert G, Hanusch S. Endoscopic surgery versus medical treatment for spontaneous intracerebral hematoma: a randomized study. J Neurosurg. 1989;70(4):530–5.
14. Moher D, Liberati A, Tetzlaff J, Altman DG. Preferred reporting items for systematic reviews and meta-analyses: the PRISMA statement. Open Med. 2009;3(3):e123–30.
15. Higgins JP, Thompson SG, Deeks JJ, Altman DG. Measuring inconsistency in meta-analyses. BMJ. 2003;327(7414):557–60.
16. Li ZY, Luo YN, Jin MS, Chen DW, Shi PQ, Xu XG. Clinical therapeutic effect of different surgical approaches on the hypertensive intracerebral. J Dalian Med Univ. 2012;34(1):60–3.
17. Yan YF, Ru DW, Du JR, Shen X, Wang ES, Yao HB. The clinical efficacy of neuronavigation-assisted minimally invasive operation on hypertensive basal ganglia hemorrhage. Eur Rev Med Pharmacol Sci. 2015;19(14):2614–20.
18. Yamamoto T, Nakao Y, Mori K, Maeda M. Endoscopic hematoma evacuation for hypertensive cerebellar hemorrhage. Minim Invasive Neurosurg. 2006;49(3):173–8.
19. Wei PB, You C, Chen H, Zhang GB, He J, Yang M. Three treatments for moderate hypertensive intracerebral hemorrhage:a comparative therapeusis. Chin J Cerebrovasc Dis. 2010;7(10):519–22.
20. Wang XY, Yang SY, Huang Y, Sun M, Zhao L, Zhuo J, Gao M. Effects of craniopuncture and drainage of intracerebral hemorrhage on brain edema and neurological outcome. Chin J Contemp Neurol Neurosurg. 2011;11(2):230–5.
21. Wang W, Zhou N, Wang C. Minimally invasive surgery for hypertensive intracerebral hemorrhage patients with large hematoma volume: a retrospective study. World Neurosurg. 2017;105:348–58.
22. Wang GQ, Li SQ, Huang YH, Zhang WW, Ruan WW, Qin JZ, Li Y, Yin WM, Li YJ, Ren ZJ, Zhu JQ, Ding YY, Peng JQ, Li PJ. Can minimally invasive puncture and drainage for hypertensive spontaneous basal ganglia hemorrhage improve patient outcome: a prospective non-randomized comparative study. Military Med Res. 2014;1(1):1–12.
23. Wang GD. Clinical effect of minimally invasive intracranial hematoma evacuation in treating hypertensive basal ganglia hemorrhage. Chin J Clin Ration Drug Use. 2017;(18).
24. Nakano T, Ohkuma H, Ebina K, Suzuki S. Neuroendoscopic surgery for intracerebral haemorrhage--comparison with traditional therapies. Minim Invasive Neurosurg. 2003;46(5):278–83.
25. Luo JB, Peng B, Quan W, Cao ZK, Xiao GC, Lu JP, Xu JM, He ZW. Therapeutic effects of aspiration with a directional soft tube and conservative treatment on mild hemorrhage in the basal ganglion. J First Military Med Univ. 2008; 28(8):1352–3, 1375.
26. Lin SW, Hu JQ, Yu SY, Dong CY, Wang J, Li J. The minimally invasive surgery on hypertensive cerebral hemorrhage. Chin J Neurol. 2004;37(4):307–10.
27. Kang HL, Zhan WW, Ding Y, Wang Y, Zhao YX, Yao GL, Cai QQ, Mei JJ, Jiang Y. Application of ultrasound guidance in performing minimally invasive removal of hypertensive intracerebral hemorrhage. J Intervent Radiol. 2016;25(1):74–7.
28. Huang B, Cheng D, Gao T. CLINCAL study of hypertensive intracerebral hemorrhage treated by minimally invasive surgery. China J Mod Med. 2003.
29. Feng Y, He J, Liu B, Yang L, Wang Y. Endoscope-assisted keyhole technique for hypertensive cerebral hemorrhage in elderly patients: a randomized controlled study in 184 patients. Turk Neurosurg. 2016;26(1):84–9.
30. Zhang HZ, Li YP, Yan ZC, Wang XD, She L, Wang XD, Dong L. Endoscopic evacuation of basal ganglia hemorrhage via keyhole approach using an adjustable cannula in comparison with craniotomy. Biomed Res Int. 2014; 2014(2):898762.
31. Hu Y, Wang J, Luo B. Epidemiological and clinical characteristics of 266 cases of intracerebral hemorrhage in Hangzhou, China. J Zhejiang Univ-Sci B (Biomedicine & Biotechnology). 2013;14(6):496–504.
32. Zhao Z, Zhang W, Zhuo LX, Yin LM, Zhong DQ, Wang WT, Xu WG. Clinical analysis on postoperative complications of minimally invasive treatment in patients with hypertensive cerebral hemorrhage. J Taishan Med College. 2014.
33. Zhou X, Chen J, Li Q, Ren G, Yao G, Liu M, Dong Q, Guo J, Li L, Guo J, Xie P. Minimally invasive surgery for spontaneous supratentorial intracerebral hemorrhage: a meta-analysis of randomized controlled trials. Stroke. 2012; 43(11):2923–30.
34. Ruiz-Sandoval JL, Chiquete E, Romero-Vargas S, Padilla-Martínez JJ, González-Cornejo S. Grading scale for prediction of outcome in primary intracerebral hemorrhages. Stroke. 2007;38(5):1641–4.

Characterization of the symptoms of neurogenic orthostatic hypotension and their impact from a survey of patients and caregivers

Daniel O. Claassen[1]*, Charles H. Adler[2], L. Arthur Hewitt[3] and Christopher Gibbons[4]

Abstract

Background: Neurogenic orthostatic hypotension (nOH) results from impaired vasoconstriction due to dysfunction of the autonomic nervous system and is commonly associated with Parkinson disease (PD), multiple system atrophy (MSA), and pure autonomic failure. nOH can increase the risk of falls due to symptoms that include postural lightheadedness or dizziness, presyncope, and syncope. The purpose of this study was to obtain information from patients and caregivers regarding the symptoms and burden of nOH to expand on limited knowledge regarding the impact of nOH on quality of life.

Methods: This author-designed survey included questions regarding nOH (e.g., frequency and impact of symptoms, management) and was conducted online by Harris Poll via distribution to individuals who agreed to participate in Harris Poll online surveys or who were members of relevant disease advocacy organizations. Eligible patients were aged ≥ 18 years with PD, MSA, or pure autonomic failure and ≥ 1 of the following: orthostatic hypotension (OH), nOH, low blood pressure upon standing, or OH/nOH symptoms. Eligible caregivers cared for such patients but were not necessarily linked to any patient participant.

Results: Survey responses were received from 363 patients and 128 caregivers. PD was the most frequent underlying disorder (90% of patients; 88% of individuals managed by the caregivers). Despite meeting survey diagnosis criteria, a formal diagnosis of OH or nOH was reported by only 36% of patients and 16% of caregivers. The most frequent symptoms of nOH were dizziness or lightheadedness, fatigue when standing, and difficulty walking. A negative impact on patient quality of life caused by nOH symptoms was reported by 59% of patients and 75% of caregivers. Most respondents (≥87%) reported that nOH symptoms adversely affected patients' ability to perform everyday activities (most frequently physical activity/exercise, housework, and traveling). Falls (≥1) in the previous year due to nOH symptoms were reported by 57% of patients and 80% of caregivers.

Conclusions: These survey results support the premise that nOH symptoms have a substantial negative impact on patient function and quality of life. The relatively low rates of formal nOH/OH diagnosis suggest the need for heightened awareness regarding the condition and its symptom burden.

Keywords: Neurogenic orthostatic hypotension, Parkinson disease, Multiple system atrophy, Quality of life, Disease burden

* Correspondence: Daniel.claassen@vanderbilt.edu
[1]Department of Neurology, Vanderbilt University Medical Center, 1161 21st Avenue South A-0118, Nashville, TN 37232, USA
Full list of author information is available at the end of the article

Background

Orthostatic hypotension (OH) is defined as a sustained reduction in systolic blood pressure (BP) of ≥20 mmHg or in diastolic BP of ≥10 mmHg upon standing [1]. OH generally results from 3 common etiologies: (1) medications such as antidepressants or antihypertensive agents, (2) non-neurologic conditions such as hypovolemia or cardiovascular disorders causing cardiac failure, or (3) impaired vasoconstriction due to dysfunction of the autonomic nervous system (also referred to as neurogenic OH [nOH]). The neurogenic form of OH is commonly associated with neurodegenerative disorders that affect the central or peripheral autonomic nervous system, such as Parkinson disease (PD), multiple system atrophy (MSA), and pure autonomic failure, or it may be secondary to conditions such as diabetic peripheral neuropathy [1–6]. Although differential diagnosis is often challenging, nOH can be distinguished from non-neurogenic forms of OH, such as medication effects and volume depletion, through autonomic testing [5, 7]. Common symptoms of nOH include postural lightheadedness or dizziness, presyncope, falls, and syncope [1, 5]. Additional symptoms can include visual disturbances, fatigue, generalized weakness, cognitive dysfunction, neck pain or discomfort in the suboccipital and paracervical region (i.e., in a "coat hanger" configuration), and orthostatic dyspnea [1, 5].

Neurogenic OH can increase the risk of falls, particularly among older patients [8, 9]. However, only limited information regarding the impact of nOH on quality of life among patients and caregivers has been published [10–12]. We designed a survey to gain a better understanding of the following areas: (1) scope of symptoms and burden of disease among patients with nOH, (2) effect of nOH symptoms on lives of patients from the perspective of caregivers, and (3) insights on the patient and caregiver journey from diagnosis to symptom management.

Methods

A survey designed by the authors was conducted online by Harris Poll on behalf of Lundbeck between August 26, 2016, and October 3, 2016. Respondents for the survey included individuals who agreed to participate in Harris Poll online surveys or who are members of certain advocacy organizations (American Parkinson Disease Association, Davis Phinney Foundation, Michael J. Fox Foundation, MSA Coalition, National Parkinson Foundation, and Parkinson's Disease Foundation) who also met eligibility criteria and agreed to participate in the current survey. For research in which participants are intended to remain anonymous, Harris Poll uses tools and methods to ensure that there is no reasonable possibility of identifying an individual participant in the reports created (e.g., individual responses collected are combined to produce "aggregated" reports). Eligible patient participants

were US residents aged ≥18 years who self-selected a diagnosis of PD, MSA, or pure autonomic failure based on a diagnosis received from their treating physicians. Individuals also met ≥1 of the following criteria: (1) received a formal diagnosis of OH or nOH, (2) were informed by a health care provider that their symptoms are caused by low blood pressure or a sudden drop in blood pressure upon standing, or (3) experience the following upon sitting up, standing up, standing for long periods of time, or with a change in position: 2 or more listed OH/nOH symptoms at least every time, daily, weekly, monthly, or a few times a year and at least 1 of the following symptoms: dizziness or lightheadedness, feeling faint, or fainting. Because of the underlying neurologic diagnosis criteria, eligible patient responders were presumed to have "nOH" for the purposes of this study, even if they did not receive a formal diagnosis. Eligible caregiver participants cared for patients who met these criteria but were not necessarily linked to any patient responders (i.e., patient and caregiver responses to surveys were not paired in the analysis of survey results). The survey included questions regarding the frequency and impact of nOH symptoms, management, and communication with health care providers regarding symptoms (see Additional File 1 for the full list of survey questions). Descriptive statistics are reported. The study was performed in accordance with ethical standards (e.g., 1964 Helsinki Declaration and later amendments or the comparable). As an anonymous survey, the study was exempt from ethics approval based on Code of Federal Regulations Title 45, Part 46, Subpart A, Section 46.101b, Category 2 criteria.

Results

Respondents

Demographic data are provided in Table 1. A total of 363 patients (mean age ± standard deviation, 63.4 ± 12.4 years) and 128 caregivers responded to the survey. Among the caregivers, the mean ± standard deviation age of the patient cared for was 70.7 ± 14.8 years; 46% provided care to a spouse or partner. Most patients experienced long-term nOH symptoms, with 48% and 21% of patient respondents reporting living with symptoms for ≥5 and ≥ 10 years, respectively (mean ± standard deviation, 7.8 ± 10.0 years). Among caregivers, 59% and 38% reported that the patient cared for lived with symptoms for ≥5 and ≥ 10 years. PD was the most frequent underlying disorder, identified by 90% of patients and 88% of caregivers reported providing care to patients with PD. A formal diagnosis of OH or nOH was reported by 36% of patients and by 16% of caregivers. A longer duration of symptoms did not increase the proportion of patients with a formal diagnosis of OH or nOH; among patients with a symptom duration of ≥10 years compared with < 10 years, 35% (27/78) versus 36% (102/285) reported a formal diagnosis of one of these conditions.

Table 1 Baseline Characteristics of Survey Respondents

Characteristic	Patients (n = 363)	Caregivers (n = 128)	
		Self	Patient Being Cared for
Men	51%	37%	54%
Mean ± SD age, y	63.4 ± 12.4	56.2 ± 14.9	70.7 ± 14.8
White	90%	92%	NA
Neurologic diagnosis[a]			
Parkinson disease	90%	NA	88%
Multiple system atrophy	10%	NA	11%
Pure autonomic failure	4%	NA	3%
Mean ± SD years experiencing nOH symptoms	7.8 ± 10.0	NA	10.0 ± 9.9
Years living with nOH symptoms			
< 1	10%	NA	5%
1–4	42%	NA	37%
5–9	27%	NA	21%
≥ 10	21%	NA	38%
Formal diagnosis of nOH or OH	36%	NA	16%

NA not available, nOH neurogenic orthostatic hypotension, OH orthostatic hypotension
[a]Multiple responses could be selected; therefore, the sum of percentages is > 100%

Among all respondents, 49% of patients reported that they were in fair or poor health, with 72% of caregivers reporting that the patients they provided care for were in fair or poor health. Among the subgroup with a diagnosis of PD or MSA, 34% of patients (121/357) and 49% of caregivers (61/125) somewhat or strongly agreed that nOH symptoms appeared before patients developed motor symptoms. Among patients diagnosed with PD (n = 328), 44% somewhat or strongly agreed that their nOH symptoms were more troublesome than their motor symptoms. Findings from caregivers of patients with PD (n = 113) were similar (47%).

nOH symptom experience and impact
nOH symptoms
The most frequently reported symptoms of nOH were dizziness or lightheadedness, fatigue when standing, and difficulty walking; a substantial proportion of patients reported that dizziness or lightheadedness (37%), fatigue when standing (33%), and difficulty walking (32%) occurred every time or multiple times a day when they sit up, stand up, are standing for long periods of time, or have a change in position (Fig. 1). Other symptoms reported as occurring multiple times a day by > 10% of patients included blurry vision, pain running down neck

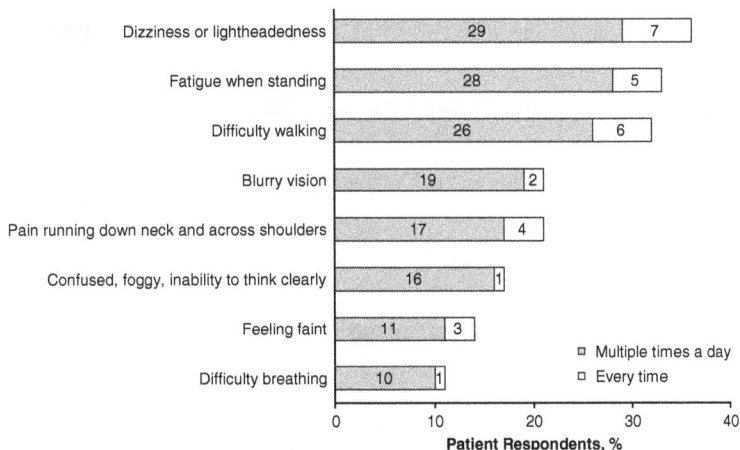

Fig. 1 Proportion of patient respondents reporting postural nOH symptoms.* nOH=neurogenic orthostatic hypotension. *Reported symptoms could be experienced upon sitting or standing up, when standing for long periods of time, or during a change in position

and across shoulders, cognitive difficulties, faintness, and difficulty breathing (Fig. 1).

No distinct pattern emerged regarding the frequency and severity of nOH symptoms throughout the day (Fig. 2). When asked about conditions that exacerbated their nOH symptoms, the majority of patients and caregivers (61% each) somewhat or strongly agreed that nOH symptoms worsened in hot and/or humid conditions. Exacerbation of nOH symptoms after meals was reported less frequently (27% of patients, 34% of caregivers). Falls due to nOH symptoms (at least 1 in the previous year) were reported by 57% of patients (mean, 5.1 falls) and 80% of caregivers (mean, 7.8 falls).

Functional impact of nOH symptoms

The majority of patients (87%) and caregivers (95%) reported that nOH symptoms had an overall negative impact on patients' ability to perform everyday activities;

this was categorized as severe or very severe by approximately one-fifth of patients and two-fifths of caregivers (Fig. 3). A substantial proportion of patients reported that nOH symptoms negatively impacted their quality of life (59%), robbed them of their independence (42%), or drastically changed their life (40%). In the caregiver cohort, 75% of respondents reported that nOH symptoms had a negative impact on the patient's quality of life, and approximately two-thirds reported that nOH symptoms had robbed patients of their independence (66%) or drastically changed their life (65%). The symptom burden of nOH did not appear to be affected by the duration of symptom experience. Similar proportions of patients with nOH symptoms for < 10 years and ≥ 10 years reported that symptoms had a negative impact on their quality of life (60% and 55%, respectively), caused a drastic change in their life (38% and 49%), or robbed them of their independence (41% and 47%).

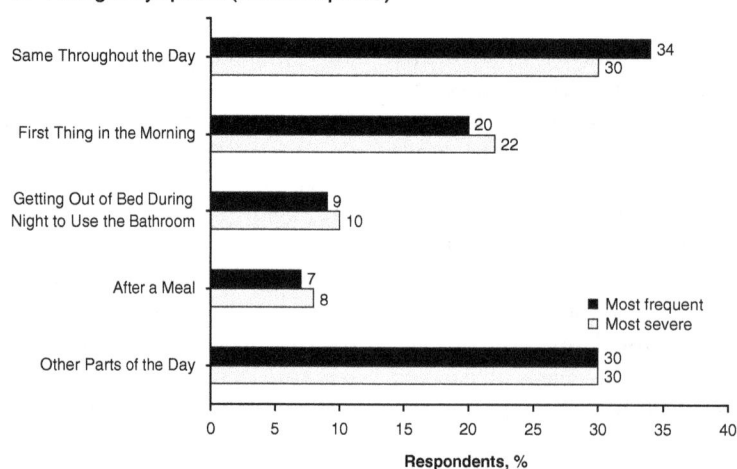
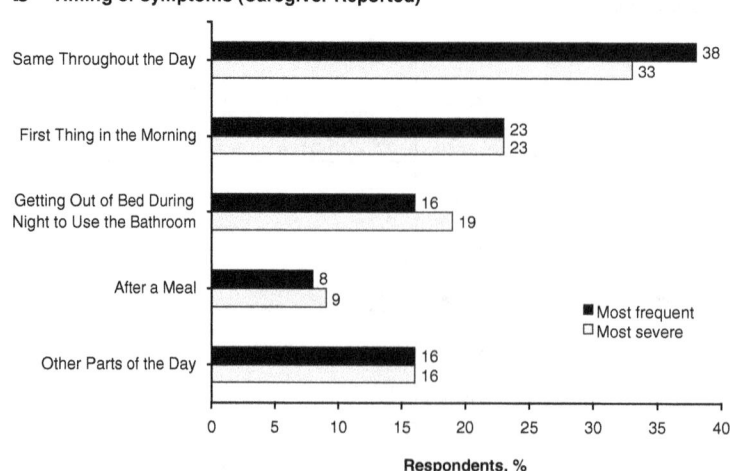

Fig. 2 Daily pattern of most frequent/severe nOH symptoms as reported by **a** patients and **b** caregivers.* nOH = neurogenic orthostatic hypotension. *Respondents in the patient and caregiver cohorts were not paired

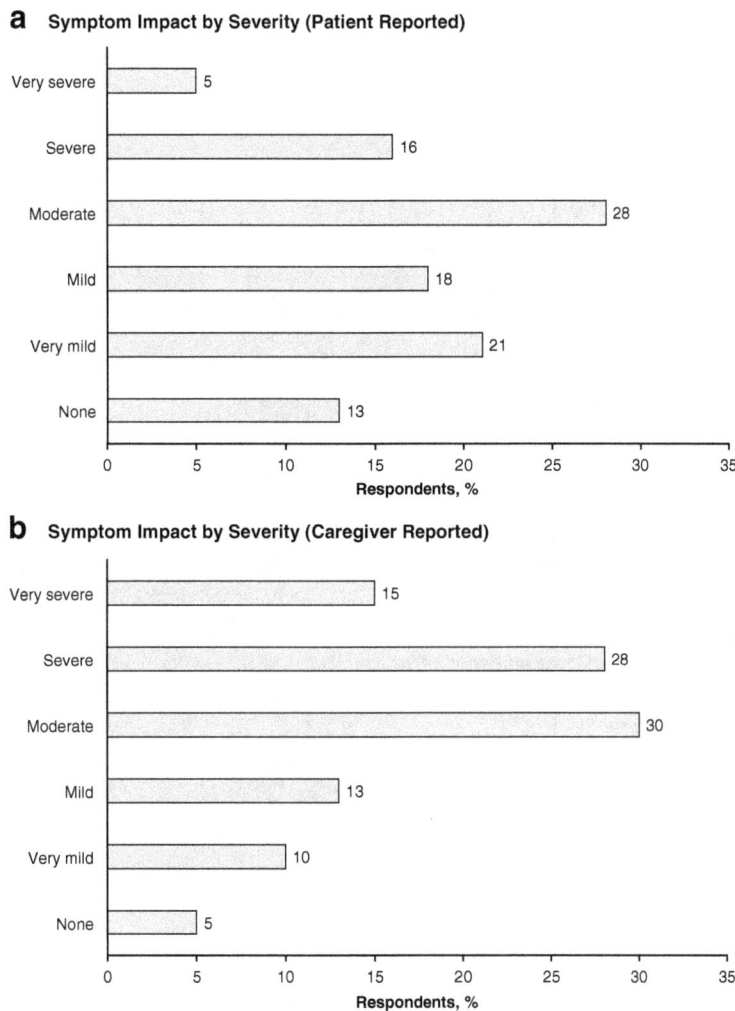

a   Symptom Impact by Severity (Patient Reported)

Severity	Respondents, %
Very severe	5
Severe	16
Moderate	28
Mild	18
Very mild	21
None	13

b   Symptom Impact by Severity (Caregiver Reported)

Severity	Respondents, %
Very severe	15
Severe	28
Moderate	30
Mild	13
Very mild	10
None	5

Fig. 3 nOH symptom impact on patient daily activities as reported by **a** patients and **b** caregivers.*,† nOH = neurogenic orthostatic hypotension. *Respondents in the patient and caregiver cohorts were not paired. †Percentages rounded to the nearest whole number

Activities that were reported as reduced or stopped because of symptoms of nOH by > 40% of patients were physical activity/exercise, housework, traveling, time spent out of the house to run errands or socialize, driving, hobbies, and entertaining at home (Fig. 4a). Caregivers reported that such activities were reduced or stopped in ≥59% of the patients they care for (Fig. 4b). More than half (56%) of patients and 85% of caregivers reported that patients needed assistance with day-to-day activities (e.g., walking, getting out of a chair) in the past month, and up to 53% of patients and 73% of caregivers reported that some daily activities were reduced or stopped because of nOH symptoms.

Half of patients (50%) somewhat or strongly agreed that nOH symptoms caused them anxiety or worry and somewhat or strongly agreed that the management of symptoms caused them to be depressed or discouraged; 39% somewhat or strongly agreed that they really struggled to

get their nOH symptoms under control. Despite the negative impact of nOH symptoms on functionality and quality of life, 60% of patients and 53% of caregivers somewhat or strongly agreed that patients often hide or minimize their nOH symptoms.

Patient/health care provider interactions and the path to diagnosis of nOH

Most patients (75%) and caregivers (77%) somewhat or strongly agreed that they were satisfied with the quality of communication with health care providers. The health care providers most commonly seen (i.e., reported by > 20% of patients or caregivers) for the management of underlying medical conditions manifesting with nOH were primary care providers, movement disorder specialists, general neurologists, and general cardiologists. A delay of 6 months or more between the time of symptom onset to discussion

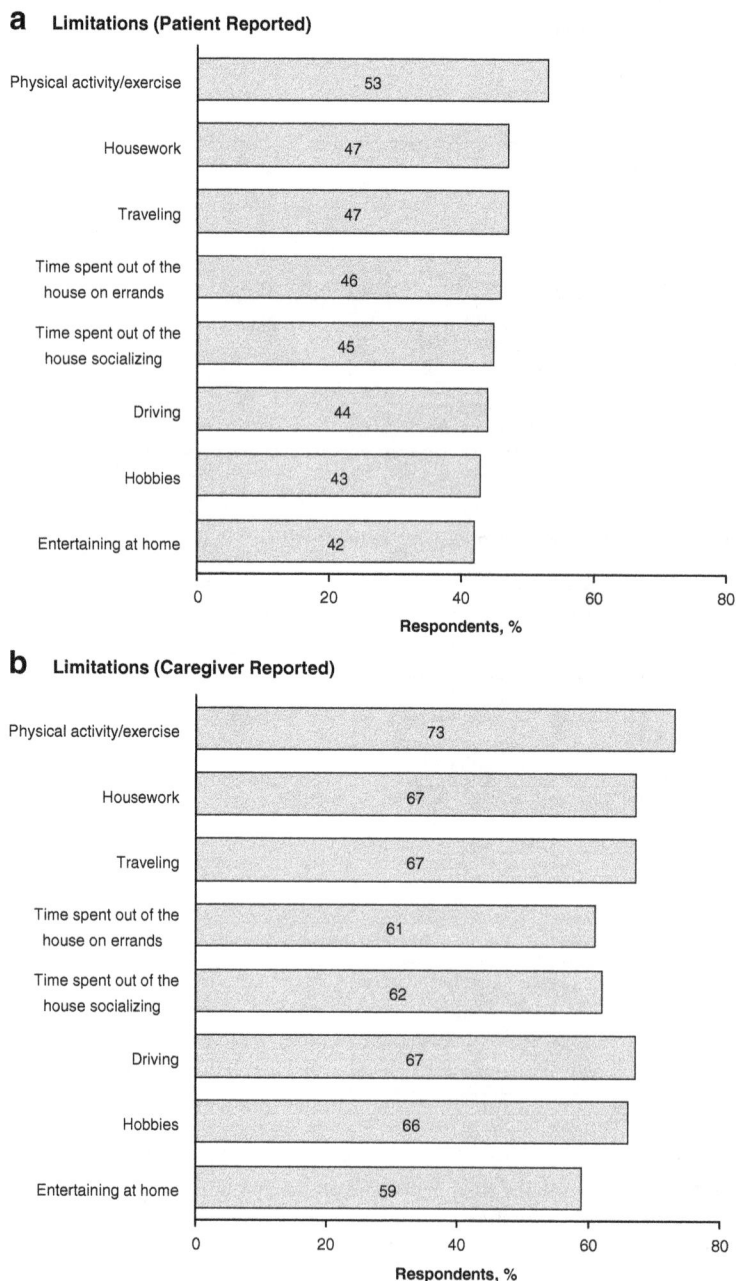

Fig. 4 nOH symptom-related limitations on patient daily activities as reported by **a** patients and **b** caregivers.* nOH = neurogenic orthostatic hypotension. *Percentages represent the proportion of respondents who reported the patient reduction or stopping of the activity. Respondents in the patient and caregiver cohorts were not paired

with a health care provider was reported by 33% of patients and 41% of caregivers. Patients and caregivers (55% each) somewhat or strongly agreed that patients did not initiate a discussion about their nOH symptoms with their health care provider unless the symptoms were severe, and 26% of patients and 39% of caregivers somewhat or strongly agreed that patients were uncomfortable talking with their health care provider about the impact of nOH symptoms.

Approximately one-fourth (26%) of patients and a third (33%) of caregivers somewhat or strongly agreed that patients had to mention their nOH symptoms repeatedly to their health care provider to draw attention to the problem. In the subgroup of 129 patients with a formal diagnosis of nOH or OH, 43% reported seeing 3 or more health care providers before being diagnosed with OH or nOH. Half (50%) of the patients who were formally diagnosed somewhat or strongly agreed that the path to diagnosis of nOH was very frustrating. However, 70% of the patients formally diagnosed with OH/nOH somewhat or strongly agreed that management of their symptoms improved after diagnosis. Only 20 caregiver responders cared for patients who had a formal diagnosis of OH/nOH, so a similar subgroup analysis was not performed.

Symptom management and treatments/interventions

Approximately half (53%) of patients and 62% of caregivers somewhat or strongly agreed that they received a solution from health care providers to better manage symptoms of nOH. Interventions recommended by health care providers were avoidance of quick positional changes, increased fluid intake, adjustment of PD medications, increased salt intake, use of compression garments, elevating the head of the bed, and avoiding hot environments. Caregivers reported the same interventions with similar frequency (Table 2). A third (34%) of patients and 45% of caregivers reported that a prescription for a medication to treat nOH symptoms was received; 25% of patients and 9% of caregivers reported that patients were not counseled to do anything to manage their nOH symptoms.

Discussion

The results of this patient and caregiver survey strongly support the premise that nOH symptoms have a substantial negative impact on patient function and quality of life. Data from both patients and caregivers suggest that nOH symptoms are associated with impaired mobility, such as difficulty with positional changes, increased frequency of falls, and decreased ability to maintain activities of daily life. Despite the high level of symptom burden and long-standing symptoms of nOH (e.g., 48% of patients with symptoms for ≥5 years), the majority of respondents did not report having a formal diagnosis of OH or nOH. Stratification of patients based on their duration of symptoms (< 10 years or ≥ 10 years) did not increase the likelihood of a formal diagnosis of OH or nOH. Further, there were minimal differences on the impact of nOH symptoms between these 2 subgroups of patients.

In this survey, the majorities of patients and caregivers did not report that nOH symptoms occurred more frequently or with greater severity first thing in the morning, after meals, or when getting out of bed during the night. Rather, more respondents indicated that nOH symptoms were more likely to occur or be more severe throughout the day. These results are contrary to the general clinical understanding that nOH symptoms are often worse in the morning and can be exacerbated after eating [13]. The lack of a distinct daily pattern for the frequency and severity of nOH symptoms emphasizes that symptoms do not always occur at a specific time or event (e.g., morning, after a meal) and is an important point of awareness for clinicians in the evaluation of patients for nOH.

This survey also revealed factors that may contribute to the relatively low rate of formal nOH diagnosis. The majority of patients reported hiding or minimizing their nOH symptoms. Further, patients indicated that they were uncomfortable discussing the impact of symptoms with health care providers and did not discuss the impact of their symptoms unless they were severe. Finally, some patients and caregivers reported that symptoms had to be discussed several times in order to draw them to the attention of the treating provider.

Reticence of patients to share symptoms with caregivers and health care providers has been observed with depression, pain, and other chronic conditions [14–16]. Patients may hide or minimize their nOH symptoms because they view symptoms as a sign of weakness or because they are embarrassed, in denial, do not want to be a "bother" to others, or other reasons [14–16]. Of note, among patients in the current survey with a diagnosis of nOH, many (70%) perceived that their symptoms had improved after

Table 2 Recommended Interventions for nOH by Health Care Providers

Intervention	Patients Reporting (n = 363)	Caregivers Reporting (n = 128)
Avoid quick positional changes	49%	48%
Increase fluid intake	47%	52%
Adjust PD medication	28%	43%
Increase salt intake	27%	20%
Wear compression stockings and/or abdominal binders	24%	27%
Elevate head of the bed	22%	28%
Avoid heated environments	16%	16%
Adjust or discontinue blood pressure or heart medications	15%	28%
Physical counter maneuvers (e.g., standing up and crossing legs, standing up and squeezing hands tightly)	12%	13%
No intervention recommended	25%	9%

nOH neurogenic orthostatic hypotension, *PD* Parkinson disease

receiving the diagnosis. However, a substantial proportion of patients were not counseled on how to manage nOH, were not prescribed medication for nOH symptoms, and felt they did not have adequate control of their nOH symptoms.

Inadequate management of nOH symptoms appears to be a cause of distress for many patients. Nonpharmaceutical treatment recommendations for nOH include ensuring adequate salt and fluid intake, avoiding rapid postural changes, adjusting medications, and sleeping with the head of the bed elevated [5, 17]. Patients and caregivers indicated that such nonpharmaceutical interventions were commonly recommended and frequently helpful. However, a substantial proportion of respondents indicated that they did not achieve symptomatic relief, and only a third of patients indicated that they received a prescription for a medication to treat symptoms of nOH. These results provide greater understanding of the disease burden of nOH. Previously, a negative impact of nOH symptoms was found in a single-center study of 141 inpatients with PD, in which 53% of patients reported that orthostatic dizziness had "a lot" or "very much" impact on daily life [11]. A 2-center study of patients with PD has suggested that both symptomatic ($n = 14$) and asymptomatic ($n = 23$) nOH were associated with worse measures of functionality and quality of life compared with patients with PD but without nOH ($n = 84$) [18]. Our study adds to the evidence by inclusion of data from a larger cohort of patients ($N = 363$) who experience nOH symptoms due to a variety of underlying conditions, including MSA and pure autonomic failure (however, most of the cohort reported a PD diagnosis). Further, to the best of our knowledge, our study is the first to investigate the impact of nOH from both the patient and caregiver perspective. nOH is one of the many manifestations of autonomic dysfunction, and patients may also have their quality of life affected by other symptoms, including gastrointestinal dysfunction (e.g., dysphagia, constipation), bladder dysfunction (e.g., urinary urgency, incontinence), sexual dysfunction (e.g., erectile dysfunction), cardiovascular dysfunction (e.g., hypertension, supine hypertension), and thermoregulation and sweating abnormalities (e.g., dyshidrosis) [19, 20].

Survey methodology has inherent limitations, such as selection bias and recall bias. Patient and caregiver responses were not paired; therefore, it is not possible to draw conclusions regarding consistency of responses between patients and their caregivers. Pairing each patient's response with their caregiver's response for each question should be considered in future studies. Many participants (64% of patients, 84% of caregivers) did not have a formal diagnosis of OH or nOH; therefore, the survey may underestimate the burden of symptoms of those formally diagnosed with OH or nOH.

Conclusions

The findings from this survey underscore a significant symptom burden associated with nOH. Many patients have a delay or lack of diagnosis of nOH, which creates diagnostic uncertainty and slows symptom management. As a consequence of this under-recognition of nOH, patients may face an increased risk of falls and associated morbidity [21, 22]. This study highlights the need for a more timely diagnosis of nOH. Improved patient/provider communication about symptoms of nOH may facilitate more timely and appropriate intervention for these patients. Overall, heightened awareness regarding nOH and its symptom burden should be an educational priority for patients, as well as for their caregivers and for health care providers.

Abbreviations
BP: blood pressure; MSA: multiple system atrophy; NA: not available; nOH: neurogenic orthostatic hypotension; OH: orthostatic hypotension; PD: Parkinson disease

Acknowledgments
The authors received editorial assistance from CHC Group (North Wales, PA), which was supported by Lundbeck.

Funding
The data reported were derived from a survey that was supported by Lundbeck. The sponsor participated in the design of this study, data analysis and interpretation, and in the preparation of the manuscript.

Authors' contributions
DOC, CHA, LAH, and CG participated in survey design and interpretation of data. Each author was involved in drafting, reviewing, and final approval of the manuscript for publication. All authors read and approved the final manuscript.

Competing interests
DOC receives grant support from the National Institutes of Health and the Michael J. Fox Foundation for Parkinson's Research; is a site investigator for clinical trials sponsored by Vaccinex, AbbVie, CHDI, and Auspex/Teva Neuroscience; and has received personal remuneration from Lundbeck, Teva Neuroscience, Acadia, and AbbVie for consulting, advisory board participation, and speaking honoraria. CHA has received research funding from the National Institutes of Health and the Michael J. Fox Foundation for Parkinson's Research and consulting fees from Acadia, Acorda, Adamas, Cynapsus, Jazz, Lundbeck, Minerva, Neurocrine, and Sunovion. LAH is an employee of Lundbeck Medical Affairs. CG has served on advisory boards for Lundbeck and Pfizer and on data safety monitoring boards for Janssen and Astellas, and has received grants from Grifols and Celgene.

Author details
[1]Department of Neurology, Vanderbilt University Medical Center, 1161 21st Avenue South A-0118, Nashville, TN 37232, USA. [2]Parkinson's Disease and Movement Disorders Center, Department of Neurology, Mayo Clinic College of Medicine, Mayo Clinic, 13400 East Shea Boulevard, Scottsdale, AZ 85259, USA. [3]Medical Affairs, Lundbeck, 6 Parkway North, Deerfield, IL 60015, USA. [4]Department of Neurology, Beth Israel Deaconess Medical Center, Harvard Medical School, 330 Brookline Avenue, Boston, MA 02215, USA.

References

1. Freeman R, Wieling W, Axelrod FB, Benditt DG, Benarroch E, Biaggioni I, et al. Consensus statement on the definition of orthostatic hypotension, neurally mediated syncope and the postural tachycardia syndrome. Clin Auton Res. 2011;21:69–72.

2. Ha AD, Brown CH, York MK, Jankovic J. The prevalence of symptomatic orthostatic hypotension in patients with Parkinson's disease and atypical parkinsonism. Parkinsonism Relat Disord. 2011;17:625–8.

3. Metzler M, Duerr S, Granata R, Krismer F, Robertson D, Wenning GK. Neurogenic orthostatic hypotension: pathophysiology, evaluation, and management. J Neurol. 2013;260:2212–9.

4. Senard JM, Rai S, Lapeyre-Mestre M, Brefel C, Rascol O, Rascol A, et al. Prevalence of orthostatic hypotension in Parkinson's disease. J Neurol Neurosurg Psychiatry. 1997;63:584–9.

5. Gibbons CH, Schmidt P, Biaggioni I, Frazier-Mills C, Freeman R, Isaacson S, et al. The recommendations of a consensus panel for the screening, diagnosis, and treatment of neurogenic orthostatic hypotension and associated supine hypertension. J Neurol. 2017;264:1567–82.

6. Goldstein DS, Sharabi Y. Neurogenic orthostatic hypotension: a pathophysiological approach. Circulation. 2009;119:139–46.

7. Shibao C, Lipsitz LA, Biaggioni I. ASH position paper: evaluation and treatment of orthostatic hypotension. J Clin Hypertens (Greenwich). 2013;15:147–53.

8. McDonald C, Pearce M, Kerr SR. Newton J. A prospective study of the association between orthostatic hypotension and falls: definition matters. Age Ageing. 2017;46:439–45.

9. Ooi WL, Hossain M, Lipsitz LA. The association between orthostatic hypotension and recurrent falls in nursing home residents. Am J Med. 2000;108:106–11.

10. Fereshtehnejad SM, Lokk J. Orthostatic hypotension in patients with Parkinson's disease and atypical parkinsonism. Parkinsons Dis. 2014;2014: 475854.

11. Magerkurth C, Schnitzer R, Braune S. Symptoms of autonomic failure in Parkinson's disease: prevalence and impact on daily life. Clin Auton Res. 2005;15:76–82.

12. McDonell KE, Shibao CA, Claassen DO. Clinical relevance of orthostatic hypotension in neurodegenerative disease. Curr Neurol Neurosci Rep. 2015;15:78.

13. Freeman R. Clinical practice. Neurogenic orthostatic hypotension. N Engl J Med. 2008;358:615–24.

14. Cagle J, Bunting M. Patient reluctance to discuss pain: understanding stoicism, stigma, and other contributing factors. J Soc Work End Life Palliat Care. 2017;13:27–43.

15. Sawada N, Uchida H, Watanabe K, Kikuchi T, Suzuki T, Kashima H, et al. How successful are physicians in eliciting the truth from their patients? A large-scale internet survey from patients' perspectives. J Clin Psychiatry. 2012;73: 311–7.

16. Clarke LH, Bennett E. "you learn to live with all the you": gender and the experience of multiple chronic conditions in later life. Ageing Soc. 2013;33: 342–60.

17. Isaacson SH, Skettini J. Neurogenic orthostatic hypotension in Parkinson's disease: evaluation, management, and emerging role of droxidopa. Vasc Health Risk Manag. 2014;10:169–76.

18. Merola A, Romagnolo A, Rosso M, Lopez-Castellanos JR, Wissel BD, Larkin S, et al. Orthostatic hypotension in Parkinson's disease: does it matter if asymptomatic? Parkinsonism Relat Disord. 2016;33:65–71.

19. Palma JA, Kaufmann H. Treatment of autonomic dysfunction in Parkinson disease and other synucleinopathies. Mov Disord. 2018;33:372–90.

20. Mathias C. Autonomic diseases: clinical features and laboratory evaluation. J Neurol Neurosurg Psychiatry. 2003;74:iii31–41.

21. Craig GM. Clinical presentation of orthostatic hypotension in the elderly. Postgrad Med J. 1994;70:638–42.

22. Shaw BH, Claydon VE. The relationship between orthostatic hypotension and falling in older adults. Clin Auton Res. 2014;24:3–13.

Targeting the Notch1 oncogene by miR-139-5p inhibits glioma metastasis and epithelial-mesenchymal transition (EMT)

Jianlong Li[1,2†], Qingbin Li[1,4,5†], Lin Lin[1,4,5], Rui Wang[3], Lingchao Chen[6], Wenzhong Du[7], Chuanlu Jiang[1,4,5*] and Ruiyan Li[1,4,5*]

Abstract

Background: Glioma metastasis, invasion, epithelial-mesenchymal transition (EMT) and chemoresistance indicate poor prognosis. Accumulating evidence reveals that Notch1 is an important factor in tumour progression. However, the role of Notch1 in glioma EMT and associated microRNAs (miRNAs) with the Notch pathway remain controversial.

Methods: Utilizing cBioPortal database to examine the gene signature of NOTCH1 (encoding Notch1), CDH2 (encoding N-cadherin) and SNAI1 (encoding Snail-1) in disease-free survival (DFS) and overall survival (OS). We analyzed the Notch1 expression from Oncomine. We used Western blot (WB), immunohistochemistry (IHC) and immunofluorescence to determine protein levels. Transcription was evaluated by quantitative real-time (qRT)-PCR. siRNA and lentivirus were used to knock down Notch1 and overexpress miR-139-5p, respectively. The migration and invasion of glioma cells were assessed by wound healing and transwell assays. Luciferase reporter assays were utilized to verify the relationship between Notch1 and miR-139-5p. A U87-implanted intracranial model was used to study the effect of miR-139-5p on tumour growth and Notch1 suppression efficacy or EMT reversion.

Results: It revealed the association of NOTCH1, CDH2, SNAI1 genomic alterations with decreases in DFS and OS. Notch1 was upregulated in classical and proneural subtypes of GBM, and associated with tumour grade. Notch1 inhibition suppressed the biological behaviours of metastasis, invasion and EMT. Notch1 was identified as a novel direct target of miR-139-5p. MiR-139-5p overexpression partially phenocopied Notch1 siRNA, whereas the forced expression of Notch1 reversed the effects of miR-139-5p on the invasion of glioma. Moreover, intracranial tumourigenicity and EMT behaviours were reduced by the introduction of miR-139-5p and partially mediated by the decreased Notch1 expression.

Conclusions: miR-139-5p was identified as a tumour suppressor by negatively targeting Notch1, and this work suggests a possible molecular mechanism of the miR-139/Notch1/EMT axis for glioma treatment.

Keywords: miR-139-5p, Notch1, EMT, Glioma

Background

Glioma is the most common primary malignant tumour of the central nervous system in adults [1, 2]. The high metastasis and invasiveness of glioma induce a high incidence of recurrence, which means a worse prognosis [3]. Epithelial-mesenchymal transition (EMT) includes molecular changes, decreased cell-cell junction and adhesion, and increased cell motility. EMT can be determined by the loss of epithelial markers (E-cadherin) along with the upregulation of mesenchymal markers (N-cadherin, Fibronectin and Vimentin) [4].

Accumulating evidence shows that Notch1 plays an important role in tumour progress. The activation of Notch signalling by tenascin-C promotes the growth of human brain tumour-initiating cells [5]. Notch1 activation is a poor prognostic factor in patients with gastric cancer [6]. Recently, β-carotene has been reported to

* Correspondence: jcl6688@163.com; ruiyanli@yeah.net
†Jianlong Li and Qingbin Li contributed equally to this work.
[1]Department of Neurosurgery, The Second Affiliated Hospital of Harbin Medical University, 246 Xuefu Road, Nangang, 150086 Harbin, People's Republic of China
Full list of author information is available at the end of the article

inhibit EMT though Notch pathway [7]. NOTCH signaling is a primary inducer of EMT in a number of epithelial cancers, including cancer of the lung, breast and pancreas [8]. D Maciaczyk et al. recently demonstrate that blocking Notch-pathway member CBF1 inhibits EMT-activator ZEB1 in glioma cells [9]. However, little is known about the Notch1 interaction with EMT in glioma. Also, the molecular mechanisms remain elusive.

MicroRNAs (miRNAs) are non-coding RNA molecules comprising 18~ 22 nucleotides [10]. They regulate the expression of genes by directly targeting the 3′-untranslated regions (3′-UTR) of corresponding messenger RNAs (mRNAs) [11]. miRNAs are involved in a variety of biological behaviours, including suppressing or promoting tumours. Among these, miR-139 inhibits the growth and metastasis of several cancers including myeloid leukaemia [12], laryngeal squamous carcinoma [13] and liver cancer through targeting, for example, c-Fos and CXCR4 [13, 14]. In particular, miR-139-5p suppresses cancer cell migration by targeting ZEB1 and ZEB2 in glioma [15]. Our previous study confirmed that miR-139 was downregulated in clinical gliomas and glioma cell lines, and miR-139 inhibits Mcl-1 expression and potentiates TMZ-induced apoptosis in glioma [16]. Few reports could be assessed until now, however, regarding the regulation of miR-139 on EMT in glioma, especially though Notch1.

In this study, we attempted to investigate the expression and functions of Notch1 in gliomas and its relationship with miR-139-5p. For the first time, we showed that miR-139-5p reverses the Notch1-mediated EMT of glioma. This suggests an alternative for multiple treatments of glioma by regulating the miR-139-5p/Notch1/EMT pathway.

Methods

Patients and specimens

Twenty-nine human glioma tissues and four brain tissues were collected from patients who underwent surgical resection between January 2016 and March 2017 at the Second Affiliated Hospital of Harbin Medical University (HMU). Informed consent was obtained from all patients before the application of their tissue samples. This study complied with the regulations of Declaration of Helsinki and was approved by the medical ethics committee of HMU. All samples were graded histologically by clinical pathologists according to WHO guidelines, and they included 5 grade I tumours, 9 grade II tumours, 5 grade III tumours, and 10 grade IV tumours (Table 1). In addition, 4 normal adult brain tissue specimens were collected from patients who underwent severe traumatic brain injury and required surgical intervention (with informed consent).

Cell culture

LN229, U87, T98G and U251 glioma cell lines (human) were purchased from the Chinese Academy of Sciences cell bank. Oligodendroglia (Olig) was a gift from Fengmin Zhang, who is a professor of Harbin Medical University. These cells were cultured in a 5% CO_2, 37 °C incubator in Dulbecco's Modified Eagle's Medium (DMEM, Corning, USA) supplemented with 10% foetal bovine serum (FBS, Biological Industries, Israel).

MicroRNAs, siRNA and plasmid transfection

MiR-139-5p mimic was purified by high-performance liquid chromatography (GenePharma, Shanghai, China). Notch1 siRNA was composed and purchased from Invitrogen (USA) [17], and the sequences are listed in Additional file 1. The plasmid of full-length Notch1 without the corresponding 3′-UTR, pEGFP-N-Notch1 (GeneChem, Shanghai, China), was amplified and cloned into the GV230 (GeneChem, Shanghai, China). The plasmid along with miR-139-5p mimics or scramble were transfected into glioma cells with Lipofectamine 2000 (Invitrogen, USA) according to the manufacturer's instructions.

Transfected cells were incubated for another 24–72 h at 37 °C with 5% CO_2 atmosphere. Afterwards, cells were harvested for RNA and protein analysis.

In silico analysis and establishing of a three-gene genomic signature

To investigate the potential miRNAs that may regulate Notch1 mRNA, we utilized four commonly used miRNA databases, including miRanda algorithm (http://34.236.212.39/microrna/home.do), miRwalk (http://zmf.umm.uni-heidelberg.de/apps/zmf/mirwalk2/), Pictar (http://www.pictar.org/), and TargetScan (http://www.targetscan.org/vert_71/).

The TCGA data set within the cBioPortal database [18, 19] (http://www.cbioportal.org/index.do) was extracted. The Glioblastoma Multiforme (GBM) cohort (TCGA, Provisional, $n = 577$), a merged cohort (TCGA, Cell 2016, $n = 1084$) of Brain Lower Grade Glioma (LGG) and GBM, the LGG cohort (TCGA, Provisional, $n = 513$) were utilized. NOTCH1 (encoding Notch1), CDH2 (encoding N-cadherin) and SNAI1 (encoding Snail-1) three-gene signature was then examined on independent cohorts above for effects on disease-free survival (DFS) and overall survival (OS).

Notch1 mRNA expression from Oncomine (https://www.oncomine.org/resource/login.html#) and the prognostic meaning of miR-139-5p in glioma from OncoLnc (http://www.oncolnc.org/) was extracted.

Table 1 Clinicopathologic parameters of 33 samples from HMU

No.	Age range	Pathology (WHO)	No.	Age range	Pathology (WHO)
01	60–69	Brain Tissue	17	20–29	Pleomorphic Xanthoastrocytoma II
02	50–59	Brain Tissue	18	30–39	Diffuse Astrocytoma II
03	70–79	Brain Tissue	19	40–49	Anaplastic Oligoastrocytoma III
04	50–59	Brain Tissue	20	20–29	Anaplastic Astrocytoma III
05	60–69	Astrocytoma I	21	40–49	Anaplastic Oligoastrocytoma III
06	30–39	Astrocytoma I	22	50–59	Anaplastic Astrocytoma III
07	30–39	Astrocytoma I	23	50–59	Anaplastic Astrocytoma III
08	60–69	Astrocytoma I	24	20–29	Glioblastoma IV
09	40–49	Astrocytoma I	25	50–59	Glioblastoma IV
10	70–79	Oligoastrocytoma II	26	40–49	Glioblastoma IV
11	30–39	Oligoastrocytoma II	27	50–59	Glioblastoma IV
12	40–49	Astrocytoma II	28	40–49	Glioblastoma IV
13	40–49	Diffuse Astrocytoma II	29	30–39	Glioblastoma IV
14	30–39	Diffuse Astrocytoma II	30	50–59	Glioblastoma IV
15	60–69	Diffuse Astrocytoma II	31	70–79	Glioblastoma IV
16	40–49	Oligodendroglioma II	32	60–69	Glioblastoma IV
33	40–49	Glioblastoma IV			

Abbreviation: *WHO* World Health Organization, *HMU* Harbin Medical University

RNA isolation and quantitative real-time (qRT-PCR) assays
Total RNA was picked up using Trizol Reagent (Invitrogen, USA) according to the manufacturer's instructions. Total cDNA was reversely transcribed from 1 μg of total RNA (Perfect Real Time, Takara, Japan). Two-step qRT-PCR was performed for quantifying gene expression. We used a FastStart Universal SYBR Green Master (ROX) in the Roche LightCycler^R Real-Time System. The expression levels were normalized to glyceraldehyde-3-phosphate dehydrogenase (GAPDH) or U6. The PCR conditions started at 95 °C for 15 s, then annealed and extended at 60 °C for 60 s. It is going on for 40 cycles followed by a melting curve analysis. The data was analysed by $2^{-\Delta\Delta Ct}$ method. All experiments were performed in triplicate. The primers used are shown in Additional file 2.

Western blotting assay
Cell lysates were harvested. Total protein of equivalent amounts were separated by 10% SDS polyacrylamide gel electrophoresis (SDS-PAGE). After that, they were transferred to polyvinylidene difluoride (PVDF) membranes. Block the membranes with 5% fat-free milk and 0.1% Tween-20 in tris-buffered saline with Tween (TBST) for 1.5 h. Next, the membranes were incubated with diluted anti-Notch1 (Abcam), E-cadherin (CST), N-cadherin (CST), Vimentin (Abcam), Fibronectin (Abcam), Snail-1 (Wanleibio), Shh (CST) and anti-GAPDH (Wanleibio) primary antibodies. Anti-rabbit or anti-mouse secondary antibodies (ZSGB-BIO), which were horseradish

peroxidase-conjugated, were used and detected by the ECL system (Fujifilm Las-4000).

Luciferase reporter assay
GV272-Notch1–3′-UTR (Genechem), a wild-type luciferase reporter plasmid was created. It contain a putative miR-139-5p binding sites as previously reported [20]. Using Lipofectamine 2000 reagent (Invitrogen) to transfect these constructs into U87 or LN229 cells, with or without miR-139-5p mimics according to the manufacturer's protocol. miRNA mimics and firefly luciferase plasmid were co-transfected into cells. For normalization, they were co-transfected with CV045 *Renilla* luciferase plasmid (Genechem, Shanghai, China). Forty hours later, we used Dual-Glo luciferase assay system (E2920, Promega, USA) to measure the luciferase activity. The ratio of Firefly Luciferase activity to that of *Renilla* was defined as normalized luciferase activity.

Wound healing assay and transwell assay
Cells were plated in 6-well plates. miR-139-5p or Notch1 siRNA were transfected into cells when confluency. A 200-μl sterile pipette tip was used to create scratches. Wash cells twice with PBS and then supply them with DMEM without FBS. Capture photographs at 0 h and after 24–36 h using an Axiovert 200 microscope (Carl Zeiss) and the data was analysed using Image pro-plus software.

Transwell membranes was coated with Matrigel (BD Biosciences, San Jose, CA). About 5×10^4 cells/well were plated in the upper chamber. These cells were treated with miRNAs or Notch1 siRNA. The medium in upper chamber was serum-free. The medium in the lower chamber was 10% FBS. After 24 h, the cells in the top well was removed. The bottom cells were fixed with 95% ethanol, stained with 0.1% crystal violet. Take photographes in three independent 10× fields for each well. Three independent experiments were repeated.

Immunohistochemistry and immunofluorescence assay

Immunohistochemistry (IHC) and immunofluorescence assays were performed as previously described [21]. IHC scores were assessed using a semiquantitative grading system [22]. The appropriate antibodies against Notch1 (Abcam), E-cadherin (CST), N-cadherin (CST), Fibronectin (Abcam) and Vimentin (Abcam) were used. Immunofluorescence assays were visualized using Goat anti-Rabbit Alexa Fluor® 594-conjugated (ZSGB-BIO) or Goat anti-Mouse Fluorescein–conjugated (ZSGB-BIO) antibodies. Cell nuclei were counterstained using Hoechst 33258 (Thermo Fisher Scientific). Representative images were captured, and they were analysed by Olympus FV1000 Digital laser scanning microscopy.

Xenograft assay

U87 cells that were co-transducted with miR-139-5p lentivirus/scramble and luciferase lentivirus were injected intracranially into 5-week–old BALB/c-nude mice (Beijing Vital River Laboratory Animal Technology Co., Ltd.) as described earlier [23, 24]. Methods of animal care-taking and feeding were carried out according to the instructions of Beijing Vital River Laboratory Animal Technology (http://www.vitalriver.com/welfare.aspx). Exactly, they were cultured in SPF-class barrier system feeding conditions. The feed was disinfected with 121 degrees, 15 min, 1 kg pressure sterilization. Drinking water was filtered by multiple layers. Each group had 5 mice. After 20 days, the mice were sacrificed exposing to carbon dioxide. Continue to input carbon dioxide at a concentration of 100% for 2 min until the mouse stops breathing and then turns off the switch on the carbon dioxide bottle. Tumours were measured by fluorescent images of whole mice using an IVIS Lumina Imaging System (Xenogen). Portions of the tumour tissues were used to measure the Notch1 and EMT markers by IHC. Cryosections (4 mm) were used for IHC [1, 22]. These procedures were performed with approval by the Harbin Medical University Institutional Animal Care and Use Committee.

Statistical analysis

SPSS version 13.0 software (Chicago, IL, USA) was used to carried out all statistical analyses. Data were exhibited as means ± SD. Differences between the means of the treatment and control groups were analyzed using student's t-test. Significance among three or more groups was analyzed by a one-way analysis of variance (ANOVA). Categorical variables were compared using the χ^2-test and Fisher's exact test. Data at $p < 0.05$ level were considered statistically significant. The survival curves were analysed using the log-rank test employing GraphPad Prism software.

Results

The three-gene signature correlated with decreases in DFS and OS in glioma

We first explored the alteration frequency of NOTCH1 in different type of brain tumors ($n = 1300$) (cBioPortal) [18, 19] and found the major type of genomic alterations in glioma was mutation or amplication (Fig. 1a and b). Then, we examined NOTCH1, CDH2 and SNAI1 three-gene signature in the Glioblastoma Multiforme (GBM) cohort (TCGA, Provisional, $n = 577$) (Fig. 1c) and demonstrated its association with decreases in DFS ($P < 0.05$) (Fig. 1d). This association was also revealed in a merged cohort (TCGA, Cell 2016, $n = 1084$) of Brain Lower Grade Glioma (LGG) and GBM ($P < 0.001$) (Fig. 1e and f). However, the association was not significant in the LGG cohort (TCGA, Provisional, $n = 513$) ($p = 0.588$) (Fig. 1g).

Notch1 was upregulated in glioma tissues and cell lines and associated with tumour grade

We first extracted the data from Oncomine. From Bredel Brain and Sun Brain data sets, we analyzed Notch1 mRNA expression. The result indicated that GBM samples overexpressed more Notch1 (Fig. 2a). Further, we analyzed the mRNA microarray data from TCGA. It suggested that Notch1 were significantly upregulated in classical and proneural subtypes of GBM (Fig. 2b). Notch1 expression was measured using an immunohistochemical analysis in 29 different grades of glioma tissues and 4 normal brain tissues. In Grade III-IV tissues, Notch1 was higher than that in low grade gliomas (WHO II) or normal brain tissues ($P < 0.05$) (Fig. 2c). Furthermore, the expression patterns of Notch1 were confirmed by Western blotting assay in 4 glioma cell lines (LN229, U87, T98G and U251). Glioma cells, especially U87 and LN229 cells, expressed more Notch1 compared with Olig (Fig. 2d). In addition, we assessed the correlation between Notch1 expression and clinicopathologic characteristics in 33 patients and found that Notch1 expression was positively correlated with tumour grade and negatively correlated with Karnofsky Performance status (KPS) score ($P < 0.05$, Table 2).

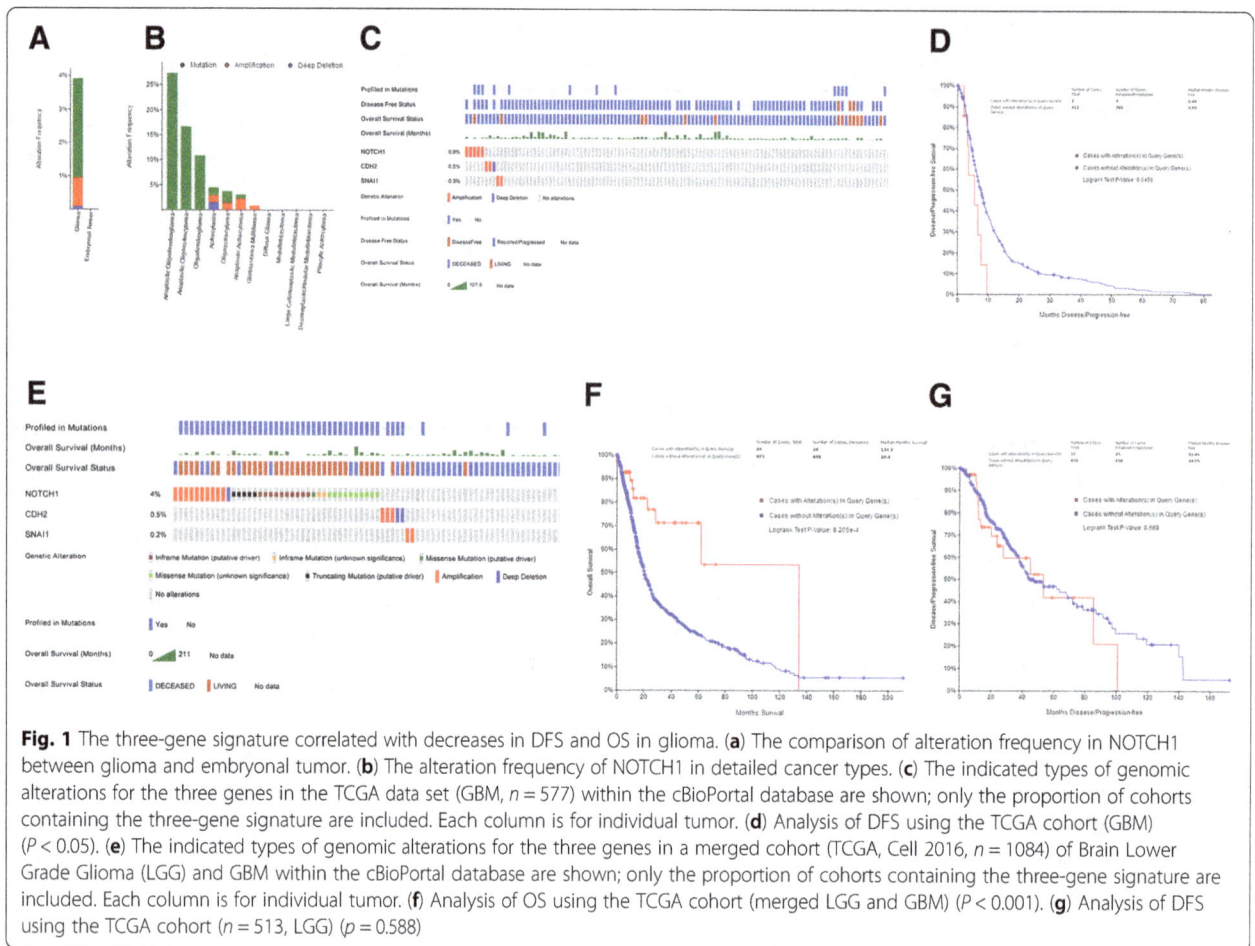

Fig. 1 The three-gene signature correlated with decreases in DFS and OS in glioma. (**a**) The comparison of alteration frequency in NOTCH1 between glioma and embryonal tumor. (**b**) The alteration frequency of NOTCH1 in detailed cancer types. (**c**) The indicated types of genomic alterations for the three genes in the TCGA data set (GBM, $n = 577$) within the cBioPortal database are shown; only the proportion of cohorts containing the three-gene signature are included. Each column is for individual tumor. (**d**) Analysis of DFS using the TCGA cohort (GBM) ($P < 0.05$). (**e**) The indicated types of genomic alterations for the three genes in a merged cohort (TCGA, Cell 2016, $n = 1084$) of Brain Lower Grade Glioma (LGG) and GBM within the cBioPortal database are shown; only the proportion of cohorts containing the three-gene signature are included. Each column is for individual tumor. (**f**) Analysis of OS using the TCGA cohort (merged LGG and GBM) ($P < 0.001$). (**g**) Analysis of DFS using the TCGA cohort ($n = 513$, LGG) ($p = 0.588$)

Notch1 knockdown suppressed metastasis and invasion capability of glioma cells

Given that Notch1 is highly expressed in glioma and a crucial regulator of epithelial-mesenchymal-transition (EMT), we subsequently investigated its biological importance on the tumourigenic property of glioma cells, including metastasis and invasion. We knocked down Notch1 in LN229 and U87 cells (Fig. 3a and b, Fig. 6c and d) and then performed a wound-healing assay and transwell assay to test invasive characteristics. The results showed that siNotch1 attenuated cell migration (Fig. 3c and e for LN229, Fig. 3d and f for U87) and

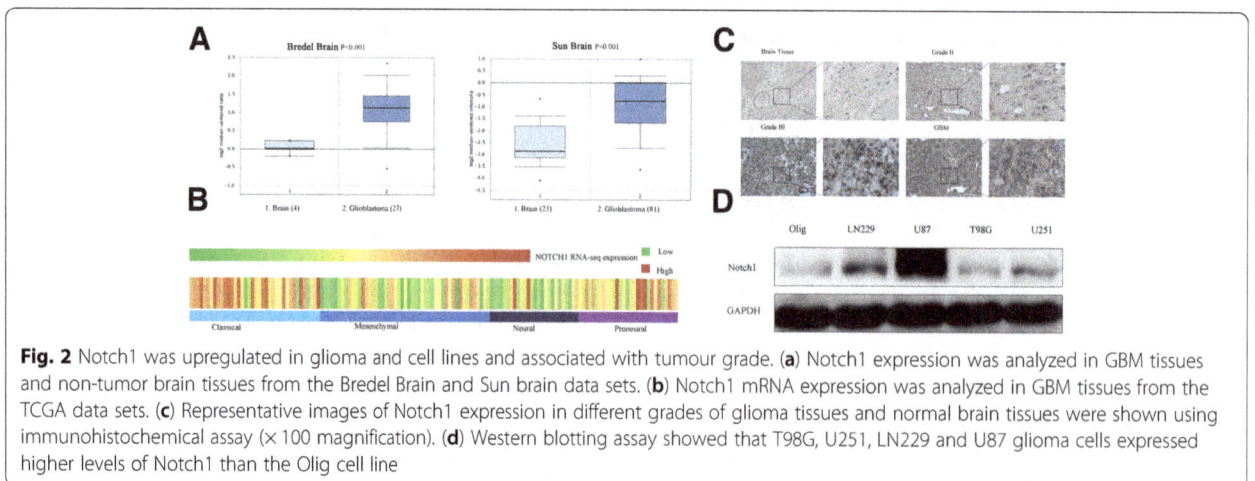

Fig. 2 Notch1 was upregulated in glioma and cell lines and associated with tumour grade. (**a**) Notch1 expression was analyzed in GBM tissues and non-tumor brain tissues from the Bredel Brain and Sun brain data sets. (**b**) Notch1 mRNA expression was analyzed in GBM tissues from the TCGA data sets. (**c**) Representative images of Notch1 expression in different grades of glioma tissues and normal brain tissues were shown using immunohistochemical assay (× 100 magnification). (**d**) Western blotting assay showed that T98G, U251, LN229 and U87 glioma cells expressed higher levels of Notch1 than the Olig cell line

Table 2 Notch1 expression and clinicopathologic characteristics of 33 cases

Variable	Notch1 low expression	Notch1 high expression	P value
Gender			0.711
Male	6	5	
Female	12	10	
Age (mean/Y)	48.7	48.3	0.391
< 50	11	7	
≥ 50	6	9	
KPS			0.023*
<80	3	10	
≥ 80	14	6	
Grade			0.002*
WHO <II	13	5	
WHO III-IV	2	13	

Abbreviation: *KPS* Karnofsky Performance Status, *WHO* World Health Organization, χ2-test or the Fisher exact test; *statistically significant ($P < 0.05$)

decreased the number of invasive glioma cells compared with the scramble siRNAs (Fig. 3g and i for LN229, Fig. 3h and j for U87).

Notch1 was a direct target of miR-139-5p

To investigate whether microRNAs were involved in regulating Notch1, we used the Targetscan, miRanda, Pictar and miRwalk databases and identified potential miR-NAs, including miR-139-5p (Fig. 4a), that target Notch1 3′-UTR. Accordingly, we transfected miR-139-5p mimics into glioma cells and evaluated the Notch1 expression level. Transfection efficiency was evaluated using qRT-PCR (Additional file 3). qRT-PCR and Western blotting showed that miR-139-5p induced an obvious decline in Notch1 expression (Fig. 4b and c). Further, we sought to confirm whether Notch1 was a direct target of miR-139-5p. GV272-Notch1–3′-UTR, luciferase reporter plasmid was constructed. It contained a putative miR-139-5p binding site (Fig. 4d). We transfected these plasmids into glioma cells with miRNAs. The data showed that luciferase activity decreased in the group of WT-Notch1–3′-UTR and miR-139-5p mimics. No significant change in any other group (Fig. 4e and f). These data suggest that miR-139-5p binds to the 3′-UTR of Notch1 directly.

Overexpressed miR-139-5p inhibited glioma metastasis, invasion and EMT

After confirming the relationship between Notch1 and miR-139-5p, we intended to test the effect of miR-139-5p on invasive activity. The wound-healing assay and transwell assay showed that miR-139-5p attenuated cell migration (Fig. 5a and b) and decreased the number of invasive

glioma cells compared with the scramble miRNAs (Fig. 5c and d). Moreover, miR-139-5p downregulated the mesenchymal markers (N-cadherin, vimentin and fibronectin) but upregulated the epithelial marker (E-cadherin) at both the mRNA and protein levels (Fig. 5e, f, g, h and i), which indicated an EMT-suppressive role of miR-139-5p.

Mir-139-5p reversed EMT via down-regulating the expression of Notch1

To further investigate the mechanism of miR-139-5p on glioma suppression, we sought to determine whether the anti-EMT effects of miR-139-5p are mediated by Notch1. To address this, we treated U87 and LN229 with Notch1 siRNA followed by a rescue experiment. The qRT-PCR and Western blotting assay confirmed specific knockdown of Notch1 by siRNA (Fig. 6a-d). Notch1 siRNA dramatically decreased the mesenchymal markers (N-cadherin, vimentin and fibronectin) while increasing the epithelial marker E-cadherin (Fig. 6a-d). Snail-1 is a zinc finger transcription factor that can repress E-cadherin transcription [25, 26]. Sonic hedgehog (Shh) is one of the stem cell-associated protein [27]. The results also showed Notch1 siRNA significantly decreased the expression of Snail-1 and Shh (Fig. 6c and d). In addition, in the treatment with full-length Notch1 without the corresponding 3′-UTR and followed by miR-139-5p mimics for 48 h, we found that miR-139-5p partially inhibits forced Notch1 expression in glioma cells (Fig. 6e and f). Furthermore, the effects of Notch1 on EMT markers after overexpression of miR-139-5p were also examined. The result showed forced expression of Notch1 reversed the effects of miR-139-5p on EMT markers (Fig. 6e and f). Accordingly, the upregulation of Notch1 significantly rescued the glioma invasion behaviour (Fig. 6g and h). Taken together, these data indicated that Notch1 was a mediator of the EMT-suppressive role of miR-139-5p.

MiR-139-5p inhibited glioma xenograft growth, metastasis and EMT in vivo and prolonged survival

To evaluate the antiglioma effect of miR-139-5p in vivo, a U87 xenograft model was used. We found that miR-139-5p-treated cells significantly reduced tumour size ($P < 0.05$, Fig. 7a and b). The Kaplan-Meier curve analysis showed a marked longer survival period of the miR-139-5p-treated group compared with the scramble group ($P < 0.05$, Fig. 7c). In the meantime, miR-139-5p decreased the expression of Notch1 as well as mesenchymal markers (N-cadherin, vimentin, fibronectin) while increasing E-cadherin (Fig. 7d).

Discussion

Glioblastoma is characterized by a high capacity to proliferate and invade. Gliomas that metastasize often

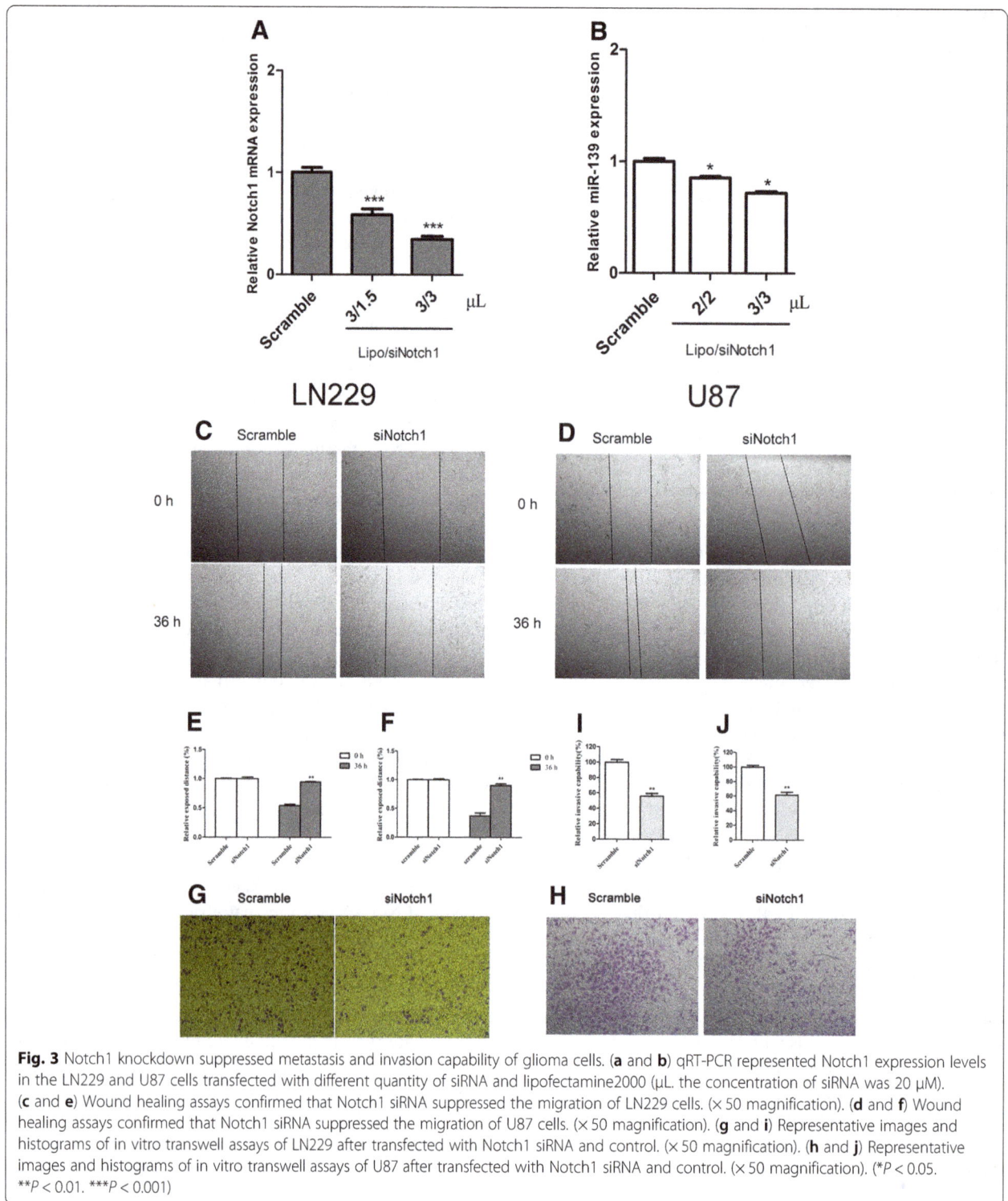

Fig. 3 Notch1 knockdown suppressed metastasis and invasion capability of glioma cells. (**a** and **b**) qRT-PCR represented Notch1 expression levels in the LN229 and U87 cells transfected with different quantity of siRNA and lipofectamine2000 (μL. the concentration of siRNA was 20 μM). (**c** and **e**) Wound healing assays confirmed that Notch1 siRNA suppressed the migration of LN229 cells. (× 50 magnification). (**d** and **f**) Wound healing assays confirmed that Notch1 siRNA suppressed the migration of U87 cells. (× 50 magnification). (**g** and **i**) Representative images and histograms of in vitro transwell assays of LN229 after transfected with Notch1 siRNA and control. (× 50 magnification). (**h** and **j**) Representative images and histograms of in vitro transwell assays of U87 after transfected with Notch1 siRNA and control. (× 50 magnification). (*P < 0.05. **P < 0.01. ***P < 0.001)

have poor prognosis [28, 29]. The search for effective drugs that can suppress glioma metastasis has been a main topic of clinician research. The Notch signalling pathway plays an important role in cell fate determination during normal development [30]. Notch1 has tumour-suppressing and promoting functions in human prostate cancer [31] or in different tumours [5, 32]. A combination of Notch1 blockade and chemotherapy synergistically reduced chemotherapy-enriched cancer stem cells (CSC) [33]. Blocking Notch-1 resulted in downregulation of NF-kappaB and its target genes (*CXCL8*, *MMP9* and *VEGF*), which suppressed invasion

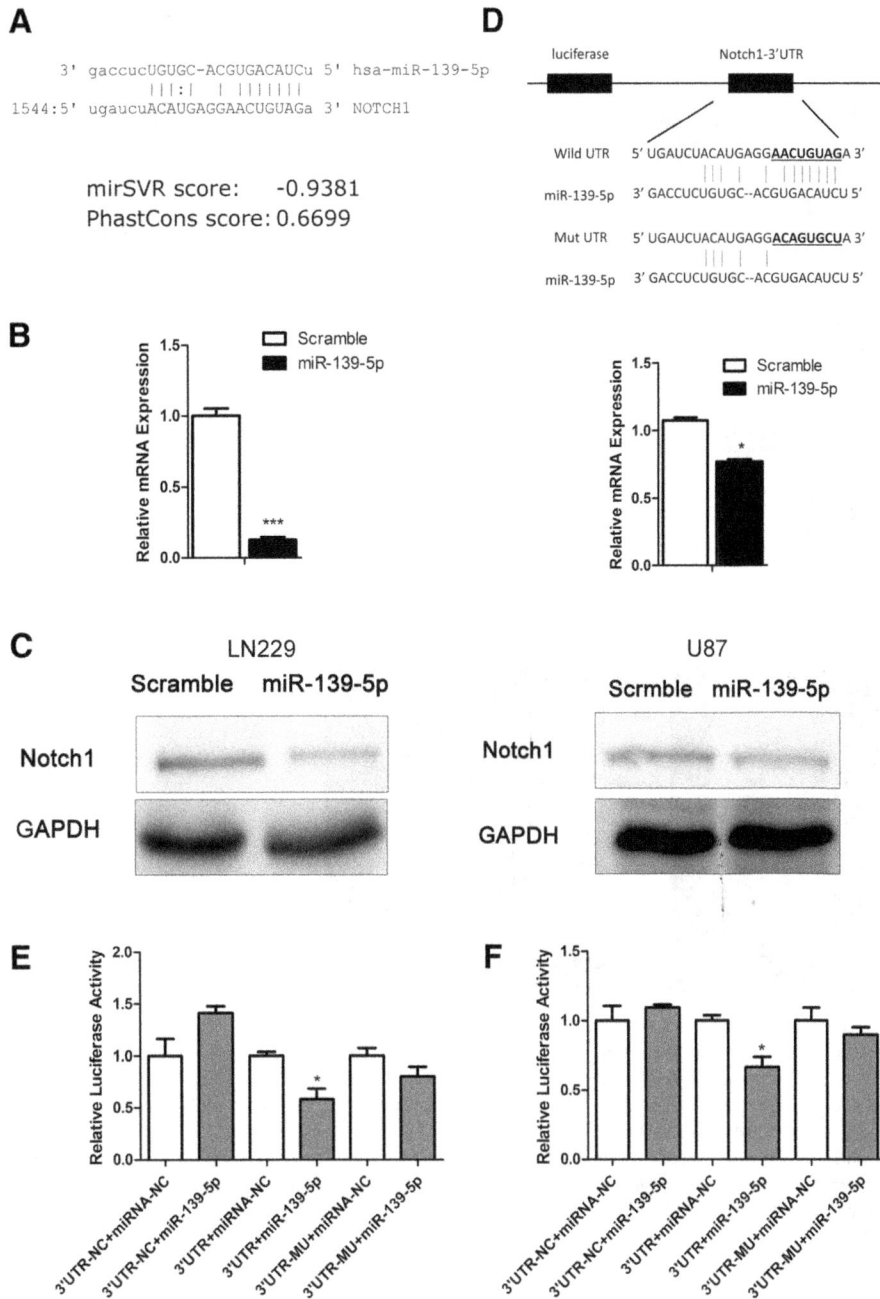

Fig. 4 Notch1 was a direct target of miR-139-5p. (**a**) Diagram of the seed sequence of miR-139-5p matched the 3'-UTR of Notch1. (**b** and **c**) qRT-PCR and Western blotting for Notch1 expression after transfection with miR-139-5p or miR-Scr. (*$P < 0.05$. ***$P < 0.001$). (**d**) Schematic diagram of the design of wild or mutant Notch1 3'-UTR containing reporter constructs. (**e** and **f**) Luciferase reporter assays in LN229 and U87 glioma cells after co-transfection with wild-type or mutant 3'-UTR Notch1 and miRNAs. 3'-UTR-NC, Negative Control of Notch1 3'-UTR. miRNA-NC, Negative Control of miR-139-5p. The data represent the fold change in the expression (means+SE) of 3 replicates (*$P < 0.05$)

and angiogenesis in breast cancer [34]; therefore, we would evaluate these targets next in glioma cell lines and in any other experiments where miR-139-5p levels are manipulated. Sonic hedgehog (Shh) could promote tumour proliferation in a Notch-dependent manner [35–38]. The Hedgehog and Notch pathways interact to control the EMT/MET [35]. However, little is

known regarding Notch1 interactions with EMT in glioma. Our study demonstrated that Notch1 was obviously upregulated in glioma tissues. Interestingly, Notch1 also expressed in normal brain tissue, which could be explained by Notch1 signalling being involved in cell fate decision during normal development while abnormal activation would promote carcinogenesis

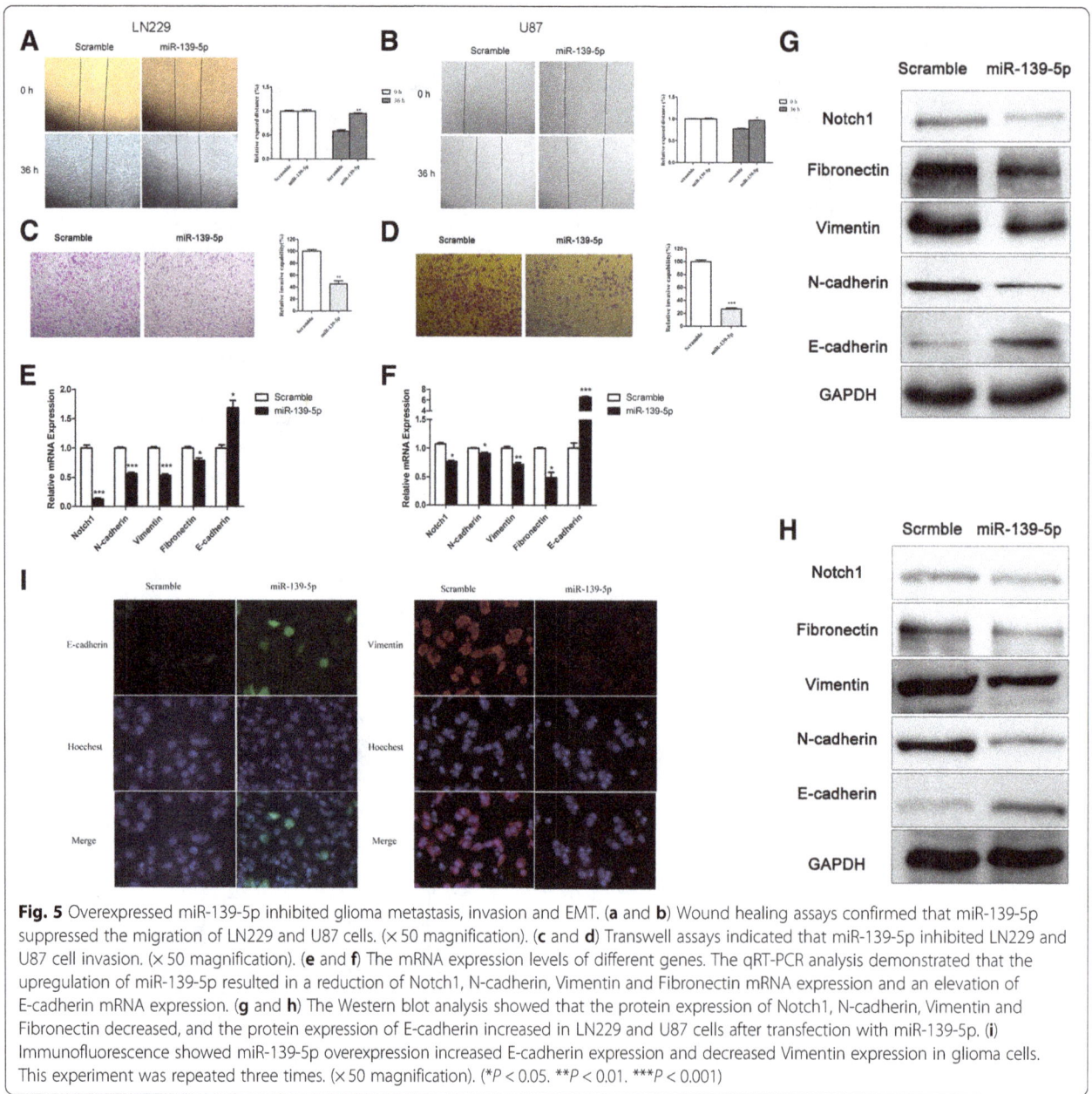

Fig. 5 Overexpressed miR-139-5p inhibited glioma metastasis, invasion and EMT. (**a** and **b**) Wound healing assays confirmed that miR-139-5p suppressed the migration of LN229 and U87 cells. (× 50 magnification). (**c** and **d**) Transwell assays indicated that miR-139-5p inhibited LN229 and U87 cell invasion. (× 50 magnification). (**e** and **f**) The mRNA expression levels of different genes. The qRT-PCR analysis demonstrated that the upregulation of miR-139-5p resulted in a reduction of Notch1, N-cadherin, Vimentin and Fibronectin mRNA expression and an elevation of E-cadherin mRNA expression. (**g** and **h**) The Western blot analysis showed that the protein expression of Notch1, N-cadherin, Vimentin and Fibronectin decreased, and the protein expression of E-cadherin increased in LN229 and U87 cells after transfection with miR-139-5p. (**i**) Immunofluorescence showed miR-139-5p overexpression increased E-cadherin expression and decreased Vimentin expression in glioma cells. This experiment was repeated three times. (× 50 magnification). (*$P < 0.05$. **$P < 0.01$. ***$P < 0.001$)

[30]. In addition, Notch1 was upregulated in glioma cell lines, especially U87 and LN229. Knocking down Notch1 in these cells effectively suppressed glioma metastasis, invasion and EMT. These results demonstrated that Notch1 plays an important role in glioma and could be a potential therapeutic target.

MiR-139-5p has been demonstrated as a tumour suppressor in a variety of tumours. Krowiorz et al. found that miR-139-5p is specifically downregulated in CN-AML with mutated FLT3 and acts as a strong tumour suppressor [12]. Wang et al. reported that miR-139 functions as an anti-oncomir to repress glioma progression through targeting IGF-1R, AMY-1, and

PGC-1beta [39]. Moreover, miR-139-5p can sensitize colorectal cancer cells to 5-fluorouracil by targeting NOTCH-1 [40]. Until now, limited information is available about the effect of miR-139-5p on EMT in glioma. miR-139-5p had prognostic meaning in LGG (Additional file 4). Our recent work demonstrates that miR-139 is downregulated in glioma tissues and negatively correlated to tumour grade [16]. In this study, we searched four databases to find that miR-139-5p may target Notch1 3′-UTR. The combination of bioinformatics prediction, luciferase reporter assays and functional experiments determined that miR-139-5p decreased Notch1 expression

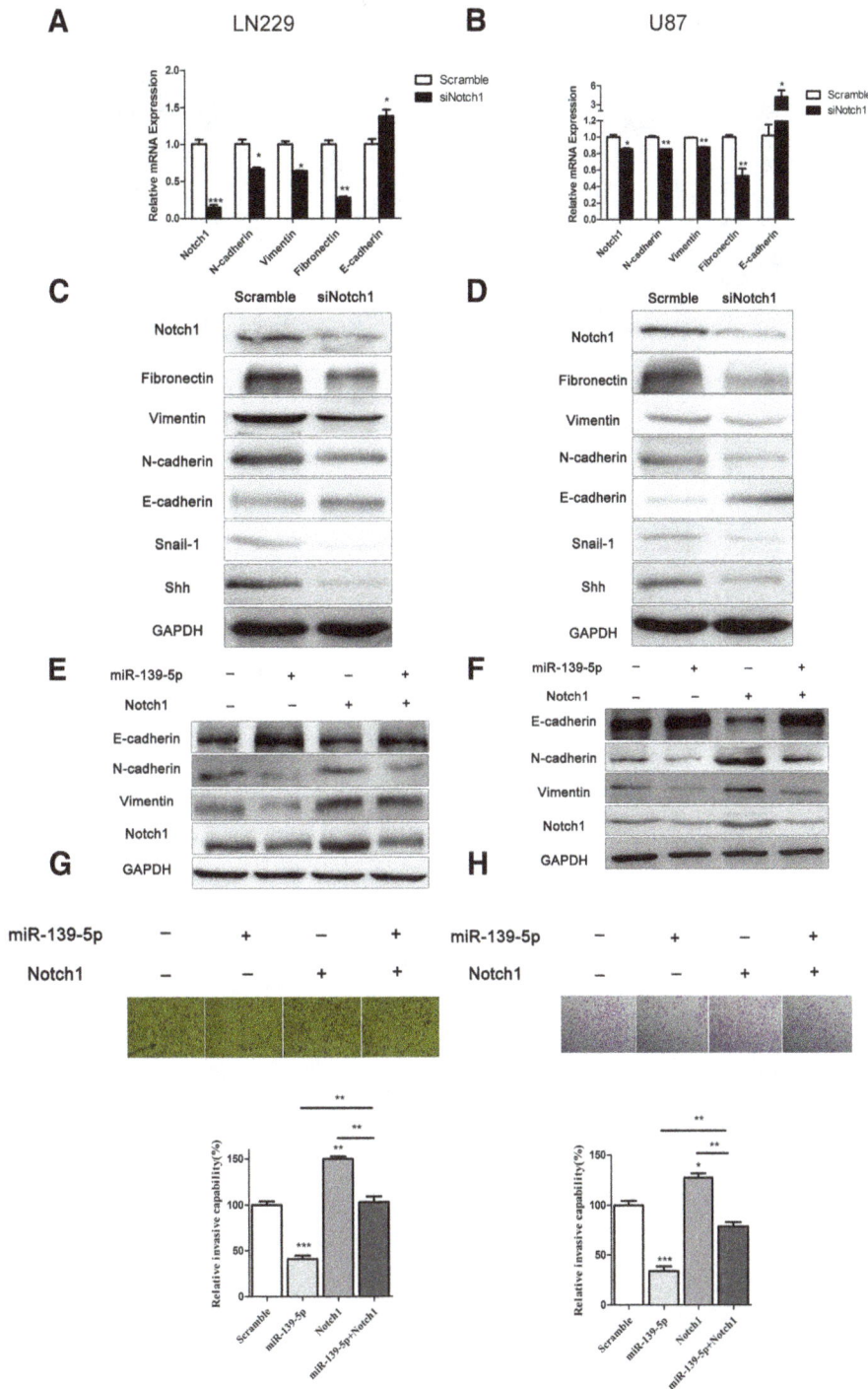

Fig. 6 Mir-139-5p reversed EMT via down-regulating the expression of Notch1. (**a** and **b**) qRT-PCR analysis demonstrated that downregulation of Notch1 resulted in a reduction of Notch1, N-cadherin, Vimentin and Fibronectin mRNA expression and an elevation of E-cadherin mRNA expression. (**c** and **d**) Western blot analysis showed that the protein expression of Notch1, N-cadherin, Vimentin, Fibronectin, Snail-1 and Shh decreased, and the protein expression of E-cadherin increased in LN229 and U87 cells treated with Notch1 siRNA. (**e** and **f**) Notch1, E-cadherin, N-cadherin and Vimentin expression levels in the LN229 and U87 cells transfected with full length Notch1 without the corresponding 3′-UTR or/ and miR-139-5p were assessed by Western blotting. (**g** and **h**) Invasiveness of LN229 and U87 glioma cells transfected with full-length Notch1 without the corresponding 3′-UTR or/and miR-139-5p were estimated by transwell assays. This experiment was repeated three times. ($\times 50$ magnification). (*$P < 0.05$. **$P < 0.01$. ***$P < 0.001$)

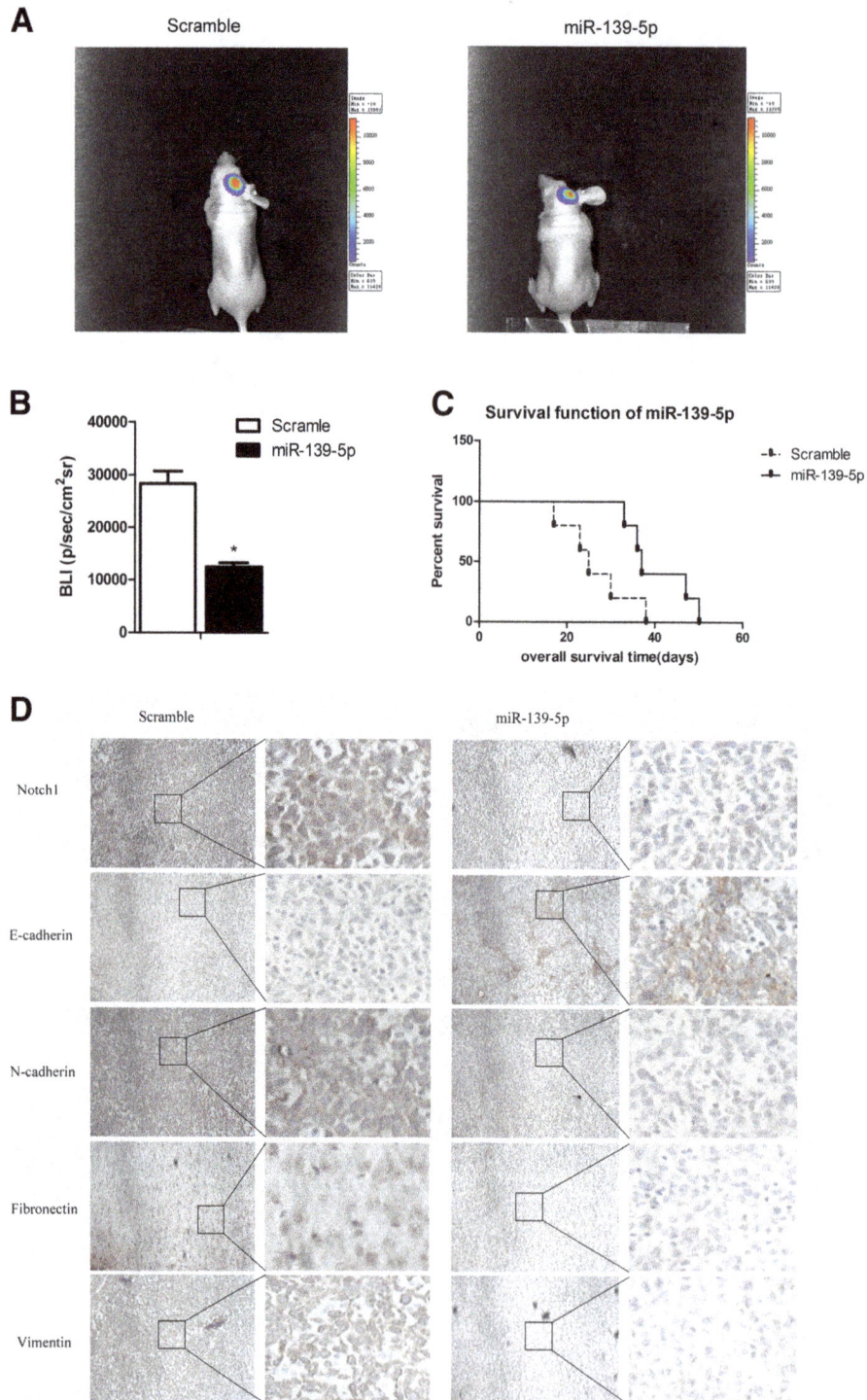

Fig. 7 MiR-139-5p inhibited glioma xenograft growth, metastasis and EMT in vivo and prolonged survival. (**a** and **b**) Luminescence imaging for miR-139-5p–treated U87-luc tumours versus scramble-treated controls. (**c**) Kaplan-Meier survival curves indicating that mice transfected with miR-139-5p showed a significantly better outcome than the miR-Scr-treated group (*$P < 0.05$). (**d**) Notch1, E-cadherin, N-cadherin, Fibronectin and Vimentin expression after transfecting miR-139-5p in tumour sections following IHC analysis. (× 100 magnification)

and suppressed Notch1-induced EMT in vitro and in vivo. Importantly, miR-139-5p reduced tumourigenicity and prolonged mouse survival. Inhibiting EMT-associated drugs in combination with traditional therapies may provide potential targets for future treatment. There are still important hurdles to overcome such as quick degradation, low efficiency in crossing the blood-brain barrier, side effects and the off-targeting of miR-139-5p.

Conclusion

Notch1 is markedly overexpressed in glioma and accelerated tumour metastasis, invasion and EMT. Upregulating miR-139-5p in cells inhibits glioma growth and reverses Notch1-induced EMT. This suggests that the miR-139-5p/Notch1/EMT pathway could be a novel target for glioma therapy.

Additional files

Additional file 1: The oligonucleotide sequences. (PDF 269 kb)

Additional file 2: Gene-specific primers for qRT-PCR analysis. (PDF 261 kb)

Additional file 3: miR-139-5p expression was quantified by qRT-PCR analysis. (PDF 297 kb)

Additional file 4: The clinical prognostic meaning of miR-139-5p in glioma patients with different grade. LGG, brain lower grade glioma. GBM, glioblastoma multiforme. (JPG 632 kb)

Abbreviations

DFS: Disease-free survival; EMT: Epithelial-to-mesenchymal transition; Hh: Hedgehog; OL: Oligodendroglia cell line; OS: Overall survival; PVDF: Polyvinylidene difluoride; qRT-PCR: Quantitative reverse transcriptase PCR; SDS-PAGE: SDS polyacrylamide gel electrophoresis; Shh: Sonic Hedgehog

Acknowledgements

We thank Professor Quan Liu and Professor Jinquan Cai (HMU) for guidance on the study.

Funding

This work was supported by the National Natural Science Foundation of China (81572743), President Foundation of Nanfang Hospital, Southern Medical University (2017B030), National Natural Scientific Fund (81372173, 81502404), the Scientific Fund Project of Hospital (KYBS2015–15) and the HLJ Province Natural Scientific Fund (QC2015128).

Authors' contributions

LR, JC and CL conceived and designed this study. LJ, LQ and LL drafted the manuscript and performed the statistical analysis. WR and DW participated in the clinical evaluation of the patients. All authors approved this manuscript to be submitted.

Competing interests

The authors declare that they have no competing interests.

Author details

[1]Department of Neurosurgery, The Second Affiliated Hospital of Harbin Medical University, 246 Xuefu Road, Nangang, 150086 Harbin, People's Republic of China. [2]Department of Orthopaedic Surgery, Nanfang Hospital, Southern Medical University, Guangzhou 510515, China. [3]Department of Neurology, The Second Affiliated Hospital of Harbin Medical University, Harbin 150086, China. [4]Neuroscience Institute, Heilongjiang Academy of Medical Sciences, Harbin 150086, China. [5]Chinese Glioma Cooperative Group (CGCG), Beijing 100050, China. [6]Department of Neurosurgery, Huashan Hospital, Fudan University, Shanghai 200040, China. [7]Department of Neurosurgery, The First Affiliated Hospital of Harbin Medical University, Harbin 150086, China.

References

1. Cai J, Zhu P, Zhang C, Li Q, Wang Z, Li G, Wang G, Yang P, Li J, Han B, et al. Detection of ATRX and IDH1-R132H immunohistochemistry in the progression of 211 paired gliomas. Oncotarget. 2016;7(13):16384–95.
2. Li J, Cai J, Zhao S, Yao K, Sun Y, Li Y, Chen L, Li R, Zhai X, Zhang J, et al. GANT61, a GLI inhibitor, sensitizes glioma cells to the temozolomide treatment. J Exp Clin Cancer Res. 2016;35(1):184.
3. Giese A, Bjerkvig R, Berens ME, Westphal M. Cost of migration: invasion of malignant gliomas and implications for treatment. J Clin Oncol. 2003;21(8):1624–36.
4. Nieto MA, Huang RY, Jackson RA, Thiery JP. EMT: 2016. Cell. 2016;166(1):21–45.
5. Sarkar S, Mirzaei R, Zemp FJ, Wu W, Senger DL, Robbins SM, Yong VW. Activation of NOTCH signaling by tenascin-C promotes growth of human brain tumor-initiating cells. Cancer Res. 2017;77:3231–43.
6. Zhang H, Wang X, Xu J, Sun Y. Notch1 activation is a poor prognostic factor in patients with gastric cancer. Br J Cancer. 2014;110(9):2283–90.
7. Blaquiere JA, Wong KKL, Kinsey SD, Wu J, Verheyen EM. Homeodomain-interacting protein kinase promotes tumorigenesis and metastatic cell behavior. Dis Model Mech. 2018;11(1):1.
8. Brabletz S, Bajdak K, Meidhof S, Burk U, Niedermann G, Firat E, Wellner U, Dimmler A, Faller G, Schubert J, et al. The ZEB1/miR-200 feedback loop controls Notch signalling in cancer cells. EMBO J. 2011;30(4):770–82.
9. Maciaczyk D, Picard D, Zhao L, Koch K, Herrera-Rios D, Li G, Marquardt V, Pauck D, Hoerbelt T, Zhang W, et al. CBF1 is clinically prognostic and serves as a target to block cellular invasion and chemoresistance of EMT-like glioblastoma cells. Br J Cancer. 2017;117:102.
10. Chen L, Zhang A, Li Y, Zhang K, Han L, Du W, Yan W, Li R, Wang Y, Wang K, et al. MiR-24 regulates the proliferation and invasion of glioma by ST7L via beta-catenin/Tcf-4 signaling. Cancer Lett. 2013;329(2):174–80.
11. Chen L, Zhang W, Yan W, Han L, Zhang K, Shi Z, Zhang J, Wang Y, Li Y, Yu S, et al. The putative tumor suppressor miR-524-5p directly targets Jagged-1 and Hes-1 in glioma. Carcinogenesis. 2012;33(11):2276–82.
12. Krowiorz K, Ruschmann J, Lai C, Ngom M, Maetzig T, Martins V, Scheffold A, Schneider E, Pochert N, Miller C, et al. MiR-139-5p is a potent tumor suppressor in adult acute myeloid leukemia. Blood Cancer Journal. 2016;6(12):e508.
13. Luo HN, Wang ZH, Sheng Y, Zhang Q, Yan J, Hou J, Zhu K, Cheng Y, Xu YL, Zhang XH, et al. MiR-139 targets CXCR4 and inhibits the proliferation and metastasis of laryngeal squamous carcinoma cells. Med Oncol. 2014;31(1):789.
14. Fan Q, He M, Deng X, Wu WK, Zhao L, Tang J, Wen G, Sun X, Liu Y. Derepression of c-Fos caused by microRNA-139 down-regulation contributes to the metastasis of human hepatocellular carcinoma. Cell Biochem Funct. 2013;31(4):319–24.
15. Yue S, Wang L, Zhang H, Min Y, Lou Y, Sun H, Jiang Y, Zhang W, Liang A, Guo Y, et al. miR-139-5p suppresses cancer cell migration and invasion through targeting ZEB1 and ZEB2 in GBM. Tumour Biol. 2015;36(9):6741–9.
16. Li RY, Chen LC, Zhang HY, Du WZ, Feng Y, Wang HB, Wen JQ, Liu X, Li XF, Sun Y, et al. MiR-139 inhibits Mcl-1 expression and potentiates TMZ-induced apoptosis in glioma. CNS Neurosci Ther. 2013;19(7):477–83.
17. Zhou Q, Wang Y, Peng B, Liang L, Li J. The roles of Notch1 expression in the migration of intrahepatic cholangiocarcinoma. BMC Cancer. 2013;13:244.
18. Cerami E, Gao J, Dogrusoz U, Gross BE, Sumer SO, Aksoy BA, Jacobsen A, Byrne CJ, Heuer ML, Larsson E, et al. The cBio cancer genomics portal: an open platform for exploring multidimensional cancer genomics data. Cancer Discov. 2012;2(5):401–4.
19. Gao J, Aksoy BA, Dogrusoz U, Dresdner G, Gross B, Sumer SO, Sun Y, Jacobsen A, Sinha R, Larsson E, et al. Integrative analysis of complex cancer genomics and clinical profiles using the cBioPortal. Sci Signal. 2013;6(269):pl1.
20. Li J, Wang F, Wang G, Sun Y, Cai J, Liu X, Zhang J, Lu X, Li Y, Chen M, et al. Combination epidermal growth factor receptor variant III peptide-pulsed dendritic cell vaccine with miR-326 results in enhanced killing on EGFRvIII-positive cells. Oncotarget. 2017;8(16):26256–68.
21. Du W, Liu X, Chen L, Dou Z, Lei X, Chang L, Cai J, Cui Y, Yang D, Sun Y, et al. Targeting the SMO oncogene by miR-326 inhibits glioma biological behaviors and stemness. Neuro-Oncology. 2015;17(2):243–53.
22. Zhu ZH, Sun BY, Ma Y, Shao JY, Long H, Zhang X, Fu JH, Zhang LJ, Su XD, Wu QL, et al. Three immunomarker support vector machines-based prognostic classifiers for stage IB non-small-cell lung cancer. J Clin Oncol. 2009;27(7):1091–9.

23. Liu X, Wang X, Du W, Chen L, Wang G, Cui Y, Liu Y, Dou Z, Wang H, Zhang P, et al. Suppressor of fused (Sufu) represses Gli1 transcription and nuclear accumulation, inhibits glioma cell proliferation, invasion and vasculogenic mimicry, improving glioma chemo-sensitivity and prognosis. Oncotarget. 2014;5(22):11681–94.

24. Du WZ, Feng Y, Wang XF, Piao XY, Cui YQ, Chen LC, Lei XH, Sun X, Liu X, Wang HB, et al. Curcumin suppresses malignant glioma cells growth and induces apoptosis by inhibition of SHH/GLI1 signaling pathway in vitro and vivo. CNS Neurosci Ther. 2013;19(12):926–36.

25. Kahlert UD, Nikkhah G, Maciaczyk J. Epithelial-to-mesenchymal(−like) transition as a relevant molecular event in malignant gliomas. Cancer Lett. 2013;331(2):131–8.

26. KU D, JJ V, KFA E. EMT- and MET-related processes in nonepithelial tumors: importance for disease progression, prognosis, and therapeutic opportunities. Mol Oncol. 2017;11(7):860–77.

27. Takebe N, Harris PJ, Warren RQ, Ivy SP. Targeting cancer stem cells by inhibiting Wnt, Notch, and hedgehog pathways. Nat Rev Clin Oncol. 2010;8:97.

28. Tobias A, Ahmed A, Moon KS, Lesniak MS. The art of gene therapy for glioma: a review of the challenging road to the bedside. J Neurol Neurosurg Psychiatry. 2013;84(2):213–22.

29. Chen L, Han L, Zhang K, Shi Z, Zhang J, Zhang A, Wang Y, Song Y, Li Y, Jiang T, et al. VHL regulates the effects of miR-23b on glioma survival and invasion via suppression of HIF-1alpha/VEGF and beta-catenin/Tcf-4 signaling. Neuro-Oncology. 2012;14(8):1026–36.

30. Koch U, Radtke F. Notch and cancer: a double-edged sword. Cell Mol Life Sci. 2007;64(21):2746–62.

31. Lefort K, Ostano P, Mello-Grand M, Calpini V, Scatolini M, Farsetti A, Dotto GP, Chiorino G. Dual tumor suppressing and promoting function of Notch1 signaling in human prostate cancer. Oncotarget. 2016;

32. Qi R, An H, Yu Y, Zhang M, Liu S, Xu H, Guo Z, Cheng T, Cao X. Notch1 signaling inhibits growth of human hepatocellular carcinoma through induction of cell cycle arrest and apoptosis. Cancer Res. 2003;63(23):8323–9.

33. Zhao ZL, Zhang L, Huang CF, Ma SR, Bu LL, Liu JF, Yu GT, Liu B, Gutkind JS, Kulkarni AB, et al. NOTCH1 inhibition enhances the efficacy of conventional chemotherapeutic agents by targeting head neck cancer stem cell. Sci Rep. 2016;6:24704.

34. Liu Y, Su C, Shan Y, Yang S, Ma G. Targeting Notch1 inhibits invasion and angiogenesis of human breast cancer cells via inhibition nuclear factor-kappaB signaling. Am J Transl Res. 2016;8(6):2681–92.

35. Xie G, Karaca G, Swiderska-Syn M, Michelotti GA, Kruger L, Chen Y, Premont RT, Choi SS, Diehl AM. Cross-talk between Notch and hedgehog regulates hepatic stellate cell fate in mice. Hepatology. 2013;58(5):1801–13.

36. Doyle AJ, Redmond EM, Gillespie DL, Knight PA, Cullen JP, Cahill PA, Morrow DJ. Differential expression of hedgehog/Notch and transforming growth factor-beta in human abdominal aortic aneurysms. J Vasc Surg. 2015;62(2):464–70.

37. Li L, Grausam KB, Wang J, Lun MP, Ohli J, Lidov HG, Calicchio ML, Zeng E, Salisbury JL, Wechsler-Reya RJ, et al. Sonic hedgehog promotes proliferation of Notch-dependent monociliated choroid plexus tumour cells. Nat Cell Biol. 2016;18(4):418–30.

38. Bertrand FE, Angus CW, Partis WJ, Sigounas G. Developmental pathways in colon cancer: crosstalk between WNT, BMP, hedgehog and Notch. Cell cycle (Georgetown Tex). 2012;11(23):4344–51.

39. Wang H, Yan X, Ji LY, Ji XT, Wang P, Guo SW, Li SZ. miR-139 functions as an Antioncomir to repress glioma progression through targeting IGF-1 R, AMY-1, and PGC-1beta. Technol Cancer Res Treat. 2016;16:497–511.

40. Liu H, Yin Y, Hu Y, Feng Y, Bian Z, Yao S, Li M, You Q, Huang Z. miR-139-5p sensitizes colorectal cancer cells to 5-fluorouracil by targeting NOTCH-1. Pathol Res Pract. 2016;

10

"Recurrent multiple cerebral infarctions related to the progression of adenomyosis"

Yasuhiro Aso*⬥, Ryo Chikazawa, Yuki Kimura, Noriyuki Kimura and Etsuro Matsubara

Abstract

Background: Benign gynecologic tumor, such as uterine adenomyosis, has been suggested to develop hypercoagulability. Although some cases of cerebral infarction associated with adenomyosis have been reported, the mechanism of hypercoagulation initiated by adenomyosis is still not clear, and the therapeutic strategy is uncertain.

Case presentation: A 44-year-old woman was presented to our department with headache, left hand weakness, and gait disturbance during her menstrual phase. She had a history of adenomyosis and infertility treatment for 18 years and heavy menstrual bleeding. Magnetic resonance imaging on admission showed multiple hyperintense lesions in cortical and subcortical areas in the cerebrum and cerebellum on diffusion-weighted imaging. Transesophageal echocardiography showed neither embolic sources nor existence of foramen ovale. Her laboratory data revealed anemia, a high D-dimer level, and elevated levels of a mucinous tumor marker. She had adenomyosis and no malignancy was detected. Anticoagulation therapy with intravenous heparin followed by rivaroxaban did not prevent recurrence of cerebral infarction. We discontinued rivaroxaban, and started warfarin therapy with pseudomenopause treatment, which prevented recurrence for 6 months. Five months after her last pseudomenopause treatment, multiple cerebral infarctions occurred. Total hysterectomy was performed, which prevented recurrence of the multiple cerebral infarctions for 2 years without anticoagulation therapy.

Conclusions: Our findings reveal for the first time that anticoagulation therapy, including novel oral anticoagulants, had no preventive effect against cerebral infarctions associated with adenomyosis in a middle-aged woman. Although pseudomenopause treatment temporarily prevented recurrence, resection of the adenomyosis might be the most effective therapy in these cases.

Keywords: Multiple cerebral infarctions, Adenomyosis, Hypercoagulagulability, Anticoagulation therapy

Background

Uterine adenomyosis is a benign gynecologic condition, defined as the presence of ectopic endometrial glands and stroma surrounded by hyperplastic smooth muscle within the myometrium. Approximately 20% of women attending a general gynecologic clinic were revealed to have adenomyosis [1]. Although common symptoms are menorrhagia, dysmenorrhea, and heavy menstrual bleeding, one-third of women are asymptomatic [2].

Some patients with adenomyosis develop multiple cerebral infarctions (CIs) [3–5] (Table 1). Almost all patients are middle-aged, with severe anemia and elevated serum carbohydrate antigen 125 (CA125). These patients are initially administered conventional anticoagulant therapy, which is often combined with gonadotropin-releasing hormone (GnRH) therapy, and in some cases the adenomyosis is subsequently resected.

Here, we report the case of a middle-aged woman with adenomyosis who developed multiple CIs in her menstrual phase. Although she received edaravone and anticoagulation treatment with rivaroxaban, the recurrence of multiple CIs was not prevented. Pseudomenopause therapy with a GnRH agonist normalized her hypercoagulation state, but multiple CIs occurred after therapy was discontinued. Finally, a hysterectomy was performed, which successfully prevented CI recurrence. We propose that treatment of

* Correspondence: yasuhiroaso@oita-u.ac.jp
Department of Neurology, Faculty of Medicine, Oita University, Yufu-city, Oita 879-5593, Japan

Table 1 Patient characteristics and therapy for CI associated with adenomyosis

Case	Age (y.o.)	D-dimer (µg/ml)	FDP (µg/ml)	CA125 (U/ml)	hemoglobin (g/dl)	treatment for CI		treatment for adenomyosis	recurrence of CI	reference
						initial treatment	subsequent treatment			
1	45	1.1	–	159	8.4	hepalin	antipletelet therapy	GnRH agonist	–	Yamashiro K et al. 2012
2	44	–	5.9	–	7	hepalin	warfalin	GnRH agonist	–	
3	50	0.57	–	42.6	6.9	aspirin	–	GnRH agonist	–	
4	42	6.0	–	1750	8.6	antiplatelet therapy	warfalin	GnRH agonist	+	
5	59	7.0	–	334.8	–	antithrombotic therapy	–	–	–	Hijikata N et al. 2016

CIs due to adenomyosis with anticoagulant therapy is not effective, and briefly discuss the underlying etiology and therapeutic strategy.

Case presentation

A 44-year-old woman experienced sudden onset of difficulty using her left hand and walking during her menstrual phase. She had a history of adenomyosis and infertility treatment for 18 years, and heavy menstrual bleeding. She complained of headache, abdominal pain, nausea, and had a fever (37.7 °C) at presentation. She is not obese (BMI of 21.5 kg/m^2), had no history of taking steroids or contraceptives. Neurologic examination revealed left spatial neglect, left facial hypoalgesia, mild paresis in her left arm, and right pyramidal signs. Brain magnetic resonance imaging (MRI) revealed bilaterally multiple infarctions in the cerebrum and cerebellum, including cortical and subcortical lesions (Fig. 1a). MR angiography presented severe stenosis in the M2, M3,

>and M4 portions of right middle cerebral artery (Fig. 1b). Contrast computed tomography revealed a splenic infarction (Fig. 1c). Blood examination revealed normocytic anemia (hemoglobin 10.3 g/dl, mean corpuscular volume 90.5 µm^3), thrombocytopenia (112,000 /µl), and low-grade elevation of C-reactive protein (2.9 mg/dl). The serum levels of D-dimer (17.0 µg/ml, normal < 0.5 µg/ml), CA125 (2115 U/ml, normal < 35.0 U/ml), and carbohydrate antigen 19–9 (CA19–9) (1824 U/ml, normal < 37.0 U/ml) were increased. Results of a hypercoagulable panel, including protein C and S, antithrombin III level, lupus anticoagulant, and anticardiolipin antibody titers, were within normal limits. Pelvic MRI revealed giant adenomyosis (Fig. 1d), but no malignancy was detected. Fluorine-18–2-fluoro-2-deoxy-d-glucose (FDG) positron emission tomography revealed FDG accumulation in the adenomyosis, but no malignancy was detected by cervical cytology. The result of continuous electrocardiography monitoring, transesophageal echocardiography with

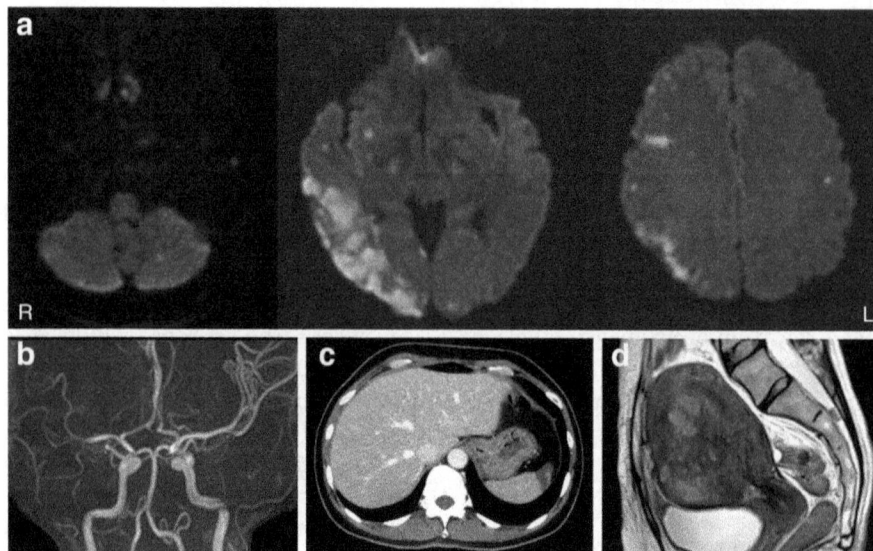

Fig. 1 Diffusion-weighted magnetic resonance imaging (MRI) scan of the brain reveals multiple infarctions in the cerebellum and cerebrum (**a**). The M2, M3, and M4 portions of the right middle cerebral artery were not well visualized by MR angiography (**b**). Contrast computed tomography revealed splenic infarction (**c**). Giant adenomyosis was revealed by a T2-weighted MRI scan of the pelvis (**d**)

agitated saline injection, carotid ultrasonography, upper gastrointestinal endoscopy, and colonoscopy were normal.

She was treated with edaravone (60 mg/day) and anticoagulated with heparin for 2 weeks. Subsequently, she was treated with rivaroxaban (15 mg/day). Her serum levels of D-dimer, CA125, and CA19–9 improved (2.7 µg/ml, 911 U/ml, and 501 U/ml, respectively), and the treatment was continued.

At day 31, a day after her menstrual phase started, she complained of numbness in her left lower limb. Brain MRI revealed a new CI in the right cerebrum (Fig. 2a). The serum levels of D-dimer, CA125, CA19–9 were 2.4 µg/ml, 561 U/ml, 417 U/ml, respectively. We discontinued the rivaroxaban treatment, and started anticoagulant therapy with warfarin. Afterwards, her menstrual bleeding increased, the anemia progressed, and the serum level of D-dimer increased (14.1 µg/ml). She started to receive pseudomenopause treatment with a GnRH agonist for the adenomyosis. Ten days after initiating the GnRH agonist treatment, her serum D-dimer level improved (2.30 µg/ml). She continued the warfarin and GnRH agonist once a month for 6 months, and showed no recurrence of CIs during that time. The serum levels of CA125, CA19–9 improved after 3 months of initiating the therapy (117 U/ml, 224 U/ml, respectively).

She presented with transient weakness of her right lower limb and visited our clinic 5 months after her last GnRH agonist therapy, when her irregular menstrual bleeding had continued for a month. Brain MRI revealed new multiple cortical and subcortical infarctions in the left occipital lobe and right parietal lobe (Fig. 2b). Her serum D-dimer, FDP, CA125, and CA19–9 levels were elevated (22.0 µg/ml, 56.5 µg/ml, 1291.6 U/ml, and 803.2 U/ml, respectively). Anticoagulant therapy with warfarin was well controlled (PT-INR 2.5), and her electrocardiographic findings were normal. We concluded that total hysterectomy would be the most effective therapy for preventing CI recurrence. She underwent total hysterectomy and bilateral salpingo-oophorectomy, which was effective in not only preventing CI recurrence, but also for normalizing the serum D-dimer, FDP, CA125, and CA19–9 levels for the last 2 years.

Discussion and conclusions

Here we report a 44-year-old woman who developed multiple CIs after her menstrual phase, when the serum D-dimer, CA125, and CA19–9 levels were markedly elevated. Neither warfarin nor novel oral anticoagulants (NOAC) prevented CI recurrence. Although GnRH agonist therapy improved the levels of the three markers and prevented CI recurrence, the CIs recurred after the therapy was discontinued. Hysterectomy finally normalized the serum levels of the markers, and prevented CI recurrence. To our knowledge, this is the first report of an attempt to use NOAC to prevent recurrence of CI associated with adenomyosis. The clinical course of this case suggests that anticoagulation therapy is not sufficient to prevent blood hypercoagulation associated with adenomyosis, and thus resection may be the most effective therapy to normalize hypercoagulation and prevent the recurrence of thrombotic events.

Although reports of CI associated with adenomyosis are rare, some similar cases were reported. Yamashiro et al. [3] reported four cases of CI associated with adenomyosis in middle-aged women. Two of the women developed CIs in their menstrual phase. All of them presented with severe anemia (hemoglobin levels 6.9–8.6 g/dl). The D-dimer levels were elevated in two cases (1.1 µg/ml and 6.0 µg/ml), and CA125 was elevated in three cases (159 U/ml, 42.6 U/ml, and 1750 U/ml). All four cases were treated with antiplatelet medicine or an anticoagulant with a GnRH agonist. One case experienced recurrent multiple CIs after discontinuation of the therapy, when the levels of D-dimer and CA125 again increased (4.1 µg/ml and 907 U/ml, respectively). Subsequently, she was treated with anticoagulant therapy and a GnRH agonist, and the D-dimer and CA125 levels normalized. These authors suggested that hypercoagulability in association with an elevated CA125 level, menstruation-related coagulopathy, or increased tissue factor (TF) expression level is a potential risk factor for developing CI. Hijikata et al. [5] reported 59-year-old woman with a 10-year history of hormone replacement therapy for menopausal symptoms who developed multiple CIs. Her laboratory tests revealed elevated CA125 (334.8 U/ml) and D-dimer (7.0 µg/ml)

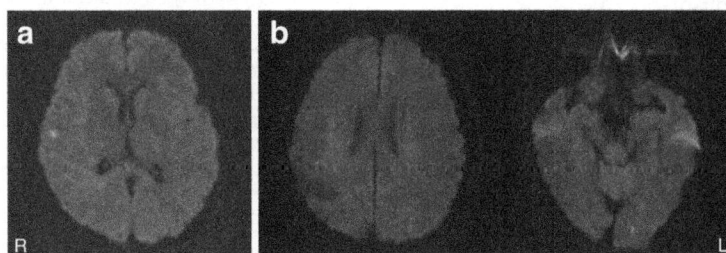

Fig. 2 Diffusion-weighted MRI revealed CIs in the right cerebrum (**a**). Multiple cortical and subcortical CIs in the left occipital lobe and right parietal lobe (**b**)

levels. Anticoagulant therapy with unfractionated heparin was started and the hormone therapy was discontinued. Although antithrombotic therapy was discontinued on day 7 because of withdrawal bleeding, the D-dimer and CA125 levels normalized. The authors concluded that both elevated CA125 levels and hormone replacement therapy are risk factors for hypercoagulability [5].

The mechanism of hypercoagulation initiated by adenomyosis remains uncertain. Several clinical studies reported an association of elevated serum CA125 and CA19–9 levels, and hypercoagulability [3–9]. CA125 is a typical mucin molecule [10], widely utilized for the diagnosis of epithelial ovarian cancer [11]. CA19–9 is a mucin-like high-molecular-weight glycoprotein utilized for the diagnosis of malignancies of the stomach, colon, and pancreas [12], and was recently reported to be associated with thrombosis in pancreatic adenocarcinoma [9]. These cancer-related-mucin molecules are suggested to play an important role in the hypercoagulative state in Trousseau's syndrome [13]. In our case, the levels of CA125 and CA19–9 were considerably high. We suppose that the high levels of these markers induced the recurrence of multiple cerebral infarctions in our case. A recent experimental study revealed that carcinoma mucin promotes thrombosis through adhesion-dependent, bidirectional signaling in neutrophils and platelets [14]. This mechanism may explain why the hypercoagulation in our case was not prevented by warfarin or NOAC.

In Trousseau's syndrome, induction of TF and its activity is postulated to promote hypercoagulability in patients with cancer [15, 16]. Expression of TF is also significantly higher in adenomyotic lesions [17], and it renders microparticles procoagulant. Increased release of TF-exposing microparticles is suggested to contribute to the development of thrombotic complications [18]. This pathology might play an important role in multiple thromboses induced by adenomyosis.

Anemia is also a suspected cardiovascular factor [19, 20]. Anemia is considered a hyperkinetic state, and it disturbs endothelial adhesion molecule genes, which may lead to thrombus formation. In addition, anemia causes blood flow augmentation and turbulence, which may result in the migration of a thrombus, thus producing artery-to-artery embolism.

In conclusion, our findings suggest that middle-aged women with adenomyosis are at high risk for CI when the serum D-dimer, CA125, and CA19–9 levels are elevated. In those patients, anticoagulant therapy including NOAC therapy could not prevent CI. Adenomyosis resection may be the most effective therapy for preventing CI in these cases.

Abbreviations

CA125: carbohydrate antigen 125; CA19–9: carbohydrate antigen 19–9; CI: cerebral infarction; FDG: Fluorine-18–2-fluoro-2-deoxy-d-glucose;

GnRH: gonadotropin-releasing hormone; MRI: magnetic resonance imaging; NOAC: novel oral anticoagulants; TF: tissue factor

Acknowledgments

The authors would like to acknowledge the following: Prof. Teruyuki Hirano at Kyorin University School of Medicine, Japan. The staff of Obstetrics and Gynecology, Oita University Faculty of Medicine, Japan.

Authors' contributions

YA, RC and YK examined and managed the patient; YA drafted the manuscript and created the figs; NK helped and revised the manuscript; EM revised the final approval of the version to be published. All authors read and approved the final manuscript.

Competing interests

The authors declare that they have no competing interests.

References

1. Naftalin J, Hoo W, Pateman K, et al. How common is adenomyosis? A prospective study of prevalence using transvaginal ultrasound in a gynaecology clinic. Hum Reprod. 2012;27:3432–9.
2. Azziz R. Adenomyosis: current perspectives. Obstet Gynecol Clin N Am. 1989;16:221–35.
3. Yamashiro K, Tanaka R, Nishioka K, et al. Cerebral infarcts associated with adenomyosis among middle-aged women. J Stroke Cerebrovasc Dis. 2005; 21:910.
4. Yamashiro K, Furuya T, Noda K, et al. Cerebral infarction developing in a patient without cancer with a markedly elevated level of mucinous tumor marker. J Stroke Cerebrovasc Dis. 2012;21:619. e1-e2
5. Hijikata N, Sakamoto Y, Nito C, et al. Multiple cerebral infarctions in a patient with adenomyosis on hormone replacement therapy: a case report. J Stroke Cerebrovasc Dis. 2016;25:e183–4.
6. Nishioka K, Tanaka R, Tsutsumi S, et al. Cerebral dural sinus thrombosis associated with adenomyosis: a case report. J Stroke Cerebrovasc Dis. 2014; 23:1985–7.
7. Jovin TG, Boosupalli V, Zivkovic SA, et al. High titers of CA-125 may be associated with recurrent ischemic strokes in patients with cancer. Neurology. 2005;64:1944–5.
8. Tas F, Killic L, Bilgin E, et al. Clinical and prognostic significance of coagulation assays in advanced epithelial ovarian cancer. Int J Gynecol Cancer. 2013;23:276–81.
9. Woei-A-Jin FJ, Tesselaar ME, Garcia Rodriguez P, et al. Tissue factor-bearing microparticles and CA19.9: two players in pancreatic cancer-associated thrombosis? Br J Cancer. 2016;115:332–8.
10. Bast RC Jr, Feeney M, Lazarus H, et al. Reactivity of a monoclonal antibody with human ovarian carcinoma. J Clin Invest. 1981;68:1331–7.
11. Maggino T, Gadducci A. Serum markers as prognostic factors in epithelial ovarian cancer: an overview. Eur J Gynaecol Oncol. 2000;21:64–9.
12. Lan MS, Bast RC Jr, Colnaghi MI, et al. Co-expression of human cancer-associated epitopes on mucin molecules. Int J Cancer. 1987;39:68–72.
13. Varki A. Trousseau's syndrome: multiple definitions and multiple mechanisms. Blood. 2007;110:1723–9.
14. Shao B, Wahrenbrock MG, Yao L, et al. Carcinoma mucins trigger reciprocal activation of platelets and neutrophils in a murine model of trousseau syndrome. Blood. 2011;118:4015–23.
15. Rickles FR. Mechanisms of cancer-induced thrombosis in cancer. Pathophysiol Haemost Thromb. 2006;35:103–10.
16. Rak J, Milsom C, May L, Klement P, et al. Tissue factor in cancer and angiogenesis: the molecular link between genetic tumor progression, tumor neovascularization, and cancer coagulopathy. Semin Thromb Hemost. 2006;32:54–70.
17. Li B, Chen M, Liu X, et al. Constitutive and tumor necrosis factor-α-induced activation of nuclear factor-κB in adenomyosis and its inhibition by andrographolide. Fertil Steril. 2013;100:568–77.
18. Van Es N, Bleker S, Sturk A, et al. Clinical significance of tissue factor-exposing microparticles in arterial and venous thrombosis. Semin Thromb Hemost. 2015;41:718–27.
19. Kaiafa G, Savopoulos C, Kanellos I, et al. Anemia and stroke: where do we stand? Acta Neurol Scand. 2017;135:596–602.
20. Kannel WB, Gordon T, Wolf PA, et al. Hemoglobin and the risk of cerebral infarction: the Framingham study. Stroke. 1972;3(4):409–20.

11

Clinical characteristics and short-term prognosis of LGI1 antibody encephalitis

Weishuai Li, Si Wu, Qingping Meng, Xiaotian Zhang, Yang Guo, Lin Cong, Shuyan Cong and Dongming Zheng[*] ⓘ

Abstract

Background: Recently, most reports of Leucine-rich glioma-inactivated 1 (LGI1) antibody encephalitis are from Europe and the US, while the short term outcome and clinical characteristics of Chinese patients are rarely reported,we study the clinical manifestations, laboratory results and brain magnetic resonance images (MRI) of eight patients who were recently diagnosed with LGI1 antibody encephalitis in our hospital to improve the awareness and knowledge of this disease.

Methods: Eight patients (five males and three females; mean age, 63.4) with LGI1 antibody encephalitis who were diagnosed and treated in the Department of Neurology of Shengjing Hospital of China Medical University from September 2016 to June 2017 were recruited for the current study. Their general information, clinical manifestations, treatment regimens, and short-term prognoses were retrospectively analyzed, as were the results from MRI and laboratory findings.

Results: Overall, patient symptoms included cognitive impairment, which manifested primarily as memory deficits (8/8), seizures (including faciobrachial dystonic seizure, (FBDS)) (8/8), psychiatric and behavioral disorders (7/8), sleep disorders (4/8), and autonomic abnormalities (3/8). Five patients also had abnormal findings on brain MRI, mainly involving the hippocampus, basal ganglia and insula. Hyponatremia occurred in six cases. All patients tested positive for LGI1 antibodies in their serum/cerebrospinal fluid (CSF)and patients were negative for tumors. Symptoms rapidly improved after treatment with immunoglobulin and/or steroid therapy. The patients were followed up for 4–13 months after discharge, and two patients relapsed.

Conclusion: Primary symptoms of LGI1 antibody encephalitis include memory impairments, seizures, FBDS, and mental and behavioral abnormalities. Increased titers of LGI1 antibodies are also present in the serum/CSF of patients. Patients often have hyponatremia, and MRIs show abnormalities in various brain regions. Finally, immunotherapy shows good efficacy and positive benefits, although patients may relapse in the short-term.

Keywords: Epilepsy, Autoimmune encephalitis, Magnetic resonance imaging, Cognitive function

Background

Leucine-rich glioma-inactivated 1 (LGI1) antibody encephalitis is a rare autoimmune voltage-gated potassium channel complex (VGKC) antibody-associated limbic encephalitis. Specifically, it is classified as an antineuronal surface antigen- or antisynaptic protein-associated autoimmune encephalitis [1]. In addition to the common symptoms of limbic encephalitis such as cognitive impairment, seizures, and psychiatric disorders, this disease is also associated with faciobrachial dystonic seizure (FBDS) and refractory hyponatremia [2]. Unlike other limbic encephalitides, LGI1 antibody encephalitis is rarely accompanied by tumors [3] and shows a good response to immunotherapy [4].

Current studies suggest two possible pathogenic mechanisms involving LGI1 antibodies: reducing the formation of the LGI1-ADAM complex and altering the dendritic spine density of neurons located in the dentate gyrus and thalamus [5–9].

* Correspondence: zhengdm@sj-hospital.org
Department of Neurology, Shengjing Hospital of China Medical University, Sanhao Street 36, Shenyang 110004, Liaoning, China

In the present study, we summarized and analyzed the clinical manifestations, laboratory results and brain magnetic resonance images (MRI) of eight patients who were recently diagnosed with LGI1 antibody encephalitis in our hospital to improve the awareness and knowledge of this disease.

Methods

Clinical data from eight patients who were diagnosed with LGI1 antibody encephalitis in the Department of Neurology of Shengjing Hospital of China Medical University from September 2016 to June 2017 were collected and analyzed. Clinical data included the following: clinical manifestations, laboratory and brain MRI results, treatment regimens, follow-up data and prognoses. All patients received a full range of laboratory tests, including standard biochemistry, thyroid function, syphilis, HIV, viral antibodies (including herpes simplex virus 1, 2, and herpes zoster virus), rheumatic indicators, tumor biomarkers and autoimmune encephalitis-related antibodies (NMDAR, LGI1, CASPR2, GABABR, AMPA1R, AMPA2R and other neuronal surface- or synaptic protein-related antibodies and classical paratuberculosis antibodies, such as CV2, Hu, Yo, Ri, Ma, and amphiphysin), as well as other laboratory tests. Some patients also received a cerebrospinal fluid (CSF) test. The blood or CSF autoimmune encephalitis-related antibodies were tested by an indirect immunofluorescence assay using standard kits (Euroimmun Medical Diagnostic (China) Co., Ltd., Beijing, People's Republic of China). All eight patients underwent brain MRI and dynamic electroencephalography (EEG) examinations; several submitted to a recheck of the titer of the LGI1 antibody during follow-up. This study was approved by the Ethics Committee of Shengjing Hospital in accordance with the Declaration of Helsinki. All participants provided written informed consent documents.

Results

Eight patients, including five males and three females between 41 and 73 years, participated in the study. The average age of onset of the disease was 63.4 years. The clinical data of all patients are shown in Table 1.

The first and core symptoms in this group of patients were seizures and cognitive disorders. Seizures included tonic-clonic seizures, partial seizures and FBDS; among them, dystonia-like episodes involving ipsilateral face or limbs (FBDS) were most common, while short-term memory impairment was the most obvious manifestation related to cognitive disorders. Spatial disorientation, hallucinations, and emotional changes were also common. Several patients suffered from sleeping disorders and autonomic dysfunctions, for example, sexual dysfunction, sweating and sinus bradycardia.

Routine CSF examination did not show abnormalities apart from a slightly increased white blood cell count and protein in one patient. All patients were positive for the LGI1 antibody in CSF, although the antibody titer was significantly lower than that in the peripheral blood; all patients tested positive for the LGI1 antibody in their blood. Blood sodium levels in six patients were below normal, and three others had refractory hyponatremia. All patients were negative for other autoimmune encephalitis antibodies. There were no abnormal results for thyroid function, rheumatism series and tumor biomarkers. Two patients had abnormal EEG signals, which presented separately as diffuse slow waves and paroxysmal spike-slow waves. No abnormal EEG signals were detected during FDBS. MRI identified abnormalities (high T2 signaling, low T1 signaling, and high fluid-attenuated inversion recovery [FLAIR] sequences) in the insula, hippocampus, and basal ganglia of five patients (Fig. 1). In one patient, the low T1 signal gradually increased during the follow-up period.

All patients received treatment with oral antiepileptic drugs (AEDs) and glucocorticoid therapy (intravenous infusion of methylprednisolone (1000,500,250,120 mg/d for 3 days each)). Four patients were also given intravenous immunoglobulin (0.4 g/kg/d for 5 days). The average length of stay was 16.8 days, and patients had significantly improved at discharge. All patients continued to take oral prednisone (prednisone tablets from 60 mg/d, decreased by 5 mg every 2 weeks) and AEDs, with a follow-up period of 4–13 months. Two patients relapsed within 3 months, but symptoms improved remarkably after immunotherapy. Primary posttreatment symptoms included mild memory impairments, spatial disorientation, and sleep disorders. Only one patient had subsequent seizures.

Discussion

Recently, encephalitis cases in which the antibodies target cell-surface or synaptic proteins are being identified with increasing frequency; the antigens include the N-methyl-D-aspartate receptor (NMDAR), the α-amino-3-hydroxy-5-methyl-4-isoxazolepropionic acid receptor (AMPAR), the γ-aminobutyric acid receptor-B (GABA$_B$ receptor), and voltage-gated potassium channels (VGKCs) [1]. VGKCs are now known to be leucine-rich glioma-inactivated protein 1 (LGI1) and contactin-associated protein-like 2 (Caspr2) [2]. Since antibody LGI1 encephalitis patients are characterized by acute or subacute onset of cognitive dysfunction, the disease has often been misdiagnosed as a mental illness in the past. Recent studies have also deepened the understanding of LGI1 antibody encephalitis. For example, Shin et al. indicated that this disease accounted for 11.2% of all autoimmune encephalitis [10]. Results from European-based

Table 1 Clinical manifestations of eight patients with LGI1 antibody encephalitis

Characteristic	Case1	Case2	Case3	Case4	Case5	Case6	Case7	case8
Sex	Male	Male	Female	Female	Male	Male	Female	Male
Age (years)	64	69	60	63	67	73	41	70
Onset to visit (days)	60	45	300	15	20	10	150	30
Initial symptoms	FBDS (50/d)	FBDS(20/d)	Tonic-clonic seizures (12 in total)	Tonic-clonic seizures(5 in total),	Memory deficit,	Memory deficit,	FBDS(100/d)	FBDS(40/d)
Other symptoms	Memory deficit, Partial seizures(arrector pili muscle contraction) Sleep disorder, Autonomic disorders (Sexual dysfunction, sinus bradycardia with chest tightness)	Memory deficit, Tonic-clonic(2 in total), partial seizures(3–5/d) Halluci nation(visual+ auditory) Spatial disorientation, Sleep disorder, Ataxia, Autonomic disorders(sweating)	Memory deficit, Hallucinations(auditory) Spatial disorientation, Sleep disorder, Emotional changes (irritability,indifference), Autonomic disorders (Bradycardia)	FBDS(70/d), Memory deficit, Spatial disorientation, Hallucination(visual+ auditory) Emotional changes (indifference)	Partial seizures (10–15/d) Hallucination(visual+ auditory), Sleep disorder	FBDS(50/d) Spatial disorientation Emotional changes (indifference)	Memory deficit, Emotional change (anxiety, irritability suspiciousness)	Memory deficit, Emotional change (anxiety)
MMSE score (0–30)(Education)	University	high school	high school	high school	University	University	University	high school
Admission misse points	26 recall (1) calculation(1) orientation(1) complex commands (1)	16 recall (3) calculation (3) orientation (3)repetition (1) complex commands (1)	18 recall (3) calculation (3) orientation (3) repetition (1) complex commands (4)	15 registration (1) recall (3) calculation (3) orientation (3) repetition (1) complex commands(3)	20 recall (2) calculation (2) orientation (3) complex commands(3)	22 recall (2) calculation (2) orientation (1) complex commands(3)	23 recall (2) calculation (2) orientation (1) complex commands(2)	14 registration (1) recall (3) calculation (3) orientation (3) repetition (1) complex commands(5)
Discharge misse points	30	23 recall (2) calculation (1) orientation (1) complex commands (3)	28 recall (1) complex commands(1)	26 recall (1) calculation (1) orientation (1) complex commands(1)	25 recall (1) calculation (1) orientation (1) complex commands(2)	28 recall (1) orientation (1)	29 recall (1)	26 recall (1) calculation (1) orientation (1) complex commands(1)
LGi1 antibody (serum)	1:10 (before admission) 1:32 (after admission)	1:32	1:32	1:10	1:32	1:32	1:100	1:32
LGi1 antibody (CSF)	1:1	–	–	1:1	1:3.2	1:1	–	–
Blood sodium (normal 135–155 mmol/L)	135.1	130	127.9	126	131.4	121.2	132	140
White blood cell (CSF) (normal 0–5 × 106/L)	4	–	–	2	10	2	–	–
Protein(CSF) (normal 0.15–0.45 g/L)	0.25	–	–	0.31	0.46	0.28	–	–
Glucose(CSF)(normal 2.5–4.5 mmol/L)	3.5	–	–	4.07	3.91	4.1	–	–
Brain MRI	Right insula	Norma	Bilateral hippocampus	Bilateral caudate nucleus+ putamen	Right hippocampus	Normal	Right caudate nucleus	Normal
EEG	Normal	Normal	Normal	Diffuse slow wave (4-6 Hz)	Paroxysmal spike-slow wave (right frontal lobe,middle and posterior temporal lobe)	Normal	Normal	Normal

Table 1 Clinical manifestations of eight patients with LGI1 antibody encephalitis (Continued)

Characteristic	Case1	Case2	Case3	Case4	Case5	Case6	Case7	case8
AEDs	Levetiracetam Lamotrigine	Sodium valproate	Sodium valproate	Sodium valproate	Levetiracetam	Levetiracetam	Sodium valproate	Sodium valproate
Immunotherapy	methylprednisolone +Gamma globulin	methylprednisolone	methylprednisolone	methylprednisolone +Gamma globulin	methylprednisolone +Gamma globulin	methylprednisolone + Gamma globulin	methylprednisolone	methylprednisolone
Symptoms at discharge	FBDS disappeared	FBDS reduction	No seizures	FBDS disappeared	No seizures	FBDS disappeared	FBDS disappeared	FBDS disappeared
Length of stay(days)	13	15	16	12	21	25	17	15
Follow up time(months)	4	4	7	6	6	13	4	4
serum antibody follow up	1:10	–	1:32	–	–	–	–	–
Relapse(months)	No	No	No	1	No	3	No	No
Remaining symptoms	amnesia	amnesia Spatial disorientation	amnesia Insomnia	amnesia	Insomnia	amnesia Spatial disorientation	No	amnesia
AEDs	No	Sodium valproate	Sodium valproate	Sodium valproate	Levetiracetam	Levetiracetam	Sodium valproate	Sodium valproate
Seizure	No	No	No	No	Occasionally(absence seizures)	No	No	No

'-', No test information;
Abbreviations: CSF cerebrospinal fluid, FBDS faciobrachial dystonic seizure, MMSE Mini-Mental State Examination, LGI1 leucine-rich glioma-inactivated 1, AEDs antiepileptic drugs, EEG electroencephalography

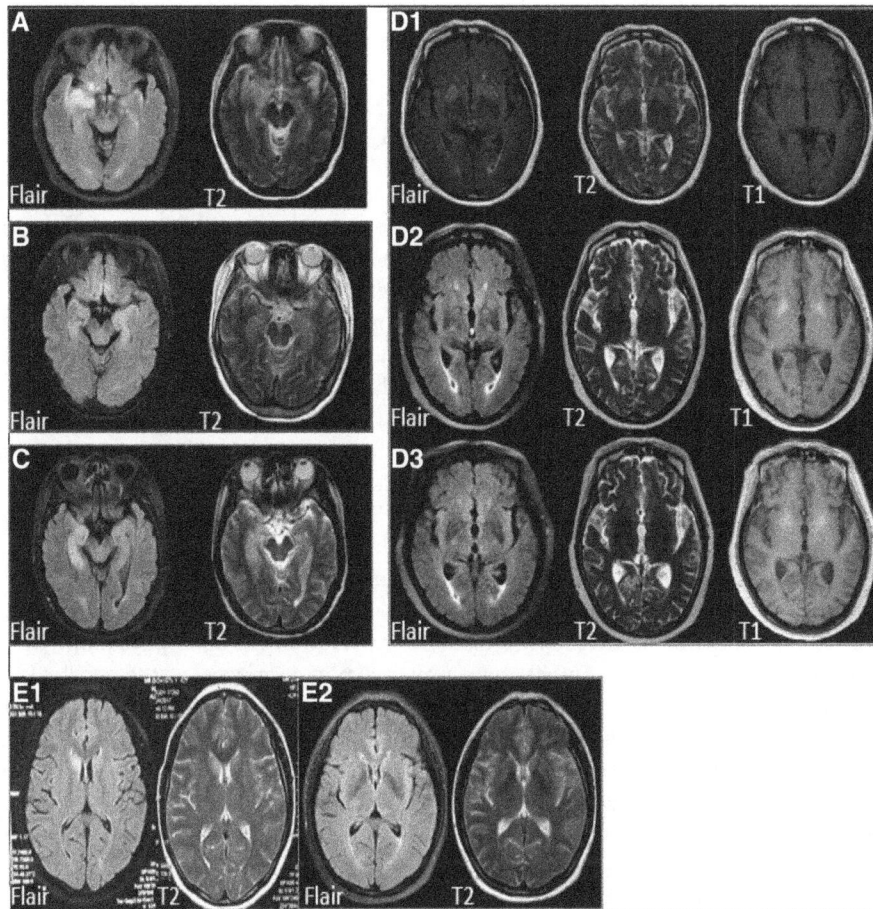

Fig. 1 MRI images of five patients with LGI1 antibody encephalitis. **a** FLAIR sequences and high T2 signal changes in the right insula in case 1; **b** FLAIR sequences and high T2 signal changes in the bilateral hippocampus in case 3; **c** FLAIR sequences and high T2 signal changes in the right hippocampus in case 5; **D**1 Abnormal signals in the bilateral caudate nucleus and putamen in case 4 at admission; MRI follow-up after 1 month (**D**2) and 2 months (**D**3) showed that the lesion signal intensity changed to a high T1 signal; (**E**1) Abnormal signals in bilateral caudate nucleus in case 7 at admission; **E**2 MRI of case 7 after 5 months. Abbreviations: MRI, magnetic resonance imaging; FLAIR, fluid-attenuated inversion recovery

studies showed that the peak age of disease onset was between 61 and 64 years and that males accounted for 55–66% of the patient population, while the annual rate of incidence was 0.63–0.83/million [11, 12]. The average age of onset of the disease of the eight cases in our study was 63.4 years old, and five were male, which was in line with the European data.

Our study also showed that epilepsy and cognitive impairments were common and prominent clinical manifestations in patients with LGI1 antibody encephalitis. Epilepsy was the initial symptom in the majority of the patients, with several patients exhibiting multiple forms of seizures. Seizures involving ipsilateral face and/or limb dystonia-like seizures (FBDS) were the most common characteristic. We also showed FBDS were short duration and high in frequency. In most cases, the seizures were not accompanied by conscious disturbances, and in several instances, they were difficult to capture by EEG. These clinical features agree with previous reports

[2, 11]; FBDS appear earlier than other symptoms in many patients [10, 13], while tonic-clonic seizures often occur concurrently or immediately after a decline in patient cognitive function [11]. Therefore, it was suggested that following initial FBDS, immediate immunotherapy treatment might prevent the development of cognitive impairments [14]. In our study, six patients had FBDS, and four patients experienced these seizures prior to cognitive impairment. Interestingly, the conditions of these patients gradually worsened. We believe this was a direct result of being administered only antiepileptic treatments and not immunotherapy treatments. Given that FBDS occur early and have a high incidence in LGI1 antibody encephalitis, we suggest that all patients with FBDS be examined for increased LGI1 antibody titers as soon as possible, and upon definitive diagnosis, immunotherapy be initiated immediately. These measures may largely prevent the onset of cognitive impairment.

Interestingly, it is still arguable whether FBDS are dystonic or epileptic seizures. Epileptic waves have been recorded in patients during FBDS [15], while studies also showed that epileptic seizures occurred if LGI1 gene expression was deficient [6, 16]. However, others believe that the causative lesions in patients with FBDS occur in the basal ganglia and do not affect EEG readings, and therefore, FBDS is a type of dystonia derived from deep brain dysfunction [17, 18]. In our study, two patients had FBDS-associated basal ganglia lesions, suggesting that FBDS may be associated specifically with these lesions. Therefore, the specific mechanisms involving the onset of FBDS need further study.

Our results regarding memory deficits and disorientation as the primary manifestations of LGI1 antibody encephalitis-associated cognitive impairment in the patients are in agreement with previous studies, as were results demonstrating changes in both personality and mood and patient hallucinations (visual and/or auditory) [11, 12, 19]. It has been proposed that memory impairment is due to the interaction of LGI1-ADAM22-AMPAR affecting long-term depression and long-term potentiation [20]. Collingridge et al. found that long-term depression was also closely associated with the formation of spatial memory [21]. In our study, two patients were first treated for dementia because in both cases, their initial symptom was memory deficit. Therefore, caution is needed when making initial diagnoses in middle-aged and elderly patients who present with memory deficit. In addition to the aforementioned typical symptoms, patients with LGI1 antibody encephalitis can also exhibit, among other symptoms, sleep or autonomic disorders and ataxias [11, 14, 22, 23]. Although less frequent, these symptoms also occurred in the patients in our study.

Over half of patients suffering from LGI1 antibody encephalitis also exhibit hyponatremia and in most cases, refractory hyponatremia [2, 12]. The pathogenic mechanism involved in the onset of hyponatremia is likely associated with lowered antidiuretic hormone levels due to the effects of LGI1 antibodies on the hypothalamic paraventricular nucleus and kidney [24]. In our study, hyponatremia occurred in six patients, and three presented with refractory hyponatremia, highlighting the prevalence of hyponatremia in patients with LGI1 antibody encephalitis.

Patients with LGI1 antibody encephalitis are often normal in routine CSF tests [25]; the positive rate of LGI1 antibody detection in CSF is lower than that in serum [26]. Even if CSF is positive for LGI1 antibodies, its titer is only 1 to 10% of a serum titer [27]. Therefore, if LGI1 antibody encephalitis is suspected, routine serum tests for autoimmune encephalitis antibodies are first performed, thus occasionally negating the need for invasive lumbar punctures. As expected, both serum and CSF LGI1 antibody titers can decrease or increase with the disease remission and relapse, respectively [3, 28]. However, Ariño et al. showed that lowered LGI1 antibody titers were not significantly associated with patient prognosis [26], and in agreement with this, one patient in our study who recovered did not have decreased LGI1 titer levels compared with disease onset levels. Taking these findings together, we speculate that antibody titer does not always correlate with disease severity and therefore needs further investigation.

Approximately 70% of patients with LGI1 antibody encephalitis have increased T2 and FLAIR MRI signals in the hippocampus or temporal lobe (unilaterally or bilaterally), and some can extend to the amygdala, insula or striatum [11, 12]. Flanagan et al. found that ~ 40% of patients also had basal ganglia lesions corresponding to FBDS, and T1 hyperintensities either occurred concurrently with or were preceded by short-lived T2 hyperintensities during the episodes, with T1 hyperintensities persisting longer than T2 hyperintensities; regarding the T1 hyperintensity pathophysiology, the authors suggest that hypoxic damage is the most likely substrate [29]. Examples of these abnormal images can be found in our study: the follow-up MRIs of 5 months showed that basal ganglia lesions completely regressed in one patient, although the condition of the patient was exacerbated (Fig. 1 E1-E2); another patient showed increased T1 signaling in the initial lesion region after 1and 2 months later (Fig. 1 D1-D3). The above results suggest that the presence or absence of abnormal MRI findings is related to the time of onset. The different MRI examination times may lead to the illusion that the imaging results and clinical symptoms are inconsistent. Therefore, the time when the T1 and T2 abnormalities occur and the time of existence requires further study.

In view of similar clinical manifestations, the diagnosis of LGI1 antibody encephalitis need to be distinguished from viral encephalitis, Hashimoto's encephalopathy, Creutzfeldt's disease (CJD), and other forms of autoimmune encephalitis [30]. In combination with clinical manifestations, laboratory tests, and imaging examinations, the diagnosis of LGI1 antibody encephalitis is usually correct; however, it should be noted that increased LGI1 antibody titers were also found in a pathologically confirmed CJD case [31]. We therefore recommend using a combination of examinations to confidently and correctly diagnose LGI1 antibody encephalitis.

First-line therapies for the disease include intravenous glucocorticoid therapy and immunoglobulin and plasma exchange, with early combinatorial treatments providing better efficacy [10, 11, 30]. In addition to these combinatorial treatments, it is sometimes necessary to supplement treatment with cyclophosphamide or rituximab [32]. Studies have shown that ~ 80% of patients had a reduction in seizures and had improvements in cognitive impairments after a 2-week first-line treatment regimen; while 70% of patients had a good prognosis after a 2-year follow up, the recurrence rate was ~ 30%, and most recurrences occurred in the first 6 months; a small number of patients needed long-term administration of oral immunomodulatory agents and AEDs; and finally, the mortality rate of LGI1 antibody encephalitis is 6–19% [11, 26].

In the present study, all eight patients showed symptom improvement after a 2-week first-line treatment regimen. Patients were followed up for 4–13 months, and the overall recovery was good. The major remaining symptoms were amnesia, spatial disorientation, and insomnia. Two patients relapsed within 3 months and presented with frequent episodes of FBDS, which were reversed after intravenous injection of glucocorticoids and immunoglobulins. In the final follow-up, seven patients still took oral AEDs, and only one patient had occasional seizures.

Limitations

We obtained the most reliable data by analyzing patients' files and interviewing patients, relatives, and treating physicians, and all MRIs were reviewed by a specialized neuroradiologist. However, given the retrospective nature of this study, the limited number of patients, the short duration of the follow-up, and the variable laboratory and brain MRI timing, the conclusions about clinical characteristics and the short-term prognosis of LGI1 antibody encephalitis have limitations.

Conclusion

The primary symptoms of LGI1 antibody encephalitis include cognitive impairment (recent memory loss or spatial disorders), seizures (typically FBDS), hyponatremia, and sleep disorders, while serum titers (and occasionally cerebrospinal fluid) of LGI1 antibodies are increased. In addition, brain MRIs may indicate abnormal signals in the temporal lobe, hippocampus, or basal ganglia.

Early immunotherapy can achieve both increased efficacy and good long-term prognosis. We believe that if patients present with recurrent epileptic seizures and cognitive dysfunctions, LGI1 antibody testing should be promptly performed and appropriate treatments given immediately. These measures will not only improve seizure control but also may improve long-term prognosis.

Abbreviations

AEDs: Antiepileptic drugs; AMPAR: α-amino-3-hydroxy-5-methyl-4-isoxazolepropionic acid receptor; Caspr2: Contactin-associated protein-like 2; CJD: Creutzfeldt's disease; CSF: Cerebrospinal fluid; EEG: Electroencephalography; FBDS: Faciobrachial dystonic seizure; FLAIR: fluid-attenuated inversion recovery; GABA-B receptor: γ-aminobutyric acid receptor-B; LGI1: leucine-rich glioma-inactivated 1; MRI: magnetic resonance imaging; NMDAR: N-methyl-D-aspartate receptor; VGKC: Voltage-gated potassium channel complex; VGKCs: Voltage-gated potassium channels

Acknowledgments
We thank all of the subjects and medical staff for their assistance with this study.

Funding
Data collection, analysis, and interpretation of the study was supported by grants from the Natural Science Foundation of Liaoning Province (Grant No. 201602883).

Authors' contributions
S-W, Q-pM, S-yC, X-tZ, C-L and Y-G collected the data and participated in the clinical evaluation of the patients, performed MRI and dynamic electroencephalography data analysis and interpretation. W-sL wrote the main manuscript text and analyzed the data, while D-mZ participated in the design and coordination of the study and has been involved in revising the manuscript for important intellectual content, All authors read and approved the final manuscript.

Competing interests
The authors declare that they have no competing interests.

References

1. ELancaster , J Dalmau. Neuronalautoantigens–pathogenesis, associated disorders and antibody testing. Nat Rev Neurol. 2012;8:380–90.
2. IraniSR AS, Waters P, Kleopa KA, Pettingill P, Zuliani L, Peles E, Buckley C, Lang B, Vincent A. Antibodies to Kv1 potassiumchannel-complex proteins leucine-rich, glioma inactivated 1 protein andcontactin-associated protein-2 in limbic encephalitis, Morvan's syndrome andacquired neuromyotonia. Brain. 2010;133:2734–48.
3. Irani SR, Gelfand JM, Al-Diwani A, Vincent A. Cell-surface central nervous system autoantibodies:clinical relevance and emerging paradigms. Ann Neurol. 2014;76:168–84.
4. Asztely F, Kumlien E. The diagnosis and treatment of limbic encephalitis. Acta Neurol Scand. 2012;126:365–75.
5. Lai M, Huijbers MG, Lancaster E, Graus F, Bataller L, Balice-Gordon R, Cowell JK, Dalmau J. Investigation of LGI1 as theantigen in limbic encephalitis previously attributed to potassiumchannels: a case series. Lancet Neurol. 2010;9:776–85.
6. Fukata Y, Lovero KL, Iwanaga T, Watanabe A, Yokoi N, Tabuchi K, Shigemoto R, Nicoll RA, Fukata M. Disruption of LGI1-linked synaptic complex causes abnormal synaptic transmission and epilepsy. Proc Natl Acad Sci U S A. 2010;107:3799–804.
7. Thomas R, Favell K, Morante-Redolat J, Pool M, Kent C, Wright M, Daignault K, Ferraro GB, Montcalm S, Durocher Y, et al. LGI1 is a Nogo receptor 1 ligand that antagonizes myelin-based growth inhibition. J Neurosci. 2010;30: 6607–12.
8. Zhou YD, Lee S, Jin Z, Wright M, Smith SE, Anderson MP. Arrestedmaturation of excitatory synapses in autosomal dominant lateral temporal lobe epilepsy. Nat Med. 2009;15:1208–14.
9. Zhou YD, Zhang D, Ozkaynak E, Wang X, Kasper EM, Leguern E, Baulac S, Anderson MP. Epilepsy gene LGI1 regulates postnatal developmental remodelingof retinogeniculate synapses. J Neurosci. 2012;32:903–10.
10. Shin YW, Lee ST, Shin JW, Moon J, Lim JA, Byun JI, Kim TJ, Lee KJ, Kim YS, Park KI, et al. VGKC-complex/LGI1-antibodyencephalitis: clinical manifestations and response to immunotherapy. J Neuroimmunol. 2013;265:75–81.
11. van Sonderen A, Thijs RD, Coenders EC, Jiskoot LC, Sanchez E, de Bruijn MA, van Coevorden-Hameete MH, Wirtz PW, Schreurs MW, Sillevis Smitt PA, Titulaer MJ. Anti-LGI1 encephalitis: Clinical syndrome and long-term follow-up. Neurology. 2016;87:1449–56.
12. Celicanin M, Blaabjerg M, Maersk-Moller C, Beniczky S, Marner L, Thomsen C, Bach FW, Kondziella D, Andersen H, Somnier F, Illes Z, Pinborg LH. Autoimmune encephalitis associated with voltage-gated

potassiumchannels-complex and leucine-rich glioma-inactivated 1 antibodies a national cohort study. Eur J Neurol. 2017;24:999–1005.

13. Irani SR, Michell AW, Lang B, Pettingill P, Waters P, Johnson MR, Schott JM, Armstrong RJ, S Zagami A, Bleasel A, et al. Faciobrachial dystonicseizures precede LGI1 antibody limbic encephalitis. Ann Neurol. 2011;69:892–900.

14. Irani SR, Stagg CJ, Schott JM, Rosenthal CR, Schneider SA, Pettingill P, Pettingill R, Waters P, Thomas A, Voets NL, et al. Faciobrachial dystonicseizures: the influence of immunotherapy on seizure control and prevention of cognitive impairment in a broadening phenotype. Brain. 2013;136:3151–62.

15. Andrade DM, Tai P, Dalmau J, Wennberg R. Tonic seizures: adiagnostic clue of anti-LGI1 encephalitis ? Neurology. 2011;76:1355–7.

16. Chabrol E, Navarro V, Provenzano G, Cohen I, Dinocourt C, Rivaud-Péchoux S, Fricker D, Baulac M, Miles R, Leguern E, Baulac S. Electroclinical characterization of epileptic seizures in leucine-rich, glioma-inactivated 1-deficient mice. Brain. 2010;133:2749–62.

17. Naasan G, Irani SR, Bettcher BM, Geschwind MD, Gelfand JM. Episodic bradycardia asneurocardiac prodrome to voltage-gated potassium channel complex/leucine-rich, glioma inactivated 1 antibody encephalitis. JAMA Neurol. 2014;71:1300–4.

18. Ramdhani RA, Frucht SJ. Isolated chorea associated with LGI1 antibody. Tremor Other Hyperkinet Mov (N Y). 2014;4

19. Wegner F, Wilke F, Raab P, Tayeb SB, Boeck AL, Haense C, Trebst C, Voss E, Schrader C, Logemann F, et al. Anti-leucine rich glioma inactivated 1 protein and anti-N-methyl-D-aspartate receptor encephalitisshow distinct patterns of brain glucose metabolism in 18F-fluoro-2-de-oxy-d-glucose positron emission tomography. BMC Neurol. 2014;20:136–47.

20. Ohkawa T, Fukata Y, Yamasaki M, Miyazaki T, Yokoi N, Takashima H, Watanabe M, Watanabe O, Fukata M. Autoantibodies to epilepsy-related LGI1 in limbic encephalitis neutralize LGI1-ADAM22 interaction and reduce synaptic AMPA receptors. J Neurosci. 2013;33:18161–74.

21. Collingridge GL, Peineau S, Howland JG, Wang YT. Long-term depression in the CNS. Nat Rev Neurosci. 2010;11:459–73.

22. Dalmau PJ, Lancaster E, Martinez-Hernandez E, Rosenfeld PMR, Balice-Gordon PR. Clinical experience and laboratory investigations in patients with anti-NMDAR encephalitis. Lancet Neurol. 2011;10:63–74.

23. Nilsson AC, Blaabjerg M. More evidence of a neurocardiac prodrome in anti-LGI1 encephalitis. J Neurol Sci. 2015;357:310–1.

24. Ellison DH, Berl T. Clinical practice The syndrome of inappropriate antidiuresis. N Engl J Med. 2007;356:2064–72.

25. Szots M, Marton A, Kover F, Kiss T, Berki T, Nagy F, Illes Z. Natural course of LGI1 encephalitis: 3-5years of follow-up without immunotherapy. J Neurol Sci. 2014;343:198–202.

26. Ariño H, Armangué T, Petit-Pedrol M, Sabater L, Martinez-Hernandez E, Hara M , Lancaster E, Saiz A, Dalmau J, Graus F.Anti-LGI1-associated cognitive impairment:Presentation and long-term outcome.Neurology2016;87:759–765.

27. Vincent A, Buckley C, Schott JM, Baker I, Dewar BK, Detert N, Clover L, Parkinson A, Bien CG, Omer S, et al. Potassium channel antibody associated encephalopathy: a potentially immunotherapy-responsive form of limbic encephalitis. Brain. 2004;127:701–12.

28. Agazzi P, Bien CG, Staedler C, Biglio V, Gobbi C. Over 10-year follow-up of limbic encephalitis associated with anti-LGI1 antibodies. J Neurol. 2015;262: 469–70.

29. Flanagan EP, Kotsenas AL, Britton JW, McKeon A, Watson RE, Klein CJ, Boeve BF, Lowe V, Ahlskog JE, Shin C, et al. Basal gangliaT1 hyperintensity in LGI1-autoantibody faciobrachial dystonic seizures. Neurol Neuroimmunol Neuroinflamm. 2015;2:1–8.

30. Wang M, Cao X, Liu Q, Ma W, Guo X, Liu X. Clinical features of limbic encephalitis with LGI1 antibody. Neuropsychiatr Dis Treat. 2017;13:1589–96.

31. Kim B, Yoo P, Sutherland T, Collins SLGI. 1 antibody encephalopathy overlapping with sporadic Creutzfeldt-Jakob disease. Neurol Neuroimmunol Neuroinflamm. 2016;3:1–5.

32. Gastaldi M, Thoui A, Vincent A. Antibody–mediated autoimmune encephalopathies and immunotherapies. Neurotherpeutics. 2016;13:147–62.

12

Altered development of dopaminergic neurons differentiated from stem cells from human exfoliated deciduous teeth of a patient with Down syndrome

Thanh Thi Mai Pham[1], Hiroki Kato[1]*(iD), Haruyoshi Yamaza[1], Keiji Masuda[1], Yuta Hirofuji[1], Hiroshi Sato[1], Huong Thi Nguyen Nguyen[1], Xu Han[1], Yu Zhang[1], Tomoaki Taguchi[2] and Kazuaki Nonaka[1]

Abstract

Background: Down syndrome (DS) is a common developmental disorder resulting from the presence of an additional copy of chromosome 21. Abnormalities in dopamine signaling are suggested to be involved in cognitive dysfunction, one of the symptoms of DS, but the pathophysiological mechanism has not been fully elucidated at the cellular level. Stem cells from human exfoliated deciduous teeth (SHED) can be prepared from the dental pulp of primary teeth. Importantly, SHED can be collected noninvasively, have multipotency, and differentiate into dopaminergic neurons (DN). Therefore, we examined dopamine signaling in DS at the cellular level by isolating SHED from a patient with DS, differentiating the cells into DN, and examining development and function of DN.

Methods: Here, SHED were prepared from a normal participant (Ctrl-SHED) and a patient with DS (DS-SHED). Initial experiments were performed to confirm the morphological, chromosomal, and stem cell characteristics of both SHED populations. Next, Ctrl-SHED and DS-SHED were differentiated into DN and morphological analysis of DN was examined by immunostaining. Functional analysis of DN was performed by measuring extracellular dopamine levels under basal and glutamate-stimulated conditions. In addition, expression of molecules involved in dopamine homeostasis was examined by quantitative real-time polymerase chain reaction and immunostaining. Statistical analysis was performed using two-tailed Student's t-tests.

Results: Compared with Ctrl-SHED, DS-SHED showed decreased expression of nestin, a neural stem-cell marker. Further, DS-SHED differentiated into DN (DS-DN) exhibiting decreased neurite outgrowth and branching compared with Ctrl-DN. In addition, DS-DN dopamine secretion was lower than Ctrl-DN dopamine secretion. Moreover, aberrant expression of molecules involved in dopaminergic homeostasis was observed in DS-DN.

Conclusions: Our results suggest that there was developmental abnormality and DN malfunction in the DS-SHED donor in this study. In the future, to clarify the detailed mechanism of dopamine-signal abnormality due to DN developmental and functional abnormalities in DS, it is necessary to increase the number of patients for analysis. Non-invasively harvested SHED may be very useful in the analysis of DS pathology.

Keywords: Down syndrome, Dopamine, Human exfoliated deciduous teeth, SHED, Stem cells, Dopaminergic neurons, Differentiation, Dopamine secretion

* Correspondence: kato@dent.kyushu-u.ac.jp
[1]Section of Oral Medicine for Child, Division of Oral Health, Growth & Development, Faculty of Dental Science, Kyushu University, Maidashi 3-1-1, Higashi-Ku, Fukuoka 812-8582, Japan
Full list of author information is available at the end of the article

Background

Down syndrome (DS) is caused by an extra copy of chromosome 21 and is one of the most common developmental disorders. Reported symptoms of DS include impairment of cognitive functions, such as learning, memory, language, and executive function [1–4]. Dopamine (DA) is an important neurotransmitter in the regulation of cognitive function. It has been suggested that disturbance of the DA signaling system causes the cognitive impairments observed in DS [5–7].

The amount of DA in the brain and cerebrospinal fluid (CSF) of patients with DS has been reported to be both higher and lower than that in healthy people [8, 9], suggesting that a disturbance in DA homeostasis is implicated in DS. It has also been reported that there is reduced expression of DA receptors D1R and D2R in the brains of patients with DS [10]. As observed in patients with DS, varied amounts of DA have also been reported in mouse models of DS [6, 7, 11, 12], suggesting that variable DA levels are associated with abnormal brain development. However, the role of the DA signaling system in DS pathology has yet to be analyzed at a cellular level.

Stem cells from human exfoliated deciduous teeth (SHED) can be acquired noninvasively and used for research [13–15]. Thus, using SHED, consent to participate in research may be obtained more readily from the parents of young patients. SHED can be differentiated into dopaminergic neurons (DN) and used for the treatment of a parkinsonian rat model [16, 17]. The authors have also previously used SHED derived from a patient with Rett syndrome to elucidate the relationship between abnormal DN development and decreased mitochondrial function in vitro [18]. Therefore, SHED are a valuable source of stem cells for DN transplantation and for in vitro disease models.

The aim of this study was to elucidate a relationship between DS and abnormal DN development and function. Here, SHED were prepared from a normal participant and a patient with DS and were then used to examine DS pathology on a cellular level. Our results demonstrate the utility of SHED as a disease model for DS.

Methods

Isolation and preparation of SHED

Human exfoliated deciduous teeth were provided by Pediatric Dentistry and Special Need Dentistry at Kyushu University Hospital in Japan. After informed parental consent was obtained, deciduous teeth were collected from a normal participant and a patient with DS at 6 and 14 years of age, respectively. The isolation procedure was completed as previously described [15]. Briefly, the pulp tissue was subjected to an enzymatic dissociation in 3 mg/mL collagenase I (Washington, NJ, USA) and 4 mg/mL dispase II (Wako, Osaka, Japan) for 1 h, and then maintained at 37 °C

in a humidified 5% CO_2 incubator in the Alpha modification of Eagle's Minimal Essential Medium (α-MEM; Sigma-Aldrich, MO, USA) containing 15% fetal bovine serum (Sigma-Aldrich), 100 μM L-ascorbic acid 2-phosphate (Wako), 2 mM L-glutamine (Life Technologies, NY, USA), 250 μg/mL Fungizone (Life Technologies), 100 U/mL penicillin (Life Technologies), and 100 μg/mL streptomycin (Life Technologies). Cells of not more than 10 passages were used, but Ctrl-SHED and DS-SHED were not always of the same passage.

Fluorescence in situ hybridization

SHED were treated with 75 mM KCl for 40 min and then fixed with 3:1 ethanol:acetic acid (v/v). Fluorescence in situ hybridization (FISH) of chromosome 21 was performed with a chromosome 21 control probe labeling the BAC probe, followed by the standard procedure with green 5-Fluorescein dUTP (CHR21–10-GR; Empire Genomics, NY, USA). Hybridization was performed by denaturing the slides in 70% formamide/2× standard saline citrate, dehydrating the slides with serial ethanol washes, and applying the probe to the slides. Post-hybridization, the slides were washed and stained with 0.1 μg/mL 4′,6-diamidino-2-phenylindole (DAPI; Dojindo, Kumamoto, Japan) to identify nuclei. Fluorescence images were taken with a Zeiss Axio Imager M2 microscope (Zeiss, Oberkochen, Germany) equipped with ApoTome2 (Zeiss).

Western blotting

Whole-cell lysates were extracted with lysis buffer (62.5 mM Tris-HCl pH 6.8, 2% SDS, 5% β-mercaptoethanol, and 10% glycerol), and the protein concentration was measured using Bradford ULTRA (Novexin, Cambridge, UK). A total of 5 μg of protein was separated by SDS-PAGE and transferred to a polyvinylidene difluoride membrane. After blocking with 5% non-fat milk for 30 min, the membrane was incubated overnight at 4 °C with anti-nestin (1:1000; Millipore, CA, USA) and anti-HSP90 (1:1000; Santa Cruz Biotechnology, CA, USA) antibodies. Membranes were washed and incubated with HRP-conjugated secondary antibody (1:5000; Santa Cruz Biotechnology) for 1 h at room temperature and visualized with ECL prime (GE Healthcare, Buckinghamshire, UK). The chemiluminescent signals were detected and quantified using LAS-1000 pro (Fuji Film, Tokyo, Japan) with Image Gauge software (Fuji Film). HSP90 was used as an internal control. To normalize the nestin expression, the chemiluminescent signal of nestin was divided by the chemiluminescent signal of HSP90.

DN differentiation

DN differentiation was induced as previously described with minor modifications (brain derived neurotrophic factor [BDNF] was excluded in the second step) [16]. In the first step, 1.5×10^5 SHED were plated onto a 6-well culture plate or glass coverslips coated with 0.01% poly-L-lysine (Sigma-Aldrich), in the same culture medium as described above. They were incubated overnight at 37 °C in the presence of 5% CO_2, and were then cultured in serum-free Dulbecco's Modified Eagle's Medium (DMEM, Sigma-Aldrich) supplemented with 20 ng/mL epidermal growth factor (Sigma-Aldrich), 20 ng/mL basic fibroblast growth factor (Peprotech, NJ, USA), and 1% N2 supplement (Life Technologies) for 2 days at 37 °C, in the presence of 5% CO_2. In the second step, DMEM was replaced with neurobasal medium (Life Technologies) supplemented with 2% B27 supplement (Life Technologies), 1 mM dibutyryladenosine 3,5-cyclic monophosphate (Sigma-Aldrich), 0.5 mM 3-isobutyl-1-methylxanthine (Sigma-Aldrich), and 200 µM ascorbic acid (Nacalai Tesque, Kyoto, Japan), and cells were incubated for 5 days, at 37 °C, in the presence of 5% CO_2.

Immunocytochemistry

The cells cultured on coverslips were fixed with 4% paraformaldehyde in 0.1 M phosphate buffer (pH 7.4) for 10 min. The cells were permeabilized with 0.1% TritonX-100 for 5 min, then blocked with 2% bovine serum albumin (BSA; Wako) in PBS for 20 min at room temperature. Next, cells were stained with primary antibodies against STRO-1 (1:100; Millipore), nestin (1:250; Millipore), β-tubulin III (1:250; Sigma-Aldrich), tyrosine hydroxylase (TH; 1:100; Millipore), N-methyl-d-aspartate receptor subunit 1 (NMDAR1; 1:100; Millipore), and DA (1:200; Abcam) for 90 min. Following this, cells were incubated with Alexa Fluor secondary antibodies (1:500; Life Technologies) for 1 h at room temperature in the dark. The cells were counterstained with 0.1 µg/mL DAPI (Dojindo) for 5 min, and then mounted with ProLong diamond (Life Technologies). The fluorescence images were taken with Nikon C2 confocal microscope (Nikon, Tokyo, Japan) in Fig. 1c and 3a, with Zeiss LSM700 confocal scanning microscope (Zeiss) in Fig. 2a and d, with Zeiss Axio Imager M2 microscope (Zeiss) equipped with ApoTome2 (Zeiss) in Fig. 4c and d.

Morphological analysis of DN

For morphological analysis, the TH-immunostained images were analyzed with MetaMorph software (Molecular Devices, CA, USA). A morphological analysis of DN was performed as previously described [19]. Briefly, neurite length and number of branches were measured from 100 TH-positive cells in 20 non-overlapping TH-immunostained images selected randomly from three experiments using the Neurite Outgrowth and Multi-Wavelength Cell Scoring module of MetaMorph software (Molecular Devices). Next, the cells were classified into 4 stages based on neurite length and cell diameter as previously described [19].

Measurement of NMDAR1 puncta in neurite

To measure the number of NMDAR1 puncta per unit length of neurite, DN were immunostained with anti-NMDAR1 and anti-TH antibodies. Thirty neurites that were in focus and clearly observed were chosen from 10 Ctrl-DN and 12 DS-DN that were positive for both NMDAR1 and TH. These cells were randomly chosen from three experiments. The number of NMDAR1 puncta per 25 µm of neurite was analyzed.

Extracellular DA measurement

Extracellular DA was measured using a Dopamine Research ELISA kit (BA E-5300, LDN, Nordhorn, Germany) according to the manufacturer's instructions. SHED were plated at a concentration of 5×10^5 cells per 6-cm dish and differentiated into DN. 500 µl of culture medium was collected to measure extracellular DA. To measure extracellular DA under glutamate stimulated conditions, the cells were treated with 30 µM L-glutamate for 1 min at 37 °C before harvesting the medium. Next, the cell culture medium was centrifuged at 20,400 g for 5 min at 4 °C to remove cell debris and immediately stored at – 80 °C until assayed. Subsequently, total protein was extracted from cells using lysis buffer (62.5 mM Tris-HCl pH 6.8 supplemented with 2% SDS, 5% β-mercaptoethanol, and 10% glycerol), and the protein concentration was measured using Bradford ULTRA (Novexin). To normalize the DA amount in each sample, the DA amount was divided by the total protein of that sample.

RNA extraction and quantitative real-time polymerase chain reaction (RT-qPCR)

Total RNA was extracted from the cells using an RNAeasy Mini Kit (Qiagen, Hilden, Germany). First-strand cDNA was synthesized using a ReverTra Ace qPCR RT Master Mix with gDNA Remover (Toyobo, Osaka, Japan). The sequences of primer sets used in this study were as follows: DAT1: 5'-TGCTGCACAGACACCGTGAG-3' (forward), 5'-AATGGTCCAGGAGCGTGAAGA-3' (reverse); VMA T2: 5'-TGAAGAGAGAGGCAACGTCA-3' (forward), 5'-CGTCTTCCCCACAAACTCAT-3' (reverse); HPRT1: 5'-CCTGGCGTCGTGATTAGTG-3' (forward), 5'-TCCC ATCTCCTTCATCACATC-3' (reverse). Real-time quantitative PCR was performed using GoTaq qPCR Master Mix (Promega, WI, USA) and analyzed with StepOnePlus Real-Time PCR Systems (Life Technologies). The threshold cycle (Ct) value of HPRT1 was subtracted from the Ct value of the target genes (ΔCt). Statistical analysis was performed using the ΔCt values from four experiments. The relative expressions of the target genes are shown as fold changes determined using the $2^{-\Delta\Delta Ct}$ method.

Statistical analysis

Values are represented as mean ± standard error of the mean (SEM) from at least three experiments. Two-tailed

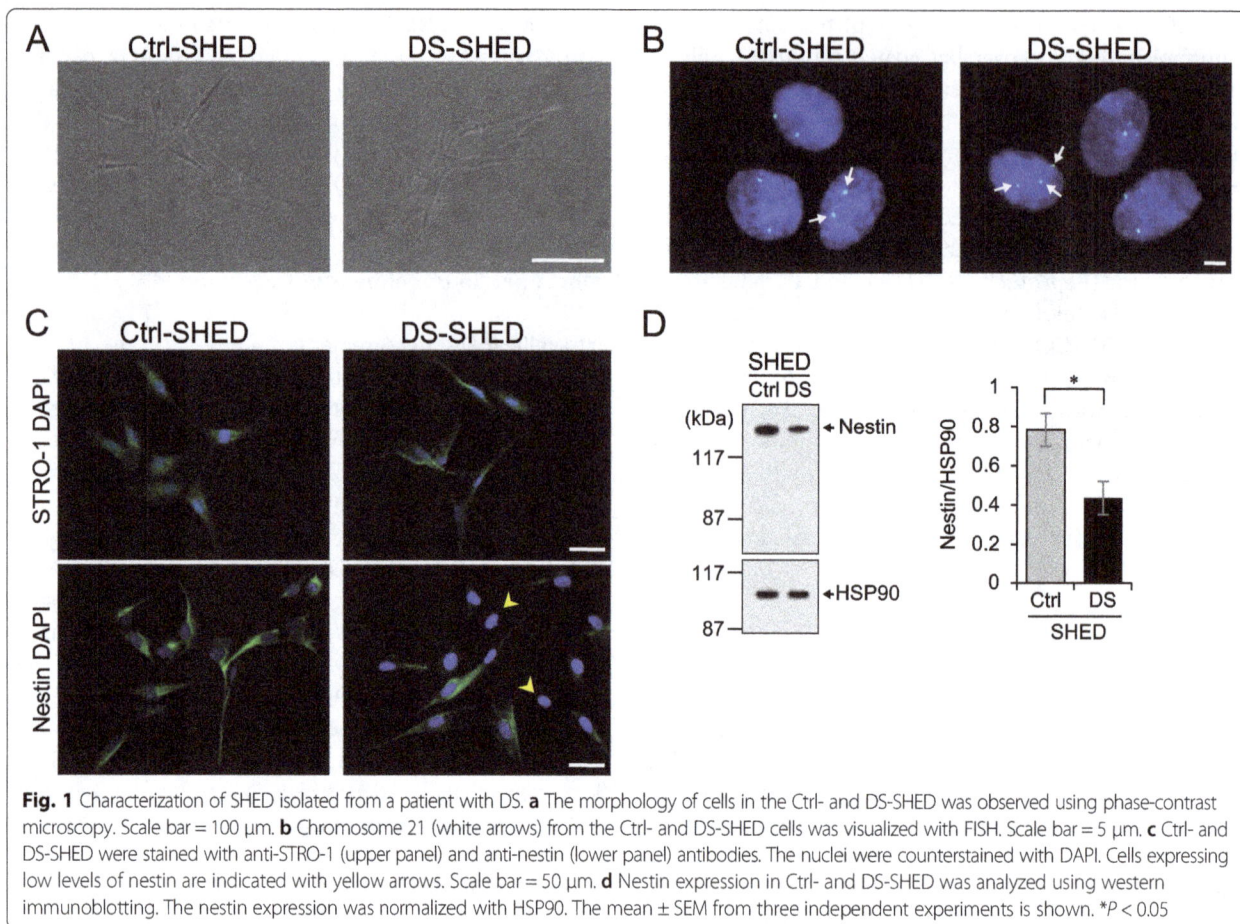

Fig. 1 Characterization of SHED isolated from a patient with DS. **a** The morphology of cells in the Ctrl- and DS-SHED was observed using phase-contrast microscopy. Scale bar = 100 μm. **b** Chromosome 21 (white arrows) from the Ctrl- and DS-SHED cells was visualized with FISH. Scale bar = 5 μm. **c** Ctrl- and DS-SHED were stained with anti-STRO-1 (upper panel) and anti-nestin (lower panel) antibodies. The nuclei were counterstained with DAPI. Cells expressing low levels of nestin are indicated with yellow arrows. Scale bar = 50 μm. **d** Nestin expression in Ctrl- and DS-SHED was analyzed using western immunoblotting. The nestin expression was normalized with HSP90. The mean ± SEM from three independent experiments is shown. *$P < 0.05$

Student's t-tests were used to compare the Ctrl and DS groups. Differences were considered significant if $p < 0.05$. JMP software (SAS Institute, NC, USA) was used for the statistical analysis.

Methods of figure S1 and S2 are described in Additional file 4.

Results

Characteristics of SHED isolated from a patient with DS

We isolated SHED from the deciduous teeth of a child with DS (DS-SHED) and a normal participant (Ctrl-SHED). DS-SHED were spindle-shaped and exhibited a fibroblastic cell morphology that was similar to Ctrl-SHED (Fig. 1a). The presence of 3 copies of chromosome 21 in the nuclei of DS-SHED was verified by FISH (Fig. 1b). Next, analysis of cell proliferation showed similar proliferation of DS-SHED and Ctrl-SHED (Additional file 1: Figure S1). SHED have multi-lineage potential and express mesenchymal and neuronal stem cell markers. To examine the stem cell characteristics of DS-SHED, immunofluorescence staining was performed using antibodies against stem cell markers. Both DS-SHED and Ctrl-SHED expressed STRO-1, a mesenchymal stem cell marker (Fig. 1c, upper panel). In contrast, expression of nestin, a neuronal stem cell marker,

was reduced in DS-SHED compared to Ctrl-SHED (Fig. 1c; lower panel; yellow arrows denote cells with weak nestin expression). Western blotting (Fig. 1d) and flow cytometry analysis (Additional file 2: Figure S2) were also used to examine nestin expression and showed reduced nestin expression in DS-SHED compared to Ctrl-SHED.

Altered differentiation of DS-SHED into DN

We differentiated Ctrl-SHED and DS-SHED into DN, and immunostained these with antibodies to the neuronal marker β-tubulin III and DN marker TH. DN differentiated from DS-SHED (DS-DN) expressed β-tubulin III and TH (Fig. 2a), but neurite length and branching were reduced compared to DN differentiated from Ctrl-SHED (Ctrl-DN). Quantitative analysis also showed that neurite length and branching were reduced in TH-expressing DS-DN compared to Ctrl-DN (Fig. 2b, c). DN development, evaluated in 4 stages according to cell morphology (Fig. 2d; based on a report by Leach et al.) [19], showed that DS-DN development was reduced compared to Ctrl-DN (Fig. 2e).

Disturbance of DA secretion in DS-DN

A functional analysis of DN was performed by examining DA expression and DA secretion. DA expression was

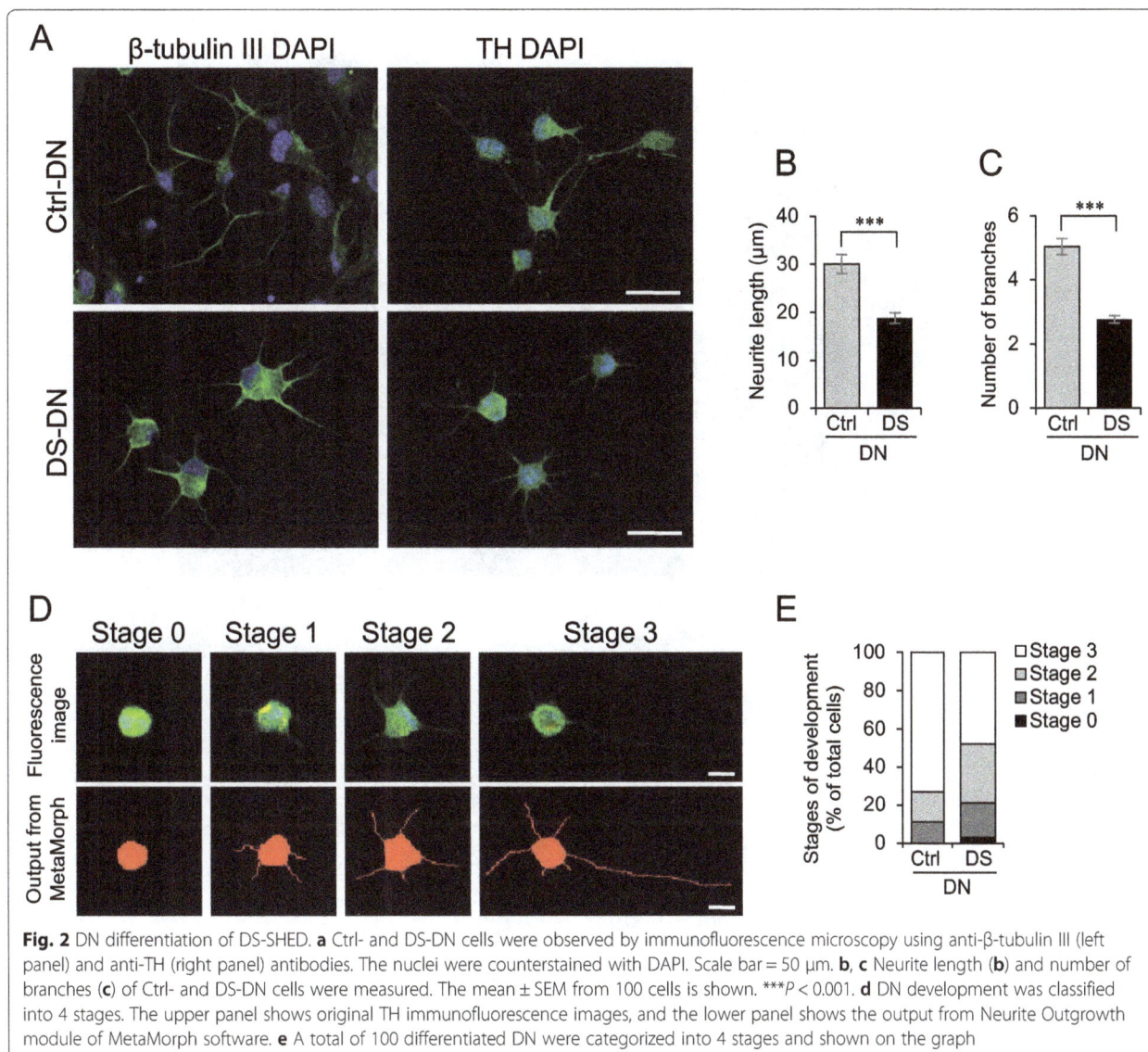

Fig. 2 DN differentiation of DS-SHED. **a** Ctrl- and DS-DN cells were observed by immunofluorescence microscopy using anti-β-tubulin III (left panel) and anti-TH (right panel) antibodies. The nuclei were counterstained with DAPI. Scale bar = 50 μm. **b, c** Neurite length (**b**) and number of branches (**c**) of Ctrl- and DS-DN cells were measured. The mean ± SEM from 100 cells is shown. ***$P < 0.001$. **d** DN development was classified into 4 stages. The upper panel shows original TH immunofluorescence images, and the lower panel shows the output from Neurite Outgrowth module of MetaMorph software. **e** A total of 100 differentiated DN were categorized into 4 stages and shown on the graph

examined by immunostaining cells, which showed that DA expression was present in both Ctrl- and DS-DN (Fig. 3a). Next, DA secretion was examined by measuring extracellular DA and it was observed that extracellular DA of DS-DN was significantly reduced compared with that of Ctrl-DN under basal conditions ($p = 0.046$; Fig. 3b). Although no significant differences between the DS- and Ctrl-DN were observed ($P = 0.506$), extracellular DA of DS-DN was lower than that of Ctrl-DN under glutamate stimulated conditions (Fig. 3c).

Aberrant expression of molecules involved in DA homeostasis in DS-DN

Possible causes of reduced DA section from DS-DN include the abnormal expression of molecules involved in DA homeostasis, such as dopamine transporter 1 (DAT1) that

mediates DA reuptake, vesicular monoamine transporter 2 (VMAT2) that mediates packaging of DA into secretory vesicles, and glutamate receptors. Analysis of DAT1 and VMAT2 mRNA expression showed that DAT1 expression was greater and VMAT2 expression was reduced in DS-DN compared to Ctrl-DN (Fig. 4a, b). Furthermore, expression of NMDAR1, a subunit of glutamate receptor, by immunostaining showed that the number of NMDAR1 puncta per unit length of neurite was reduced in DS-DN compared to Ctrl-DN (Fig. 4c-e).

Discussion

In this study, various tests on SHED derived from a patient with DS suggest that DN development is reduced and DN function is disturbed in DS. Previous studies have implicated abnormal neuronal cell development in DS based on

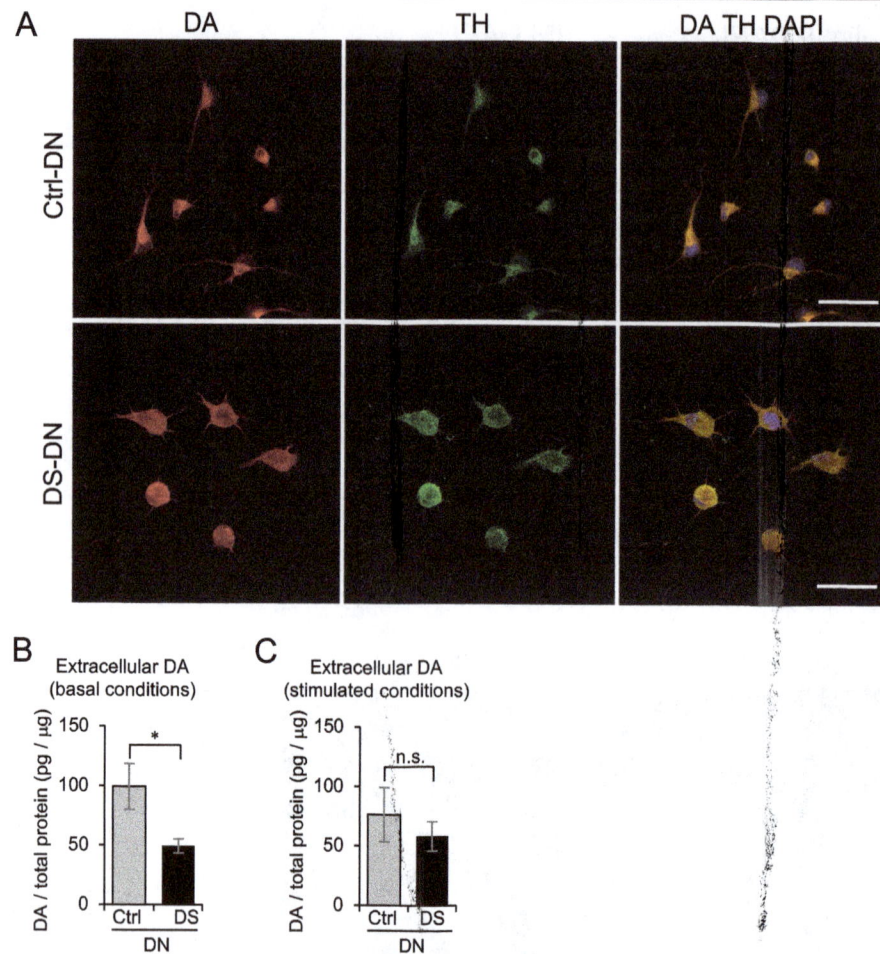

Fig. 3 Altered DA secretion in DS-DN. **a** DA expression in Ctrl- and DS-DN cells was observed by immunofluorescence microscopy. Ctrl- and DS-DN cells were stained with anti-DA and anti-TH antibodies, and fluorescence images were captured using the same acquisition settings. Nuclei were counterstained with DAPI; merged images are shown in the right panels. Scale bar = 50 μm. **b**, **c** Extracellular DA amount under basal conditions **b** and glutamate-stimulated conditions **c** were measured by ELISA. The DA amount was normalized with total protein extracted from each cell. Graphs show the mean ± SEM from four experiments. *$P < 0.05$; n.s., not significant

the examination of induced pluripotent stem cells (iPSCs) and neurospheres derived from the fetal brains of DS patients [20, 21]; however, these studies did not involve the differentiation of stem cells into a specific type of neuronal cell. Thus, the present study focused on DN and is the first to elucidate a relationship between DS and abnormal DN development and function.

Compared to Ctrl-SHED, the expression of the neuronal stem cell marker nestin was reduced in DS-SHED. It has been reported that when iPSCs from a patient with DS are induced to become neural progenitor cells (NPCs), nestin expression, neuronal cell differentiation capacity, neurite length, and synapse formation are reduced compared to controls [20]. In these NPCs, glia markers as well as the differentiation into glia were enhanced over the differentiation into neurons [20]. Although glia were not examined in the present study, because nestin expression

was reduced in SHED derived from the patient with DS, it is possible that differentiation into glia was also enhanced, though further investigation is required to confirm this.

A reduction in DA secretion was observed from DS-DN compared to Ctrl-DN. Expression of DAT1, which mediates DA reuptake, was increased and expression of VMAT2, which is involved in packaging DA into secretory vesicles, was decreased in DS-DN compared to Ctrl-DN. An increase in DA reuptake and reduction of DA packaging into secretory vesicles may have led to the observed reduction in extracellular DA of DS-DN. Furthermore, though no significant differences between the DS- and Ctrl-DN were observed, extracellular DA of DS-DN was reduced under glutamate stimulated conditions. The amount of NMDAR1 in neurites was reduced in DS-DN, which could explain the observed reduction in extracellular DA under glutamate

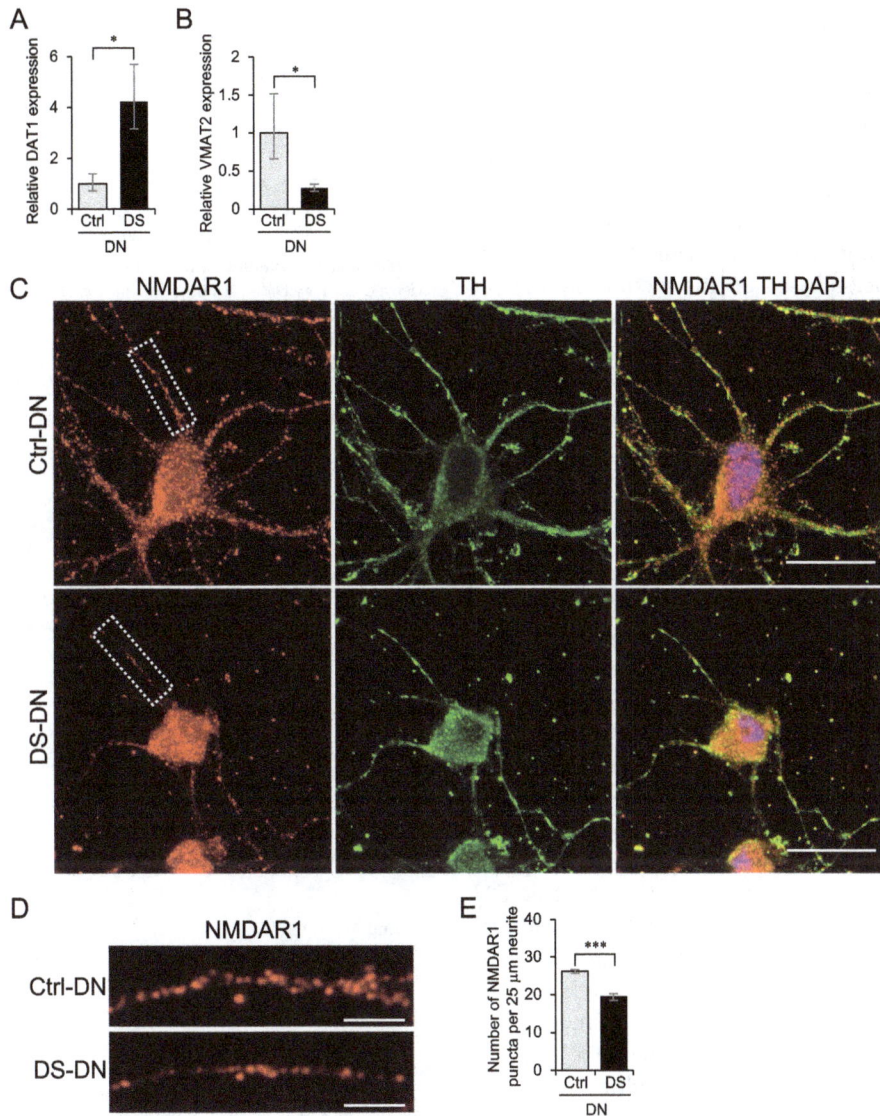

Fig. 4 Aberrant expression of molecules involved in DA homeostasis in DS-DN. **a**, **b** The mRNA expression of DAT1 (**a**) and VMAT2 (**b**) was measured by RT-qPCR. The relative expression of each gene was calculated with the $2^{-\Delta\Delta Ct}$ method. Graphs show the mean ± SEM from four experiments. *$P < 0.05$. **c-e** NMDAR1 and TH in Ctrl- and DS-DN cells were observed by immunofluorescence microscopy (**c**). Cells were counterstained with DAPI. Scale bar = 25 μm. Details of the boxed region in (**c**) are shown (**d**). Scale bar = 5 μm. The number of NMDAR1 puncta per 25 μm of neurite was counted (**e**). Graph shows the mean ± SEM of NMDAR1 puncta from 30 neurites. ***$P < 0.001$

stimulated conditions. In addition, DAT1 is important for basal extracellular levels of DA [22] and the dramatic change observed in DAT1 could have caused the cause of the greater difference in DA under basal conditions compared to glutamate stimulated conditions.

DS is caused by an extra copy of chromosome 21 and overexpression of the *DYRK1a* and *DSCR1* genes encoded by chromosome 21 are considered to have particularly important roles in the manifestation of DS symptoms [23, 24]. Overexpression of *DYRK1a* and *DSCR1* in mouse brains is reported to delay differentiation of neuronal precursor cells, causing reduced neuronal development [25]. In our study,

neurite length and branching as well as development were reduced in DN derived from DS-SHED. We anticipate that *DYRK1a* and *DSCR1* are involved in this reduced DN development. Further investigation into the expression of these genes and the effects of inhibitors [26, 27] and siRNA in SHED and DN from DS patients are required.

This study used SHED to investigate DS. The stem cell potential of mesenchymal stem cells is reported to change with repeated passages [28]. The present study used SHED of no more than 10 passages. There was no significant difference in cell proliferation and nestin expression between SHED of fewer passages (6 passages) and 10 passages

(Additional file 1: Figure S1 and Additional file 2: Figure S2); for this reason, passage-related differences were considered to have a minimal effect on our data. Nevertheless, to increase the utility of the SHED disease model, it will be necessary to determine how many passages of SHED can be used by performing repeated passages and obtaining an accurate understanding of its effect on stem cell marker expression and cell proliferation capacity.

In the present study, we differentiated SHED into DN using a 2-step process based on the method by Fujii et al. [16]; they added brain-derived neurotrophic factor (BDNF) to differentiation media in the second step, but we omitted this addition. Aberrant expression of BDNF is reported in DS patients and mouse models of DS [29–31], suggesting a relationship between neuronal development and BDNF in DS. BDNF is secreted extracellularly and mediates neuronal development and survival. BDNF serves autocrine and paracrine functions [32, 33]. If BDNF exhibits abnormal autocrine function in DS, adding BDNF to the media would conceal DS-SHED pathology. For this reason, BDNF was not added to the media in the present study. It will be necessary to examine BDNF and BDNF receptor expression in future studies to elucidate the involvement of BDNF in DN development of DS.

Fujii et al. reported that *Ngn2* and *Mash1* expression are important as they are activated in the first step of the process that involves differentiation of SHED into early stage DN [16]. In the second step, Fujii et al. speculated that BDNF promotes maturation of early stage DN to DN. When the authors differentiated SHED into DN and performed immunostaining with MAP2 and Tau antibodies, both Ctrl-DN and DS-DN expressed both proteins in whole-cells (Additional file 3: Figure S3). Previous immunostaining studies utilizing mature neuronal cells revealed that the MAP2 antibody stains dendrites, while the Tau antibody stains axons [34, 35]. This suggests that the DN in this study are still developing and have thus not fully matured. This is a limitation of our study. Further studies involving the addition of BDNF are needed to examine synapse formation and other phenomena in mature DN.

Conclusion

SHED were prepared from a patient with DS and differentiated into DN, revealing abnormal DN development and function. We predict that this DS patient has abnormal DA signaling, but further investigations, such as analyzing cognitive function and DA levels in this DS patient, are necessary. In the future, it will also be necessary to increase the number of patients for analysis to clarify the disturbance in dopaminergic neurodevelopment implicated in the pathophysiology of DS. SHED, which can be prepared noninvasively, offers an effective disease model for this research.

Additional files

Additional file 1: Figure S1. Cell proliferation of SHED in different passage. Ctrl- and DS-SHED were cultured for 24 h and 48 h. The number of cells were counted, and the means ± SEMs from three experiments are shown in the graph. P6; passage 6. P10; passage 10. n.s., not significant. (PDF 10 kb)

Additional file 2: Figure S2. Nestin expression in different passages of SHED. Nestin expression in Ctrl- and DS-SHED cells was analyzed with flow cytometry at different passages. P6; passage 6. P10; passage 10. (PDF 186 kb)

Additional file 3: Figure S3. Distribution of Tau and MAP2 in DN derived from SHED in this study. Ctrl- and DS-DN were stained with anti-Tau (1:100; Wako) and anti-MAP2 (1:100; Sigma-Aldrich) antibodies. The cells were counterstained with DAPI. The distribution of Tau and MAP2 was observed with Zeiss Axio Imager M2 microscope (Zeiss) equipped with ApoTome2 (Zeiss). Scale bar = 25 μm. (PDF 7737 kb)

Additional file 4: Supplemental methods. Methods for Figure S1 and S2. (DOCX 30 kb)

Abbreviations
DA: Dopamine; DN: dopaminergic neurons; DS: Down Syndrome; NMDAR1: *N*-methyl-D-aspartate receptor subunit NR1; SHED: stem cells from human exfoliated deciduous teeth; TH: tyrosine hydroxylase

Acknowledgments
We thank Drs. Takahiro Kato, Yasunari Sakai and Takayoshi Yamaza (Kyushu University) for their valuable suggestions and technical support. We appreciate the technical assistance provided by the Research Support Center, Research Center for Human Disease Modeling, Kyushu University Graduate School of Medical Sciences.

Funding
This work was supported by JSPS KAKENHI Grant Numbers JP25670877 and JP16K15839 to KN.

Authors' contributions
TP, HK: contribution to conception and design the study; acquisition of the data; analysis and interpretation of the data; drafting the manuscript; revising the manuscript; final approval of the version to be published. HY, KM: contribution to conception and design the study; acquisition of the data; revising the manuscript; final approval of the version to be published. YH, HS, HN, XH, YZ: acquisition of the data; drafting the manuscript; final approval of the version to be published. TT, KN: contribution to conception and design the study; analysis and interpretation of the data; revising the manuscript; final approval of the version to be published.

Competing interests
The authors declare that they have no competing interests.

Author details
[1]Section of Oral Medicine for Child, Division of Oral Health, Growth & Development, Faculty of Dental Science, Kyushu University, Maidashi 3-1-1, Higashi-Ku, Fukuoka 812-8582, Japan. [2]Department of Pediatric Surgery, Reproductive and Developmental Medicine, Graduate School of Medical Sciences, Kyushu University, Maidashi 3-1-1, Higashi-Ku, Fukuoka 812-8582, Japan.

References

1. Edgin JO, Mason GM, Spano G, Fernandez A, Nadel L. Human and mouse model cognitive phenotypes in Down syndrome: implications for assessment. Prog Brain Res. 2012;197:123–51. https://doi.org/10.1016/B978-0-444-54299-1.00007-8.

2. Edgin JO. Cognition in Down syndrome: a developmental cognitive neuroscience perspective. Wiley Interdiscip Rev Cogn Sci. 2013;4(3):307–17. https://doi.org/10.1002/wcs.1221.

3. Fidler DJ, Nadel L. Education and children with Down syndrome: neuroscience, development, and intervention. Ment Retard Dev Disabil Res Rev. 2007;13(3):262–71. https://doi.org/10.1002/mrdd.20166.

4. Lott IT, Dierssen M. Cognitive deficits and associated neurological complications in individuals with Down's syndrome. Lancet Neurol. 2010; 9(6):623–33. https://doi.org/10.1016/S1474-4422(10)70112-5.

5. Mason GM, Spano G, Edgin J. Symptoms of attention-deficit/hyperactivity disorder in Down syndrome: effects of the dopamine receptor D4 gene. Am J Intellect Dev Disabil. 2015;120(1):58–71. https://doi.org/10.1352/1944-7558-120.1.58.

6. Shimohata A, Ishihara K, Hattori S, Miyamoto H, Morishita H, Ornthanalai G, et al. Ts1Cje Down syndrome model mice exhibit environmental stimuli-triggered locomotor hyperactivity and sociability concurrent with increased flux through central dopamine and serotonin metabolism. Exp Neurol. 2017;293:1–12. https://doi.org/10.1016/j.expneurol.2017.03.009.

7. London J, Rouch C, Bui LC, Assayag E, Souchet B, Daubigney F, et al. Overexpression of the DYRK1A gene (dual-specificity tyrosine phosphorylation-regulated kinase 1A) induces alterations of the serotoninergic and dopaminergic processing in murine brain tissues. Mol Neurobiol. 2018;55(5):3822–31. https://doi.org/10.1007/s12035-017-0591-6.

8. Kay AD, Schapiro MB, Riker AK, Haxby JV, Rapoport SI, Cutler NR. Cerebrospinal fluid monoaminergic metabolites are elevated in adults with Down's syndrome. Ann Neurol. 1987;21(4):408–11. https://doi.org/10.1002/ana.410210416.

9. Whittle N, Sartori SB, Dierssen M, Lubec G, Singewald N. Fetal Down syndrome brains exhibit aberrant levels of neurotransmitters critical for normal brain development. Pediatrics. 2007;120(6):e1465–71. https://doi.org/10.1542/peds.2006-3448.

10. Falsafi SK, Dierssen M, Ghafari M, Pollak A, Lubec G. Reduced cortical neurotransmitter receptor complex levels in fetal Down syndrome brain. Amino Acids. 2016;48(1):103–16. https://doi.org/10.1007/s00726-015-2062-6.

11. Singer HS, Tiemeyer M, Hedreen JC, Gearhart J, Coyle JT. Morphologic and neurochemical studies of embryonic brain development in murine trisomy 16. Brain Res. 1984;317(2):155–66.

12. Dekker AD, Vermeiren Y, Albac C, Lana-Elola E, Watson-Scales S, Gibbins D, et al. Aging rather than aneuploidy affects monoamine neurotransmitters in brain regions of Down syndrome mouse models. Neurobiol Dis. 2017;105: 235–44. https://doi.org/10.1016/j.nbd.2017.06.007.

13. Miura M, Gronthos S, Zhao M, Lu B, Fisher LW, Robey PG, et al. SHED: stem cells from human exfoliated deciduous teeth. Proc Natl Acad Sci U S A. 2003;100(10):5807–12. https://doi.org/10.1073/pnas.0937635100.

14. Kato H, Thi Mai Pham T, Yamaza H, Masuda K, Hirofuji Y, Han X, et al. Mitochondria Regulate the Differentiation of Stem Cells from Human Exfoliated Deciduous Teeth. Cell Struct Funct. 2017;42(2):105–16. https://doi.org/10.1247/csf.17012.

15. Kato H, Han X, Yamaza H, Masuda K, Hirofuji Y, Sato H, et al. Direct effects of mitochondrial dysfunction on poor bone health in Leigh syndrome. Biochem Biophys Res Commun. 2017;493(1):207–12. https://doi.org/10.1016/j.bbrc.2017.09.045.

16. Fujii H, Matsubara K, Sakai K, Ito M, Ohno K, Ueda M, et al. Dopaminergic differentiation of stem cells from human deciduous teeth and their therapeutic benefits for parkinsonian rats. Brain Res. 1613;2015:59–72. https://doi.org/10.1016/j.brainres.2015.04.001.

17. Wang J, Wang X, Sun Z, Wang X, Yang H, Shi S, et al. Stem cells from human-exfoliated deciduous teeth can differentiate into dopaminergic neuron-like cells. Stem Cells Dev. 2010;19(9):1375–83. https://doi.org/10.1089/scd.2009.0258.

18. Hirofuji S, Hirofuji Y, Kato H, Masuda K, Yamaza H, Sato H, et al. Mitochondrial dysfunction in dopaminergic neurons differentiated from exfoliated deciduous tooth-derived pulp stem cells of a child with Rett

syndrome. Biochem Biophys Res Commun. 2018;498(4):898–904. https://doi.org/10.1016/j.bbrc.2018.03.077.

19. Leach MK, Naim YI, Feng ZQ, Gertz CC, Corey JM. Stages of neuronal morphological development in vitro--an automated assay. J Neurosci Methods. 2011;199(2):192–8. https://doi.org/10.1016/j.jneumeth.2011.04.033.

20. Hibaoui Y, Grad I, Letourneau A, Sailani MR, Dahoun S, Santoni FA, et al. Modelling and rescuing neurodevelopmental defect of Down syndrome using induced pluripotent stem cells from monozygotic twins discordant for trisomy 21. EMBO Mol Med. 2014;6(2):259–77. https://doi.org/10.1002/emmm.201302848.

21. Bahn S, Mimmack M, Ryan M, Caldwell MA, Jauniaux E, Starkey M, et al. Neuronal target genes of the neuron-restrictive silencer factor in neurospheres derived from fetuses with Down's syndrome: a gene expression study. Lancet. 2002;359(9303):310–5. https://doi.org/10.1016/s0140-6736(02)07497-4.

22. Gainetdinov RR, Jones SR, Fumagalli F, Wightman RM, Caron MG. Re-evaluation of the role of the dopamine transporter in dopamine system homeostasis. Brain Res Brain Res Rev. 1998;26(2–3):148–53.

23. Guimera J, Casas C, Estivill X, Pritchard M. Human minibrain homologue (MNBH/DYRK1): characterization, alternative splicing, differential tissue expression, and overexpression in Down syndrome. Genomics. 1999;57(3): 407–18. https://doi.org/10.1006/geno.1999.5775.

24. Fuentes JJ, Genesca L, Kingsbury TJ, Cunningham KW, Perez-Riba M, Estivill X, et al. DSCR1, overexpressed in Down syndrome, is an inhibitor of calcineurin-mediated signaling pathways. Hum Mol Genet. 2000;9(11):1681–90.

25. Kurabayashi N, Sanada K. Increased dosage of DYRK1A and DSCR1 delays neuronal differentiation in neocortical progenitor cells. Genes Dev. 2013; 27(24):2708–21. https://doi.org/10.1101/gad.226381.113.

26. Ogawa Y, Nonaka Y, Goto T, Ohnishi E, Hiramatsu T, Kii I, et al. Development of a novel selective inhibitor of the Down syndrome-related kinase Dyrk1A. Nat Commun. 2010;1:86. https://doi.org/10.1038/ncomms1090.

27. Kim H, Lee KS, Kim AK, Choi M, Choi K, Kang M, et al. A chemical with proven clinical safety rescues down-syndrome-related phenotypes in through DYRK1A inhibition. Dis Model Mech. 2016;9(8):839–48. https://doi.org/10.1242/dmm.025668.

28. Zhuang Y, Li D, Fu J, Shi Q, Lu Y, Ju X. Comparison of biological properties of umbilical cord-derived mesenchymal stem cells from early and late passages: immunomodulatory ability is enhanced in aged cells. Mol Med Rep. 2015;11(1):166–74. https://doi.org/10.3892/mmr.2014.2755.

29. Dogliotti G, Galliera E, Licastro F, Corsi MM. Age-related changes in plasma levels of BDNF in Down syndrome patients. Immun Ageing. 2010;7:2. https://doi.org/10.1186/1742-4933-7-2.

30. Troca-Marin JA, Alves-Sampaio A, Montesinos ML. An increase in basal BDNF provokes hyperactivation of the Akt-mammalian target of rapamycin pathway and deregulation of local dendritic translation in a mouse model of Down's syndrome. J Neurosci. 2011;31(26):9445–55. https://doi.org/10.1523/JNEUROSCI.0011-11.2011.

31. Parrini M, Ghezzi D, Deidda G, Medrihan L, Castroflorio E, Alberti M, et al. Aerobic exercise and a BDNF-mimetic therapy rescue learning and memory in a mouse model of Down syndrome. Sci Rep. 2017;7(1):16825. https://doi.org/10.1038/s41598-017-17201-8.

32. Cheng PL, Song AH, Wong YH, Wang S, Zhang X, Poo MM. Self-amplifying autocrine actions of BDNF in axon development. Proc Natl Acad Sci U S A. 2011;108(45):18430–5. https://doi.org/10.1073/pnas.1115907108.

33. Wang L, Chang X, She L, Xu D, Huang W, Poo MM. Autocrine action of BDNF on dendrite development of adult-born hippocampal neurons. J Neurosci. 2015;35(22):8384–93. https://doi.org/10.1523/JNEUROSCI.4682-14.2015.

34. Dehmelt L, Halpain S. The MAP2/Tau family of microtubule-associated proteins. Genome Biol. 2005;6(1):204. https://doi.org/10.1186/gb-2004-6-1-204.

35. Kosik KS, Finch EA. MAP2 and tau segregate into dendritic and axonal domains after the elaboration of morphologically distinct neurites: an immunocytochemical study of cultured rat cerebrum. J Neurosci. 1987;7(10): 3142–53.

Electroclinical characteristics of seizures arising from the precuneus based on stereoelectroencephalography (SEEG)

Yanfeng Yang[1,2], Haixiang Wang[3], Wenjing Zhou[3], Tianyi Qian[4], Wei Sun[1*] and Guoguang Zhao[2*]

Abstract

Background: Seizures arising from the precuneus are rare, and few studies have aimed at characterizing the clinical presentation of such seizures within the anatomic context of the frontoparietal circuits. We aimed to characterize the electrophysiological properties and clinical features of seizures arising from the precuneus based on data from stereoelectroencephalography (SEEG).

Methods: The present retrospective study included 10 patients with medically intractable epilepsy, all of whom were diagnosed with precuneal epilepsy via stereoelectroencephalography (SEEG) at Yuquan Hospital and Xuan Wu Hospital between 2014 and 2016. Clinical semiology, scalp electroencephalography (EEG) findings, magnetic resonance images (MRI), and positron emission tomography (PET) images were analyzed during phase I preoperative evaluations. Following electrode implantation, the semiological sequence, ictal SEEG evolution, and anatomy of the relevant brain structures were analyzed for each seizure.

Results: Seven of ten patients reported auras, including body image disturbance (2/7), vestibular responses (2/7), somatosensory auras (1/7), visual auras (1/7), and non-specific auras (1/7). Primary motor manifestations included bilateral asymmetric tonic seizures (BATS) (7/10) and hypermotor seizures (HMS) (3/10). In one patient, epileptiform discharge on interictal EEG occurred ipsilateral to the side of the epileptogenic zone (EZ). Discharge was non-lateralized in the remaining nine patients. In six patients, interictal EEG signals were primarily localized in the temporal–parietal–occipital area. In two patients, ictal onset occurred ipsilateral to the EZ, which was mainly located in the temporal–parietal–occipital area. Two patterns of seizure spread were observed. The first pattern was characterized by BATS activity with ictal spread to the supplementary motor area (SMA), paracentral lobule (PCL), precentral gyrus (PrCG), or postcentral gyrus (PoCG). The second pattern was characterized by HMS activity with ictal spread to middle cingulate cortex (MCC) and posterior cingulate cortex (PCC).

Conclusion: Aura type (e.g., body image disturbance and vestibular response), BATS, and HMS are the main indicators of precuneal epilepsy. Scalp EEG is of little use when attempting to localize precuneal seizures. Our findings indicate that the clinical characteristics of precuneal epilepsy vary among patients, and that the final electro–clinical phenotype depends on the pattern of seizure spread.

Keywords: Precuneal epilepsy, SEEG, Electroclinical characteristics, Anatomical-electrical-clinical correlations

* Correspondence: bmusunnyw@163.com; ggzhao@vip.sina.com
[1]Department of Neurology, Xuan Wu Hospital, Capital Medical University, No 45, Changchun Street, Xicheng District, Beijing 100053, China
[2]Department of Neurosurgery, Xuan Wu Hospital, Capital Medical University, No 45, Changchun Street, Xicheng District, Beijing 100053, China
Full list of author information is available at the end of the article

Background

The precuneus is a discrete area located in the posterior region of the medial parietal cortex, neighbored anteriorly by the marginal branch of the cingulate cortex, posteriorly by the parietal-occipital fissure, and inferiorly by the subparietal sulcus [1]. Anatomical and connectivity studies have indicated that the precuneus belongs to a widespread network of cortical and subcortical structures [2]. Primary connections of the precuneus include the posterior cingulate and retrosplenial cortices, other regions of the parietal cortex, the frontal cortex, and the temporal-parietal-occipital area [1]. Among these connections, we focus on the frontoparietal circuits, as they are regarded as the main elements of the cortical motor system [3]. Each motor area receives afferents from a specific set of parietal territories. Studies have shown that area 5ci [4], which is in the anterior medial region of the precuneus, is essentially the secondary somatosensory area due to its close association with the supplementary motor area (SMA), and that areas 5 L and 5 M are connected to the superior parietal lobule (SPL), medial primary somatosensory area (SI), and motor cortex. The central region of the precuneus exhibits overlap with the mesial 7A and is connected to the dorsolateral and dorsomedial prefrontal cortices [5, 6].

Seizures arising from the precuneus are rare, and few studies have aimed to characterize the clinical presentation of such seizures within the anatomic context of the frontoparietal circuits. Previous studies are limited in that their analyses focused on parietal lobe epilepsy as a general entity [7]. These studies showed that an important feature of parietal lobe epilepsy is the polymorphism of ictal manifestation [8]. Parietal lobe epilepsy is usually associated with various auras, including somatosensory impairments; disturbances of body image; vertiginous sensations; and visual, auditory, or aphasic auras [9, 10]. Focal motor clonic activity, tonic posturing, and oral-gestural automatisms occur in 57, 28, and 17% of patients, respectively [11]. More recent studies have investigated seizures arising from subregions of the parietal lobe, including the precuneus. Seizures arising from the precuneus are more frequently associated with body movement sensations, visual auras, eye movements, vestibular manifestations, asymmetric tonic posturing, and hypermotor activity [1]. Precuneal epilepsy is difficult to differentiate from other types of epilepsy—particularly frontal lobe epilepsy—because seizure onset occurs at an anatomically deep and semiologically silent area [12]. As such seizures may spread to the frontal cortex, misinterpretation of the clinical manifestations can lead to incorrect localization. False localization has been reported in up to 16% of cases [13]. Hence, it is important to improve our understanding of the clinical and neurophysiological features of precuneal epilepsy to improve pre-operative evaluation and surgical strategies.

Stereoelectroencephalography (SEEG) offers distinct advantages over conventional noninvasive approaches, which may be insufficient due to the deep origin of precuneal epilepsy. First introduced by Talairach and Bancaud in the early 1960's [14], SEEG is an invasive approach that can be used to reliably identify deeply buried anatomic structures, allowing one to construct a dynamic, three-dimensional (3D) spatiotemporal picture of epileptic activity [15]. Indeed, previous studies have utilized SEEG to precisely investigate the electrical activity of different brain structures involved in seizure generation and propagation [10, 16] .

In focal epilepsy, the symptoms are determined by the dynamic evolution of epileptic discharge from the initial seizure onset zone to the adjacent/distant cortical or subcortical areas. Therefore, characterizing the temporospatial evolution of seizure propagation and symptoms is crucial for improving our understanding of different clinical phenotypes [17, 18]. In the present study, we investigated the electroclinical characteristics of epilepsy originating from the precuneus, as well as the correlation between clinical phenotypes and the ictal pattern of seizure propagation.

Methods

Participants

The present retrospective study included 10 patients (9 men, 1 woman) with medically intractable epilepsy, all of whom underwent evaluation for surgical treatment at Yuquan Hospital and Xuan Wu Hospital between 2014 and 2016. The strategy for SEEG electrode implantation was decided upon during a multidisciplinary patient management conference at the Epilepsy Center. SEEG electrodes were implanted following comprehensive evaluation of each patient, which included a detailed history, video-EEG recording, MRI, PET, and other noninvasive localization methods. Patients with precuneal epilepsy were selected based on the following criteria: (a) SEEG-confirmed seizure onset from the precuneus; (b) extent of surgical excision limited or mostly limited within the precuneus; (c) post-operative follow-up at least every 6 months and ILAE Class 1–2 [19]; (d) no evidence of progressive brain disorders or systemic diseases. All included patients and caregivers provided written informed consent to participate and for publication. Patients in whom multiple epileptogenic zones or possible epileptogenic lesions were identified (e.g., tuberous sclerosis, multiple cavernous hemangioma) and those in whom independent epileptogenic cortical areas beyond the precuneus were confirmed using SEEG were excluded.

We began with 13 cases of electrodes embedded in the precuneus, but two of them were excluded due to diffuse electrodecremental events observed in the SEEG and uncertain seizure onset zones. An additional case was excluded due to bilateral epileptic foci and rejection of surgical treatment by the patient and family. Finally, we enrolled 10 patients. The clinical characteristics of the included patients are shown in Table 1. The mean age at seizure onset was 6.15 ± 6.2 years. The mean age at consultation was 13.6 ± 5.6 years. Our analyses focused on clinical semiology, as well as scalp EEG/SEEG findings.

Analysis of long-term scalp EEG monitoring and clinical semiology

Clinical characteristics and the results of scalp EEG monitoring are shown in Table 2. Prolonged EEG data were acquired via video-EEG monitoring (Nihon Kohdon, Japan or Bio-logic, USA). All patients underwent at least three typical seizures while awake and during sleep. The recording parameters were as follows: sampling rate = 1024 Hz, low filter setting = 0.16 Hz, high filter setting =70 Hz (Nihon Kohdon, Japan) or sampling rate = 256 Hz, low filter setting = 0.16 Hz, and high filter setting = 70 Hz (Bio-logic, USA). Each EEG sample was analyzed and classified according to the following criteria: (a) lateralization: (i) left, (ii) right, or (iii) not applicable (NA, when bilateral, generalized, or non-lateralized); (b) site: (i) frontal, (ii) temporal, (iii) parietal, (iv) occipital, (v) vertex, or (vi) not applicable (NA, when generalized or non-localized).

Three independent clinicians utilized Lüders' semiological seizure classification to evaluate ictal semiology and determine the semiological evolution sequence [18, 20]. For patients who experienced auras, aura information was derived from their previous medical history if

disturbance of consciousness or postictal amnesia occurred during monitoring.

Implantation of electrodes and analysis of anatomic-electrical-clinical correlations based on SEEG findings

A T1-weighted MRI scan and magnetic resonance angiography data were integrated to construct three-dimensional images using Neurotech stereotactic software (Neurotech, China). SEEG electrode implantation was based on a preimplantation hypothesis regarding the possible location of the epileptogenic zone (EZ). A Leksell headstock was installed on the morning of surgery, following which MRI scans were obtained and combined with previous MRI results to calculate the target position of each electrode (x, y, and z axes; α angle; β angle). Based on the calculated target positions, the electrodes were implanted using the Leksell stereotactic system. Postoperative high-resolution computed tomography (CT) scans were obtained to verify the exact location of each contact and to screen for postoperative complications. FreeSurfer (http://www.surfer.nmr.mgh.harvard.edu) was used to generate three-dimensional (3D) surface images of the brain, in order to determine the relationships of electrode position, the corresponding cortex, and surface vessels. Postoperative CT images were then co-registered with preoperative MR images using 3D Slicer (http://www.slicer.org) to confirm the actual locations of the SEEG electrodes.

The number of implanted SEEG electrodes ranged from 8 to 16 (median: 11.5) per patient, and the locations of the SEEG electrodes varied among patients.

Table 1 Demographics and clinical features of patients ($n = 10$)

Patient	Age/Sex (M/F)	Age at onset (Y)	MRI	PET hypometabolism	Hypothesis	Surgery	Pathology	ILAE class/ Outcome (M)	Complication
1	17 M	8	Normal	Rt. F, rt. P	Rt. P, rt. F	Rt. PrC	FCD	1 (29)	None
2	6 M	2.5	Lt. P PG	Lt. F, lt. P	Lt. P, lt. F, lt. T	Lt. PrC, lt. SPL	PG	1 (23)	None
3	19 M	7.5	Normal	Rt. P	Rt. P, rt. F, rt. T	Rt. PrC, rt. PCC	FCD	2 (30)	None
4	20 M	16	Lt. P, lt. O	Lt. P	Lt. P, lt. O, lt. T	Lt. PrC, lt. Cu	EM	1 (35)	Rt. Inf. quadranopsia
5	8 M	3	Normal	Lt. T, lt. P	Rt. P, rt. T	Rt. PrC, rt. RSC, rt. PCC	FCD	2 (34)	None
6	17 M	3	Normal	Lt. T	Lt. P, lt. O, lt. T	Lt. PrC, lt. Cu	FCD	2 (33)	Rt. Inf. quadranopsia
7	19 M	19	Lt. P lesion	Normal	Lt. P, lt. F	Lt. PrC, lt. PCL	EM	1 (26)	Transient Rt. LE paresthesia
8	4 M	0.5	Normal	Bil. T	Lt.P, lt. T, lt. O, lt, I	Lt. PrC, lt. PCC	FCD	1 (18)	Upper respiratory infection
9	15F	1.5	Bil. P and bil. O lesion	Lt. T	Lt. P, lt. O, lt. F	Lt. PrC, lt. PCC, lt. Cu	EM	2 (37)	Rt. Inf. quadranopsia
10	11 M	0.5	Lt. P and bil. O lesion	Lt. T, lt. P	Lt. P, lt. O, lt. T	Lt. PrC, lt. PCC, lt. Cu, lt.RSC	EM	2 (37)	Rt. Inf. quadranopsia

Bil bilateral, *Lt* left, *Rt* right, *Inf* inferior, *F* frontal, *T* temporal, *P* parietal, *O* occipital, *I* insula, *PrC* precuneus, *SPL* superior parietal lobule, *PCC* posterior cingulate cortex, *Cu* cuneus, *RSC* retrosplenial cortex, *PCL* paracentral lobule, *FCD* focal cortical dysplasia, *PG* pachygyria, *EM* encephalomalacia, *LE* lower extremity

Table 2 Features of scalp EEG and semiology in patients ($n = 10$)

No	Interictal		Ictal		Semiology sequence	Seizure number	Seizure duration/frequence
	Lateralization	Site	Lateralization	Site			
1	NA	Central-parietal	NA	NA	Left limb tonic→hypermotor	13	20–30s; 2–3/d
2	NA	Temporal-parietal-occipital	NA	NA	Aura(indescribable discomfort) → eyes right deviation→bilateral asymmetric tonic seizure	6	90s–150s; 1–2/m
3	NA	Temporal-parietal-occipital	Rt	Temporal-parietal-occipital	Aura(vestibular response) → left versive→bilateral asymmetric tonic seizure→GTCS	3	2-7 min; 2–3/m
4	NA	NA	Lt	Temporal-parietal-occipital	Aura(vestibular response) → bilateral asymmetric tonic seizure→right versive→GTCS	5	90s–110s; 1–2/m
5	NA	Temporal-parietal-occipital	NA	NA	Aura(body image disturbance) → dyleptics→rapid eyes blinking→ bilateral asymmetric tonic seizure	3	150 s-5 min; 1–2/w
6	NA	Temporal-parietal-occipital	NA	NA	Aura(blur vision of eyes) → right version→bilateral asymmetric tonic seizure	10	15S-1min; 3–4/d
7	Left	Parietal	NA	NA	Aura(body image disturbance) → hypermotor	12	30s; 3–4/d
8	NA	NA	NA	NA	Dialeptic→bilateral asymmetric tonic seizure	4	15–30s; 5–6/d
9	NA	Diffused	NA	NA	Aura(somatosensory aura) → bilateral asymmetric tonic seizure	5	1 min 2–3/w
10	NA	Diffused	NA	NA	Right version→hypermotor→GTCS	6	3 min 3–4/w

Signals were recorded by 5–18 contacts per intracranial electrode. SEEG data were recorded at a sampling rate of 2000 Hz and band-pass filtered between 0.16 Hz and 600 Hz (Nihon Koden, Japan), or at a sampling rate of 256 Hz and band-pass filtered between 0.16 Hz and 100 Hz (Bio-logic, USA). SEEG electrodes were referenced to screw electrodes placed at the vertex or to white matter electrodes.

Ictal onset and propagation were retrospectively analyzed by three clinicians based on the SEEG data. Following implantation, the clinicians analyzed the semiological sequence, ictal SEEG evolution, and the underlying anatomical structures for each seizure. As the seizure evolved, we marked the time points corresponding to each symptom and the electrode contacts exhibiting fast SEEG rhythms, following which we determined the corresponding anatomical locations on MR images. Finally, we analyzed the relationship between the anatomical position of the fast rhythm and the appearance of symptoms based on seizure evolution, as well as the anatomical-electrical-clinical relationship of each seizure.

Surgery and pathology

The surgical procedure was performed with controlled respiration under general inhalation anesthesia. The extent of surgical resection was based on a review of the interictal and ictal changes, extraoperative cortical stimulation functional map, and imaging data collected, which were used to reach consensus at a multidisciplinary patient management conference. Areas of the brain targeted for resection were removed using a microneurosurgical technique. During the surgery, the earlier video EEG findings and intraoperative ECoG information were

used to help to further identify the area targeted for resection, which typically included the ictal onset area and adjacent areas where frequent interictal spikes were demonstrated. Surgical specimens were fixed in 10% buffered formalin, embedded in paraffin, and then stained.

Results
Semiological characteristics
Aura

Seven of the 10 included patients experienced auras. Two patients experienced body image disturbance (Pt. 4 and 7) (i.e., a feeling that an extremity has spatial displacement), two patients experienced vestibular responses (Pt. 3 and 5), and one patient experienced a somatosensory aura (Pt. 9) (i.e., numbness in the bottom of the right foot spreading upwards toward the knee). One patient experienced a visual aura (Pt. 6) (i.e., blurred vision in both eyes), while one patient experienced a non-specific aura characterized by discomfort in the heart (Pt. 2).

Motor manifestations

Seven of the 10 included patients experienced BATS (Pt. 2, 3, 4, 5, 6, 8, and 9), while the remaining three experienced HMS (Pt. 1, 7, and 10). Patient 1 exhibited horizontal movement of the trunk and hips accompanied by stiffness in the contralateral limbs. Patient 7 exhibited trunk and hip movement accompanied by pedaling motions in the bilateral lower extremities. Patient 10 exhibited right upper limb flapping accompanied by pedaling motions in the bilateral lower extremities and exaggerated facial expressions. In addition, four patients exhibited continuous and vigorous bilateral conjugated eye movements towards the side contralateral to the epileptic region, which were accompanied by synchronous head movements.

Interictal and ictal EEG data

All patients underwent video-EEG monitoring. In Patient 7, interictal epileptiform discharge occurred ipsilateral to the side of the EZ. Discharge was non-lateralized in eight patients, and one patient (Pt. 4) exhibited no interictal discharge. In six patients, interictal EEG signals were mainly localized to the temporal-parietal-occipital area. In the remaining four patients, interictal discharge was generalized or non-localized.

In two patients (Pt. 3, 4), the ictal onset occurred ipsilateral to the EZ, and the site of seizure onset was primarily localized in the temporal-parietal-occipital area. In the remaining patients, ictal EEG signals were generalized or non-localized.

Anatomic-electrical-clinical correlations based on SEEG findings

Two patterns of anatomic–electrical–clinical correlations were observed. The first pattern was characterized by BATS activity with ictal spread to the supplementary motor area (SMA), paracentral lobule (PCL), postcentral gyrus (PoCG), or precentral gyrus (PrCG) of the ipsilateral hemisphere. Seven of the ten included patients

exhibited BATS (Fig. 1a). However, due to limitations in the number and scope of the electrodes, data from only three patients were used to explore the frontoparietal circuits.

The ictal SEEG trace of Patient 2 revealed that seizure onset was characterized by the appearance of fast, low-voltage discharge (gamma band) in the precuneus (mesial contacts of electrode C1–3). After 5 s, an indescribable aura appeared. Approximately 20 s later, seizure activity spread to the PCC (mesial contacts of electrode D1–3), intraparietal sulcus (IPS) (middle contacts of electrode D8–10), and PoCG (lateral contacts of electrode E12–16). At this time, rightward deviation of the eyes was observed. A BATS was observed only when ictal activity had propagated to the PCL (mesial contacts of electrode J1–3), PrCG (lateral contacts of electrode K10–14), and SMA (mesial contacts of electrode L1–2) (Fig. 2).

The ictal SEEG recording of Patient 9 revealed that seizure onset occurred in the precuneus (mesial contacts of electrode D1–3). Two seconds later, a somatosensory aura was observed. BATS activity appeared once the seizure had spread to the SMA (mesial contacts of electrode F1–2), PrCG (lateral contacts of electrode F8–12), PCL (mesial contacts of electrode K1–3), and PoCG (lateral contacts of electrode K10–14) (Fig. 3).

The ictal SEEG recording of Patient 3 revealed that seizure onset occurred within a relatively focal region of the

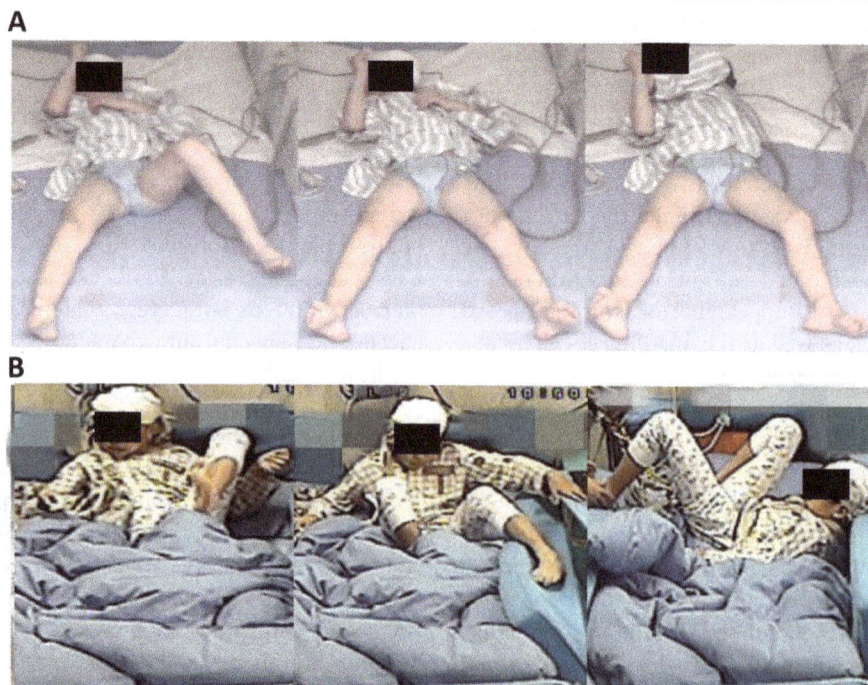

Fig. 1 Seizure samples. Video samples of the BATS of patient 2 (**a**) and the HMS of patient 10 (**b**). Signed consent forms authorizing publication have been obtained for all identifiable patients

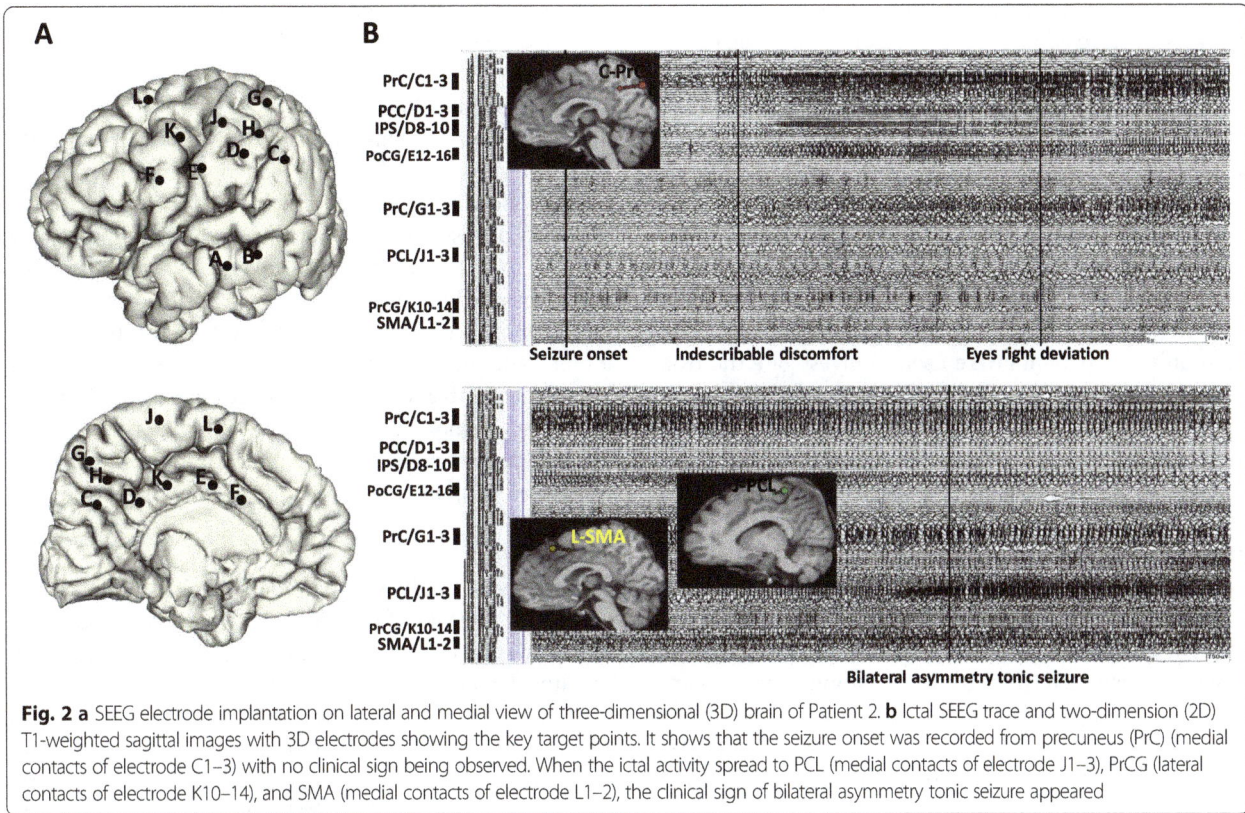

Fig. 2 a SEEG electrode implantation on lateral and medial view of three-dimensional (3D) brain of Patient 2. **b** Ictal SEEG trace and two-dimension (2D) T1-weighted sagittal images with 3D electrodes showing the key target points. It shows that the seizure onset was recorded from precuneus (PrC) (medial contacts of electrode C1–3) with no clinical sign being observed. When the ictal activity spread to PCL (medial contacts of electrode J1–3), PrCG (lateral contacts of electrode K10–14), and SMA (medial contacts of electrode L1–2), the clinical sign of bilateral asymmetry tonic seizure appeared

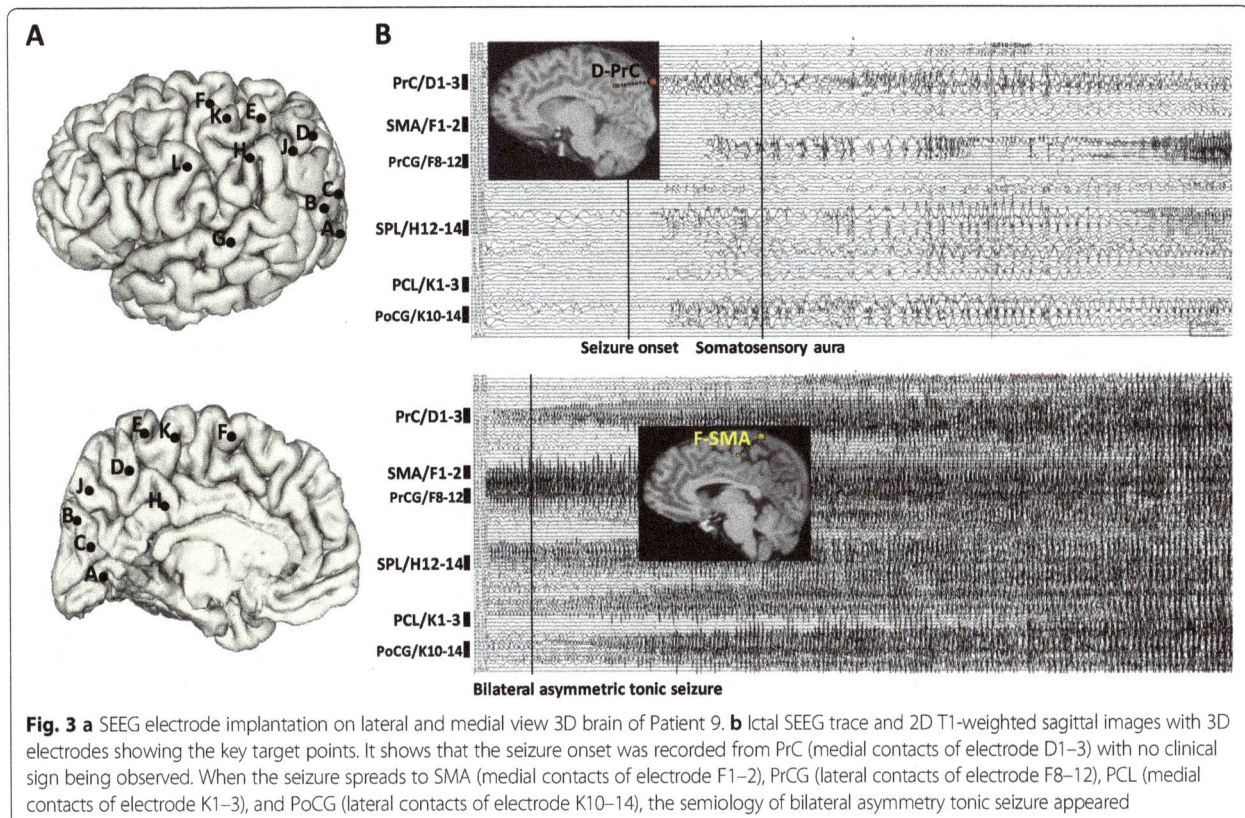

Fig. 3 a SEEG electrode implantation on lateral and medial view 3D brain of Patient 9. **b** Ictal SEEG trace and 2D T1-weighted sagittal images with 3D electrodes showing the key target points. It shows that the seizure onset was recorded from PrC (medial contacts of electrode D1–3) with no clinical sign being observed. When the seizure spreads to SMA (medial contacts of electrode F1–2), PrCG (lateral contacts of electrode F8–12), PCL (medial contacts of electrode K1–3), and PoCG (lateral contacts of electrode K10–14), the semiology of bilateral asymmetry tonic seizure appeared

precuneus (middle contacts of electrode C4–7 and mesial contacts of electrode E1–3). Ten seconds later, seizure activity had spread to the PCC (mesial contacts of electrode J1–3) and IPS (middle contacts of electrode G4–6). A BATS was observed only once seizure activity had spread to the PoCG (lateral contacts of electrode H11–14) and SMA (medial contacts of electrode L1–3) (Fig. 4).

The second pattern was characterized by HMS activity with ictal spread to the PCC and MCC of the ipsilateral hemisphere, which was observed in three patients (Fig. 1b). However, due to electrode limitations, data from only two patients were used to investigate the frontoparietal circuits. The ictal SEEG trace of Patient 7 revealed that seizure onset occurred within the precuneus (medial contacts of electrode G1–3 and H1–3), in the absence of clinical signs. Hypermotor signs were observed once seizure activity had spread to the MCC (medial contacts of electrode C1–3), PCC (medial contacts of electrode F1–3), and PoCG (lateral contacts of electrode D8–12) (Fig. 5).

The ictal SEEG trace of Patient 1 revealed that seizure onset was characterized by a transition from preictal rhythmic spiking to fast discharge (gamma band) in the precuneus (medial contacts of electrode C1–3 and electrode D1–3), which occurred over the course of approximately 6 s, in the absence of clinical signs. Hypermotor signs were observed only once seizure activity had

spread to the MCC (medial contacts of electrode F2–5) and PCC (medial contacts of electrode G3–5) (Fig. 6).

Surgical complications

Surgical complications were observed in six patients. Four (Pt. 4, 6, 9, and 10) showed right inferior quadranopsia following resection, which was considered a complication of resection of the precuneus and cuneus. One (Pt. 7) had a transient contralateral lower extremity paresthesia, which was considered a result of postoperative edema causing transient damage to the paracentral lobule, and the symptom resolved 2 weeks later. One (Pt. 8) had upper respiratory infection on the third day after operation. This may be related to the patient's young age and weak resistance; the patient returned to normal after appropriate anti-inflammatory treatment.

Discussion

In the present study, we analyzed semiological characteristics and EEG/SEEG data in order to identify anatomic–electrical–clinical relationships in 10 patients with precuneal epilepsy. Previous studies have revealed that precuneal epilepsy is associated with several types of premonitory auras [1]. In one such study, visual auras were reported in three patients (50%), vestibular responses in two patients (33%), and sensations of falling or movement in one patient [10]. Previous studies have

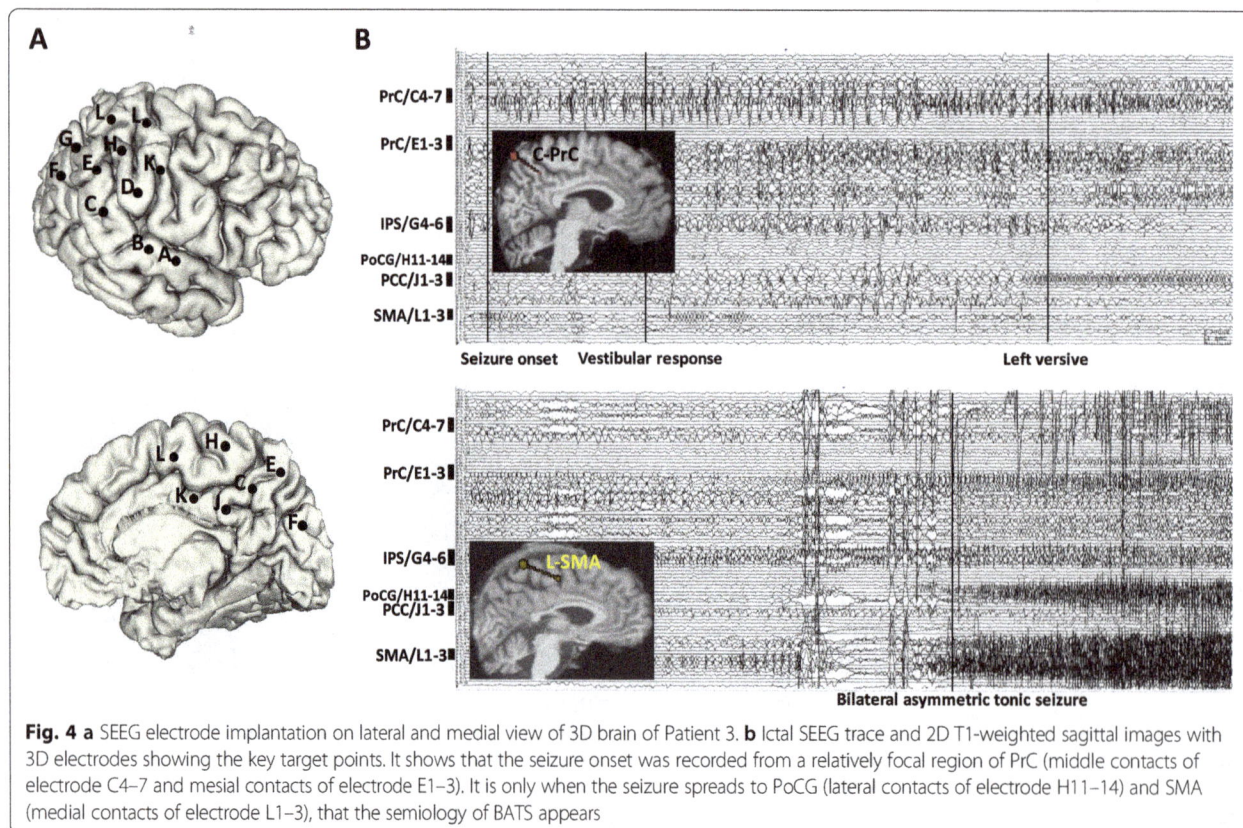

Fig. 4 a SEEG electrode implantation on lateral and medial view of 3D brain of Patient 3. b Ictal SEEG trace and 2D T1-weighted sagittal images with 3D electrodes showing the key target points. It shows that the seizure onset was recorded from a relatively focal region of PrC (middle contacts of electrode C4–7 and mesial contacts of electrode E1–3). It is only when the seizure spreads to PoCG (lateral contacts of electrode H11–14) and SMA (medial contacts of electrode L1–3), that the semiology of BATS appears

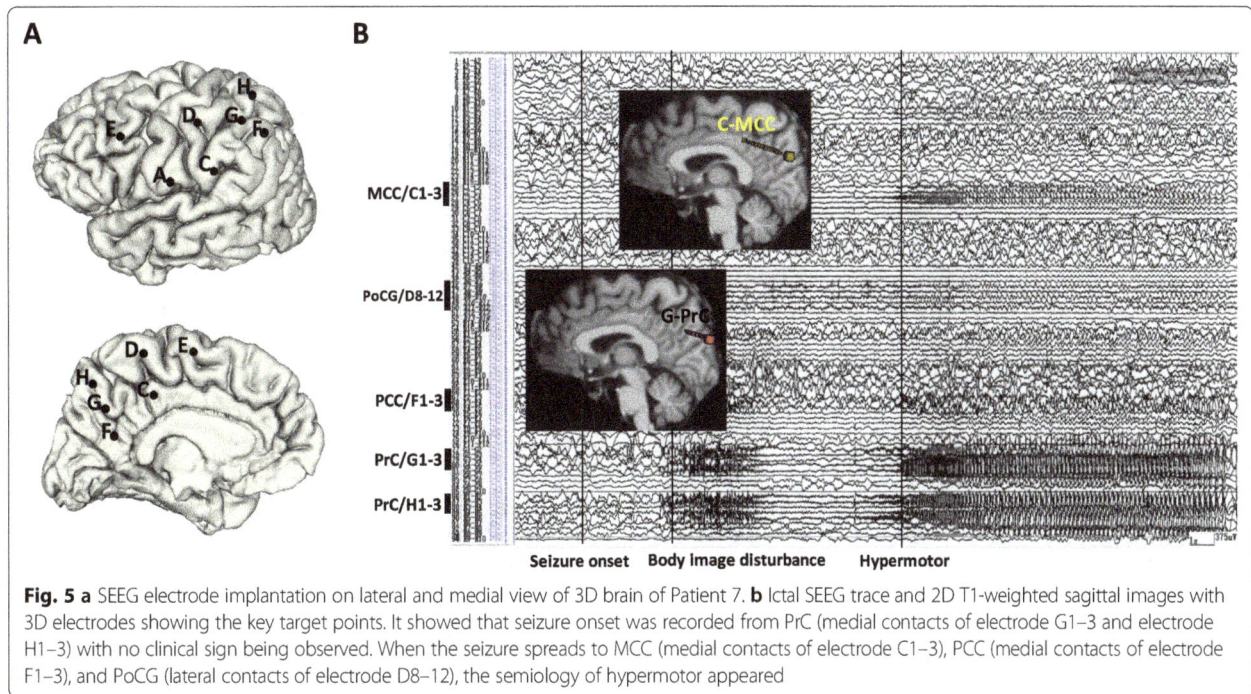

Fig. 5 a SEEG electrode implantation on lateral and medial view of 3D brain of Patient 7. **b** Ictal SEEG trace and 2D T1-weighted sagittal images with 3D electrodes showing the key target points. It showed that seizure onset was recorded from PrC (medial contacts of electrode G1–3 and electrode H1–3) with no clinical sign being observed. When the seizure spreads to MCC (medial contacts of electrode C1–3), PCC (medial contacts of electrode F1–3), and PoCG (lateral contacts of electrode D8–12), the semiology of hypermotor appeared

demonstrated that stimulation of the anterior portion of the precuneus results in body image disturbance, while stimulation of the posterior portion results in visuo-motor illusions [21, 22]. Additional studies have reported that stimulation of the precuneus evokes vestibular responses [23]. Our findings are mostly consistent with these previous studies, although body image disturbance occurred more frequently in our patient group, perhaps because most patients exhibited seizure activity in the anterior precuneus.

We observed two major patterns of activity in patients of the present study: BATS and HMS. BATS is often associated with seizure activity in the mesial parietal region [24], similar to patterns observed in patients with mesial frontal lobe epilepsy. However, seizures originating from the precuneus are typically briefer than those

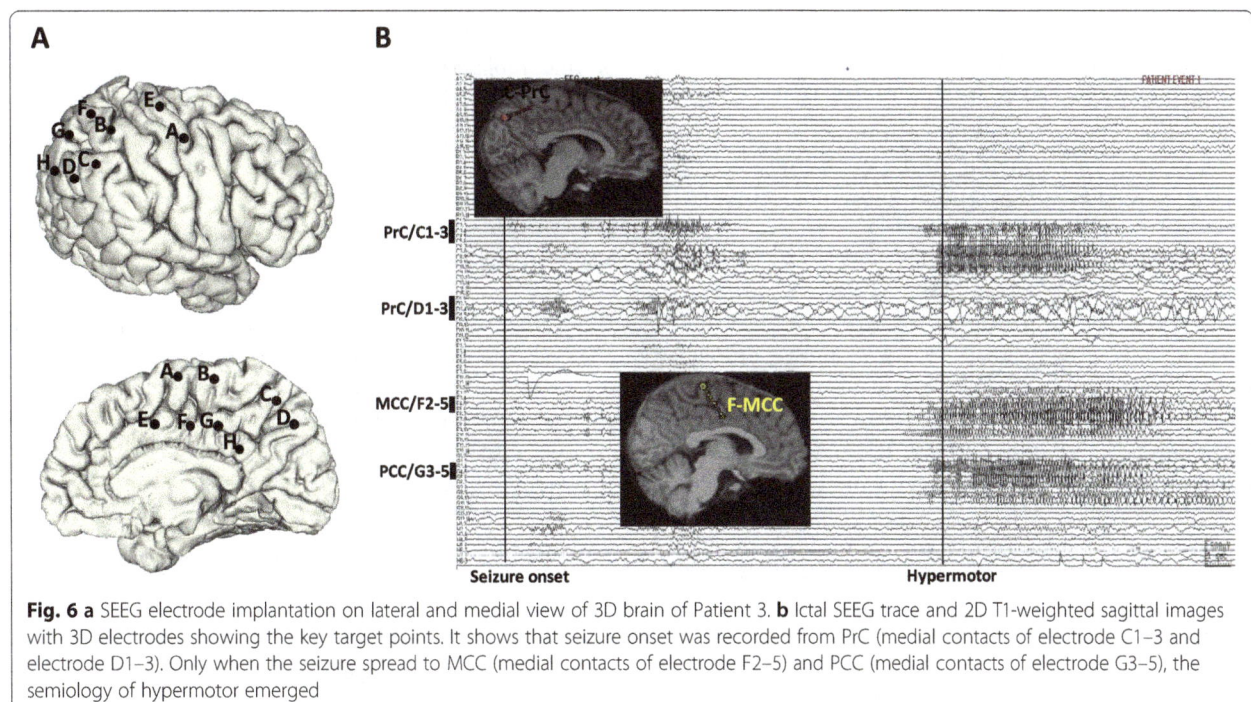

Fig. 6 a SEEG electrode implantation on lateral and medial view of 3D brain of Patient 3. **b** Ictal SEEG trace and 2D T1-weighted sagittal images with 3D electrodes showing the key target points. It shows that seizure onset was recorded from PrC (medial contacts of electrode C1–3 and electrode D1–3). Only when the seizure spread to MCC (medial contacts of electrode F2–5) and PCC (medial contacts of electrode G3–5), the semiology of hypermotor emerged

with an SMA onset, and patients with precuneal seizures are typically quicker to regain awareness [25]. These features were also observed in our patients who experienced BATS.

Some studies have reported that seizures originating from the lateral and mesial parietal regions may manifest as hypermotor activity [26]. Such hypermotor activity was also observed in some patients of the present study. However, HMS typically has a frontal lobe onset and occur in 15–27% of patients with frontal lobe epilepsy, in which seizures primarily rise from the orbitofrontal or mesial frontal cortex [27–29]. In such cases, it is difficult to distinguish seizures arising from the parietal lobe from those arising from the frontal lobe. However, some studies have indicated that the type of aura and the delay between seizure onset and hypermotor activity can be used to make this distinction [26]. As previously mentioned, precuneal HMS is often preceded by unique auras (e.g., body image disturbance and vestibular responses). In addition, patients with frontal lobe seizures almost always experience hypermotor activity at seizure onset or during the first third of the seizure [30]. However, in patients with precuneal seizures, there is usually a substantial delay between seizure onset and the appearance of hypermotor activity, which may represent the time required for the seizure to propagate from the precuneus to the frontal lobe or to subcortical structures [31, 32].

In precuneal epilepsy, the interictal EEG provides little clue to the lateralization and localization of seizure activity [9], as discharge is prone to spread to other cerebral lobes and induce an error in localization. The widespread connectivity between the precuneus and other cerebral regions may represent the underlying cause of errors in localization. Hence, it is difficult to distinguish precuneal from non-precuneal seizures via scalp EEG, particularly those arising from the mesial frontal lobe. SEEG represents a unique method for identifying and characterizing the underlying physiologic mechanisms of precuneal seizures.

In SEEG methodology, the EZ is defined as the site of origin for epileptic seizures [33]. Therefore, we focused our SEEG analyses mainly on the identification of the brain regions in which specific ictal patterns developed during seizures [34, 35]. The region associated with the primary organization of ictal discharge and subsequent propagation is correlated with the anatomical positions of the electrodes that display maximal abnormal activity, and with the evolution of clinical seizure signs. At present, however, the identification of the EZ is based on the ability of experienced clinical neurophysiologists to identify the relevant anatomic–electrical–clinical correlations and SEEG patterns.

In the present study, we analyzed the ictal SEEG of five patients in whom the relevant electrodes involved the frontoparietal network. In three cases, BATS was observed only once the ictal activity had spread to the SMA, PCL, PrCG, or PoCG. Our results indicated that abnormal ictal activity is easily propagated from the precuneus to these regions, suggesting that the precuneus is functionally connected to the SMA and other central areas. Some previous studies have reported that the medial aspect of the posterior parietal lobe is connected to the SMA and premotor areas [4, 36]. Therefore, seizures occurring within the medial side of the parietal lobe may spread to the SMA, causing bilateral asymmetric tonic manifestations [24].

In two patients of the present study, HMS was observed only when ictal activity had spread to the PCC and MCC. Some studies have reported that the middle cingulate gyrus receives afferent connections from the medial surface of the parietal lobe, particularly the precuneus. Such connections provide information regarding noxious stimulation in the body, directing the motor area of the cingulate gyrus to initiate evasive actions/behaviors. Thus, seizure activity originating from the precuneus may induce hypermotor movements [37]. In one case series, two patients with electrodes implanted in the motor aspect of the MCC exhibited fast discharge in this region during hypermotor movements [26]. Thus, hypermotor activity associated with precuneal seizures may be due to the ease with which abnormal ictal activity propagates from the precuneus to the PCC and MCC. Taken together, the accumulated evidence suggests that the precuneus is functionally connected with the PCC and MCC.

The present study possesses several limitations of note. First, the study was limited by the number and coverage of the implanted electrodes. The spatial limitations of recording may have caused difficulties in identifying all possible pathways of seizure propagation. The study was also limited by the small number of included cases and its retrospective design. Nonetheless, our study provides valuable evidence regarding the electroclinical characteristics of precuneal epilepsy, as well as the possible mechanisms underlying variations in semiology based on SEEG findings within frontoparietal circuits. Such findings may represent clinical indicators of precuneal epilepsy. Future studies should investigate further subdivisions of the precuneus using a greater number of electrodes in order to provide a more complete characterization of precuneal epilepsy.

Conclusion

The clinical characteristics of precuneal epilepsy are complex and various. Aura type (e.g., body image disturbance and vestibular response), BATS, and HMS are the main indicators of precuneal epilepsy. Scalp EEG is of little use when attempting to localize precuneal seizures. Analysis of high-quality SEEG data can help to identify the relevant anatomic-electrical-clinical correlations. Our findings indicate that the clinical characteristics of precuneal epilepsy are different among patients, and that the final electro–clinical phenotype depends on the pattern of seizure spread.

Abbreviations
2D: Two-dimensional; 3D: Three-dimensional; BATS: Bilateral asymmetric tonic seizure; CT: Computed tomography; EEG: Electroencephalography; EZ: Epileptogenic zone; HMS: Hypermotor seizure; IPS: Intraparietal sulcus; MCC: Middle cingulate cortex; MRI: Magnetic resonance imaging; PCC: Posterior cingulate cortex; PCL: Paracentral lobule; PET: Positron emission tomography; PoCG: Postcentral gyrus; PrC: Precuneus; PrCG: Precentral gyrus; SEEG: Stereoeletroencephalography; SMA: Supplementary motor area; SPL: Superior parietal lobule

Funding
This work supported by National Natural Science Foundation of China (81571267) and the capital health research and development of special (2016-2-2013).

Authors' contributions
YY contributed to the data acquisition and analysis of the manuscript. WS and GZ contributed to the data acquisition, analysis and redaction of the manuscript, and also the interpretation of the data. WZ and HW contributed to the data acquisition. TQ contributed to redaction of the manuscript. All authors read and approved the final manuscript.

Competing interests
None of the authors has any conflict of interest to disclose. We confirm that we have read the Journal's position on issues involved in ethical publication and affirm that this report is consistent with those guidelines.

Author details
[1]Department of Neurology, Xuan Wu Hospital, Capital Medical University, No 45, Changchun Street, Xicheng District, Beijing 100053, China. [2]Department of Neurosurgery, Xuan Wu Hospital, Capital Medical University, No 45, Changchun Street, Xicheng District, Beijing 100053, China. [3]Epilepsy Center, Yuquan hospital, Tsinghua University, Beijing 100049, China. [4]Department of Radiology, Beijing Key Lab of magnetic resonance imaging (MRI) and Brain Informatics, Xuan Wu Hospital, Capital Medical University, Beijing 100053, China.

References
1. Harroud A, Boucher O, Tran TPY, Harris L, Hall J, Dubeau F, Mohamed I, Bouthillier A, Nguyen DK. Precuneal epilepsy: clinical features and surgical outcome. Epilepsy Behav. 2017;73:77–82.
2. Cavanna AE, Trimble MR. The precuneus: a review of its functional anatomy and behavioural correlates. Brain. 2006;129(Pt 3):564–83.
3. Rizzolatti G, Luppino G, Matelli M. The organization of the cortical motor system: new concepts. Electroencephalogr Clin Neurophysiol. 1998;106(4):283–96.
4. Scheperjans F, Eickhoff SB, Homke L, Mohlberg H, Hermann K, Amunts K, Zilles K. Probabilistic maps, morphometry, and variability of cytoarchitectonic areas in the human superior parietal cortex. Cerebral Cortex (New York : 1991). 2008;18(9):2141–57.
5. Caminiti R, Innocenti GM, Battaglia-Mayer A. Organization and evolution of parieto-frontal processing streams in macaque monkeys and humans. Neurosci Biobehav Rev. 2015;56:73–96.
6. Margulies DS, Vincent JL, Kelly C, Lohmann G, Uddin LQ, Biswal BB, Villringer A, Castellanos FX, Milham MP, Petrides M. Precuneus shares intrinsic functional architecture in humans and monkeys. Proc Natl Acad Sci U S A. 2009;106(47):20069–74.
7. Salanova V, Andermann F, Rasmussen T, Olivier A, Quesney LF. Parietal lobe epilepsy. Clinical manifestations and outcome in 82 patients treated surgically between 1929 and 1988. Brain. 1995;118(Pt 3):607–27.
8. Francione S, Liava A, Mai R, Nobili L, Sartori I, Tassi L, Scarpa P, Cardinale F, Castana L, Cossu M, Russo GL. Drug-resistant parietal epilepsy: polymorphic ictal semiology does not preclude good post-surgical outcome. Epileptic Disord. 2015;17(1):32–46.
9. Salanova V. Parietal lobe epilepsy. J Clin Neurophysiol. 2012;29(5):392–6.
10. Bartolomei F, Gavaret M, Hewett R, Valton L, Aubert S, Regis J, Wendling F, Chauvel P. Neural networks underlying parietal lobe seizures: a quantified study from intracerebral recordings. Epilepsy Res. 2011;93(2–3):164–76.
11. Salanova V, Andermann F, Rasmussen T, Olivier A, Quesney LF. Tumoural parietal lobe epilepsy. Clinical manifestations and outcome in 34 patients treated between 1934 and 1988. Brain. 1995;118(Pt 5):1289–304.
12. Enatsu R, Bulacio J, Nair DR, Bingaman W, Najm I, Gonzalez-Martinez J. Posterior cingulate epilepsy: clinical and neurophysiological analysis. J Neurol Neurosurg Psychiatry. 2014;85(1):44–50.
13. Foldvary N, Klem G, Hammel J, Bingaman W, Najm I, Luders H. The localizing value of ictal EEG in focal epilepsy. Neurology. 2001;57(11):2022–8.
14. Talairach J, Bancaud J, Bonis A, Szikla G, Tournoux P. Functional stereotaxic exploration of epilepsy. Confin Neurol. 1962;22:328–31.
15. McGonigal A, Bartolomei F, Regis J, Guye M, Gavaret M, Trebuchon-Da Fonseca A, Dufour H, Figarella-Branger D, Girard N, Peragut JC, et al. Stereoelectroencephalography in presurgical assessment of MRI-negative epilepsy. Brain. 2007;130(Pt 12):3169–83.
16. Gavaret M, Trebuchon A, Bartolomei F, Marquis P, McGonigal A, Wendling F, Regis J, Badier JM, Chauvel P. Source localization of scalp-EEG interictal spikes in posterior cortex epilepsies investigated by HR-EEG and SEEG. Epilepsia. 2009;50(2):276–89.
17. Chauvel P, Kliemann F, Vignal JP, Chodkiewicz JP, Talairach J, Bancaud J. The clinical signs and symptoms of frontal lobe seizures. Phenomenology and classification. Adv Neurol. 1995;66:115–25. discussion 125-116
18. Bonini F, McGonigal A, Trebuchon A, Gavaret M, Bartolomei F, Giusiano B, Chauvel P. Frontal lobe seizures: from clinical semiology to localization. Epilepsia. 2014;55(2):264–77.
19. Wieser HG, Blume WT, Fish D, Goldensohn E, Hufnagel A, King D, Sperling MR, Luders H, Pedley TA. ILAE commission report. Proposal for a new classification of outcome with respect to epileptic seizures following epilepsy surgery. Epilepsia. 2001;42(2):282–6.
20. Luders H, Acharya J, Baumgartner C, Benbadis S, Bleasel A, Burgess R, Dinner DS, Ebner A, Foldvary N, Geller E, et al. Semiological seizure classification. Epilepsia. 1998;39(9):1006–13.
21. Richer F, Martinez M, Cohen H, Saint-Hilaire JM. Visual motion perception from stimulation of the human medial parieto-occipital cortex. Exp Brain Res. 1991;87(3):649–52.
22. Richer F, Martinez M, Robert M, Bouvier G, Saint-Hilaire JM. Stimulation of human somatosensory cortex: tactile and body displacement perceptions in medial regions. Exp Brain Res. 1993;93(1):173–6.
23. Kahane P, Hoffmann D, Minotti L, Berthoz A. Reappraisal of the human vestibular cortex by cortical electrical stimulation study. Ann Neurol. 2003; 54(5):615–24.
24. Khan SA, Carney PW, Archer JS. Brief asymmetric tonic posturing with diffuse low-voltage fast activity in seizures arising from the mesial parietal region. Epilepsy Res. 2014;108(10):1950–4.
25. Baumgartner C, Flint R, Tuxhorn I, Van Ness PC, Kosalko J, Olbrich A, Almer G, Novak K, Luders HO. Supplementary motor area seizures: propagation pathways as studied with invasive recordings. Neurology. 1996;46(2):508–14.
26. Montavont A, Kahane P, Catenoix H, Ostrowsky-Coste K, Isnard J, Guenot M, Rheims S, Ryvlin P. Hypermotor seizures in lateral and mesial parietal epilepsy. Epilepsy Behav. 2013;28(3):408–12.
27. Jobst BC, Siegel AM, Thadani VM, Roberts DW, Rhodes HC, Williamson PD. Intractable seizures of frontal lobe origin: clinical characteristics, localizing signs, and results of surgery. Epilepsia. 2000;41(9):1139–52.
28. Rheims S, Ryvlin P, Scherer C, Minotti L, Hoffmann D, Guenot M, Mauguiere F, Benabid AL, Kahane P. Analysis of clinical patterns and underlying epileptogenic zones of hypermotor seizures. Epilepsia. 2008;49(12):2030–40.
29. Gibbs SA, Figorilli M, Casaceli G, Proserpio P, Nobili, L. Sleep related hypermotor seizures with a right parietal onset. J Clin Sleep Med. 2015;11(8): 953–5.
30. Kotagal P, Arunkumar G, Hammel J, Mascha E. Complex partial seizures of frontal lobe onset statistical analysis of ictal semiology. Seizure. 2003; 12(5):268–81.

31. Ryvlin P, Minotti L, Demarquay G, Hirsch E, Arzimanoglou A, Hoffman D, Guenot M, Picard F, Rheims S, Kahane P. Nocturnal hypermotor seizures, suggesting frontal lobe epilepsy, can originate in the insula. Epilepsia. 2006;47(4):755–65.

32. Dobesberger J, Ortler M, Unterberger I, Walser G, Falkenstetter T, Bodner T, Benke T, Bale R, Fiegele T, Donnemiller E, et al. Successful surgical treatment of insular epilepsy with nocturnal hypermotor seizures. Epilepsia. 2008;49(1):159–62.

33. Munari C, Bancaud J. The role of stereo-electro-encephalography (SEEG) in the evaluation of partial epileptic patients. London: Butterworths; 1987. p. 267–306.

34. Bancaud J, Angelergues R, Bernouilli C, Bonis A, Bordas-Ferrer M, Bresson M, Buser P, Covello L, Morel P, Szikla G, et al. Functional stereotaxic exploration (SEEG) of epilepsy. Electroencephalogr Clin Neurophysiol. 1970;28(1):85–6.

35. Engel J Jr. Epilepsy surgery. Curr Opin Neurol. 1994;7(2):140–7.

36. Scheperjans F, Hermann K, Eickhoff SB, Amunts K, Schleicher A, Zilles K. Observer-independent cytoarchitectonic mapping of the human superior parietal cortex. Cereb Cortex (New York,: 1991). 2008;18(4):846–67.

37. Vogt BA. Pain and emotion interactions in subregions of the cingulate gyrus. Nat Rev Neurosci. 2005;6(7):533–44.

Wearables for gait and balance assessment in the neurological ward - study design and first results of a prospective cross-sectional feasibility study with 384 inpatients

Felix P. Bernhard[1,2†], Jennifer Sartor[1,2†], Kristina Bettecken[1,2†], Markus A. Hobert[1,2,3], Carina Arnold[1,2], Yvonne G. Weber[4], Sven Poli[5], Nils G. Margraf[3], Christian Schlenstedt[3], Clint Hansen[3*] and Walter Maetzler[1,2,3]

Abstract

Background: Deficits in gait and balance are common among neurological inpatients. Currently, assessment of these patients is mainly subjective. New assessment options using wearables may provide complementary and more objective information.

Methods: In this prospective cross-sectional feasibility study performed over a four-month period, all patients referred to a normal neurology ward of a university hospital and aged between 40 and 89 years were asked to participate. Gait and balance deficits were assessed with wearables at the ankles and the lower back. Frailty, sarcopenia, Parkinsonism, depression, quality of life, fall history, fear of falling, physical activity, and cognition were evaluated with questionnaires and surveys.

Results: Eighty-two percent ($n = 384$) of all eligible patients participated. Of those, 39% ($n = 151$) had no gait and balance deficit, 21% ($n = 79$) had gait deficits, 11% ($n = 44$) had balance deficits and 29% ($n = 110$) had gait and balance deficits. Parkinson's disease, stroke, epilepsy, pain syndromes, and multiple sclerosis were the most common diseases. The assessment was well accepted.

Conclusions: Our study suggests that the use of wearables for the assessment of gait and balance features in a clinical setting is feasible. Moreover, preliminary results confirm previous epidemiological data about gait and balance deficits among neurological inpatients. Evaluation of neurological inpatients with novel wearable technology opens new opportunities for the assessment of predictive, progression and treatment response markers.

Keywords: Accelerometer, Inertial sensor, Postural control, Neurological diseases

Background

Gait and balance deficits occur in many neurological diseases. The evaluation of these deficits at the wards of hospitals is often based on qualitative parameters collected by the treating physicians and allied health professionals or on semi-quantitative scoring tools. For example, in Parkinson's disease (PD), the Unified Parkinson Disease Rating Scale (MDS-UPDRS) is regularly used to rate motor symptoms including gait and postural stability [1]. While such scales, questionnaires and surveys have been subject to multiple validation studies, they have limitations regarding inter-rater variability and subjectivity [2–5].

With the recent and ongoing development of wearables (mainly in the sport and fitness sectors), this technology has reached a sophisticated level making it interesting for medical purposes [6–16]. A particularly relevant field is the complementary assessment of inpatients at neurological wards, as wearables are specifically

* Correspondence: C.Hansen@neurologie.uni-kiel.de
[†]Felix P. Bernhard, Jennifer Sartor and Kristina Bettecken contributed equally to this work.
[3]Department of Neurology, University Hospital Schleswig-Holstein, Campus Kiel, Arnold-Heller-Str. 3, Haus 41, 24105 Kiel, Germany
Full list of author information is available at the end of the article

capable of assessing gait and balance deficits which are common in neurological patients [15, 17].

Only a small number of studies have investigated feasibility and acceptability of wearables in an inpatient setting, with limitations such as small sample sizes [18] and the investigation of only one disease [19]. This study aims to investigate the feasibility and usefulness of wearables during clinical evaluation in a large sample of neurological inpatients.

Methods

Participants

All inpatients referred to the three normal wards of the Neurology Center at the University Hospital of Tübingen between 09/2014 and 04/2015 (16-week assessment periods for each ward) were asked to take part in the study if they were between 40 to 89 years of age (this selection criterion was chosen due to feasibility issues) and were able to walk with or without walking aid. Exclusion criteria were the inability to give informed consent, a fall frequency of more than one fall per week (risk of falls during the assessment too high), and impaired cognition as defined by a Mini Mental State Examination (MMSE) score below 10 points. Participants who had at least one fall during the last 2 years were defined as fallers. The ethics committee of the medical faculty of the University of Tübingen approved the study (No. 356/2014BO2) and all participants gave written informed consent prior to participation.

Quantitative gait and balance assessment

Participants were equipped with a wearable sensor system (Rehawatch®, Hasomed, Magdeburg, Germany) consisting of three sensor-units worn at both ankles and at the lower back (L4-L5) [20]. Each sensor-unit contains 3D accelerometers (±8 g), 3D gyroscopes (±2000°/s) and 3D magnetometers (±1.3Gs) resulting in nine degrees of freedom and the raw data was processed and analyzed using validated and company provided algorithms [21]. The assessment included the following tasks: Participants walked seven times a 20 m distance under single (slow, comfortable, and fast speed) and dual tasking conditions (checking boxes and subtracting serial 7 s during comfortable and fast walking) [22, 23]. Static balance during quiet standing at the center of stability was tested on flat ground with four different positions of the feet for 30 s each: open stance with feet placed in parallel position with 5–10 cm in between, closed stance (parallel position), semi-tandem stance, and tandem stance [24]. The task one difficulty level below the one successfully performed on flat ground was then performed for 30 s on a foam pad (Airex balance pad, 50x41x6 cm). Static balance at the limit of

stability was tested with an adapted version of the Functional Reach Test [25] over a 15 s period. Overall mobility and transfer was tested with the Timed-Up-and-Go test (TUG) under comfortable and fast speed conditions [26–28]. Muscle strength was assessed with a hydraulic hand dynamometer (DanMic Global®, San Jose, USA) and muscle mass with bioimpedance (Akern Bia 101, SMT medical GmbH&Co. KG, Würzburg, Germany).

Assessments with scales and questionnaires

Fear of falling was assessed with the German version of the Falls Efficacy Scale-International (FES-I) [29]. Self-concepts of health, activity, cognition, social support and risk factors for age-associated diseases were assessed [30]. Depression was evaluated with the German version of the Beck's Depression Inventory II (BDI-II) [31, 32]. Health-related quality of life was assessed with the EQ-5D-5 L. This scale addresses mobility, autonomy, pain, fear, despondence, daily living activities and health [33]. The MMSE [34] and the Trail Making Test (TMT) [35] were used to assess cognition, and part III of the Movement Disorders Society-sponsored Unified Parkinson's Rating Scale (MDS-UPDRS) [1] was used for the assessment of motor symptoms. Function of the sensory nerves was assessed at the medial malleoli of the lower extremities and the basal joint of each thumb with a Rydel Seiffer tuning fork.

Classification of impaired gait and balance

A gait deficit was defined as > 15% lower walking speed compared to mean age-corrected speed according to [36, 37]. Presence of a balance deficit was considered when tandem stance could be performed no longer than 10 s [38, 39].

Statistical analysis

Statistical analysis was conducted with JMP 11.1.1 (SAS). Demographic data of the different groups were compared with Kruskal-Wallis-test (or Fisher's exact test for categorical data). Post hoc testing was performed with Mann-Whitney-U test. P values below 0.05 were considered significant. Bonferroni correction for multiple testing was applied for post-hoc tests ($p < 0.0083$).

Results

Of 468 inpatients eligible for the study (i.e., fulfilled all inclusion criteria and no exclusion criterion, and were not excluded due to logistic reasons), 384 (82%) participated. Of those, 60% were male. Mean age of the cohort was 62 years. The 10 most common diagnoses (69% of all investigated patients) were Parkinson's disease (PD, n = 51), stroke (n = 50), epilepsy (n = 30), pain syndromes (n = 26), multiple sclerosis (MS, n = 23), CNS tumours

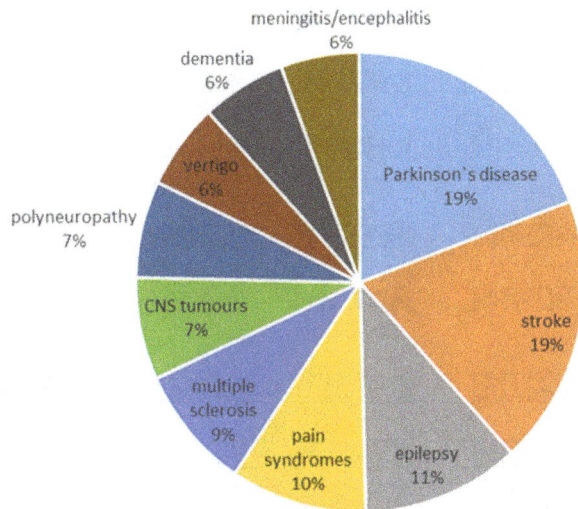

Fig. 1 Graphical representation of the ten most common diagnoses within the 384 study participants

($n = 19$), polyneuropathy ($n = 18$), vertigo ($n = 16$), dementia ($n = 16$), and meningitis/encephalitis ($n = 15$). During the study, no severe adverse events occurred (Fig. 1).

One hundred and 51 participants (39%) had no gait and balance deficit (control group), 79 (21%) had a gait deficit, 44 (11%) had a balance deficit and 110 (29%) had a gait and balance deficit. The highest proportion of patients with gait deficits (33%) was found in the meningitis/encephalitis cohort, the highest proportion of patients with balance deficits (17%) in the MS cohort, and the highest proportion of participants with gait and balance deficits (41%) in the PD cohort. Patients with pain syndromes had rarely gait and/or balance deficits.

Patients complied well with the quantitative gait and balance assessment and descriptive results from the balance, gait and postural transitions are shown in Figs. 2, 3 and 4.

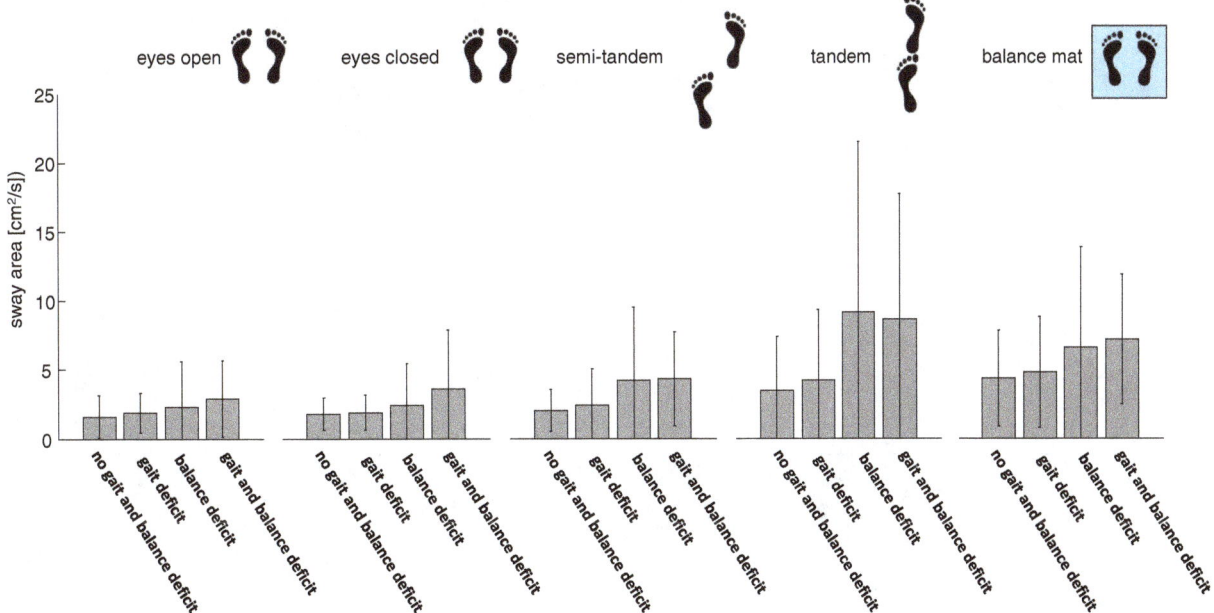

Fig. 2 During the balance assessment the participants with a balance or gait and balance deficit show the largest sway area compared to the controls and the patients with the gait deficit

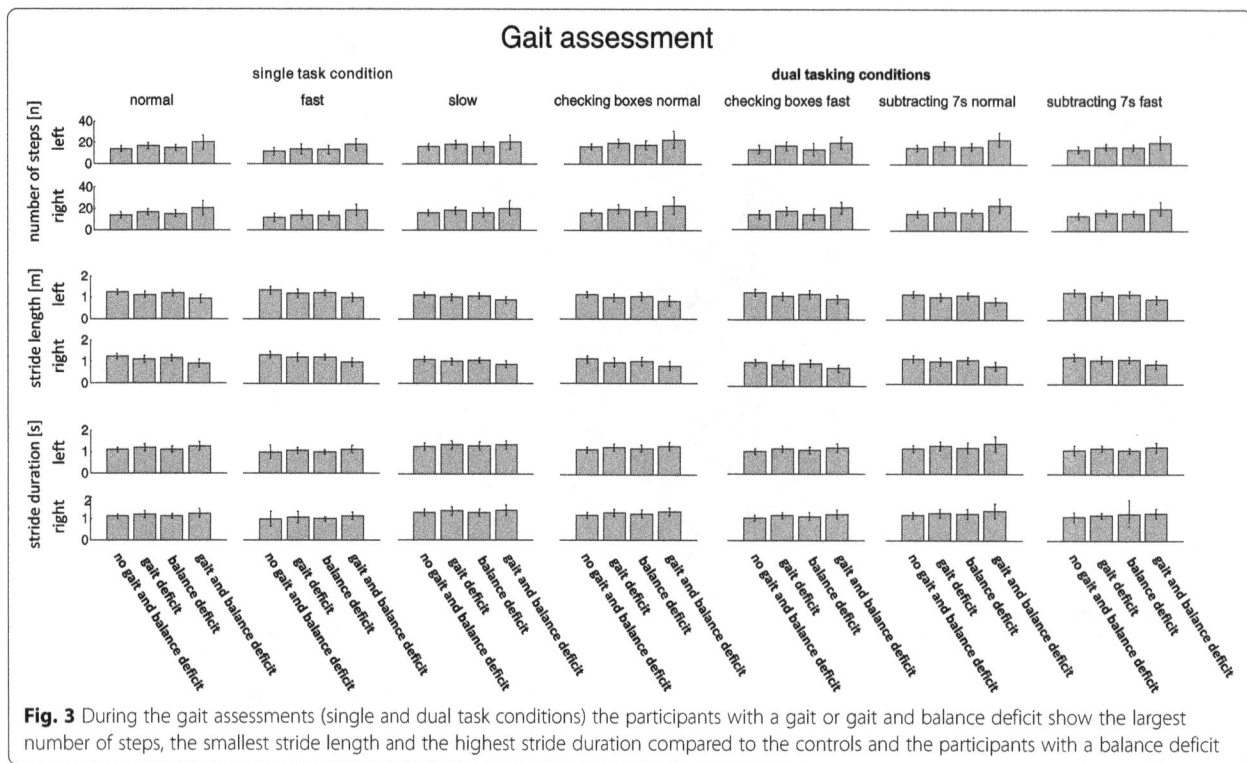

Fig. 3 During the gait assessments (single and dual task conditions) the participants with a gait or gait and balance deficit show the largest number of steps, the smallest stride length and the highest stride duration compared to the controls and the participants with a balance deficit

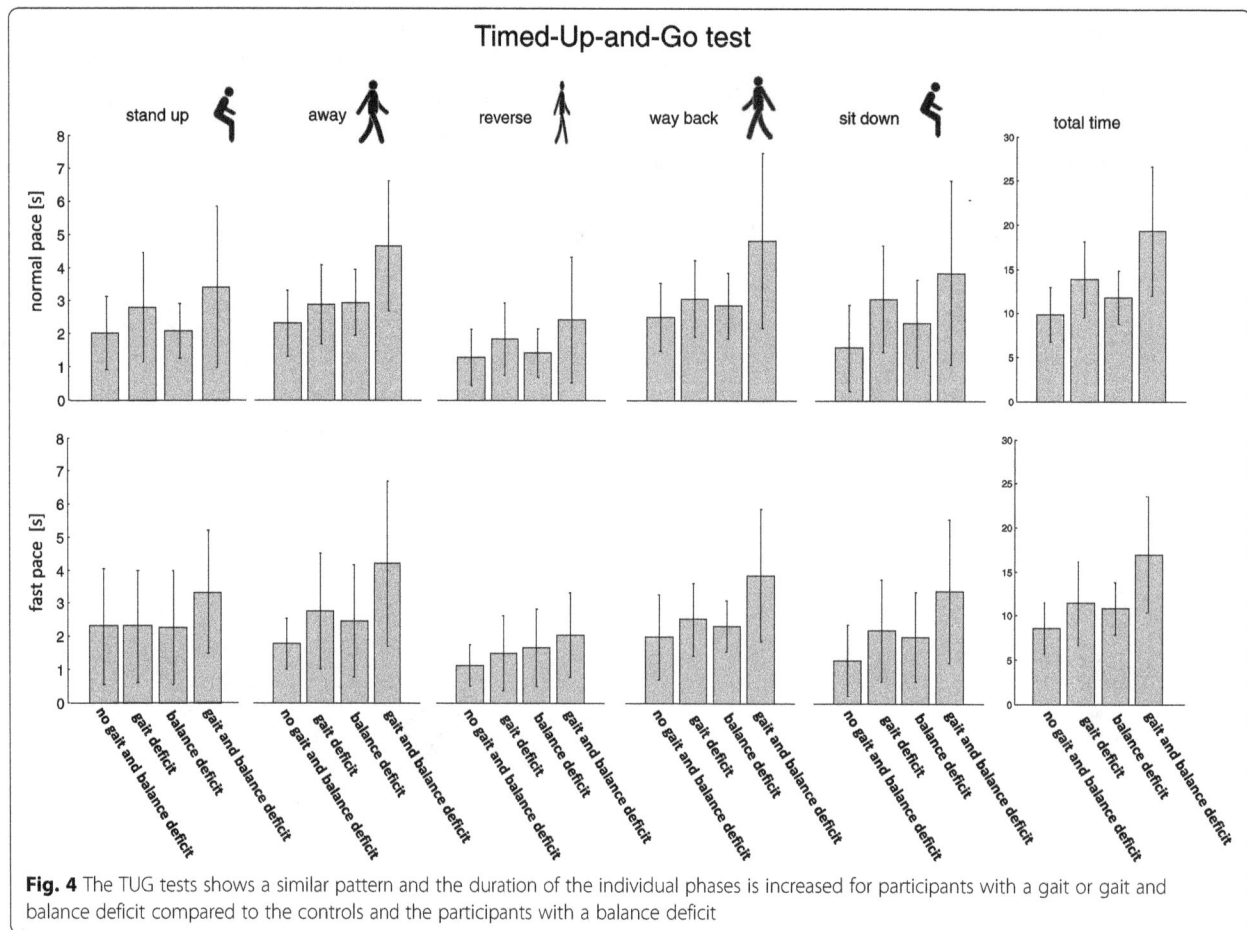

Fig. 4 The TUG tests shows a similar pattern and the duration of the individual phases is increased for participants with a gait or gait and balance deficit compared to the controls and the participants with a balance deficit

MMSE and TMT performances were significantly worse in all cohorts with gait and/or balance deficits, compared to the control cohort. Moreover, the cohort with gait and balance deficits performed worse in the TMT compared to the group with gait deficits. TUG durations were slower in the cohort with gait and balance deficits than in both the gait deficit cohort and the balance deficit cohort, and fastest in the control cohort. The same pattern was observed with regard to fear of falling, with highest FES-I values (i.e. the highest fear of falling) in the gait and balance deficits cohort. BDI II values were higher in the cohort with gait and balance deficits, compared to the control cohort. The cohort with gait and balance deficits had lower grip force when compared to the cohort with gait deficits and the control cohort. A more detailed description of the inter-cohort comparisons is presented in Table 1.

Discussion

In the presented study, we performed routine clinical gait and balance assessments complemented by an exhaustive evaluation of geriatric parameters in a neurological department at a university hospital. To the best of our knowledge, this is the first sensor-based cross-sectional study in a clinical environment of a university hospital, covering a wide range of neurological diseases. Our overall cohort represents a wide range and representative number of neurological diseases. A study with a similar setting but without sensor-unit-based assessments displayed a comparable composition of neurological diseases [17] with the five most common diagnoses completely overlapping.

Acceptance of sensor-unit-based assessments in our study was high. Only 18% of eligible patients refused to take part in the study. We did not experience any logistical issues during the assessments. The sensor system

Table 1 Demographic, clinical, and semiquantitative/quantitative study outcomes of the whole cohort, as well as of the subcohorts with and without gait and balance deficits

	Whole cohort (N = 384)		Controls (N = 151)		Gait deficits (N = 79)		Balance deficits (N = 44)		Gait and balance deficits (N = 110)		P-Value
	Median	Range	Median	Range	Median	Range	Median	Range	Median	Range	
Age [years]	64	40–90	57	40–86	60	40–89	70*#	44–89	69.5*#	41–90	< 0.0001
Gender [% female]	42.4		43.0		36.7		43.2		45.5		0.67
Height [m]	1.72	1.48–2.01	1.73	1.49–2.01	1.73	1.48–1.98	1.70	1.58–1.88	1.70	1.49–2.00	0.04
Weight [kg]	79	37–134	80	50–134	82	46–117	79	55–115	74	37–123	0.13
BMI [kg/m²]	26.2	14.9–43.0	26.3	19.4–41.8	26.4	17.3–41.6	26.8	19.4–38.4	25.9	14.9–43.0	0.77
Falls in the last 24 months [N]	0	0–100	0	0–50	0	0–50	1*	0–55	1*#	0–100	< 0.0001
At least one fall in the last 24 months [%]	46		29		42		62*		65*#		< 0.0001
LACHS (0–15)	3	0–10	2	0–8	3*	0–6	3*	1–9	4*#	0–10	< 0.0001
MMSE (0–30)	28	13–30	29	24–30	28*	13–30	28*	13–30	27*	13–30	< 0.0001
TMT-A [s]	49	13–300	38	13–300	48*	23–300	55*	26–300	72*#	17.7–300	< 0.0001
TMT-B [s]	149	34–300	101	34–300	129*	38–300	174*	60–300	300*#	38.8–300	< 0.0001
ΔTMT [s]	85	−30–280	60	−30–280	78*	0–253	98	0–257	149*	0–270	< 0.0001
Timed up and go convenient speed [s]	12	6–92	10	6–25	12*	8–28	11*	8–18	16*#+	8–92	< 0.0001
Timed up and go fast speed [s]	9	5–47	7	5–15	10*	6–22	11*	6–15	14*#+	7–47	< 0.0001
BDI II (0–63)	10	0–51	8	0–51	10	0–28	10	0–38	12*	0–51	0.0004
FES-I (0–64)	20	0–64	18	0–63	21*	0–44	20*	14–48	27*#+	14–64	< 0.0001
EQ5D VAS (0–100)	60	1–100	70	20–100	55	10–95	50*	5–90	50*#	1–95	< 0.0001
Functional Reach [cm]	23	3–82	27	8–45	23*	3–82	20*	5–35	18*#	5–34	< 0.0001
Gait speed [m/s]	1.10	0.27–2.33	1.34	0.95–2.33	0.99*	0.56–1.67	1.15*#	0.81–2.03	0.80*#+	0.27–1.5	< 0.0001
Grip force [kg]	27	3–76	29	10–76	29	7–56	28	15–51	23*#	3–51	< 0.0001

Data is presented with median and range. P-values were calculated using the Kruskal-Wallis-test, with post hoc Mann-Whitney-U-Test and Chi² test. For post hoc testing Bonferroni correction for multiple testing was applied. * p < 0.0083 for comparison with the control cohort group, # p < 0.0083 for comparison with the gait deficit cohort, + p < 0.0083 for comparison with the balance deficit cohort. BDI II Beck's depression inventory II, BMI Body mass index, EQ5D VAS Visual analog scale of the EuroQol-5 dimension questionnaire, FES-I Falls efficacy scale international, LACHS Geriatric screening according to Lachs et al., MMSE Mini-mental state examination, TMT Trail making test (part A, B, and B-A = ΔTMT)

was easy and quick to apply and none of the patients felt restricted by the sensor system. Moreover, no serious adverse events, e.g. falls, occurred. These results bode well for the clinical uptake of wearable sensors into regular care.

Not surprisingly, frequencies of gait and balance deficits of neurological inpatients are higher compared to observations in the community and in outpatient clinics. However, these deficits are ubiquitously observed. In a community-based study investigating 467 participants, the prevalence of gait deficits was 14% in those between 67 and 74 years of age, 29% in those between 75 and 84 years and 49% in those 85 years and older [40]. In a cross-sectional investigation of 488 community residing adults aged between 60 and 97 years, 32% of the cohort presented with impaired gait and the prevalence increased with age. However, 38% of the subjects aged 80 years and older still had a normally preserved gait [41]. In outpatients clinics, gait deficits occur in 35% of patients, most of them having neurological causes [42].

It is of note that, in our study, the cohort with gait (but not balance) deficits was of similar age as the control cohort. This suggests that the slower gait speed of this group was not induced by an overall decline in performance due to aging, but rather due to the underlying disease processes. This could be an interesting observation in the light of ongoing studies investigating gait speed as a relevant outcome parameter for disease and disability. Moreover, groups with gait and/or balance deficits showed impaired cognitive performance compared to the control group, supporting the association between motor performance and cognition [43–45]. It is also of note that not only the balance deficit cohort but also the gait deficit cohort performed worse than the controls in the functional reach test. This finding supports the link between static balance and gait and reflects the various aspects of postural control which should be further investigated in future studies.

The current study has several limitations. First, only gait velocity was used to define gait deficits. Although reduced gait speed impacts patients' mobility, there are several additional gait variables (e.g. gait variability, asymmetry) which are important features as they are associated with fall risk [46–49]. However, numerous more sophisticated algorithms are currently developed and validated allowing investigation of the multidimensional aspects of postural control (e.g., [20, 50, 51]) in more detail. Including dynamic, proactive, and reactive postural control parameters will give a broader view of the multidimensional aspects of balance control and help understand different pathologies of the diseases. This aspect is currently the focus of a more detailed sensor-unit-based analysis of the dataset.

Conclusion

In conclusion, this study shows that the use of inertial sensors in a clinical setting by investigating patients in neurological wards of a university hospital over a time of 16 weeks is feasible. These results should motivate to further design inpatient assessments using wearable technology, and of collaborative projects using such datasets for further in-depth analyses.

Abbreviations
BDI-II: Beck's Depression Inventory II; EQ-5D-5 L: Instrument to assess health-related quality of life; FES-I: Falls Efficacy Scale-International; MDS-UPDRS: Movement Disorders Society-sponsored Unified Parkinson's Rating Scale; MMSE: Minimal Mental State Examination; PD: Parkinson's disease; TMT: Trail Making Test; TUG: Timed-Up-and-Go test

Acknowledgements
We thank all participants who took part in the study and the financial support by Land Schleswig-Holstein within the funding programme Open Access Publikationsfonds.

Funding
We acknowledge financial support by Land Schleswig-Holstein within the funding programme Open Access Publikationsfonds.

Authors' contributions
WM, FPB, and KB, conceived and planned the experiments. FPB, JS, KB, MAH, CA, YGW, and SP carried out the experiments. FPB, NMG, CS, CH, and WM contributed to the interpretation of the results and took the lead in writing the manuscript. All authors provided critical feedback and helped shape the research, analysis and manuscript. All authors read and approved the final manuscript.

Competing interests
The authors declare that they have no competing interests.

Author details
[1]Department of Neurology and Neurodegenerative Diseases and Hertie Institute for Clinical Brain Research, University Tübingen, 72076 Tübingen, Germany. [2]DZNE, German Center for Neurodegenerative Diseases, Tuebingen, Germany. [3]Department of Neurology, University Hospital Schleswig-Holstein, Campus Kiel, Arnold-Heller-Str. 3, Haus 41, 24105 Kiel, Germany. [4]Department of Neurology and Epileptology, University Tübingen, 72076 Tübingen, Germany. [5]Department of Neurology & Stroke, University Hospital Tübingen, Tübingen, Germany.

References
1. Goetz CG, Tilley BC, Shaftman SR, Stebbins GT, Fahn S, Martinez-Martin P, et al. Movement Disorder Society-sponsored revision of the unified Parkinson's disease rating scale (MDS-UPDRS): scale presentation and clinimetric testing results. Mov Disord. 2008;23:2129–70.
2. Parry SW, Deary V, Finch T, Bamford C, Sabin N, McMeekin P, et al. The STRIDE (strategies to increase confidence, InDependence and energy) study: cognitive behavioural therapy-based intervention to reduce fear of falling in older fallers living in the community - study protocol for a randomised controlled trial. Trials. 2014;15:210.
3. Canning C, Sherrington C, Lord S, Fung V, Close J, Latt M, et al. Exercise therapy for prevention of falls in people with Parkinson's disease: a protocol for a randomised controlled trial and economic evaluation. BMC Neurol. 2009;9:4.
4. Wong TH, Nguyen HV, Chiu MT, Chow KY, Ong MEH, Lim GH, et al. The low fall as a surrogate marker of frailty predicts long-term mortality in older trauma patients. PLoS One. 2015;10:1–14.

5. Veuas BJ, Wayne SJ, Romero LJ, Baumgartner RN, Garry P. Fear of falling and restriction of mobility in elderly fallers. Age Ageing. 1997;26:189–93.

6. Starkstein SE, Merello M. The unified parkinson's disease rating scale: validation study of the mentation, behavior, and mood section. Mov Disord. 2007;22:2156–61. Available from: http://www.ncbi.nlm.nih.gov/pubmed/17721877 .

7. Rampp A, Barth J, Schuelein S, Gassmann K-G, Klucken J, Eskofier BM. Inertial sensor-based stride parameter calculation from gait sequences in geriatric patients. IEEE Trans Biomed Eng. 2015;62:1089–97. Available from: http://ieeexplore.ieee.org/document/6949634/ .

8. Schülein S, Barth J, Rampp A, Rupprecht R, Eskofier BM, Winkler J, et al. Instrumented gait analysis: a measure of gait improvement by a wheeled walker in hospitalized geriatric patients. J Neuroeng Rehabil. 2017;14:18. Available from: http://jneuroengrehab.biomedcentral.com/articles/10.1186/s12984-017-0228-z .

9. Klucken J, Barth J, Kugler P, Schlachetzki J, Henze T, Marxreiter F, et al. Unbiased and mobile gait analysis detects motor impairment in Parkinson's disease. PLoS One. 2013;8:e56956. Available from: http://dx.plos.org/10.1371/journal.pone.0056956 .

10. Bianchi MT. Sleep devices: wearables and nearables, informational and interventional, consumer and clinical. Metabolism. 2018;84:99–108. https://doi.org/10.1016/j.metabol.2017.10.008.

11. Torous J, Firth J, Mueller N, Onnela JP, Baker JT. Methodology and reporting of mobile heath and smartphone application studies for schizophrenia. Harv Rev Psychiatry. 2017;25:146–54.

12. Pevnick JM, Birkeland K, Zimmer R, Elad Y, Kedan I. Wearable technology for cardiology: an update and framework for the future. Trends Cardiovasc Med. 2018;28:144–50.

13. Haghi M, Thurow K, Stoll R. Wearable devices in medical internet of things: scientific research and commercially available devices. Healthc Inform Res. 2017;23:4–15.

14. Cahn A, Akirov A, Raz I. Digital health technology and diabetes management. J Diabetes. 2018;10:10–7.

15. Vienne A, Barrois RP, Buffat S, Ricard D, Vidal P-P. Inertial sensors to assess gait quality in patients with neurological disorders: a systematic review of technical and analytical challenges. Front Psychol. 2017;8:817.

16. Maetzler W, Klucken J, Horne M. A clinical view on the development of technology-based tools in managing Parkinson's disease. Mov Disord. 2016;31:1263–71.

17. Stolze H, Klebe S, Baecker C, Zechlin C, Friege L, Pohle S, et al. Prevalence of gait disorders in hospitalized neurological patients. Mov Disord. 2005;20:89–94.

18. Arora S, Venkataraman V, Zhan A, Donohue S, Biglan KM, Dorsey ER, et al. Detecting and monitoring the symptoms of Parkinson's disease using smartphones: a pilot study. Parkinsonism Relat Disord. 2015;21:650–3. Available from: https://www.sciencedirect.com/science/article/pii/S1353802015000814 .

19. Silva de Lima AL, Hahn T, Evers LJW, de Vries NM, Cohen E, Afek M, et al. Feasibility of large-scale deployment of multiple wearable sensors in Parkinson's disease. PLoS One. 2017;12:e0189161. Available from: http://dx.plos.org/10.1371/journal.pone.0189161 .

20. Pham MH, Elshehabi M, Haertner L, Din SD, Srulijes K, Heger T, et al. Validation of a step detection algorithm during straight walking and turning in patients with Parkinson's disease and older adults using an inertial measurement unit at the lower back. Front Neurol. 2017;8:457.

21. Donath L, Faude O, Lichtenstein E, Nüesch C, Mündermann A. Validity and reliability of a portable gait analysis system for measuring spatiotemporal gait characteristics: comparison to an instrumented treadmill. J Neuroeng Rehabil. 2016;13:6. Available from: http://www.ncbi.nlm.nih.gov/pubmed/26790409 .

22. Hobert MA, Niebler R, Meyer SI, Brockmann K, Becker C, Huber H, et al. Poor Trail making test performance is directly associated with altered dual task prioritization in the elderly - baseline results from the TREND study. PLoS One. 2011;6:e27831.

23. Elshehabi M, Maier KS, Hasmann SE, Nussbaum S, Herbst H, Heger T, et al. Limited effect of dopaminergic medication on straight walking and turning in early to moderate Parkinson's disease during single and dual tasking. Front Aging Neurosci. 2016;8:4.

24. Maetzler W, Mancini M, Liepelt-Scarfone I, Müller K, Becker C, van Lummel RCRC, et al. Impaired trunk stability in individuals at high risk for Parkinson's disease. PLoS One. 2012;7:e32240. 2012/03/30

25. Hasmann SE, Berg D, Hobert MA, Weiss D, Lindemann U, Streffer J, et al. Instrumented functional reach test differentiates individuals at high risk for Parkinson's disease from controls. Front Aging Neurosci. 2014;6:286.

26. Podsiadlo D, Richardson S. The timed "up & go": a test of basic functional mobility for frail elderly persons. 1991.

27. Van Uem JMT, Walgaard S, Ainsworth E, Hasmann SE, Heger T, Nussbaum S, et al. Quantitative timed-up-and-go parameters in relation to cognitive parameters and health-related quality of life in mild-to-moderate Parkinson's disease. PLoS One. 2016;11:e0151997. Available from: http://dx.plos.org/10.1371/journal.pone.0151997 .

28. Weiss A, Herman T, Plotnik M, Brozgol M, Maidan I, Giladi N, et al. Can an accelerometer enhance the utility of the timed up & go test when evaluating patients with Parkinson's disease? Med Eng Phys. 2010;32:119–25.

29. Dias N, Kempen GIJM, Beyer N, Freiberger E, Yardley L. Die Deutsche Version der Falls Efficacy Scale-International Version. Z Gerontol Geriatr. 2006;39:297. https://doi.org/10.1007/s00391-006-0400-8.

30. Lachs MS, Becker M, Siegal AP, Miller RL, Tinetti ME. Delusions and behavioral disturbances in cognitively impaired elderly persons. J Am Geriatr Soc. 1992;40:768–73.

31. Kühner C, Bürger C, Keller F, Hautzinger M. Reliabilität und Validität des revidierten Beck-Depressionsinventars (BDI-II). Nervenarzt. 2007;78:651–6.

32. Beck AT, Beamesderfer A. Assessment of depression: the depression inventory. Mod Probl Pharmacopsychiatry. 1974;7:151–69. Cited 22 Mar 2018. Available from: http://www.ncbi.nlm.nih.gov/pubmed/4412100.

33. EuroQol Group. EuroQol--a new facility for the measurement of health-related quality of life. Health Policy. 1990;16:199–208. Available from: http://www.ncbi.nlm.nih.gov/pubmed/10109801 .

34. Folstein MF, Folstein SE, McHugh PR. Mini-mental state: a practical method for grading the state of patients for the clinician. J Psychiatr Res. 1975;12:189–98.

35. Brown EC, Casey A, Fisch RI, Neuringer C. Trial making test as a screening device for the detection of brain damage. J Consult Psychol. 1958;22:469–74. Available from: http://www.ncbi.nlm.nih.gov/pubmed/13611107 .

36. Bohannon RW, Williams AA. Normal walking speed: a descriptive meta-analysis. Physiotherapy. 2011;97:182–9.

37. Studenski S, Perera S, Patel K, Rosano C, Faulkner K, Inzitari M, et al. Gait speed and survival in older adults. JAMA. 2011;305:50–8.

38. Amadori K, Püllen R, Steiner T. Gangstörungen im Alter. Nervenarzt. 2014;85:761–72.

39. Guralnik JM, Ferrucci L, Simonsick EM, Salive ME, Wallace RB. Lower-extremity function in persons over the age of 70 years as a predictor of subsequent disability. N Engl J Med. 1995;332:556–61.

40. Odenheimer G, Funkenstein HH, Beckett L, Chown M, Pilgrim D, Evans D, et al. Comparison of neurologic changes in "successfully aging" persons vs the Total aging population. Arch Neurol. 1994;51:573–80. American Medical Association

41. Mahlknecht P, Kiechl S, Bloem BR, Willeit J, Scherfler C, Gasperi A, et al. Prevalence and burden of gait disorders in elderly men and women aged 60–97 years: a population-based study. PLoS One. 2013;8:e69627. Available from: http://dx.plos.org/10.1371/journal.pone.0069627 .

42. Verghese J, LeValley A, Hall CB, Katz MJ, Ambrose AF, Lipton RB. Epidemiology of gait disorders in community-residing older adults. J Am Geriatr Soc. 2006;54:255–61.

43. Fitzpatrick AL, Buchanan CK, Nahin RL, Dekosky ST, Atkinson HH, Carlson MC, et al. Associations of gait speed and other measures of physical function with cognition in a healthy cohort of elderly persons. J Gerontol A Biol Sci Med Sci. 2007;62:1244–51. Available from: http://www.ncbi.nlm.nih.gov/pubmed/18000144 .

44. Parihar R, Mahoney JR, Verghese J. Relationship of gait and cognition in the elderly. Curr Transl Geriatr Exp Gerontol Rep. 2013;2:167–73. Available from: http://link.springer.com/10.1007/s13670-013-0052-7 .

45. Verghese J, Lipton RB, Katz MJ, Hall CB, Derby CA, Kuslansky G, et al. Leisure activities and the risk of dementia in the elderly. N Engl J Med. 2003;348:2508–16. Available from: http://www.nejm.org/doi/abs/10.1056/NEJMoa022252 .

46. Hausdorff JM, Rios DA, Edelberg HK. Gait variability and fall risk in community-living older adults: a 1-year prospective study. Arch Phys Med Rehabil. 2001;82:1050–6. Available from: http://linkinghub.elsevier.com/retrieve/pii/S0003999301632155 .

47. Johansson J, Nordström A, Nordström P. Greater fall risk in elderly women than in men is associated with increased gait variability during multitasking. J Am Med Dir Assoc. 2016;17:535–40. Available from: http://www.ncbi.nlm.nih.gov/pubmed/27006336 .

48. Dadashi F, Mariani B, Rochat S, Büla CJ, Santos-Eggimann B, Aminian K. Gait and foot clearance parameters obtained using shoe-worn inertial sensors in a large-population sample of older adults. Sensors (Basel). 2013;14:443–57. Available from: http://www.mdpi.com/1424-8220/14/1/443 .

49. Del Din S, Godfrey A, Rochester L. Validation of an accelerometer to quantify a comprehensive battery of gait characteristics in healthy older adults and Parkinson's disease: toward clinical and at home use. IEEE J Biomed Heal Informatics. 2016;20:838–47.

50. Mancini M, Chiari L, Holmstrom L, Salarian A, Horak FB. Validity and reliability of an IMU-based method to detect APAs prior to gait initiation. Gait Posture. 2016;43:125–31. Available from: http://www.ncbi.nlm.nih.gov/pubmed/26433913 .

51. Pham MH, Elshehabi M, Haertner L, Heger T, Hobert MA, Faber GS, et al. Algorithm for turning detection and analysis validated under home-like conditions in patients with Parkinson's disease and older adults using a 6 degree-of-freedom inertial measurement unit at the lower back. Front Neurol. 2017;8:135. Available from: http://journal.frontiersin.org/article/10.3389/fneur.2017.00135/full.

Intracranial pressure responsiveness to positive end-expiratory pressure is influenced by chest wall elastance: a physiological study in patients with aneurysmal subarachnoid hemorrhage

Han Chen[1,2], Kai Chen[2], Jing-Qing Xu[2], Ying-Rui Zhang[2], Rong-Guo Yu[2] and Jian-Xin Zhou[1]*

Abstract

Background: Respiratory system elastance (E_{RS}) is an important determinant of the responsiveness of intracranial pressure (ICP) to positive end-expiratory pressure (PEEP). However, lung elastance (E_L) and chest wall elastance (E_{CW}) were not differentiated in previous studies. We tested the hypothesis that patients with high E_{CW} or a high E_{CW}/E_{RS} ratio have greater ICP responsiveness to PEEP.

Methods: An esophageal balloon catheter was placed to measure esophageal pressure. PEEP was increased from 5 to 15 cmH_2O. Airway pressure and esophageal pressure were measured and E_L, E_{CW} and E_{RS} were calculated at the two PEEP levels. Patients were classified into either an ICP responder group or a non-responder group based on whether the change of ICP after PEEP adjustment was greater than or less than the median of the overall study population.

Results: The magnitude of the increase in esophageal pressure (median [interquartile range]) at end-expiratory occlusion was significantly increased in the responder group compared with that in the non-responder group (4.1 [2.7–4.1] versus 2.7 [0.0–2.7] cmH_2O, $p = 0.033$) after PEEP adjustment. E_{CW} and the E_{CW}/E_{RS} ratio were significantly higher in ICP responders than in non-responders at both low PEEP ($p = 0.021$ and 0.017) and high PEEP ($p = 0.011$ and 0.025) levels. No significant differences in E_{RS} and E_L were noted between the two groups at both PEEP levels.

Conclusions: Patients with greater ICP responsiveness to increased PEEP exhibit higher E_{CW} and a higher E_{CW}/E_{RS} ratio, suggesting the importance of ECW monitoring.

Keywords: Respiratory mechanics, Chest wall elastance, Intracranial pressure, Positive end-expiratory pressure, Esophageal pressure

Background

Acute lung injury is prevalent in patients with acute brain injury [1–4]. Mechanical ventilation is needed in this population, and positive end-expiratory pressure (PEEP) is often used to improve oxygenation and prevent or recruit alveolar collapse [5–7]. However, there have long been concerns that the use of PEEP in brain-injured patients could reduce cerebral perfusion pressure due to both

increased intracranial pressure (ICP) and decreased mean arterial pressure [8, 9]. Previous studies yielded inconsistent effects of PEEP on ICP [10] and diverse individual responsiveness [11–13], suggesting that the mechanism of action might be multifactorial. Several possible determinants for the influence of PEEP on ICP have been proposed, including baseline ICP [14], intracranial compliance [15, 16], respiratory mechanics [16, 17], dead space change and alveolar recruitment by PEEP [18].

Theoretically, PEEP may increase ICP by reducing venous return via elevating intrathoracic pressure [9]. Thus, ICP responsiveness to PEEP might largely depend

* Correspondence: zhoujx.cn@icloud.com
[1]Department of Critical Care Medicine, Beijing Tiantan Hospital, Capital Medical University, No 6, Tiantan Xili, Dongcheng District, Beijing, China
Full list of author information is available at the end of the article

on pressure transmission from the lung to the pleural cavity, which is determined by the distribution of lung elastance (E_L) and chest wall elastance (E_{CW}) in respiratory system elastance (E_{RS}). Although clinical studies have suggested that an increased E_{RS} might attenuate the effect of PEEP on ICP, E_L and E_{CW} were not differentiated in these studies [16, 17]. A given increased E_{RS} might mainly contribute to the increase in E_L due to pulmonary causes, such as acute respiratory distress syndrome (ARDS), or the increase in E_{CW} due to the chest wall impairment, such as intra-abdominal hypertension or massive pleural effusion [19]. In mechanical ventilated patients, the reported E_{CW} to E_{RS} ratio (E_{CW}/E_{RS} ratio) varied from 0.2 to 0.8 [19]. To date, no study has been performed to determine the different effects of E_L and E_{CW} on ICP responsiveness to PEEP, which is worthy of investigation.

We hypothesized that the patients with high E_{CW} or a high E_{CW}/E_{RS} ratio might exhibit more significant ICP responsiveness to PEEP. In the present study, patients with aneurysmal subarachnoid hemorrhage after clipping surgeries were enrolled, and two different levels of PEEP were applied. Changes in ICP after PEEP adjustment were monitored. Esophageal pressure was measured as a surrogate for pleural pressure, and the distribution of E_L and E_{CW} in E_{RS} was determined. The aim was to investigate the possible influencing factors in ICP responsiveness to PEEP, especially for E_{CW} and the E_{CW}/E_{RS} ratio.

Methods
Ethics and setting
This study was conducted in the Surgical Intensive Care Unit of Fujian Provincial Hospital, Fuzhou, China. The study protocol was approved by the Institutional Review Board of Fujian Provincial Hospital (K2015–023-01) on September 30, 2015, and the study was registered at ClinicalTrials.org (NCT02670733) on January 26, 2016 [20]. Because the study enrolled patients that were in a coma state, written informed consent was obtained from patient's appropriate substitute decision maker designated to provide consent upon admission to the hospital.

Patients
All adult patients receiving aneurysm clipping after aneurysmal subarachnoid hemorrhage were consecutively screened daily. The inclusion criteria included 1) Glasgow Coma Scale (GCS) ≤ 8; 2) ventricular ICP monitor previously placed for ICP monitoring and cerebrospinal fluid drainage during the operation; and 3) need for mechanical ventilation with PEEP. The exclusion criteria were 1) age under 18 years; 2) after decompressive craniectomy; 3) ICP > 25 mmHg; 4) hemodynamic instability requiring greater than 10 μg/kg/min dopamine or more than 0.5 μg/kg/min norepinephrine; 5) history of esophageal

surgery or chronic obstructive pulmonary disease; 6) evidence of active air leak from the lung or existing chest tube; and 7) expected to survive less than 24 h.

Given the lack of a widely accepted threshold to identify the responsiveness of ICP to increased PEEP levels, we classified each patient into two groups according to the median change of ICP after PEEP adjustment in the overall study population: above the median value was considered the "responder" group and below the median value was considered the "non-responder" group. This was an unblinded study, but the researchers were not aware of the patients' allocation until all data were collected (the median can only be determined by then).

ICP monitoring and intracranial ventricular compliance measurements
ICP was measured using a ventricular ICP monitor (Codman, Johnson & Johnson, Raynham, MA, USA). Ventricular drainage was blocked during the procedure as long as tolerated by the patient (i.e. without an ICP > 25 mmHg). To measure the ventricular compliance, 2 mL of cerebrospinal fluid was drained, and immediate changes in ICP values were recorded. Ventricular compliance was calculated as the ratio of the cerebrospinal fluid drainage volume to the decrease in ICP after the drainage (mL/mm Hg) [15, 16].

Study procedure
During the study, the patient remained in a supine position with the head of the bed elevated to 30°. Esophageal pressure was measured by a SmartCath-G adult esophageal balloon catheter (7,003,300, CareFusion Co., Yorba Linda, CA, USA). An occlusion test was used to confirm the proper balloon position [21, 22]. Esophageal pressure and airway pressure were measured by two KT 100D-2 pressure transducers (KleisTEK di CosimoMicelli, Italy, range: +/– 100 cm H_2O), and flow was measured with a Fleisch pneumotachograph (Vitalograph Inc., Lenexa, KS, USA). The pressure and flow signals were displayed continuously and saved (ICU-Lab 2.5 Software Package, ICU Lab, KleisTEK Engineering, Bari, Italy) on a laptop for further analysis. Details on esophageal pressure monitoring and data collection are presented in the Additional file 1.

After the establishment of esophageal pressure monitoring, the patient was sedated and paralyzed via the intravenous infusion of 5 mg of midazolam, 0.1 mg of fentanyl, and 50 mg of rocuronium. Mechanical ventilation was set as volume-controlled ventilation with a constant flow, an inspiratory to expiratory ratio of 1:2, and a tidal volume (V_T) of 6 to 8 mL/kg of predicted body weight. The initial respiratory rate was set to maintain the $PaCO_2$ at 35 to 45 mmHg. End-tidal carbon dioxide partial pressure ($P_{ET}CO_2$) was also measured (CAPNOSTAT®, Maquet,

Solna, Sweden). Pulse oxygen saturation was maintained above 92% by adjusting the FiO_2.

Two PEEP levels were tested. The PEEP level was first set to 5 cm H_2O. After a 30-min stabilization, PaO_2, $PaCO_2$ and $P_{ET}CO_2$ were simultaneously measured, and the ratio of the alveolar dead space to the tidal volume (V_{Dalv}/V_T) was calculated. ICP, mean blood pressure, cerebral perfusion pressure, central venous pressure and ventricular compliance were measured. End-expiratory and end-inspiratory occlusions were performed for 3 s each, and the airway pressure and the esophageal pressure during the last second of occlusion were recorded. Thereafter, the PEEP level was increased to 15 cm H_2O and maintained for 30 min without changes in other ventilation settings. The same sequence of measurements was repeated, with the exception that the ventricular compliance measurement was not performed because cerebrospinal fluid drainage might influence ICP monitoring.

E_{RS}, E_L and E_{CW} were calculated using a standard formula [19, 23]. The E_{CW}/E_{RS} ratio was documented. Detailed procedures, measurements and parameter derivations are presented in the Additional file 1.

The procedure was emergently terminated if ICP increased above 25 mmHg or cerebral perfusion pressure decreased below 50 mmHg.

Statistical analysis

The primary endpoint was the difference in E_{RS}, E_L, E_{CW} and the E_{CW}/E_{RS} ratio in patients with different ICP responsiveness to PEEP. We did not calculate sample size because the differences in these elastance parameters between the two groups remain unknown. Instead, we chose 30, a widely accepted minimal sample size for a physiological study, as the sample size in the present study.

Categorical variables are presented as numbers and percentages and were analyzed by Fisher's exact test. Continuous variables are presented as the median and inter-quartile range (IQR) and were compared using the Mann-Whitney U test or Wilcoxon matched-pair signed-rank test as appropriate. We used the Scheirer-Ray-Hare test to compare the parameters between the responder and the non-responder groups at low and high PEEP levels [24]. All tests of significance were at the 5% significance level and were two-sided. Analyses were performed with SPSS statistics software (V.20.0 IBM Corporation, New York, USA).

Results

From February to November 2016, 30 patients were studied. No emergent termination occurred during the procedures. Table 1 presents the main characteristics of the enrolled patients at the low (5 cm H_2O) and high (15 cm H_2O) PEEP levels. After the PEEP level was increased, ICP significantly increased ($p < 0.001$). The median (IQR) change in ICP was 2.5 (1.0–4.0) mm Hg. According

to the predefined criterion, each of the 15 patients was allocated to the "responder" group or the "non-responder" group, which had respective ICP changes of 4.0 (3.0–5.0) and 1.0 (1.0–2.0) mm Hg. Baseline characteristics were comparable between the two groups except for responders with an older age and a lower body mass index (Table 2).

Detailed data of respiratory mechanics, ICP and hemodynamic parameters and blood gas analysis are presented in the Additional file 2 (Table E1 to E6).

Esophageal pressure at end-expiratory occlusion increased significantly after PEEP adjustment (5.4 [4.1–8.2] versus 9.5 [6.8–12.2] cm H_2O, $p < 0.001$), and the magnitude of the increase was significantly higher in the responder group than in the non-responder group (4.1 [2.7–4.1] versus 2.7 [0.0–2.7] cm H_2O, $p = 0.033$, Fig. 1). At the low PEEP level, there were no significant differences in E_{RS} ($p = 0.136$) and E_L ($p = 0.863$) between two groups, but E_{CW} and the E_{CW}/E_{RS} ratio were significantly higher in responders than in non-responders ($p = 0.021$ and 0.017) (Fig. 2a). As the PEEP level increased, no significant difference existed in the magnitude of change in E_{RS}, E_L, and E_{CW} between the two groups ($p = 0.468$ to 0.787, Fig. 2b). Thus, significant differences in E_{CW} and the E_{CW}/E_{RS} ratio between the two groups remained at the high PEEP level ($p = 0.011$ and 0.025, Fig. 2c).

No significant difference was found in baseline ICP (3.0 [2.0–6.0] versus 4.0 [4.0–10.0] mm Hg, $p = 0.163$) and intracranial ventricular compliance (1.0 [0.7–1.0] versus 1.0 [0.7–1.0] mL/mm Hg, $p = 0.723$) between the ICP responder and non-responder groups. Although central venous pressure increased significantly after the PEEP level was increased in all enrolled patients (Table 1, $p < 0.001$), no significant difference was observed in the change of central venous pressure between ICP responders and non-responders (5.0 [4.0–5.0] versus 3.0 [1.0–6.0] mm Hg, $p = 0.077$, Fig. 3). Similarly, significant decreases in mean blood pressure were observed after PEEP increase in all enrolled patients (81.0 [75.6, 92.1] versus 76.2 [67.4, 90.0], $p = 0.002$), but no difference in the change of mean blood pressure between groups (Table E3 and E4). Cerebral perfusion also decreased after PEEP was increased, the responder had a significantly greater decrease in cerebral perfusion pressure than the non-responder (− 13.0 [− 18.3, − 6.7] versus − 6.7 [− 11.3, 1.0], $p = 0.011$; Table E3 and E4).

There was no significant difference in PaO_2, PaO_2/FiO_2 and $PaCO_2$ after PEEP adjustment ($p = 0.052$ to 0.061, Table 1). $P_{ET}CO_2$ significantly decreased (29.5 [27.8–31.2] versus 29.0 [25.8–30.3] mm Hg, $p = 0.003$); thus, V_{Dalv}/V_T significantly increased (13.2 [8.5–19.9] versus 18.8 [11.9–27.7] %, $p < 0.001$). No significant differences were observed in $P_{ET}CO_2$ and V_{Dalv}/V_T between ICP responders and non-responders at either the low or high PEEP levels.

Table 1 Patients characteristics at low and high positive end-expiratory pressure

	Low PEEP (5 cmH₂O)	High PEEP (15 cmH₂O)	p
ICP and hemodynamic parameters			
ICP (mmHg)	4.0 (2.0–10.0)	7.0 (5.8–11.0)	< 0.001
MAP (mmHg)	81.0 (75.6–92.1)	76.2 (67.4–90.0)	0.002
CPP (mmHg)	74.7 (69.6–86.8)	68.7 (60.6–82.7)	< 0.001
CVP (mmHg)	8.0 (5.0–10.0)	12.0 (10.0–14.0)	< 0.001
Respiratory mechanics parameters			
V_T (mL/kg)	7.7 (7.1–8.3)	7.7 (7.1–8.2)	0.304
ΔP_{AW} (cmH₂O)	6.8 (6.5–9.5)	9.5 (7.8–10.9)	< 0.001
ΔP_{CW} (cmH₂O)	2.7 (1.4–3.1)	2.7 (2.7–4.1)	0.003
ΔP_L (cmH₂O)	4.8 (4.1–5.8)	6.8 (4.1–8.2)	0.003
E_{RS} (cmH₂O/L)	15.3 (12.5–18.6)	20.1 (16.2–23.9)	< 0.001
E_{CW} (cmH₂O/L)	5.5 (2.9–6.9)	6.2 (5.4–10.2)	0.001
E_L (cmH₂O/L)	9.4 (7.9–12.1)	12.9 (8.5–15.6)	0.004
E_{CW}/E_{RS} ratio	0.33 (0.25–0.43)	0.40 (0.29–0.47)	0.247
Resistance (cmH₂O/L/sec)	13.0 (9.9–14.2)	12.6 (10.1–15.0)	0.894
Blood gas analysis parameters			
pH	7.40 (7.36–7.44)	7.42 (7.38–7.45)	0.951
PaO_2 (mmHg)	105.5 (78.0–153.5)	115.5 (78.4–163.5)	0.058
PaO_2/FiO_2	264 (180–384)	289 (185–388)	0.061
$PaCO_2$ (mmHg)	35.3 (32.6–36.7)	35.3 (33.6–38.2)	0.052
$P_{ET}CO_2$ (mmHg)	29.5 (27.8–31.2)	29.0 (25.8–30.3)	0.003
V_{Dalv}/V_T (%)	13.2 (8.5–19.9)	18.8 (11.9–27.7)	< 0.001

Data are shown as median (interquartile range)

ICP intracranial pressure; *MAP* mean arterial pressure; *CPP* cerebral perfusion pressure; *CVP* central venous pressure; V_T tidal volume; ΔP_{AW} airway driving pressure; ΔP_{CW} chest wall driving pressure; ΔP_L: transpulmonary driving pressure; E_{RS} respiratory system elastance; E_{CW} chest wall elastance; E_L lung elastance; *PETCO₂* end-tidal carbon dioxide partial pressure; V_{Dalv}/V_T: ratio of the alveolar dead space to the tidal volume

Table 2 Patients characteristics at study entry

	All patients (n = 30)	Responders (n = 15)	Non-responders (n = 15)	p^*
Age (years)	55 (37–66)	66 (42–73)	42 (37–57)	0.045
Male	21 (70)	10 (67)	11 (73)	0.500
BMI (kg/m²)	22.8 (22.0–24.2)	22.0 (21.2–23.6)	23.6 (22.0–24.2)	0.039
GCS	5.5 (4.0–6.3)	5.0 (4.0–7.0)	6.0 (5.0–6.0)	0.513
SAPS II	49.5 (46.3–54.6)	49.7 (44.0–57.0)	49.0 (47.0–54.0)	0.400
MV duration (days)[a]	1.0 (1.0–2.0)	1.0 (1.0–2.0)	2.0 (1.0–2.0)	0.345
ARDS diagnosis	6 (20)	4 (27)	2 (13)	0.361
PaO_2	105.5 (78.0–153.5)	95.0 (76.7–130.0)	129.0 (78.4–168.0)	0.242
PaO_2/FiO_2	264 (180–384)	274 (156–325)	323 (196–420)	0.144
$PaCO_2$ (mmHg)	35.3 (32.6–36.7)	35.4 (32.7–38.1)	35.1 (30.9–36.1)	0.307

Data are presented as median (interquartile range) for continuous variables and counts (percentages) for categorical variables

ARDS acute respiratory distress syndrome, *BMI* body mass index, GCS Glasgow Coma Scale, *MV* mechanical ventilation, *SAPS II* Simplified Acute Physiology Score II

[*]p value in comparison between the responder and non-responder group

[a]MV duration before enrolment

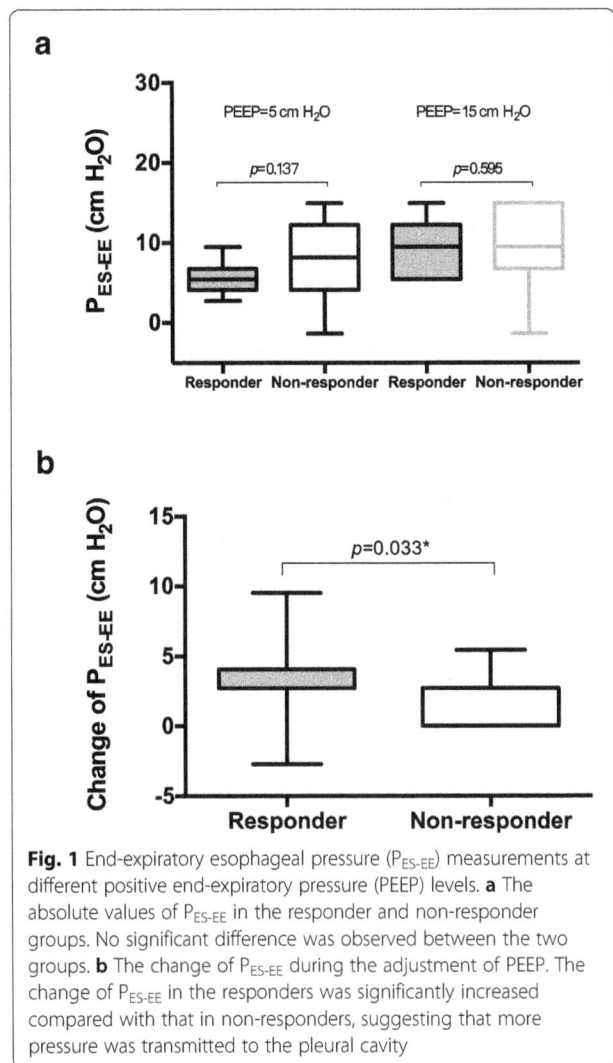

Fig. 1 End-expiratory esophageal pressure (P_{ES-EE}) measurements at different positive end-expiratory pressure (PEEP) levels. **a** The absolute values of P_{ES-EE} in the responder and non-responder groups. No significant difference was observed between the two groups. **b** The change of P_{ES-EE} during the adjustment of PEEP. The change of P_{ES-EE} in the responders was significantly increased compared with that in non-responders, suggesting that more pressure was transmitted to the pleural cavity

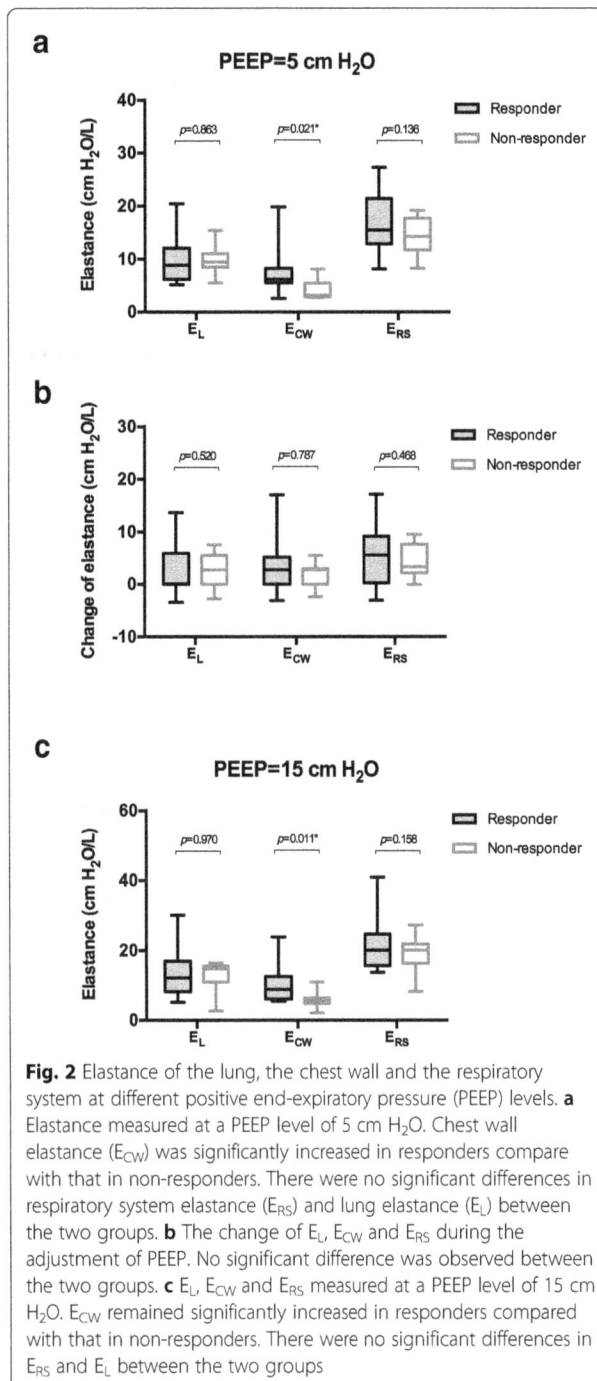

Fig. 2 Elastance of the lung, the chest wall and the respiratory system at different positive end-expiratory pressure (PEEP) levels. **a** Elastance measured at a PEEP level of 5 cm H_2O. Chest wall elastance (E_{CW}) was significantly increased in responders compare with that in non-responders. There were no significant differences in respiratory system elastance (E_{RS}) and lung elastance (E_L) between the two groups. **b** The change of E_L, E_{CW} and E_{RS} during the adjustment of PEEP. No significant difference was observed between the two groups. **c** E_L, E_{CW} and E_{RS} measured at a PEEP level of 15 cm H_2O. E_{CW} remained significantly increased in responders compared with that in non-responders. There were no significant differences in E_{RS} and E_L between the two groups

Discussion

The main finding of our study was that patients with a greater ICP responsiveness to increased PEEP exhibit a higher E_{CW} and E_{CW}/E_{RS} ratio. This finding was consistent with our hypothesis.

Regarding the influence of PEEP on ICP, clinical studies have reported conflicting results, with ICP increasing [14–18], not markedly changing [25–27] or even decreasing [28] after the application of PEEP. In patients with increased ICP, the effect of PEEP on ICP becomes evident whenever the elevation of the intrathoracic pressure induced by applied PEEP exceeds the ICP [14]. This mechanism was referred to as the Starling resistor model, which represented the role of damaged venous outflow in the response of ICP to PEEP [29]. In a study conducted by McGuire et al., 15 mmHg was used as the upper limit of the normal baseline value of ICP at zero PEEP [14]. ICP increased at PEEP levels of 10 and 15 cm

H_2O in patients with normal baseline ICP but did not significantly change at PEEP levels of 5 to 15 cm H_2O in patients with elevated baseline ICP. In our group of patients, all ICP values were less than 15 mmHg at 5 cm H_2O PEEP (4.0 [2.0–10.0] mm Hg) and increased after the PEEP level was adjusted to 15 cm H_2O (7.0 [5.8–11.0] mm Hg). The difference in ICP at the two PEEP levels (2.5 [1.0–4.0] mm Hg) in our patients was comparable to those previously reported [13, 14].

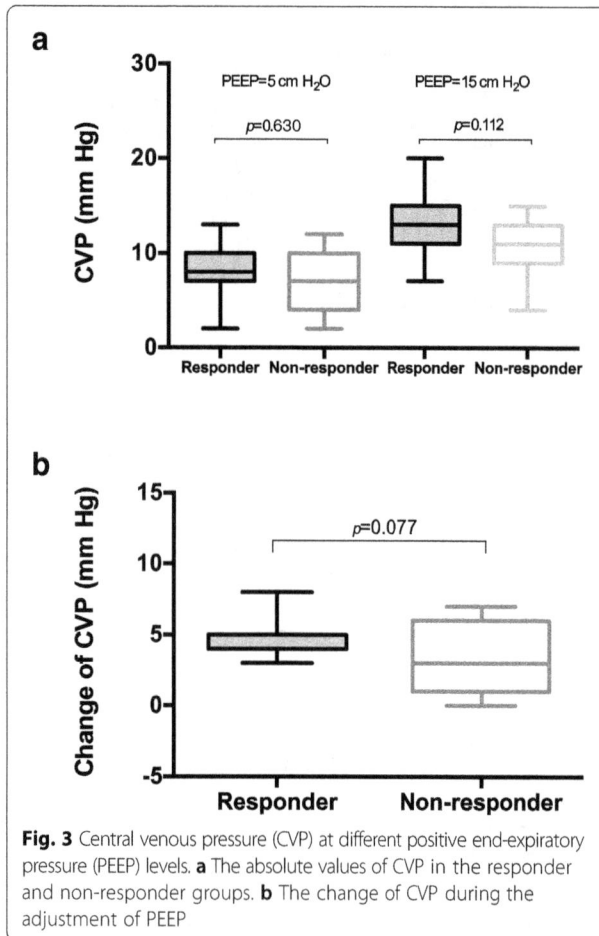

Fig. 3 Central venous pressure (CVP) at different positive end-expiratory pressure (PEEP) levels. **a** The absolute values of CVP in the responder and non-responder groups. **b** The change of CVP during the adjustment of PEEP

The PEEP-induced increase of pleural pressure may reduce cerebral venous drainage and eventually increase ICP [9]. The pleural pressure serves as an intermediate link from the lung to the cranium. In the present study, we measured esophageal pressure as a surrogate of pleural pressure and found that esophageal pressure increased more significantly in ICP responders than in non-responders (Fig. 1). This finding suggested a role of pressure transmitted to the pleural cavity in ICP responsiveness. In addition, central venous pressure increased significantly at the high PEEP level (Table 1), indicating the impairment of venous return by PEEP, which eventually resulted in reduced mean blood pressure and cerebral perfusion pressure. ICP responders had a higher tendency to have elevated central venous pressure (Fig. 3); however, statistical significance was not achieved, potentially due to the limited sample size.

The elastic properties of the respiratory system may be a key factor in determining the effect of PEEP on pleural pressure and subsequently ICP [9]. Pressure transmission from the lung to the pleural cavity depends on the distribution of E_L and E_{CW} in E_{RS}. The higher the proportion of E_{CW} is, the greater the impact of PEEP on pleural pressure [19]. Therefore, E_{CW} and the E_{CW}/E_{RS} ratio may be a more important determinant of ICP responsiveness to PEEP. In previous clinical studies, only E_{RS} was used to explore the influence of respiratory mechanics in the PEEP and ICP relationship [16, 17]. After distinguishing E_L and E_{CW} from E_{RS}, we found that the effect of PEEP on ICP was more profound in patients with higher E_{CW} and a higher E_{CW}/E_{RS} ratio (Fig. 2). Although patients with brain injury exhibited higher E_{CW} (without detailed values) in previous studies [30], E_{CW} and the E_{CW}/E_{RS} ratio measured in our group of patients were relatively "normal" (Table 1). Our results were comparable to those reported in patients under general anesthesia [31] but higher than those reported in ARDS patients [32]. However, even a slightly higher E_{CW} and E_{CW}/E_{RS} ratio might contribute to ICP responsiveness (Fig. 2). Our data suggested the importance of separate E_L and E_{CW} monitoring during the clinical application of high PEEP in brain-injured patients.

There are two consequences after the application of PEEP: recruitment of collapsed alveoli and/or overdistention of normal alveoli. In patients with severe brain injury and acute lung injury or ARDS, Mascia et al. defined two groups based on recruitment volume: ≥ 110 mL as recruiters and < 110 mL as non-recruiters [18]. As the PEEP level increased, E_{RS} and $PaCO_2$ significantly increased in non-recruiters, indicating hyperinflation. On the contrary, E_{RS} significantly decreased, and $PaCO_2$ remained unchanged in recruiters. ICP increased only in non-recruiters. In their patient population, the PaO_2/FiO_2 ratio was 95–141 mmHg, and E_{RS} was 24–25 cm H_2O/L at 5 cm H_2O PEEP [18]. In our group of patients, only six ARDS cases (20%) were enrolled, and the overall severity of lung injury was mild, as represented by the median PaO_2/FiO_2 ratio of 264 and an E_{RS} of 15.3 cm H_2O/L at the low PEEP level. Alveolar collapse might also be minor; therefore, increases in the PEEP level produced increases in E_{RS} (15.3 to 20.1 cm H_2O/L) and V_{Dalv}/V_T (13.2 to 18.8%). Despite lacking statistical significance, $PaCO_2$ and V_{Dalv}/V_T were high in ICP responders. Therefore, PEEP-induced hyperinflation might also contribute to ICP responsiveness in our patients.

The effect of PEEP on ICP might be affected by ventricular compliance [15, 16]. Apuzzo et al. reported that a significant increase in ICP was only observed in patients who manifested increased cerebral elastance when PEEP was applied [15]. Similarly, Burchiel et al. reported that PEEP increased ICP in patients with decreased intracranial compliance and that decreased lung compliance may buffer this effect [16]. In the present study, given that patients with normal ICP were enrolled and that cerebrospinal fluid was continuously drained before the start of the study, the ventricular compliance was "normal" in all patients. Additionally, for ethical reasons, we cannot measure the ventricular compliance by injecting normal saline into the ventricle instead of draining the cerebrospinal fluid. Because intracranial hypertension and ventricular compliance impairment are prevalent in patients with severe brain injury, further animal experiments should be performed to validate the role of ventricular compliance in the ICP and PEEP relationship.

Increase in PEEP decreases systematic venous return and potentially lowers the cardiac output, this will lower blood pressure and cerebral perfusion pressure. If the cerebral perfusion pressure break through the lower limit of cerebral autoregulation, cerebral perfusion will not be maintained and thus decrease cerebral blood flow, cerebral blood volume and ICP. In this case, the decrease of cerebral perfusion (and thereby decrease in ICP) will somehow contaminate the effect of PEEP on the venous side. In our study, blood pressure and cerebral perfusion pressure were maintained in a normal range, even in a high PEEP level. Therefore, although without cerebral blood flow being measured, we assumed that the cerebral perfusion was comparable between the two groups.

The responders were significant older in this study. It has been reported that the elders have higher E_{CW} due to structural changes to the thoracic cage [33, 34], which is the result of age-related osteoporosis and calcification of the rib cage that reduce the ability of the thoracic cage to expand. Our data also showed higher E_{CW} in the elders, probably due to the same reason. The responders also had significantly lower BMI. Although obesity people have higher E_{RS}, it can be the result of either increased E_L or increased E_{CW}, or even both [35]. This makes the E_{CW} unpredictable simply base on BMI. Moreover, our patients had relatively normal BMI, the small difference of BMI between the two group (although statistically significant) is unlikely the determinant of the difference of E_{CW}.

The main strength of the present study was that the contribution of the chest wall and the lung in ICP responsiveness to PEEP was distinguished. The adverse effect of PEEP on ICP may be amplified in patients with higher E_{CW} and a higher E_{CW}/E_{RS} ratio. Our data suggest the potential necessity of respiratory mechanics monitoring when applying PEEP in brain-injured patients, especially in patients with a risk of chest wall impairment.

There were several limitations of the study. First, we used the median of the increased value rather than other physiological parameters to define the ICP responders and non-responders. Given that no widely accepted standard is available to discriminate whether the patient's ICP is responsive to increased PEEP, the division of patients into two groups is reasonable and enables us to compare potential determinants between the two

groups. Second, we only included postoperative subarachnoid hemorrhage patients with relatively normal ICP and respiratory mechanics. Therefore, our results might not be directly applied to other populations. Third, although esophageal pressure has been employed as a surrogate of pleural pressure, the use of the absolute value of esophageal pressure remains questionable [19]. However, in the calculation of E_{CW}, we used the change in esophageal pressure between end-inspiration and end-expiration occlusion, which has been shown to reliably reflect the change in pleural pressure [23, 36, 37].

Conclusions

Patients with greater ICP responsiveness to increased PEEP had higher E_{CW} and a higher E_{CW}/E_{RS} ratio. Potential factors contributing to the increase in E_{CW} and the E_{CW}/E_{RS} ratio should be assessed and eliminated if possible to avoid the adverse effects of high PEEP levels on the brain.

Additional files

Additional file 1: Detailed methods of the study procedures, measurements and parameter derivations. (PDF 186 kb)

Additional file 2: Detailed results of respiratory mechanics, intracranial pressure, hemodynamics parameters and blood gas. Values of respiratory mechanics (Table E1), intracranial pressure and hemodynamics parameters (Table E3) and blood gas (Table E5) at low and high positive end-expiratory pressure (PEEP) levels were provided. Changes in respiratory mechanics (Table E2), intracranial pressure and hemodynamics parameters (Table E4) and blood gas (Table E6) from low to high PEEP were also provided. (PDF 177 kb)

Abbreviations
ARDS: Acute respiratory distress syndrome; CPP: Cerebral perfusion pressure; CVP: Central venous pressure; E_{CW}: Chest wall elastance; E_L: Lung elastance; E_{RS}: Respiratory system elastance; ICP: Intracranial pressure; MAP: Mean arterial pressure; P_{AW}: Airway pressure; PEEP: Positive end-expiratory pressure; P_{ES}: Esophageal pressure; $P_{ET}CO_2$: End-tidal carbon dioxide partial pressure; V_{Dalv}/V_T: Alveolar dead space to the tidal volume ratio; V_T: Tidal volume

Funding
The study was funded by the Beijing Municipal Administration of Hospital (grant number ZYLX201502). The sponsors had no role in the design of the study and collection, analysis, and interpretation of data and in writing the manuscript.

Authors' contributions
HC, JXZ and RGY participated in the design of the study and drafted the manuscript. HC, KC, JQX and YRZ participated in the study and data collection. All authors participated in review and revision of the manuscript. All authors read and approved the final manuscript.

Competing interests
The authors declare that they have no competing interests.

Author details
[1]Department of Critical Care Medicine, Beijing Tiantan Hospital, Capital Medical University, No 6, Tiantan Xili, Dongcheng District, Beijing, China. [2]Surgical Intensive Care Unit, Fujian Provincial Clinical College, Fujian Medical University, Fuzhou, Fujian, China.

References

1. Hoesch RE, Lin E, Young M, Gottesman RF, Altaweel L, Nyquist PA, et al. Acute lung injury in critical neurological illness. Crit Care Med. 2012;40:587–93.
2. Kahn JM, Caldwell EC, Deem S, Newell DW, Heckbert SR, Rubenfeld GD. Acute lung injury in patients with subarachnoid hemorrhage: incidence, risk factors, and outcome. Crit Care Med. 2006;34:196–202.
3. Aisiku IP, Yamal JM, Doshi P, Rubin ML, Benoit JS, Hannay J, et al. The incidence of ARDS and associated mortality in severe TBI using the berlin definition. J Trauma Acute Care Surg. 2016;80:308–12.
4. Mascia L, Sakr Y, Pasero D, Payen D, Reinhart K, Vincent JL. Extracranial complications in patients with acute brain injury: a post-hoc analysis of the SOAP study. Intensive Care Med. 2008;34:720–7.
5. Pelosi P, Ferguson ND, Frutos-Vivar F, Anzueto A, Putensen C, Raymondos K, et al. Management and outcome of mechanically ventilated neurologic patients. Crit Care Med. 2011;39:1482–92.
6. Tejerina E, Pelosi P, Muriel A, Penuelas O, Sutherasan Y, Frutos-Vivar F, et al. Association between ventilatory settings and development of acute respiratory distress syndrome in mechanically ventilated patients due to brain injury. J Crit Care. 2017;38:341–5.
7. Luo XY, Hu YH, Cao XY, Kang Y, Liu LP, Wang SH, et al. Lung-protective ventilation in patients with brain injury: a multicenter cross-sectional study and questionnaire survey in China. Chin Med J. 2016;129:1643–51.
8. Mascia L. Ventilatory setting in severe brain injured patients: does it really matter? Intensive Care Med. 2006;32:1925–7.
9. Koutsoukou A, Katsiari M, Orfanos SE, Kotanidou A, Daganou M, Kyriakopoulou M, et al. Respiratory mechanics in brain injury: a review. World J Crit Care Med. 2016;5:65–73.
10. Borsellino B, Schultz MJ, Gama de Abreu M, Robba C, Bilotta F. Mechanical ventilation in neurocritical care patients: a systematic literature review. Expert Rev Respir Med. 2016;10:1123–32.
11. Shapiro HM, Marshall LF. Intracranial pressure responses to PEEP in head-injured patients. J Trauma. 1978;18:254–6.
12. Georgiadis D, Schwarz S, Baumgartner RW, Veltkamp R, Schwab S. Influence of positive end-expiratory pressure on intracranial pressure and cerebral perfusion pressure in patients with acute stroke. Stroke. 2001;32:2088–92.
13. Zhang XY, Yang ZJ, Wang QX, Fan HR. Impact of positive end-expiratory pressure on cerebral injury patients with hypoxemia. Am J Emerg Med. 2011;29:699–703.
14. McGuire G, Crossley D, Richards J, Wong D. Effects of varying levels of positive end-expiratory pressure on intracranial pressure and cerebral perfusion pressure. Crit Care Med. 1997;25:1059–62.
15. Apuzzo JL, Wiess MH, Petersons V, Small RB, Kurze T, Heiden JS. Effect of positive end expiratory pressure ventilation on intracranial pressure in man. J Neurosurg. 1977;46:227–32.
16. Burchiel KJ, Steege TD, Wyler AR. Intracranial pressure changes in brain-injured patients requiring positive end-expiratory pressure ventilation. Neurosurgery. 1981;8:443–9.
17. Caricato A, Conti G, Della Corte F, Mancino A, Santilli F, Sandroni C, et al. Effects of PEEP on the intracranial system of patients with head injury and subarachnoid hemorrhage: the role of respiratory system compliance. J Trauma. 2005;58:571–6.
18. Mascia L, Grasso S, Fiore T, Bruno F, Berardino M, Ducati A. Cerebro-pulmonary interactions during the application of low levels of positive end-expiratory pressure. Intensive Care Med. 2005;31:373–9.
19. Gattinoni L, Chiumello D, Carlesso E, Valenza F. Bench-to-bedside review: chest wall elastance in acute lung injury/acute respiratory distress syndrome patients. Crit Care. 2004;8:350–5.
20. Chen H, Xu M, Yang YL, Chen K, Xu JQ, Zhang YR, et al. Effects of increased positive end-expiratory pressure on intracranial pressure in acute respiratory distress syndrome: a protocol of a prospective physiological study. BMJ Open. 2016;6:e012477.
21. Baydur A, Behrakis PK, Zin WA, Jaeger M, Milic-Emili J. A simple method for assessing the validity of the esophageal balloon technique. Am Rev Respir Dis. 1982;126:788–91.
22. Chiumello D, Consonni D, Coppola S, Froio S, Crimella F, Colombo A. The occlusion tests and end-expiratory esophageal pressure: measurements and comparison in controlled and assisted ventilation. Ann Intensive Care. 2016;6:13.
23. Mauri T, Yoshida T, Bellani G, Goligher EC, Carteaux G, Rittayamai N, et al. Esophageal and transpulmonary pressure in the clinical setting: meaning, usefulness and perspectives. Intensive Care Med. 2016;42:1360–73.
24. Scheirer CJ, Ray WS, Hare N. The analysis of ranked data derived from completely randomized factorial designs. Biometrics. 1976;32:429–34.
25. Frost EA. Effects of positive end-expiratory pressure on intracranial pressure and compliance in brain-injured patients. J Neurosurg. 1977;47:195–200.
26. Cooper KR, Boswell PA, Choi SC. Safe use of PEEP in patients with severe head injury. J Neurosurg. 1985;63:552–5.
27. Koutsoukou A, Perraki H, Raftopoulou A, Koulouris N, Sotiropoulou C, Kotanidou A, et al. Respiratory mechanics in brain-damaged patients. Intensive Care Med. 2006;32:1947–54.
28. Huynh T, Messer M, Sing RF, Miles W, Jacobs DG, Thomason MH. Positive end-expiratory pressure alters intracranial and cerebral perfusion pressure in severe traumatic brain injury. J Trauma. 2002;53:488–92. discussion 92-3
29. Luce JM, Huseby JS, Kirk W, Butler J. A Starling resistor regulates cerebral venous outflow in dogs. J Appl Physiol Respir Environ Exerc Physiol. 1982;53:1496–503.
30. Gamberoni C, Colombo G, Aspesi M, Mascheroni C, Severgnini P, Minora G, et al. Respiratory mechanics in brain injured patients. Minerva Anestesiol. 2002;68:291–6.
31. Cinnella G, Grasso S, Spadaro S, Rauseo M, Mirabella L, Salatto P, et al. Effects of recruitment maneuver and positive end-expiratory pressure on respiratory mechanics and transpulmonary pressure during laparoscopic surgery. Anesthesiology. 2013;118:114–22.
32. Chiumello D, Colombo A, Algieri I, Mietto C, Carlesso E, Crimella F, et al. Effect of body mass index in acute respiratory distress syndrome. Br J Anaesth. 2016;116:113–21.
33. Sharma G, Goodwin J. Effect of aging on respiratory system physiology and immunology. Clin Interv Aging. 2006;1:253–60.
34. Mittman C, Edelman N, Norris a SN. Relationship between chest wall and pulmonary compliance with age. J Appl Physiol. 1965;20:1211–6.
35. Littleton SW. Impact of obesity on respiratory function. Respirology. 2012;17:43–9.
36. Chiumello D, Carlesso E, Cadringher P, Caironi P, Valenza F, Polli F, et al. Lung stress and strain during mechanical ventilation for acute respiratory distress syndrome. Am J Respir Crit Care Med. 2008;178:346–55.
37. Chiumello D, Cressoni M, Colombo A, Babini G, Brioni M, Crimella F, et al. The assessment of transpulmonary pressure in mechanically ventilated ARDS patients. Intensive Care Med. 2014;40:1670–8.

Planning for an uncertain future in progressive neurological disease: a qualitative study of patient and family decision-making with a focus on eating and drinking

Gemma Clarke[1]* ⓘ, Elizabeth Fistein[1], Anthony Holland[2], Jake Tobin[3], Sam Barclay[1] and Stephen Barclay[1]

Abstract

Background: Dysphagia and other eating and drinking difficulties are common in progressive neurological diseases. Mealtimes can become a major source of difficulty and anxiety for patients and their families. Decisions about eating, drinking and care can become challenging as disease progresses, and the person in question loses the capacity to participate in decisions about their own care. We sought to investigate how patients and their family members make decisions about their future care as their condition deteriorates, with a particular focus on mealtimes, eating and drinking.

Methods: Longitudinal qualitative in-depth interviews were undertaken with patients and their family members ($N = 29$) across a range of disease groups, including: dementia, Parkinson's Disease, Huntington's Disease, Progressive Supranuclear Palsy, Motor Neurone Disease, Multiple Sclerosis. Patients had varying degrees of eating and drinking difficulties, and levels of decision-making capacity. Interviews were 'participant led' and undertaken in the patients' own homes or a place of their choosing. Follow-up interviews were three months to one year later depending upon disease trajectory. Interviews were audio recorded and analysed in NVivo using a Thematic Analysis approach.

Results: Twenty-nine participants were interviewed between 2015 and 2017. Two key themes emerged from the analysis: 1) *Health Literacy:* the extent to which patients and relatives appeared to know about the condition and its treatment. Patients and their family members varied in their ability to speak and communicate about their condition and prognosis. 2) *Planning style:* the extent to which participants appeared to value involvement in advance care-planning. Patients and their family members varied in the way in which they made decisions: some preferred to 'take each day as it comes', while others wished to plan extensively for the future.

Conclusions: Issues with eating and drinking are often overlooked. Clinicians need to understand both the patient's level of health literacy and their style of planning before communicating with patients and their families about these sensitive issues.

Keywords: Decision-making capacity, Dysphagia, Care planning, Mealtimes, Dementia, Parkinson's disease, Huntington's disease, Progressive Supranuclear palsy, Motor Neurone disease, Multiple sclerosis

* Correspondence: gcc29@medschl.cam.ac.uk
[1]Primary Care Unit, Department of Public Health and Primary Care, Cambridge Institute of Public Health, University of Cambridge School of Clinical Medicine, Box 113 Cambridge Biomedical Campus, Cambridge CB2 0SR, UK
Full list of author information is available at the end of the article

Background

Mealtimes are usually an important part of everyday life, with opportunities for pleasure and socialising [1, 2]. Social meanings attached to mealtimes are connected to deep experiences of self, childhood, care and identity [2–4]. People with progressive neurological diseases experience complex and unpredictable changes in their physical, cognitive, emotional and behavioural functions which can affect their decision-making capacity and their abilities at mealtimes, including changes in swallowing ability. These vary between individuals and across disease groups [5–11].

Estimates of the prevalence of dysphagia range from: 13–57% in dementia [12]; 32–85% in Parkinson's Disease (PD) [13]; 37% in Huntington's Disease (HD) [14]; 30–100% in Motor Neurone Disease (MND) [15]; 34–81% in Multiple Sclerosis (MS) [16, 17]; and 16–80% in Progressive Supranuclear Palsy (PSP) [18–20]. Difficulties with eating and drinking may arise from: physical impairments (impaired neuromuscular coordination of swallowing, tremor, rigidity, impaired coordination); cognitive difficulties (not recognising food, forgetting to chew or swallow, forgetting mealtimes); and behavioural difficulties (refusing to chew or swallow, spitting out food, or mealtime aggression) [21–23]. These can cause weight-loss, malnutrition, dehydration and aspiration pneumonia [24]. Mealtimes can become a major source of difficulty and anxiety for patients and their families [25], with emotional distress from loss of selfhood, social isolation and fear of becoming a burden to others [26].

Pharmacological and non-drug interventions aim to improve patients' quality of life through disease management and symptom control [27–30]. Support and interventions to address swallowing difficulties include; sitting with the individual at mealtimes, spooning food into the mouth, thickened food and drinks, nutritional supplements, and tube feeding by percutaneous endoscopic gastrostomy (PEG) or nasogastric (NG) tube [31, 32].

Tailoring these interventions to best suit the individual needs and wishes of each patient is an important part of the care-planning process. However, as illness progresses, decision-making capacity and communication ability may become impaired or lost, making shared decision-making more challenging. Early decisions are needed for some conditions, such as MND, as progression may be rapid with a short survival time and potential loss of decision-making capacity [10, 30]. For other conditions, such as dementia, PD and MS, the disease trajectory is typically longer, though unpredictable and uncertain, potentially allowing more time to make decisions [7, 8, 28]. If asked to make decisions in advance, patients are considering an uncertain and unknown future that may be difficult to contemplate at a time when they are adjusting to living with and coping with progressive and life-limiting illness.

Aims

We therefore undertook a study of patients and their families with a range of progressive neurological diseases. We investigated their experiences and views on decision-making concerning their care as their disease progressed, with a focus on problems with eating and drinking. The key research question was:

How do patients and their family members make decisions about their future care, with a particular focus on mealtimes, eating and drinking?

Methods

Design and recruitment

Longitudinal qualitative interviews were used to collect data from people with progressive neurological disease, their carers and healthcare professionals. A purposive sampling strategy was used to recruit a maximum variety sample of participants by disease group, decision-making capacity and degrees of eating and drinking difficulties.

Patient 'clusters' were recruited comprising up to four participants: the patient (if they had the decision-making capacity to consent to participate); a friend or relative ("informal carer"); a healthcare professional; and a paid carer (if they had one). In the first instance, (Time one - T1) in-depth qualitative interviews lasting 20 to 90 min were conducted with each participant. The length of the interview was determined by each participant's health and their responses to the questions. At a second optional 'mealtime interview' approximately one week later; the patient, relative and interviewer shared a meal in the participant's home. Subsequent follow-up interviews (Time two - T2), were undertaken three to twelve months later depending upon the trajectory of the disease.

Clinical collaborators initially approached potential patient participants with a study pack containing: a cover letter, an information sheet, a reply slip and a 'freepost' return envelope. Upon receipt of a reply slip, a member of the study team arranged a meeting at which the study was further explained, decision-making capacity was assessed, and if the participant chose to participate, informed consent was obtained. Patient participants were invited to nominate a relative or friend, a healthcare professional and a paid carer, who were all approached to participate.

Ethical issues

Capacity to consent to participation was assessed before each interview by the interviewer, who had received training in assessing decision-making capacity. Participants with capacity gave written consent, or verbal audio-recorded consent if they had communication or physical difficulties. If capacity was in doubt, a consultee was asked to provide written informed assent in accordance with the Mental Capacity Act 2005.

To minimise the potential for distress during discussion of possible future feeding difficulties, clinical collaborators only approached patients they judged suitable for such discussion and raised the research topic at that time. Further details were included in the participant information sheet. The interview schedule was participant-led; although the interviewer raised eating and drinking and deterioration in the condition in broad terms; these topics were only discussed in more detail if raised by participants. For example, PEG was only discussed if participants had already mentioned tube feeding. Participants were given contact details for support, including their GP, district nurse, specialist nurse, consultant and condition-relevant support groups or networks. None requested that the researcher contact these on their behalf. Ethical approval was given by the London South East Research Ethics Committee (REC reference: 14/LO/1156, IRAS project ID: 156054).

Research sample

Forty-two participants were interviewed between one to three times each between January 2015 and April 2017. This paper focuses on the findings from the interviews with patients and their relatives ($N = 29$). Disease groups represented were Parkinson's Disease (PD), Huntington's Disease (HD), Motor Neurone Disease (MND), Progressive Supranuclear Palsy (PSP), Corticobasal Degeneration (CBD), Multiple Sclerosis (MS) and dementia (including both Alzheimer's Disease and Frontotemporal Dementia). (Table 1) Gender identifiers have been removed from the text for reasons of confidentiality.

Data analysis

The interviews were audio-recorded, transcribed, anonymised and entered into NVivo 11 for analysis. Thematic analysis was used for data analysis and interpretation [33]. Coding was undertaken by GC, SaB and JT. Initial open inductive data driven coding was refined into broader themes that were further reviewed, refined and discussed between the coders to develop higher level analytical themes. Themes were refined on the basis of salience of content, as well as frequency of appearance.

Results

Themes relating to the research question ('what matters to patients and their carers when planning for the future, with a focus on eating and drinking?') emerged in two groups: those relating to the extent to which patients and carers appeared to know about the condition and its treatment (*health literacy*), and those relating to the extent to which they appeared to value involvement in advance care-planning (*planning style*). These are

presented in more detail below, with illustrative excerpts from the dataset.

Theme one: Health literacy

Most participants characterised themselves as sufficiently informed about what may lie ahead for them:

I: *Are there any issues that you would like, or would have liked, more information on?*

P: *No, because at the time they told us there was nothing. So they were quite up front about that, weren't they* [laughs] *and so everything plus has been a bonus ever since, hasn't it?* [Carer of HD patient. **R622**].

P: *No, I think everyone's been honest. Yes, even in terms of the timeframes you've got, I think everyone has been very honest, yes* [MS patient. **P412**]

However, this satisfaction was not universal. Some wanted more information on their condition and its likely progression, or about options for managing eating difficulties, particularly information about percutaneous endoscopic gastrostomy (PEG):

P: *If we'd have had more information then, we would have been more prepared for things as time goes on* [Carer of PD patient. **R223**].

P: *They could do a bit more to be progressive in trying to explain to people what they're about to experience. It's quite shocking if you, you know, you're looking at it for the first time* [Carer of MND patient. **R322**].

P: *Well I think I would have probably gone for the PEG earlier, if I'd have known. Obviously when the PEG was going in I weren't that sure because I didn't really know about it then, but actually having it done has made my job a lot easier. I mean, it was difficult feeding him/her before that, you know* [Carer of HD patient. **R622**].

Participants' ability to speak about their condition and potential future progression varied by disease group. Knowledge of prognosis appeared greatest in the HD, MND and PSP/CBD groups, with those in the Dementia and PD groups seemingly less able to articulate what lay in store.

Experts by experience

The HD group felt they had good knowledge of the condition because they had seen how it affected family members. They characterised this experience, rather

Table 1 Cross-tabulation of participants, disease groups and decision-making capacity (*N* = 29 participants consented)

Cluster code	Primary participant disease group	Primary participant decision-making capacity[a]	Primary participant age group in years	Years since diagnosis	Nominated relative or friend	Total no. of patients and relatives within cluster	No. of participants consented for interview[b]
A	Frontotemporal Dementia	Partial	65–80	6	Wife	2	2
B	Alzheimer's Disease	No	65–80	3	Friend	2	1
C	Parkinson's Disease	Yes	65–80	2	Partner	2	2
D	Parkinson's Disease	Yes	65–80	1	Daughter	2	2
E	Multiple Sclerosis	Yes	40–64	19	N/A	1	1
F	Multiple Sclerosis	Yes	40–64	8	Husband	2	2
G	Motor Neurone Disease	Yes	65–80	< 1	Wife	2	2
H	Motor Neurone Disease	No	65–80	2	Husband	2	1
I	Motor Neurone Disease	Yes	40–64	2	N/A	1	1
J	Progressive Supranuclear Palsy	Yes	65–80	5	[Relative relationship redacted]	2	2
K	Huntington's Disease	No	65–80	3	Husband	2	1
L	Huntington's Disease	Yes	40–64	15	Husband	2	2
M	Multiple Sclerosis	No	65–80	23	Wife	2	1
N	Progressive Supranuclear Palsy	Partial	65–80	1	Husband	2	2
O	Motor Neurone Disease	Yes	65–80	< 1	Wife	2	2
P	Progressive Supranuclear Palsy	Yes	40–65	3	Husband	2	2
Q	Alzheimer's Disease	No	65–80	12	Wife	2	1
R	Parkinson's Disease	Yes	65–80	6	Husband	2	2
Totals						34	29

[a]Decision-making capacity assessed at time of interview by the interviewer in relation to the capacity to participate in a qualitative interview
[b]Where the primary participant (patient participant) had partial or variable decision-making capacity, assent for interview participation was taken from a consultee by the interviewer. Where the primary participant did not have the capacity to participate in an interview, interviews were not undertaken with them

than anything they had been told by healthcare professionals, as the source of their health literacy:

I: And at that point did they explain to you how the illness would progress?

P: Well I already knew that from his/her mother and his/her aunties and uncles and it was, you know, family members really.

I: So they didn't need to explain anything...

P: Not really, no.

I: Did they talk about issues with eating and drinking or is that something that you...?

P: Well no, because you didn't really see that bit, you know, you didn't really see that part of the relatives, you used to go and visit them but you didn't really consider that and his/her aunty didn't want a PEG, s/he stipulated that s/he didn't want a PEG and obviously s/he had swallowing problems and died.

I: *Yeah. So his/her aunty knew early on but s/he just didn't want...?*

P: *Yeah, s/he didn't want nothing like that, no, s/he didn't want to be messed about* [Carer of HD patient. **R622**].

I: *So, at the time s/he was first diagnosed, did anyone talk to you about how the condition would progress?*

P: *We were quite aware of that ... no, we haven't really been told by anyone* [Carer of HD patient. **R621**].

Well informed from the outset

Participants in the MND and PSP/CBD groups spoke confidently and fluently about prognosis, often using medical vocabulary. They identified the information provided by health professionals as the source of their health literacy:

I: *...and did they speak to you about how the condition would progress?*

P: *Yeah. I mean that's obviously part of the condition and that was always one of the things that* [Consultant] *and* [Consultant 2] *talked about in terms of the ability to swallow through the deterioration with the muscles. That was one of their biggest concerns about, obviously which would cause aspirational pneumonia, so they were very adamant about, you know, making sure that we did everything possible to ensure that we didn't cause that. And they spoke obviously about the PEG and, you know, the benefits of the PEG* [Carer of CBD patient. **R523**].

I: *So when you saw the doctors at* [Clinic] *did they outline for you how the disease would progress?*

P: *Yeah. Yeah, I mean you get the kind of assessment that you would expect from a Consultant, and of course they have a Care Team there which you may be familiar with, so the moment they begin to think about something as serious as Motor Neurone, or whatever else it is, the Care Team are involved and they of course, they're made up of a dietician, a speech therapist ... there's three of them, and you know, they go through the whole business in great detail. So, you know, you can't fail to understand what's going on and*

the support was very good at [Hospital] *seen very regularly* [Carer of MND patient. **R322**].

I: *At that time, were you told about the progression of his/her condition?*

P: *Yeah, yeah, straight away he told us how, how it does progress but this seems to be progressing in a lot of ways different to the other people we see at the meetings, yeah? S/he still walks, most of the people we know are in wheelchairs and that, and s/he gets on quite well* [Carer of PSP patient. **R521**].

However, being 'well informed' by clinicians did not predict the participants' choices. For example, within the group of four participants diagnosed with MND, all four had discussed PEG with their care team but: one chose PEG feeding; one was strongly considering PEG feeding but died unexpectedly during the course of the study, and two were early stage and undecided.

Mixed picture

In MS clusters, responses were more mixed. Some, much like the MND and PSP/CBD groups, appeared to have been kept fully informed by healthcare professionals:

I: *At that point, did they explain to you how the disease would progress?*

P: *Yes, it was, progressing was quite rapidly, and, but they did explain the care needs for the future, and what would be needed. Yes, yes, they did explain it quite harshly, and that's what I want, you know, they did explain it fully* [MS patient. **P412**].

Others reported receiving little information from healthcare professionals, but were able to use other sources to develop their health literacy:

I: *So who first told you that you may or may not get, swallowing disorders in the first place?*

P: *Well, it's part of the progression of the disease.*

I: *And when did they first raise that with you? Was that at the time of your diagnosis or was that later on?*

P: *Nothing was given to me at the time of diagnosis, it's all been picked up as it's gone along. Various online chat rooms about MS, talking to other people with MS, common sense on these things and also I always have to treat my MS as something I'm going to look forward in the future dealing with, rather than leaving it, how you deal* *with it on a catch-up basis so it's best to be informed* [MS patient. **P411**].

However, others in the MS group described an apparent choice to remain uninformed, although information was available:

I: *And at that point did any healthcare professionals talk to you about how the disease would progress?*

P: *The information was there,* [Patient] *chose not to want to know really, s/he... I think it took her/him ten years to take it in, and that was her/him. I obviously looked up what was going to happen and had much more of an idea but s/he chose to not know* [Carer of MS patient. **R423**].

Still unaware

In contrast, participants in the dementia and PD clusters were less able to articulate their prognosis, rarely used technical language, and were sometimes hesitant in speaking. Unlike those in the MS group, who described choosing not to find out what lay in store; these participants appeared to have been offered less information than those in the other groups:

I: *And Dr* [Consultant] *has explained how the condition will evolve in the future?*

P: *Um, not really, I haven't really asked. At least I did ask, you know, I know that s/he's on the lower scale of dementia, sort of, you know, not up here but down here. I've no idea, I think it's different for... I don't think they can say. I think that's why I haven't been told, they can't really say ... Because, you know, I'm not sure if s/he will lose his mobility or if s/he will become rigid or shaky or you know, like Parkinson's or something like that, I don't know* [Carer of dementia patient. **R121**].

I: *So when you were there* [Clinic], *did they talk about how the dementia would progress? Or the eating and drinking would either?*

P: *No. Nothing* [Lay carer dementia patient. **R122**].

I: *So has he talked to you about how the condition will progress in the future? Has the doctor explained......?*

P: *No. As far as he is concerned he doesn't have an appointment with me for another six months* [PD patient. **P211**].

I: *And when they told you about that, did they tell you how about it might develop in the future?*

P: *No, not, it might not, it might just stay like it, so you know, I just carry on, and luckily it's me left hand, me left arm, so I'm right-handed so it doesn't affect me, it doesn't keep me awake at night or nothing* [PD patient. **P212**].

Theme two: Planning style

The extent to which participants expressed a wish to be involved in advance care-planning varied within and between the condition groups. Two main themes emerged: those who wanted to plan ahead and make their own decisions about care and treatment in advance, and those who preferred to live in the present, deferring decisions about future care. Some participants described using a mixture of those two approaches (with some switching preference as the condition progressed). For a small group of participants, the concept of care planning held little meaning as they did not perceive that there were any decisions to make.

'Advance planning'

Advance planning was used by some participants as a way of extending the zone of personal autonomy and involvement in decision-making beyond the stage when their ability to make decisions or communicate their wishes would be lost:

P: *In the early days of the diagnosis we obviously discussed his/her thoughts, his/her wishes going forward, s/he made her end of life wishes well known, they're documented. I think I understand everything that* [Name] *wants and I totally agree with some of the things that s/he wants but yes, we have discussed that* [Carer of CBD patient. **R523**].

This group described a need for information about the kinds of interventions to support nutritional intake that might be considered as the condition progressed:

P: *We needed it* [information on PEG] *as far as I'm concerned, I mean it's all bad news....you can mope around but there is the practical side to the whole business, even if it's your wife or husband, you need to know what, what's about to happen and what can be done* [Carer of MND patient. **R322**].

Some participants expressed a desire to be more engaged in the planning of care and were frustrated by the lack of information on offer:

P: *That's where it becomes quite frustrating 'cos I'm doing my utmost to do the best for the wife, naturally, and there doesn't seem to be that outside help to guide you and put you on a little bit further and with a bit more help* [Carer of PD patient. **R223**].

However, the relationship between adoption of an 'advance planning' strategy and the need and desire for information was not straightforward. Some participants acknowledged a need for information but nonetheless did not want to be told everything:

P: *We got information mainly at* [Hospital] *but it was very sort of top level and; 'Here's some information but we don't have to talk about it yet, you know, we'll talk about it when you're ready and unless we have to talk about it before'. So it was handed to me, for me to decide when I wanted to talk about it..... I think we needed to know what lay ahead, but only at top level, and not to go into too much detail about anything that didn't have an immediate or a near impact on me, certainly in the earlier days when you're taking everything on board* [MND patient. **P313**].

Furthermore, information from health professionals did not always seem to be an important factor in the advance planning process. Some participants made all their own care decisions in advance, in keeping with their personality and based on long-term values:

P: *I mean that's the way* [Name] *was, it may not be everybody's way of doing things, but you know, as I said to you, s/he was very independent and s/he made his/her own decisions ... so you know, s/he's not the sort of person that's going to, s/he's going to rely on specialists to help him/her but s/he will be making his/her own decisions* [Carer of MND patient. **R322**].

These decisions were not always consistent with the advice and information offered by healthcare professionals. One participant planned to seek assisted suicide. Despite receiving information about options to alleviate their concerns about a distressing death, they chose to end their own life before the condition's natural conclusion:

I: *So is there something particular that you're frightened of in the progression, that makes you think you would like to end your life sooner? Or is there another reason you decided that you wanted to make the visit to Dignitas?*

P: *I don't know because I spoke to* [Consultant] *last time about it. I was frightened of drowning in my own*

secretions, of choking to death. And he said it wasn't like that, people usually slip away but, so, but I'm quite pragmatic about it because of this condition isn't going to get any better. So I can't see why prolonging it.

[Patient identity withheld for reasons of confidentiality].

For this participant, reassurance that the dysphagia that they feared most would not arise did not have any impact upon the decision to seek assisted suicide. The provision of additional information to correct a possible misunderstanding did not change the decision. The inference that the decision was actually grounded in deep-seated values, rather than anxiety based on a potentially mistaken belief about the way the condition would progress, was expressed by their relative:

P: *S/he's very practical, s/he'll see it as the best thing all round for everybody, including her/himself; s/he said 'I'm fed up with being like this'. S/he's always sort of had her/his independence, s/he's always worked, you know, had a good job* [Carer of patient who chose assisted dying; identity withheld for reasons of confidentiality].

'Take each day as it comes'

Some participants were hesitant to engage with, or discuss, decisions concerning their future care. Particularly in the early stages of illness they preferred to focus on the 'here and now', rather than thinking about problems that might lie ahead. Decisions about future care were deferred to a later date, sometimes in the apparent hope that the eventualities that they could plan for may never arise:

I: *Did they discuss about how it* [PD] *might develop in the future?*

P: *No, not, it might not, it might just stay like it, so you know, I just carry on* [PD patient. **P212**].

P: *So, I mean, that's going to be an ongoing problem now I suppose? Unless something happens in... I don't know. I don't know if that happens in the brain, that things stop functioning and they start up again?* [Carer of Dementia patient. **R121**].

Some participants appeared to be aware of their prognosis, and of their developing problems with eating and drinking, but preferred not to focus on them. Sometimes this coping strategy was characterised as an active decision:

P: *I work out how to cope with it; don't go thinking too much in the future. But of course we all have people like Stephen Hawking in our minds, and think, 'is that where we're going to end up, looking like him?'.... 'And if that's what people visualise us as, where we're going to end up, it's a bit of a daunting prospect'* [MND patient. **P314**].

Others discussed their swallowing difficulties in a way that suggested they were aware of the problem but, perhaps unconsciously minimising or attempting to ignore it:

P: *When I'm very tired I have to be more careful about my swallowing, and make sure that I chew my food thoroughly, but at the moment it doesn't really affect me greatly ... I do have episodes of choking when I'm drinking but other than that, no, it's not a problem* [MS patient. **P411**].

Finally, some participants characterised their reluctance to be involved in future care planning as normal or expected for people of an older generation:

I: *So.... a will, but no plans about his/her care?*

P: *No, s/he said s/he knew I'd look after him/her, so I just left it at that. I don't think people of that age like to talk about that, you know, it wasn't done then, was it? It just happened* [Carer of Dementia patient. **R122**].

For participants who did not wish to engage in planning for the future, information about prognosis was not always welcome. Some wished that the information about diagnosis and prognosis had never been given:

P: *I would have rather they hadn't told [patient] he had MND ... If nobody told s/he'd got MND because s/he'd have just carried on thinking well, I'm getting old, I've got rheumatism, I can't lift my arm, I can't do this, can't do that and s/he wouldn't be stressed out and upset like s/he is, so* [Carer of MND patient. **R321**].

However, the relationship between this strategy and satisfaction with the amount of information provided was not straightforward. For some, it was information about prognosis that prompted them to choose this strategy:

I: *Did they talk to you then about how the illness would develop, or did they just sort of.......?*

P: *Well they did, a little bit, but in those days with Alzheimer's Society, you know they don't do it the same nowadays, there was a lovely lady ... and she just said*

to me, she says [Name], "I'm going to be brutal", and I said "Right, go on", she said "[Patient]'s fine now", she says "Enjoy your time that you've got with him/her now because it will get worse and worse and worse" [Carer of Dementia patient. **R123**].

For others, awareness of the complex and uncertain future lay behind their reluctance to engage in advance care planning. They expressed a preference for delaying important decisions until they had to be made, because it would be too difficult to make them without contextual information:

P: *I'd have to think about it at the time, because that means I wouldn't want someone to cure me of pneumonia during a visit to A&E, if it's just one of a succession of weekly visits to A&E, no, I wouldn't want to be cured of pneumonia. But again, a person's wishes should be taken into account* [PD patient. **P211**].

P: *No, I was asked about that [making advance care decisions] and I didn't want to do it. I really don't know how you can decide something like that* [MS patient. **P411**].

Mixed strategies

Participants did not always use a single coping strategy. As their disease progressed, some moved between 'taking each day as it comes' and 'advance planning'.

P: *Well I did contact the MND Association up in [Place], I said, "Look, send me your pack and I'll have a read," and it was page after page, and as I explained to a doctor at [Hospital], it can be quite overwhelming, and he said, "Well that's typical of charitable organisations, that they sort of paint a blacker picture, or tell you everything and you have to stand back and say, well is that relevant to me today, if that's in the future we'll worry about it in the future," and this is how I think my wife and I have sort of come to terms with it, let's live a day at a time, and we'll navigate through sticky patches when we come to them* [MND patient. **P314**].

An added complexity was that patients and their carers sometimes adopted different strategies:

P: *I've started the Power of Attorney process but it's with my husband now to finish it off, he's a little bit of an ostrich, I think that's fair to say* [MND patient. **R313**].

P: *Ah, me personally, yes, I would have done* [made advance care plans], *if that had happened to me I would have definitely chosen to do that, I don't think* [Name] *is the type of person that would have done unfortunately* [Carer of MS patient. **R423**].

Some participants expressed regret that they had not engaged with care planning earlier in the course of their condition. For decisions concerning PEG feeding, this lack of advance planning appeared to be connected with a lack of information about the options. Two participants had PEGs fitted at a late, or crisis stage, and both of their carers wished they had made decisions earlier:

I: *So do you wish you'd had yours* [PEG tube] *fitted a bit earlier to stop those?*

P: *Yeah, it's still a frightening thing but it could have been done in an easier time for his/her body* [Carer of PSP patient. **R521**].

P: *It was in the hospital, yeah, we made the decision. S/he went in, s/he had an abscess on his/ her lung where s/he'd been swallowing food down the wrong hole ... well basically s/he nearly died but the antibiotics kicked in and s/he was okay and then we had the PEG fitted in there, we had a lot of swallow tests and that done and then it was decided that the only way really was a PEG.... If I'd have known and s/he would have known I think we'd have had it a lot earlier* [Carer of HD patient. **R622**].

No decision to be made

For some participants the concept of care planning did not make any sense, as they viewed the progression of their condition, and the need to accept increasingly invasive treatment in order to stay alive, as part of an inexorable process. Consequently, there was no sense that they were choosing between planning in advance, or living in the present and delaying making decisions about care until they could be put off no longer. These participants described just doing what it took to survive:

I: *So is thickening your food and drink something that you would consider, despite the horrible taste?*

P: *Well, I'll do that when I've got no choice really.*

I: *And what about PEG feeding?*

P: *It might be the only way to feed me* [MS patient. **P411**].

Discussion

These results have clear implications for health professionals attempting to deliver person-centred care for people affected by progressive neurological conditions. One of the most striking findings is the variation, between diagnostic groups, in the degree to which participants appeared to be aware of what the future may hold for them, and the treatment options that may be available. It is unclear why those in the Parkinson's disease and dementia groups were, in comparison with those affected by other conditions, less able to describe their prognosis. It may be that they had been provided with information but were unable to recall it at the time of the interview, perhaps as a result of cognitive impairment. However, it is possible that health professionals had decided to provide the most detailed information about prognosis, including the possibility of developing dysphagia, to people with MND, PSP and CBD, as these are conditions with a relatively rapid progression and a high likelihood of developing dysphagia. Thus, patients with these conditions may be seen as having a greater need for information as they are more likely to be faced with a need to make a decision about tube feeding in the near future. In contrast, patients with dementia and Parkinson's disease, which have a slow and uncertain trajectory, may be perceived as less likely to have to make such a decision. The potential risks of giving them information about treatment for a distressing symptom that they may never develop may therefore appear to outweigh the potential advantage of enabling them to be involved in the decision to use tube-feeding, should this decision need to be made in the future after they have lost decision-making capacity. This approach could be characterised as 'physician-centred': the physician makes a decision about the patient's information needs, based on his or her expert knowledge of the natural history of the patient's condition and the likelihood of particular treatments becoming appropriate in the foreseeable future.

However, the findings of this study suggest that this approach may not be the most effective way of meeting the needs of individual patients. An understanding of their attitude to advance care planning may provide a more useful guide. The majority of participants were divided into two groups: those who wanted to deal with healthcare issues as they arose, live for the moment and not think about the future; and those who asked questions of healthcare professionals, researched their condition on their own and wanted to participate in shared decision-making and advance planning. Furthermore, the degree of health literacy demonstrated in the interviews did not predict participants' approach to care planning.

For both groups, their approach could be seen as a mechanism for coping with the emotional burden and magnitude of their diagnosis and its implications. Charmaz has suggested that the suffering of chronic illness involves the psychological suffering of the loss of selfhood. She argues that, as disease progresses, individuals may develop visible disabilities resulting in stigmatised identities, or may suffer from discreditation of their identity due to reduced participation in everyday life [26]. Being unable to participate in mealtimes or having visible problems with eating and drinking are such an example. Participants choosing a strategy of 'taking each day as it comes' can use this to resist stigmatisation, and maintain their self-image as a 'healthy person' for as long as possible. This avoids disrupting the narrative of their life which could be psychologically destructive to their sense of self, alongside the distress of the damage the illness is doing to their body. Conversely, engaging in active planning and taking control of the situation, may help the person to distance their own self-image, from the image of 'a sick person' who lacks autonomy and self-possession. Charmaz argues that the self-discreditation of the chronically ill occurs when individuals can no longer take for granted an attribute they view as fundamental. This could include the power to make one's own decisions.

The information needs of the two groups were not straightforward. The group who preferred to 'take each day as it comes' sometimes chose to do so because of the information they had received regarding prognosis, and some who had not made advance plans concerning the use of PEG feeding came to regret not doing so. Conversely, not everyone who engaged in advance planning wished to know everything about the condition or its treatment, with some expressing a wish for healthcare professionals to filter the information provided, to avoid overwhelming them, and others taking information provided by healthcare professionals into account but ultimately basing their decisions on other factors. However, an understanding of the strategy that each individual patient is adopting could usefully guide healthcare professionals to engage in sensitive, nuanced conversations that provide their patients with the information that the need to know. Furthermore, the evidence that people may switch between groups as the condition progresses suggests a need for healthcare professionals to remain alert to this possibility and adjust accordingly.

Potential limitations of the study

One limitation of the research design of this study is that it may have over-represented participants who were 'planners', as only participants who were judged willing to talk about the future were approached. Those who wanted to not think about their condition could be underrepresented: the population may include a larger number of individuals who are less engaged with healthcare and prefer not to discuss about their condition.

Some participants suggested their approach to the management of their own disease was a continuation of their personality. However, these approaches may just have been about the participants using the psychological and emotional tools available to them at the time, and not indicative of an underlying essential difference. In fact, some participants used a mixed strategy approach to their disease management, engaging at certain times and selectively ignoring symptoms at others.

Conclusions

This longitudinal qualitative study of patients with progressive neurological disease and their families investigated planning for the future and decision-making concerning eating and drinking. The thematic analysis revealed two key themes: 1) *Health literacy:* the extent to which patients and carers appeared to know about the condition and its treatment; and 2) *Planning style:* the extent to which they appeared to value involvement in advance care-planning.

Issues around eating and drinking are often overlooked by doctors and seen as the remit of speech and language therapists and nurses. However, the findings from this study showed the key role of eating and drinking in care-planning and the need for all clinicians to understand both the patient's level of health literacy and their style of planning for the future before communicating about these sensitive issues.

Abbreviations

HD: Huntington's Disease; ID: Identification/Identifier; IRAS: Integrated Research Approval System; MND: Motor Neurone Disease; MS: Multiple Sclerosis; NG: Nasogastric; PD: Parkinson's Disease; PEG: Percutaneous Endoscopic Gastrostomy; PSP: Progressive Supranuclear Palsy; REC: Research Ethics Committee; T1: Time One; T2: Time Two

Funding

This work was funded by The Dunhill Medical Trust [grant number R317/1113]. AH and SB are supported by the National Institute for Health Research (NIHR) Collaboration for Leadership in Applied Health Research and Care (CLAHRC) East of England at Cambridgeshire and Peterborough NHS Foundation Trust. AH is also supported by the Health Foundation. The funders had no role in the design, undertaking or writing of this paper, and no part in the decision to submit for publication. This paper presents independent research partly funded by the National Institute for Health Research (NIHR). The views expressed are those of the authors and not necessarily those of the NHS, the NIHR or the Department of Health. We are grateful to Angela Harper for her administrative support for this study, funded by the Dunhill Trust.

Authors' contributions
GC, EF, AH, SB conceptualised the study and designed the methodology. GC undertook the qualitative interviews. GC, JT and SaB undertook initial data coding and analysis. GC, EF, SaB and AH undertook secondary analysis of the data to produce the analytical themes. GC, EF, AH, JT, SaB and SB wrote and edited the paper. All authors read and approved the final manuscript.

Competing interests
The authors declare that they have no competing interests.

Author details
[1]Primary Care Unit, Department of Public Health and Primary Care, Cambridge Institute of Public Health, University of Cambridge School of Clinical Medicine, Box 113 Cambridge Biomedical Campus, Cambridge CB2 0SR, UK. [2]The Health Foundation, Chair in Learning Disabilities, Cambridge Intellectual and Developmental Disabilities Research Group, Department of Psychiatry, University of Cambridge, Cambridge, UK. [3]University of Cambridge, Cambridge, UK.

References
1. Coveney J. Food, morals and meaning: the pleasure and anxiety of eating. London: Routledge; 2002.
2. Counihan C, Van Esterik P. Food and culture: a reader. London: Routledge; 2012.
3. Ochs E, Shohet M. The cultural structuring of mealtime socialization. New Dir Child Adolesc Dev. 2006;2006(111):35–49. https://doi.org/10.1002/cd.154.
4. Philpin S, Merrell JOY, Warring J, Hobby D, Gregory VIC. Memories, identity and homeliness: the social construction of mealtimes in residential care homes in South Wales. Ageing and Soc. 2013;34(5):753–789. Epub 01/03. https://doi.org/10.1017/S0144686X12001274.
5. Alzheimer's Association. 2016 Alzheimer's disease facts and figures. Alzheimers Dement. 2016;12(4):459–509. Epub 2016/08/30. PubMed PMID: 27570871
6. Lyketsos CG, Carrillo MC, Ryan JM, Khachaturian AS, Trzepacz P, Amatniek J, et al. Neuropsychiatric symptoms in Alzheimer's disease. Alzheimers Dement. 7(5):532–9. https://doi.org/10.1016/j.jalz.2011.05.2410.
7. Cosh DA, Carslaw DH. Multiple sclerosis: symptoms and diagnosis. InnovAiT. 2014;7(11):651–7. https://doi.org/10.1177/1755738014551618.
8. Davie CA. A review of Parkinson's disease. Br Med Bull. 2008;86(1):109–27. https://doi.org/10.1093/bmb/ldn013.
9. Lubarsky M, Juncos JL. Progressive Supranuclear Palsy: A Current Review. The Neurologist. 2008;14(2):79–88. https://doi.org/10.1097/NRL. 0b013e31815cffc9. PubMed PMID: 00127893-200803000-00001
10. McDermott CJ, Shaw PJ. Diagnosis and management of motor neurone disease. BMJ. 2008;336(7645):658–62. https://doi.org/10.1136/bmj.39493. 511759.BE. PubMed PMID: PMC2270983
11. Kirkwood S, Su JL, Conneally P, Foroud T. Progression of symptoms in the early and middle stages of Huntington disease. Arch Neurol. 2001;58(2): 273–8. https://doi.org/10.1001/archneur.58.2.273.
12. Alagiakrishnan K, Bhanji RA, Kurian M. Evaluation and management of oropharyngeal dysphagia in different types of dementia: a systematic review. Arch Gerontol Geriatr 2013;56(1):1–9. Epub 2012/05/23. https://doi. org/10.1016/j.archger.2012.04.011. PubMed PMID: 22608838.
13. Kalf JG, de Swart BJM, Bloem BR, Munneke M. Prevalence of oropharyngeal dysphagia in Parkinson's disease: A meta-analysis. Parkinsonism Relat Disord. 2012;18(4):311–5. https://doi.org/10.1016/j.parkreldis.2011.11.006
14. de Tommaso M, Dello Monaco A, Nuzzi A, Caputo S, Sciruicchio V, Serpino C, et al. I05 Dysphagia In Huntington's Disease: A Study With Bedside Swallowing Assessment Scale. J Neurol Neurosurg Psychiatry. 2014;85(Suppl 1):A59-A5A. https://doi.org/10.1136/jnnp-2014-309032.167.
15. Haverkamp LJ, Appel V, Appel SH. Natural history of amyotrophic lateral sclerosis in a database population. Validation of a scoring system and a model for survival prediction. Brain 1995;118 (Pt 3):707–719. Epub 1995/06/01. PubMed PMID: 7600088.
16. Calcagno P, Ruoppolo G, Grasso MG, De Vincentiis M, Paolucci S. Dysphagia in multiple sclerosis - prevalence and prognostic factors. Acta Neurol Scand 2002;105(1):40–43. Epub 2002/03/21. PubMed PMID: 11903107.
17. Guan XL, Wang H, Huang HS, Meng L. Prevalence of dysphagia in multiple sclerosis: a systematic review and meta-analysis. Neurol Sci 2015;36(5): 671–681. Epub 2015/02/04. https://doi.org/10.1007/s10072-015-2067-7. PubMed PMID: 25647290.
18. O'Sullivan SS, Massey LA, Williams DR, Silveira-Moriyama L, Kempster PA, Holton JL, et al. Clinical outcomes of progressive supranuclear palsy and multiple system atrophy. Brain. 2008;131(5):1362–72. https://doi.org/10.1093/ brain/awn065.
19. Litvan I. Diagnosis and management of progressive supranuclear palsy. Semin Neurol 2001;21(1):41–48. Epub 2001/05/11. PubMed PMID: 11346024.
20. Varanese S, Di Ruscio P, Ben m' Barek L, Thomas A, Onofrj M. Responsiveness of dysphagia to acute L-Dopa challenge in progressive supranuclear palsy. J Neurol 2014;261(2):441–442. Epub 2014/01/15. https:// doi.org/10.1007/s00415-013-7232-4. PubMed PMID: 24413640.
21. Easterling CS, Robbins E. Dementia and Dysphagia. Geriatric Nursing. 2008; 29(4):275–85. https://doi.org/10.1016/j.gerinurse.2007.10.015.
22. Stavroulakis T, Baird WO, Baxter SK, Walsh T, Shaw PJ, McDermott CJ. Factors influencing decision-making in relation to timing of gastrostomy insertion in patients with motor neurone disease. BMJ Support Palliat Care. 2014;4(1): 57–63. https://doi.org/10.1136/bmjspcare-2013-000497.
23. Chang C-C, Lin Y-F, Chiu C-H, Liao Y-M, Ho M-H, Lin Y-K, et al. Prevalence and factors associated with food intake difficulties among residents with dementia. PLoS One. 2017;12(2):e0171770. https://doi.org/10.1371/journal.pone.0171770.
24. Sura L, Madhavan A, Carnaby G, Crary MA. Dysphagia in the elderly: management and nutritional considerations. Clin Interv Aging. 2012;7: 287–298. Epub 2012/09/08. https://doi.org/10.2147/cia.s23404. PubMed PMID: 22956864; PubMed Central PMCID: PMCPmc3426263.
25. Keller HH, Edward HG, Cook C. Mealtime Experiences of Families With Dementia. Am J Alzheimers Dis Other Demen. 2007;21(6):431–8. https://doi. org/10.1177/1533317506294601.
26. Charmaz K. Loss of self: a fundamental form of suffering in the chronically ill. Sociol Health Illn. 1983;5(2):168–95. Epub 1983/06/10. PubMed PMID: 10261981
27. Robinson L, Tang E, Taylor J-P. Dementia: timely diagnosis and early intervention. BMJ. 2015;350 https://doi.org/10.1136/bmj.h3029.
28. Connolly BS, Lang AE. Pharmacological treatment of parkinson disease: a review. JAMA. 2014;311(16):1670–83. https://doi.org/10.1001/jama.2014.3654.
29. Torkildsen Ø, Myhr KM, Bø L. Disease-modifying treatments for multiple sclerosis – a review of approved medications. Eur J Neurol. 2016;23(Suppl 1): 18–27. https://doi.org/10.1111/ene.12883. PubMed PMID: PMC4670697
30. Orrell RW. Motor neuron disease: systematic reviews of treatment for ALS and SMA. Br Med Bull. 2010;93(1):145–59. https://doi.org/10.1093/bmb/ldp049.
31. Rahnemai-Azar AA, Rahnemaiazar AA, Naghshizadian R, Kurtz A, Farkas DT. Percutaneous endoscopic gastrostomy: indications, technique, complications and management. World J Gastroenterol. 2014;20(24): 7739–51. https://doi.org/10.3748/wjg.v20.i24.7739. Epub 2014/07/01. PubMed PMID: 24976711; PubMed Central PMCID: PMCPmc4069302
32. Gomes CA Jr, Andriolo RB, Bennett C, Lustosa SA, Matos D, Waisberg DR, et al. Percutaneous endoscopic gastrostomy versus nasogastric tube feeding for adults with swallowing disturbances. Cochrane Database Syst Rev. 2015;5:Cd008096. https://doi.org/10.1002/14651858.CD008096. pub4. Epub 2015/05/23. PubMed PMID: 25997528
33. Braun V, Clarke V. Using thematic analysis in psychology. Qual Res Psychol. 2006;3(2):77–101. https://doi.org/10.1191/1478088706qp063oa.

17

Surgical treatment and perioperative management of intracranial aneurysms in Chinese patients with ischemic cerebrovascular diseases

Yangrui Zheng and Chen Wu[*]

Abstract

Background: Patients with ischemic cerebrovascular diseases are more likely to suffer from intracranial aneurysms, and their surgical treatment has a growing controversy in this condition. The current case series was aimed at exploring surgical treatment and perioperative management of intracranial aneurysms in Chinese patients with ischemic cerebrovascular diseases.

Methods: Minimally invasive surgical approach through small pterion or inferolateral forehead was applied in 31 patients. Anti-platelet drugs were withdrawn 1 week before surgical operation. Systolic blood pressure was controlled to be more than 110 mmHg and increased by 20% after the clipping of intracranial aneurysms. Branches of external carotid artery were spared to ensure collateral circulation. Temporary blocking was minimized and ischemic time was shortened during surgical operation.

Results: Patients had an average age of 66 (46–78) years, and proportion of males was 39% (12 males). There were 35 unruptured intracranial aneurysms with a diameter more than 5 mm. There were 20 posterior communicating and anterior choroidal aneurysms (57%), seveb middle cerebral aneurysms (20%), and eight anterior communicating aneurysms (23%), with 21 lobular aneurysms (60%). Twenty-nine patients had normal neurological function (Glasgow Outcome Scale [GOS] 5), one patient with mild neurological defect (GOS 4), and one patient with severe neurological defect (GOS 3) at discharge. Meanwhile, there were 26 patients with modified Rankin Scale (MRS) 0–1, 4 patient with MRS 2, and one patient with MRS 3 at discharge. There were four patients lost during the follow-up. During the follow-up, 26 patients had normal neurological function (GOS 5), and one patient with severe neurological defect (GOS 3). Meanwhile, there were 25 patients with MRS 0–1, one patient with MRS 2, and one patient with MRS 3. All patients had no recurrence of intracranial aneurysms after operation.

Conclusions: The current case series found that minimally invasive surgical approach and intraoperative monitoring, supplemented by effective management of cerebrovascular perfusion, circulation and coagulation, can promote the treatment of intracranial aneurysms and prevent the development of cerebral ischemia and aneurysm rupture in Chinese patients with ischemic cerebrovascular diseases. Future studies with large sample size will be needed to confirm the results from the current case series.

Keywords: Intracranial aneurysms, Ischemic cerebrovascular diseases, Perioperative management, Surgical treatment

* Correspondence: 13671007509@163.com
Department of Neurosurgery, Hainan Branch of Chinese People's Liberation
Army General Hospital, Sanya, China

Background

Ischemic cerebrovascular diseases lead to transient ischemic attack (TIA) and irreversible cerebral infarction, and cerebral infarction has a mortality rate of 30–40% [1]. Meanwhile, intracranial aneurysms are one kind of severe intracranial disease mainly responsible for subarachnoid hemorrhage, and the rupture of intracranial aneurysms results in a similar mortality rate of 30–40% [2–4]. Concurrence rate of intracranial aneurysms and ischemic cerebrovascular diseases was 0.5–5% [5, 6]. Patients with ischemic cerebrovascular diseases are more likely to suffer from intracranial aneurysms because of the change in arterial structure and function [7].

Intracranial aneurysms and ischemic cerebrovascular diseases have different disease characteristics and treatment methods, and therefore, when patients with ischemic cerebrovascular diseases had intracranial aneurysms, their surgical treatment is at the center of a growing controversy [8]. If the treatment of intracranial aneurysms precedes that of ischemic cerebrovascular diseases, perioperative hypoperfusion can induce the ischemic events and even fatal cerebral infarction with a large area [9]. If the treatment of ischemic cerebrovascular diseases precedes that of intracranial aneurysms, rapid increase in intracranial blood flow can induce the rupture of intracranial aneurysms [10]. The current case series was aimed at exploring surgical treatment and perioperative management of intracranial aneurysms in Chinese patients with ischemic cerebrovascular diseases.

Methods

Patients

In the current case series, all patients with not only intracranial aneurysms with a diameter more than 5 mm, but also cervical or intracranial arterial stenosis or occlusion (> 50%), were diagnosed on the basis of computed tomography angiography (CTA) or digital substraction angiography (DSA), and received surgical treatment of intracranial aneurysms in our hospital between April 2010 and April 2014. The existence of symptoms and signs, such as dizziness, headache and nerve localization signs, also supported clinical diagnosis. Patients with recurrent TIA, soft atherosclerotic plaques or ulcer formation were excluded from the current case series. Therefore, there were 31 patients in the current case series.

Surgical treatment

In the current case series, patients were treated based on clinical practice but not as part of a prospective, controlled study. Minimally invasive surgical approach through small pterion or inferolateral forehead was applied in all patients. Intracranial aneurysms were treated with clipping.

Surgical operation was monitored by electroencephalogram and somatosensory evoked potential.

During surgical operation, blood flow and its patency were evaluated by microvascular Doppler ultrasound. Fluorescence angiography was applied to evaluate the patency of parental artery and perforating artery. Contralateral aneurysms and ipsilateral aneurysms were defined according to the locations of intracranial aneurysms and arterial stenosis or occlusion. For communicating aneurysms, contralateral aneurysms and ipsilateral aneurysms were defined based on the advantage of blood supply.

Perioperative management

Anti-platelet drugs were applied until 1 week before surgical operation and resumed on the second day after surgical operation. In order to satisfy cerebral blood perfusion of patients with ischemic cerebrovascular diseases, systolic blood pressure was controlled to be more than 110 mmHg and increased by 20% after the clipping of intracranial aneurysms. Postoperative blood pressure was controlled to be not lower than daily level. Branches of external carotid artery, such as superficial temporal artery and middle meningeal artery, were spared to ensure collateral circulation. Temporary blocking was minimized and ischemic time was shortened during the operation.

In order to avoid the rupture of atherosclerotic plaques, these plaques should be kept away from and surgical operation should be light and soft to the largest extent when clipping intracranial aneurysms. Papaverine soaking was locally applied after the clipping of intracranial aneurysms. Low molecular weight dextran and nimodipine were applied to improve the microcirculation. Before surgical operation and during the follow-up, CTA or DSA was applied to observe arterial stenosis and intracranial aneurysms, and assess ischemic cerebrovascular capacity and tolerance. Glasgow Outcome Scale (GOS) and Modified Rankin Scale (MRS) were applied to evaluate neurological function and prognostic performance.

Postoperative follow-up

All patients were followed up at the first month, third months and sixth months, and then once a year after surgical operation. There were 4 patients lost during the mean follow-up period of 18 (6–40) months.

Results

Patients had an average age of 66 (46–78) years, and proportion of males was 39% (12 males). As shown in Table 1, percentages of dizziness, headache and nerve localization signs were 77, 52 and 29%, respectively. There were 28 patients with a long-term use of anti-platelet drugs. There were 35 intracranial aneurysms in 31 patients, and all intracranial aneurysms had a diameter more than 5 mm. There were 20 posterior communicating and anterior

Table 1 Characteristics of patients, aneurysms and prognoses

Characteristics	Descriptions
Age (year)	66 (46–78)
Males, n (100%)	12 (39%)
Appearance, n (100%)	
Dizziness	24(77%)
Headache	16(52%)
Nerve localization signs	9(29%)
Number of aneurysms, n	35
Location of aneurysms, n (100%)	
Posterior communicating and anterior choroidal aneurysm	20 (57%)
Middle cerebral aneurysm	7 (20%)
Anterior communicating aneurysm	8 (23%)
Diameter of aneurysms > 5 mm, n (100%)	35 (100%)
Aneurysm rupture, n	0
Lobular aneurysm, n (100%)	21 (60%)
Contralateral aneurysm, n (100%)	17(49%)
Ipsilateral aneurysm, n (100%)	18(51%)
Carotid arterial stenosis, n (100%)	18(58%)
Internal carotid arterial occlusion of intracranial segment, n (100%)	3(10%)
Internal carotid arterial stenosis of intracranial segment, n (100%)	4(13%)
Middle cerebral arterial stenosis, n (100%)	2(7%)
Middle cerebral arterial occlusion, n (100%)	1(3%)
Glasgow Outcome Scale at discharge, n (100%)	
5	29(94%)
4	1(3%)
3	1(3%)
Modified Rankin Scale at discharge, n (100%)	
0–1	26(84%)
2	4(13%)
3	1(3%)
Glasgow Outcome Scale at follow-up, n (100%)	
5	26(84%)
3	1(3%)
Lost	4(13%)
Modified Rankin Scale at follow-up, n (100%)	
0–1	25(81%)
2	1(3%)
3	1(3%)
Lost	4(13%)

choroidal aneurysms (57%), seven middle cerebral aneurysms (20%), and eight anterior communicating aneurysms (23%). All aneurysms had no rupture, and there were 21 lobular aneurysms (60%). There were 17

contralateral aneurysms (49%) and 18 ipsilateral aneurysms (51%). Besides, there were 18 patients with carotid arterial stenosis (> 50%, nine patients with stenosis > 75%), three patients with internal carotid arterial occlusion of cervical segment, three patients with internal carotid arterial occlusion of intracranial segment, four patients with internal carotid arterial stenosis of intracranial segment (> 50%), two patients with middle cerebral arterial stenosis (> 50%), and one patients with middle cerebral arterial occlusion.

One early awake patient became unconsciousness and had contralateral hemiplegia on the second day after surgical operation. Massive cerebral infarction was diagnosed according to CT scan in this patient. In spite of big bone flap excised and dura matter enlarged, hemiplegia and aphasia still existed in this patient (Fig. 1). Minor cerebral infarction in posterior limb of internal capsule occurred in another patient. Twenty-nine patients had normal neurological function (GOS 5), one patient with mild neurological defect (GOS 4), and one patient with severe neurological defect (GOS 3) at discharge. Meanwhile, there were 26 patients with MRS 0–1, four patients with MRS 2, and one patients with MRS 3 at discharge. During the follow-up, 26 patients had normal neurological function (GOS 5), and one patient with severe neurological defect (GOS 3). Meanwhile, there were 25 patients with MRS 0–1, one patient with MRS 2, and one patients with MRS 3. There were three patients with carotid arterial stenting, and one patients with carotid endarterectomy at the third month after surgical operation. All patients had no recurrence of intracranial aneurysm.

Discussion

Prevalence of intracranial aneurysms is obviously higher in patients with ischemic cerebrovascular diseases compared with general population [7]. Carotid arterial stenosis or occlusion on one side increases blood flow of contralateral carotid artery and cerebral arterial circle, aggravates the impact force and shear force of blood flow on the vessel wall, and results in the occurrence and development of intracranial aneurysms [11]. In South Korean patients with ischemic cerebrovascular diseases, 47.4 and 52.6% of intracranial aneurysms located on the same and other side of arterial stenosis or occlusion, respectively [7]. These results are close to our data (49 and 51%) in the current case series. Moreover, ischemic cerebrovascular diseases and intracranial aneurysms have similar etiology and pathogenesis [8]. Aging, metabolic disturbance (elevated blood pressure, glucose and lipids), and poor vessel condition accelerates the occurrence and development of intracranial aneurysms and arterial plaques [12]. Inflammatory reaction and other mechanisms should be responsible for the occurrence and development of intracranial aneurysms and arterial plaques [7].

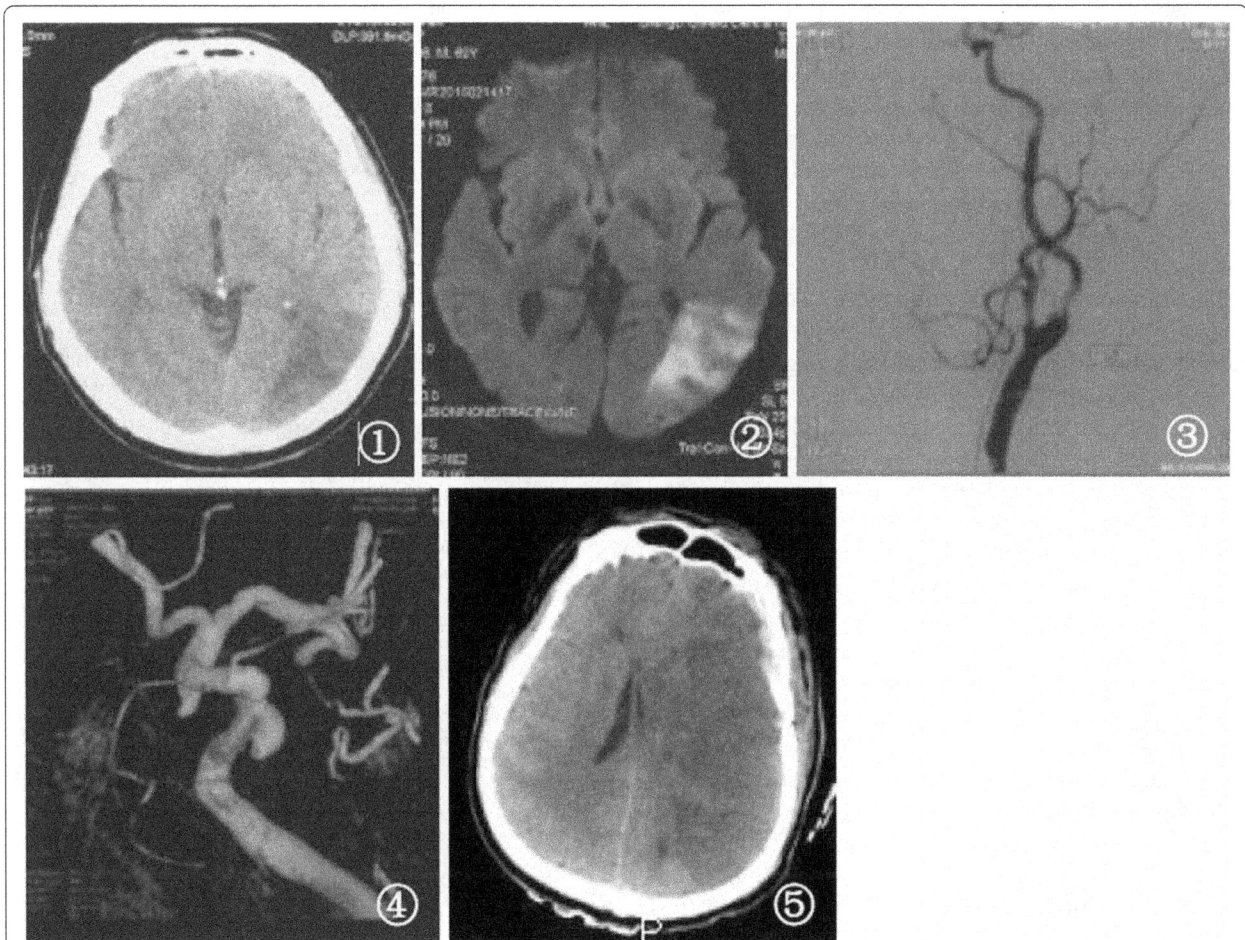

Fig. 1 One patient, 65–70 years old. ① cerebral infarction (left occipital lobe) shown in Computed Tomography scan before surgical operation; ② cerebral infarction (left occipital lobe) shown in Magnetic Resonance Imaging before surgical operation; ③left carotid arterial stenosis (> 75%) shown in Digital Subtraction Angiography before surgical operation; ④ left posterior communicating aneurysms with a diameter of 5.6 mm shown in Digital Subtraction Angiography before surgical operation; ⑤ cerebral infarction (left hemisphere) with a large area shown in Computed Tomography scan after operation

Since it is very difficult to balance the risk of aneurysm rupture and cerebral infarction, surgical treatment of intracranial aneurysms without rupture in patients with ischemic cerebrovascular diseases has been highly controversial [8]. If the treatment of ischemic cerebrovascular diseases precedes that of intracranial aneurysms, rapid increase in intracranial blood flow can induce the rupture of intracranial aneurysms [10]. If the treatment of intracranial aneurysms precedes that of ischemic cerebrovascular diseases, perioperative hypoperfusion can induce ischemic events and even fatal cerebral infarction with a large area [9]. One meta-analysis has shown no increased risk of aneurysm rupture caused by carotid endarterectomy [13]. Other study has also suggested that carotid arterial stenting and carotid endarterectomy are not related to increased aneurysm rupture [14]. It is worth noting that 82% of intracranial aneurysms have a diameter less than 5 mm in that study [14]. Thus,

ischemic cerebrovascular diseases were generally believed to receive surgical treatment before that of intracranial aneurysms with a diameter less than 5 mm.

Due to a lack of related studies, there has been debatable about sequential order of surgical treatment for ischemic cerebrovascular diseases and intracranial aneurysms with a diameter more than 5 mm. One study has found no increased prevalence of ischemic events in patients without high risk of cerebrovascular accident caused by the clipping of intracranial aneurysms with a diameter more than 5 mm [15]. Thus, surgical indications of intracranial aneurysms before ischemic cerebrovascular diseases include: 1) unruptured aneurysms with a diameter more than 5 mm; 2) without recurrent TIA, soft atherosclerotic plaques or ulcer formation; 3) aneurysm rupture and its caused subarachnoid hemorrhage.

Minimally invasive surgical approach through small pterion or inferolateral forehead is very suitable for the treatment of unruptured aneurysms in patients with ischemic cerebrovascular diseases [16]. Branches of external carotid artery, such as superficial temporal artery and middle meningeal artery, should be spared to ensure collateral circulation [9]. It is essential to minimize temporary blocking, shorten ischemic time and avoid plaque rupture. Papaverine soaking can be locally applied after the clipping of intracranial aneurysms to avoid the vasospasm.

Blood pressure is of great importance to the success of surgical operation, and should be controlled within reasonable range to avoid perioperative hypoperfusion and aneurysm rupture [4]. Preoperative communication with anesthesiologists can play a significant role in effective management of blood pressure. Postoperative blood pressure should be monitored to approach daily level to improve cerebral perfusion [2].

Patients with ischemic cerebrovascular diseases often have a long-term use of anti-platelet drugs [17]. These drugs should be withdrawn 1 week before surgical treatment, and applied on the second day after surgical treatment. Low molecular weight dextran and nimodipine can be applied to improve the microcirculation [18]. If there is an ischemic attack during the withdrawal of drugs, surgical operation should be performed with a great deal of caution.

The current case series had strength and limitation. Its strength was to explore surgical treatment and perioperative management of intracranial aneurysms in Chinese patients with ischemic cerebrovascular diseases. However, as a case series, it had a small sample size (31 patients).

Conclusions

The current case series found that minimally invasive surgical approach and intraoperative monitoring, supplemented by effective management of cerebrovascular perfusion, circulation and coagulation, can promote the treatment of intracranial aneurysms and prevent the development of cerebral ischemia and aneurysm rupture in Chinese patients with ischemic cerebrovascular diseases. Future studies with large sample size will be needed to confirm the results from the current case series.

Abbreviations

CTA: Computed tomography angiography; DSA: Digital substraction angiography; GOS: Glasgow outcome scale; MRS: Modified rankin scale; TIA: Transient ischemic attack

Acknowledgments
We are grateful to all participants for their participation in the case series.

Funding
Not applicable.

Authors' contributions
Conceived the study: YZ, CW. Performed the study: YZ, CW. Analyzed the data: YZ, CW. Contributed reagents/materials/analysis tools: YZ, CW. Wrote the paper: YZ, CW. Both authors have read and approve of the final version.

Competing interests
The authors declare that they have no competing interests.

References
1. Murray CJ, Vos T, Lozano R, et al. Disability-adjusted life years (DALYs) for 291 diseases and injuries in 21 regions, 1990–2010: a systematic analysis for the Global Burden of Disease Study 2010. Lancet. 2012; 380(9859):2197–223.
2. Connolly ES Jr, Rabinstein AA, Carhuapoma JR, et al. Guidelines for the management of aneurysmal subarachnoid hemorrhage: a guideline for healthcare professionals from the American Heart Association/American Stroke Association. Stroke. 2012;43(6):1711–37.
3. Wiebers DO, Whisnant JP, Huston J, et al. Unruptured intracranial aneurysms: natural history, clinical outcome, and risks of surgical and endovascular treatment. Lancet. 2003;362(9378):103–10.
4. Greving JP, Wermer MJ, Brown RD Jr, et al. Development of the PHASES score for prediction of risk of rupture of intracranial aneurysms: a pooled analysis of six prospective cohort studies. Lancet Neurol. 2014; 13(1):59–66.
5. Heman LM, Jongen LM, van der Worp HB, et al. Incidental intracranial aneurysms in patients with internal carotidartery stenosis: a CT angiography study and a metaanalysis. Stroke. 2009;40(4):1341–6.
6. Kappelle LJ, Eliasziw M, Fox AJ, et al. Small, unruptured intracranial aneurysms and management of symptomatic carotid artery stenosis. North American symptomatic carotid Endarterectomy trial group. Neurology. 2000; 55(2):307–9.
7. Cho YD, Jung KH, Roh JK, et al. Characteristics of intracranial aneurysms associated with extracranial carotid artery disease in South Korea. Clin Neurol Neurosurg. 2013;115(9):1677–81.
8. Ferrer I, Vidal N. Neuropathology of cerebrovascular diseases. Handb Clin Neurol. 2017;145:79–114.
9. Pereira BJ, Holanda VM, Giudicissi-Filho M, et al. Assessment of cerebral blood flow with micro-Doppler vascular reduces the risk of ischemic stroke during the clipping of intracranial aneurysms. World Neurosurg. 2015;84(6): 1747–51.
10. Mowla A, Singh K, Mehla S, et al. Is acute reperfusion therapy safe in acute ischemic stroke patients who harbor unruptured intracranial aneurysm? Int J Stroke. 2015;10(Suppl A100):113–8.
11. Jou LD, Shaltoni HM, Morsi H, et al. Hemodynamic relationship between intracranial aneurysm and carotid stenosis: review of clinical cases and numerical analyses. Neurol Res. 2010;32(10):1083–9.
12. Liang Y, Wang J, Li B. Coexistence of internal carotid artery stenosis with intracranial aneurysm. Int J Stroke. 2014;9(3):306–7.
13. Khan UA, Thapar A, Shalhoub J, et al. Risk of intracerebral aneurysm rupture during carotid revascularization. J Vasc Surg. 2012;56(6):1739–47.
14. Borkon MJ, Hoang H, Rockman C, et al. Concomitant unruptured intracranial aneurysms and carotid artery stenosis: an institutional review of patients undergoing carotid revascularization. Ann Vasc Surg. 2014;28(1):102–7.
15. Pappadà G, Fiori L, Marina R, et al. Management of symptomatic carotid stenoses with coincidental intracranial aneurysms. Acta Neurochir. 1996; 138(12):1386–90.
16. Cheng WY, Shen CC. Minimally invasive approaches to treat simultaneous occurrence of glioblastoma multiforme and intracranial aneurysm-case report. Minim Invasive Neurosurg. 2004;47(3):181–5.
17. Brewer L, Mellon L, Hall P, et al. Secondary prevention after ischaemic stroke: the ASPIRE-S study. BMC Neurol. 2015;15:216.
18. Diener HC. Stroke prevention: anti-platelet and anti-thrombolytic therapy. Neurol Clin. 2000;18(2):343–55.

The management of common recurrent headaches by chiropractors: a descriptive analysis of a nationally representative survey

Craig Moore[1]* (iD), Andrew Leaver[2], David Sibbritt[1] and Jon Adams[1]

Abstract

Background: Headache management is common within chiropractic clinical settings; however, little is yet known about how this provider group manage headache sufferers. The aim of this study is to report on the prevalence of headache patients found within routine chiropractic practice and to assess how chiropractors approach key aspects of headache management applicable to primary care settings.

Methods: A 31-item cross-sectional survey was distributed to a national sample of chiropractors ($n = 1050$) to report on practitioner approach to headache diagnosis, interdisciplinary collaboration, treatment and outcome assessment of headache patients who present with recurrent headache disorders.

Results: The survey attracted a response rate of 36% ($n = 381$). One in five new patients present to chiropractors with a chief complaint of headache. The majority of chiropractors provide headache diagnosis for common primary (84.6%) and secondary (90.4%) headaches using formal headache classification criteria. Interdisciplinary referral for headache management was most often with CAM providers followed by GPs. Advice on headache triggers, stress management, spinal manipulation, soft tissue therapies and prescriptive neck exercises were the most common therapeutic approaches to headache management.

Conclusion: Headache patients make up a substantial proportion of chiropractic caseload. The majority of chiropractors managing headache engage in headache diagnosis and interdisciplinary patient management. More research information is needed to understand the headache types and level of headache chronicity and disability common to chiropractic patient populations to further assess the healthcare needs of this patient population.

Keywords: Chiropractic, Migraine, Tension headache, Cervicogenic headache, Manual therapy, Practice-based research network, Spinal manipulation

Background

Tension headache and migraine are the most common recurrent primary headaches globally [1] and cervicogenic headache is one of the most common recurrent secondary headaches [2, 3]. While less information is available regarding the burden and economic impact associated with cervicogenic headache [4, 5], the societal impact of tension headache and migraine are significant and well documented [6–8].

In the collaborative study between the World Health Organisation (WHO) and the *'Lifting The Burden'* campaign, survey information was collected from neurologists and general practitioners in order to better understand how these providers approach headache diagnosis and management [9]. The findings of the report provided important insights into the use of headache diagnostic criteria, headache assessment tools, headache treatment and interdisciplinary collaboration.

* Correspondence: craigsmoore@mac.com
[1]Faculty of Health, University of Technology Sydney, Level 8, Building 10, 235-253 Jones Street Ultimo, Sydney, NSW 2007, Australia
Full list of author information is available at the end of the article

While headache is most often managed by general practitioners and neurologists, the report also found headache patients report a clear preference for the use of complementary and alternative treatments for headaches including physical based therapies and acupuncture.

The use of chiropractors for headache management appears to be significant. In a recent national US study, manipulative-based physical therapies were reported to be the most frequently used complementary and alternative treatments for migraine and headache patients [10]. In North America, a general population study reported between 25.7–36.2% of migraine headache patients had sought help from chiropractors at some time [11]. In Australia, chiropractic utilisation by those with headache was reported to be 9.3% in the preceding 12 months [12]. Notably, one international study found chiropractors to be the second and third most common health care provider by those with migraine in Australia and the United States respectively [13].

While the use of chiropractors for the management of headache disorders appears to be significant, little is understood about how this provider group manage this substantial patient population. With increasing research examination on interdisciplinary headache management [14, 15], more information is needed to understand the role of chiropractors within the interdisciplinary headache management landscape. Gathering this information can offer important insights that may help to guide more effective and coordinated healthcare delivery between providers and improve the management of headache patients. In direct response to this important research gap, this paper reports on a) the prevalence of patients who present to chiropractors with headache and b) how chiropractors approach keys aspects of headache patient management appropriate to primary care settings including the use of headache diagnostic criteria, headache assessment tools, approach to headache treatment and interdisciplinary engagement with other headache providers.

Methods

The study collected data via an online cross-sectional survey (Additional file 1) distributed to Australian practicing chiropractors who were recruited members of the Australian Chiropractic Research Network (ACORN) - a national practice-based research network (PBRN) [16]. Those recruited to the ACORN PBRN database are broadly representative of the wider national population of Australian chiropractors in terms of the key indicators of gender distribution, age distribution and practice location [17]. Full details of the original recruitment of chiropractors to join the national-based ACORN PBRN has been reported elsewhere [16]. This ACORN PBRN sub-study was approved by the Human Research Ethics Committee at the University of Technology Sydney (Approval number: ETH16–0639).

Recruitment and participants

Practitioner recruitment for the sub-study was a random sample of chiropractors taken from the nationally representative ACORN database. A sample of 1050 participants was selected using the random number generator function in Microsoft Excel 2016. Recruitment was conducted between August and November 2016 with participants invited to complete a 31-item online headache questionnaire using the SurveyMonkey™ platform. An embedded link to the headache questionnaire was emailed to invited participants who received three reminders during the recruitment period.

Instrument

The questionnaire introduction explained the approximate duration, purpose and contents of the study and that survey completion was voluntary, and that respondent information was anonymous. Consent was implied by completing the survey and no incentives were offered to participate in the study. As there are no previously validated instruments for the assessment of provider headache management across several clinical areas, the key themes and questions adopted for our study questionnaire were developed after consideration of the 'WHO: Lifting the Burden' report [9] and other surveys examining primary care management of headache patients [18, 19]. The headache disorders selected for the study were based upon headache types previously reported as common to chiropractic headache patient populations [20–22].

The questionnaire collected information on practitioner characteristics (i.e. gender, years in practice, place of education and practice location). Practitioner reporting of headache patient prevalence were based on practitioner consultations over the previous two weeks. Questions about the use of headache diagnostic criteria were based on the International Classification of Headache Disorders (ICHD-3 Beta) criteria for primary and secondary recurrent headaches [23]. Preceding the questions on primary headaches, the online questionnaire provided a direct link to ICHD-3 Beta diagnostic criteria. Preceding the questions on secondary headaches, a direct link was similarly provided to the ICHD-3 Beta diagnostic criteria. Questions regarding the use of headache assessment instruments were based on the use of the Migraine Disability Assessment questionnaire (MIDAS) [24], Headache Disability Inventory (HDI) [25] and the use of patient headache diaries [26]. For headache management, the questionnaire included questions on multi-disciplinary engagement with other providers (sending and receiving headache patient referrals) and questions on chiropractor's approach to headache management including treatment aims, therapeutic methods and treatment volume. For questions regarding headache management by chiropractors, headaches were divided into headaches of less than 3 months' duration and headaches of more than 3 months' duration.

The questionnaire was pilot tested with 10 chiropractors in private clinical practice from different socio-demographic backgrounds who provided feedback on content, wording and survey length. Feedback from pilot testing resulted in further changes to the length and wording of the instrument. The final version of the online survey was estimated to take around 15 min to complete. All questionnaire items were either dichotomous (yes/no) or reported as ratings on a 4-point or 5-point Likert scale.

Statistical analyses

Participant perceptions regarding the role of ICHD diagnostic criteria for primary and secondary headaches are re-categorized into 3 groups: strongly disagree/disagree; neutral and agree/strongly agree and the reporting of participant collaboration with other healthcare providers for the management of headache are re-categorised into 2 groups: never/rarely; and sometimes/often. This was due to the very low number of responses reported within some of the Likert categories provided for these questions. A minimum mean agreement score is used to report participant headache treatment aims (very unimportant/somewhat unimportant/neutral/somewhat important/very important). The reporting of chiropractic headache management provided by chiropractors are categorized as: often/almost every headache patient compared to never/rarely. Descriptive statistics are used to describe responses by participants. Continuous descriptive data are presented using means and standard deviations and categorical data presented using numbers and percentages. Statistical analysis was based upon the total number of completed surveys ($n = 321$) and conducted using software Stata 14.2.

Results

Practitioner characteristics

The questionnaire was completed by 381 practitioners, giving a response rate of 36.2%. This number represents 12.1% of the total number of practicing chiropractors in Australia at the time of recruitment. Participants mean number of years in practice was 18.1 years (SD = 10.9). When comparing survey participants to the ACORN data-base, survey respondents are generally representative for gender (64% male vs 63%) ($p = 0.379$), and place of practice: New South Wales (35.1% vs 34%), Victoria (23.2% vs 25%), Queensland (15.2% vs 15.0%), Western Australia (14.7% vs 13%), South Australia (8.5% vs 9.0%), Australian Capital Territory (1.6% vs 2%), Tasmania (0.9% vs 1%) and Northern Territory (0.5% vs 1%) ($p = 0.916$) [16]. These non-significant p values show no difference in distributions between samples for gender

and place of practice, suggesting survey respondents are generally representative of the ACORN database participants. The distribution of these participant demographic characteristics are consistent with national registration records reported by the Chiropractic Board of Australia [27].

Headache prevalence

In the previous two-week period the mean total number of new consultations reported by participants was 7.1 (SD = 4.8) where a chief complaint of headaches accounted for 1.5 (SD = 1.7) new consultations and a secondary complaint of headaches accounted for 2.5 (SD = 2.3) new consultations. In the previous two-week period the mean number of total patient consultations (new and routine treatment visits) was 170.9 (SD = 107.3) where a chief complaint of headaches accounted for 21.5 (SD = 28.6) total consultations and a secondary complaint of headaches accounted for 28.2 (33.8) total consultations.

Headache treatment plans

In terms of the number of initial treatment visits normally provided for a new patient presenting with headaches of less than 3 months duration for each of migraine, tension headache and cervicogenic headache, between 28 and 29.6% of participants reported providing less than 5 treatments, 54.2–55.5% provided between 5 and 10 visits and 14.9–16.5% reported providing more than 10 visits across all 3 headache types. For the duration of an initial headache treatment plan for a new patient presenting with headaches of less than 3 months duration - migraine, tension headache and cervicogenic headache (grouped); 11.8% of participants reported providing treatment for less than 2 weeks, 50.3% reported 2–4 weeks, 33.0% reported 4–8 weeks and 4.4% reported treatment for more than 8 weeks. With regards to the frequency of treatment during an initial headache treatment plan for a new patient presenting with headaches of less than 3 months duration (i.e. migraine, tension headache and cervicogenic), 16.0% of participants reported providing one treatment per week, 72.5% two treatments per week, 11.0% three treatments per week and 0.5% reported providing more than three visits per week. In terms of the number of initial treatment visits for a new patient presenting with headaches for more than 3 months duration for each of migraine, tension headache and cervicogenic headache, between 10.7–12.0% of participants reported providing less than 5 treatments, 46.3–50.3% provided between 5 and 10 visits and between 38.0–43.0% reported providing more than 10 visits across all 3 headache types. For the duration of an initial headache treatment plan for a patient presenting with headaches for more than 3 months duration - migraine, tension headache and cervicogenic headache (grouped), 4.7% of participants reported providing treatment for less than 2 weeks, 32.2%% reported 2–4 weeks, 46.9% reported 4–8 weeks and 16.2% reported an initial treatment period of more than 8 weeks.

Headache classification

The majority of participants reported being familiar with ICHD headache criteria for primary (98.3%; $n = 411$) and secondary (81.2%; $n = 324$) headaches and using these criteria for classifying primary (84.6%; $n = 334$) and secondary (90.4%; $n = 291$) headaches. Figure 1 provides the mean score for participants' perceptions regarding ICHD criteria for the diagnosis and management of primary and secondary headaches independently. The mean scores (0 = no agreement, 5 = high agreement) across all domains were high for participant agreement on the clinical utility of ICHD classification for a range of listed clinical purposes. There was a strong agreement amongst participants that ICHD criteria were easy to follow for primary (mean = 4.00; SD = 0.76) and secondary headaches (mean = 3.88; SD = 0.76) and represent distinct criteria for primary (mean = 3.92; SD = 0.76) and secondary headaches (mean = 3.89; SD = 0.76) and helps communication with other providers for primary (mean = 3.95; SD = 0.76) and secondary headaches (mean = 3.96; SD = 0.76). There was relatively less agreement amongst participants that patients easily fit into ICHD criteria for primary (mean = 3.29; SD = 0.76) and secondary headaches (mean = 3.39; SD = 0.76).

Multidisciplinary care

The level of interdisciplinary collaboration between chiropractors and other healthcare providers in managing patients with headaches is reported in Table 1. The most frequent collaboration between chiropractors and other providers for headache management was reported to be with other Complementary and Alternative Medicine (CAM) providers, followed by GPs for both referring and receiving headache patient referrals. The frequency of chiropractors referring headache patients to GPs was reported as substantially higher than the frequency of chiropractors receiving headache patient referrals from GPs.

The reasons chiropractors 'sometimes' or 'often' refer headache patients to other providers was to: investigate headache red-flags (83.4%; $n = 324$); assist with acute headache pain (57.1%; $n = 224$); assist with headache-related coping skills (53.8%; $n = 211$); assist with headache prevention (44.9%; $n = 176$); and confirm headache diagnosis (32.9%; $n = 129$).

Chiropractic headache management

The mean scores (0 = no agreement, 5 = high agreement) across all domains were high for participant agreement

on the importance of a range of headache treatment outcomes. There was a minimum mean agreement score of 4.23 out of 5 for: the importance of treatment providing headache prevention; improving headache recovery and headache pain relief; improving headache-related coping skills; and patient health and well-being.

The most frequent therapeutic approach by participants for migraine management was advice on headache triggers (94.1%), stress management (89.4%) and non-thrust spinal mobilisation (88.4%). The most frequent therapeutic approach by participants for tension headache management was advice on headache triggers (90.9%), stress management (90.1%) and soft tissue therapies (massage, myofascial, stretching or trigger point therapy) to the neck/shoulder area (88.1%). The most frequent therapeutic approach by participants for cervicogenic headache management was prescription exercises for the neck/shoulders (91.7%), spinal manipulation (90.6%) and soft tissue therapies (massage, myofascial, stretching or trigger point therapy) to the neck/shoulder area (88.3%) (Table 2).

When asked about the use of headache assessment instruments, a significant percentage of participants reported 'never' or 'rarely' using MIDAS (96.2%) and HDI (87.3%) headache instruments. The use of headache diaries was reported as 'sometimes' or 'almost every headache patient' by 41% of the chiropractors (data not shown).

Discussion

Results from our study suggest that a large percentage of new and routine chiropractic patient consultations are related to headache management with around one in five new patients presenting to chiropractors with a chief complaint of headache and more than one in three presenting with a secondary complaint of headache. This substantial level of headache caseload within chiropractic clinical settings raises questions about the factors that influence the preference and use of chiropractors for the management of headache compared to the use of other headache providers and treatments. Previous evidence suggests that patient dissatisfaction with preventative headache drug treatments are likely to be an important predictor for headache patient use of manual therapy providers [21]. However, there is a need for more robust research to assess the effectiveness of manual therapies for the prevention of recurrent headaches. To date, systematic reviews report significant methodological short-comings for clinical trials that aim to assess the prevention of migraine with manual therapies [28, 29], while limited, moderate quality evidence appears to support the potential role of manual therapies for the prevention of tension-type headache [30, 31] and cervicogenic headache [32, 33].

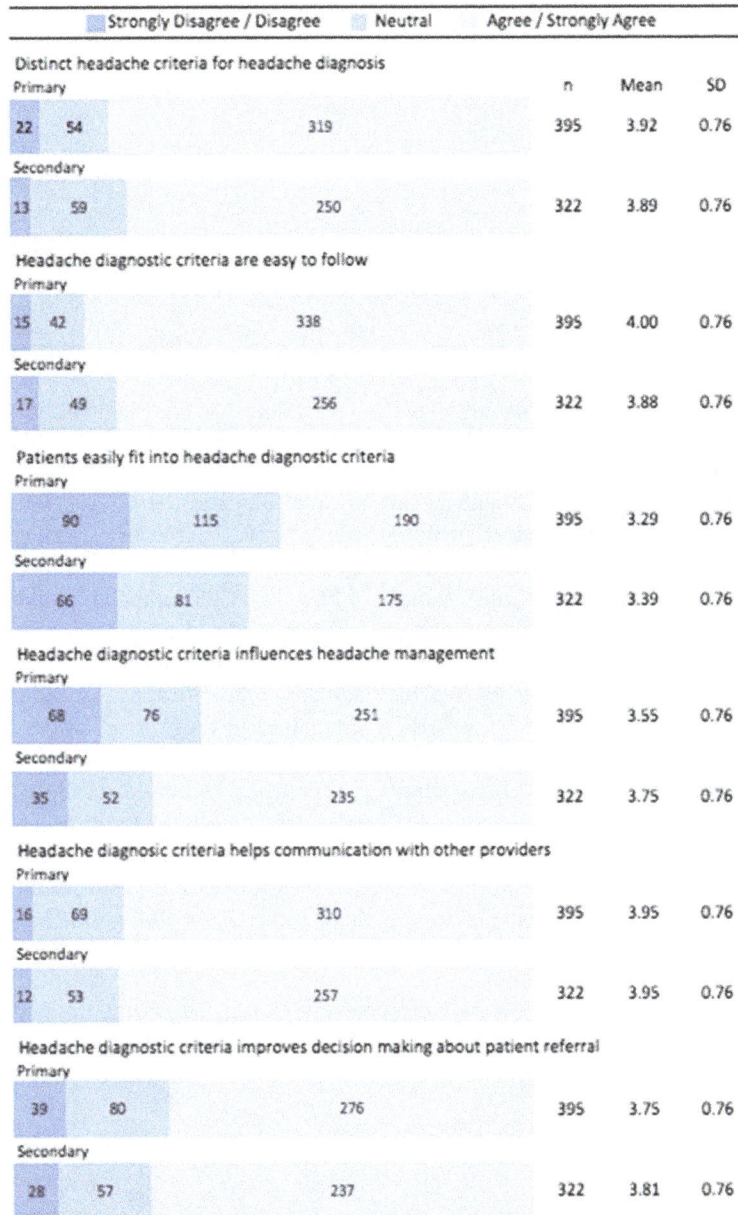

Fig. 1 Chiropractors views regarding ICHD diagnostic criteria for primary and secondary headaches (strongly disagree/disagree/neutral/agree/strongly agree)

Our study results suggest some aspects of headache patient management by chiropractors are consistent with that of medical providers. For example, the proportion of chiropractors reporting the use of primary and secondary headache diagnostic criteria in our study (84.6% and 90.4% respectively) compares favourably with the use of headache diagnosis found within medical care [9, 18]. While headache diagnosis is likely to improve clinical decision-making when managing the healthcare needs of headache sufferers [34], there is currently limited, poor quality information reporting on the proportion of migraine [13], tension headache [22], and

cervicogenic headache within chiropractic clinical settings. As such, more information is needed to better understand the types of headaches and level of headache burden more common to chiropractic clinical settings and how the management of headache patients is influenced by headache diagnosis including approaches to patient examination, education, referral and treatment.

Of note, practitioner use of secondary headache criteria for cervicogenic and medication over-use headache was reported slightly more often than practitioner familiarity with these secondary headache criteria. Poor familiarity with secondary headache criteria raises concerns

Table 1 Interdisciplinary collaboration by chiropractors with other healthcare providers for headache management (sometimes/often compared to never/rarely)

Provider	Receiving (sometimes/often) n = 392	Referring (sometimes/often) n = 392
CAM practitioner	66.1% (n = 259)	66.3% (n = 260)
General practitioner	29.6% (n = 116)	59.9% (n = 235)
Medical specialist (via GP)	3.8% (n = 15)	42.6% (n = 167)
Dentist	25% (n = 98)	40.3% (n = 158)
Psychologist	10.9% (n = 43)	16.6% (n = 65)
Physiotherapist	11.7% (n = 46)	13.3% (n = 52)
Osteopath	5.3% (n = 21)	3.8% (n = 15)

Survey key: Medical specialist (via GP) e.g. neurologist, psychiatrist. CAM practitioner e.g. acupuncturist, herbalist, naturopath, massage therapist, counsellor

about the risk to patient outcomes should chiropractors fail to appropriately diagnose secondary headaches. Such concerns could have serious consequences for secondary headaches needing urgent medical management [35]. While fully understanding this finding requires further empirical investigation, another explanation may be that some chiropractors are less familiar with at least some secondary headache diagnostic criteria listed, a finding that may relate to medication overuse headache, a secondary headache condition that can go unrecognized in clinical settings [36]. Additionally, this finding may also relate to practitioner concerns regarding the clinical utility of the diagnostic criteria associated with cervicogenic headache, an issue that has been reported elsewhere [3, 37, 38]. If so, these results may add weight to the need for further research examination into provider understanding, use and acceptance of cervicogenic headache criteria within primary care clinical settings.

The high rate of headache referral (receiving/referring) between chiropractors and other CAM providers in our study is consistent with findings from previous research in Australia and the US [39, 40]. The pattern of high referral between chiropractors and other CAM providers may be influenced by a number of factors including the influence of chiropractic organisations who sometimes promote a drugless approach to patient care [41, 42] or the higher percentage of chiropractors working at the same practice location as other CAM providers when compared to those practicing alongside other healthcare providers [40].

Our study identified that less than one in three chiropractors sometimes or often receive headache referrals from GPs. While the implication of these findings requires further empirical inquiry, this low rate of headache referral from GPs may be due to factors including GP concerns about the current level of evidence to

Table 2 Headache management characteristics by chiropractors (often/almost every headache patient compared to never/rarely)

Treatment approach	Migraine (often/almost all) (n = 387)	Tension headache (often/almost all) (n = 382)	Cervicogenic headache (often/almost all) (n = 382)
Joint-based manipulative therapies			
Spinal manipulation	318(82.2%)	337(87.5%)	349(90.6%)
Non-thrust spinal mobilisations	264(88.4%)	252(65.5%)	252(65.5%)
Instrument adjusting	279(72.1%)	270(70.1%)	273(70.9%)
Drop-piece methods	133(34.4%)	148(38.4%)	153(39.7%)
Soft-tissue based and exercise therapies			
Soft tissue to neck/shoulders	331(85.3%)	339(88.1%)	340(88.3%)
Electro-physical therapies	30(7.8%)	30(7.8%)	30(7.8%)
Soft-tissue/exercise to temporomandibular	252(65.1%)	249(64.7%)	233(60.5%)
Exercises – neck/shoulders	311(81.6%)	337(87.5%)	353(91.7%)
Patient advice and education			
Advice on headache triggers	364(94.1%)	350(90.9%)	338(87.8%)
Advice on diet and fitness	331(85.6%)	336(87.3%)	327(84.9%)
Stress management	346(89.4%)	347(90.1%)	337(87.5%)

Survey key: Spinal manipulation (manual adjusting/manipulation (including Diversified, Gonstead); Drop piece methods (drop-piece/Thompson or similar); Soft tissue – neck/shoulders (massage, myofascial, stretching or trigger points to neck/shoulders); Electro-physical therapies (including TENS, ultrasound) support the effectiveness of manual therapies for the management of headache or a less favourable GP attitude toward chiropractors as reported in a recent survey which found that 60% of Australian GPs never referred patients to a chiropractor [43]. With systematic reviews reporting evidence to support the potential role of manual therapies for some headache types [31, 32, 44], further research may be needed to better understand the current barriers to collaborative headache management that may exist between these providers. This research priority would seem important given the unmet needs remaining for some headache sufferers under medical care [45–48] and the high use of manipulative therapy providers by headache patients [10, 13, 21].

While the low frequency of headache patient referral between chiropractors and physiotherapy and osteopathic providers in our study may be partly explained by the use of similar approaches to headache treatment [49, 50], the low frequency of headache patient referral between chiropractors and psychologists deserves further consideration. Psychologists are a significant healthcare provider for the management of headache pain [51, 52] and for the management of headache-related comorbidities such as anxiety and depression. [53, 54]. As such, this finding raises questions about whether chiropractors managing headache are fully aware of the psycho-behavioural approaches available to assist in the management of headache. In comparison, the higher frequency of headache patient referral to GPs and medical specialists (via the GP) by chiropractors appears to suggest there are circumstances where chiropractors are working together with medical providers for the management of headache, a finding further supported by the high frequency of referral for the investigation of headache red-flags reported in our study. More information reporting on the types of headaches, level of headache chronicity and disability found within chiropractic headache populations would further help researchers and clinicians to better comprehend the related healthcare needs of this patient population and the clinical circumstances where greater interdisciplinary collaboration is warranted between chiropractors and other headache-related healthcare providers.

The most common therapeutic approaches reported by chiropractors in our study for the management of headache was providing advice on headache triggers, stress management, spinal manipulation, soft tissue therapies and prescriptive neck exercises. Helping patients both identify and manage headache triggers is recognised as an important aspect of headache patient management for those who present with migraine and tension headache within primary care settings [55]. However, the role of manual and exercise therapies for the management of those with recurrent headaches remains less certain with systematic reviews reporting stronger evidence for manual

therapies for the prevention of cervicogenic and tension headache [31, 32] and limited and conflicting evidence for the prevention of migraine [29]. As such, more robust research is needed to assess the effectiveness of both unimodal and multi-modal approaches to headache management by chiropractors, including for the management of both acute and chronic headache sub-types.

The chiropractors in our study most often provided between 5 and 10 treatments during an initial headache treatment plan while a slightly higher average number of treatments were provided for those with headaches of longer duration (more than 3 months). This number of treatments is similar to the number of treatments associated with significant improvement in headache outcomes for spinal mobilisation and manipulation reported in previous tension headache and cervicogenic headache studies [56, 57]. While information is limited regarding the relative costs associated with chiropractic headache management, one recent US study compared the cost of headache care using risk-adjusted scores that would otherwise affect the level of healthcare utilization [58]. This study found headache treatment costs were significantly higher both for medical doctor-only care when compared to chiropractic-only care and for medical doctor care combined with physical therapy care compared to medical doctor care combined with chiropractic care.

Our study found chiropractors more frequently engage the use of patient headache diaries, an approach to headache assessment that can help to reduce patient difficulty in recalling headache characteristics and their response to headache treatment [59]. However, the use of formal headache instruments such as MIDAS and HDI was comparatively low, a finding reported within other primary care settings [9, 60]. These validated headache instruments can assist health care providers to better understand headache disability, exacerbations and remissions and circumstances that indicate the need for specialty care [25, 61, 62]. As such, the low use of validated headache instruments reported in our study raises questions about best practice with regards to chiropractors more fully assessing headache patients to better understand clinical findings associated with more complex headache patient presentations.

A key strength of our study is the nationally representative cross-sectional sample of chiropractors in order to provide important preliminary information on the current state of chiropractic headache practice. It is however important to acknowledge several limitations to our study. While the online survey provided a direct reference and link to the ICHD-3 classification criteria for primary and secondary headaches, a comprehensive list of the headache criteria was not provided within the survey prior to asking respondents if they were familiar with the diagnostic criteria for the primary and secondary headaches listed.

Furthermore, the survey has not aimed to explore diagnosis and management of chronic headache types (15 or more days per month over a 3-month period). The response rate for our sample (36%), while similar to other studies of this type, is limited to 12% of the total practitioner population nationally. As a result, there may be important differences in the headache management characteristics between survey respondents and non-respondents. This would include the risk of selection bias that may result from the random selection of chiropractors within a PBRN compared to outside the PBRN. The Likert categories utilized in parts of the survey questionnaire are open to practitioner interpretation and findings are based upon self-report and retrospective recall and subject to recall bias. In addition, our study did not provide any assessment of adverse events that may result from manual therapies for the management of headaches. However, these findings draw upon a national sample of chiropractors in order to provide valuable insights for future investigation to further our understanding of the management of headache patients by this provider group.

Conclusions

Our national-based sample suggests headache is a substantial proportion of chiropractic caseload. While some aspects of chiropractic headache management, including the acceptance and use of headache diagnostic criteria, appears to be consistent with good clinical practice, other aspects of chiropractic headache management raise questions worthy of further research enquiry. Critically, there is a need for more detailed information on the proportion of headache types and level of headache chronicity and disability found within chiropractic headache patient populations. This information will help practitioners, researchers and policy-makers to better understand the healthcare needs associated with headache patients who seek help from this common provider of headache management.

Abbreviations
ACORN: Australian chiropractic research network; CAM: Complementary and alternative medicine; HDI: Headache disability inventory; ICHD: International classification of headache disorders; MIDAS: Migraine disability assessment questionnaire; PBRN: Practice-based research network

Acknowledgements
The authors would like to thank the Chiropractors' Association of Australia for their financial support for the ACORN PBRN. The research reported in this paper is the sole responsibility of the authors and reflects the independent ideas and scholarship of the authors alone. The authors wish to acknowledge and thank the Australian chiropractors who participated in this study.

Funding
This research received no specific grant from any funding agency in the public, commercial or not-for-profit sectors.

Authors' contributions
CM, AL, DS and JA designed the paper. CM and DS carried out the data collection, analysis and interpretation. CM wrote the drafts with revisions made by AL, DS and JA. All authors contributed to the intellectual content. All authors read and approved the final manuscript.

Competing interests
All the authors declare that they have no competing interests related to the contents of this manuscript. Furthermore, all authors declare that they have received no direct or indirect payment in preparation of this manuscript.

Author details
[1]Faculty of Health, University of Technology Sydney, Level 8, Building 10, 235-253 Jones Street Ultimo, Sydney, NSW 2007, Australia. [2]Faculty of Health Science, University of Sydney, Sydney, Australia.

References
1. Vos T, Flaxman AD, Naghavi M, Lozano R, Michaud C, Ezzati M, et al. Years lived with disability (YLDs) for 1160 sequelae of 289 diseases and injuries 1990–2010: a systematic analysis for the global burden of disease study. Lancet. 2012;380:2163–96.
2. Sjaastad O, Fredriksen T. Cervicogenic headache: criteria, classification and epidemiology. Clin Exp Rheumatol. 2000;18:S-3.
3. Sjaastad O, Bakketeig LS. Prevalence of cervicogenic headache: Vågå study of headache epidemiology. Acta Neurol Scand. 2008;117:173–80.
4. HAv S, Lamé I, van den Berg SGM S, AGH K, WEJ W. Quality of life of patients with cervicogenic headache: a comparison with control subjects and patients with migraine or tension-type headache. Headache. 2003;43: 1034–41.
5. Gesztelyi G, Bereczki D. Determinants of disability in everyday activities differ in primary and cervicogenic headaches and in low back pain. Psychiatry Clin Neurosci. 2006;60:271–6.
6. Zebenholzer K, Andree C, Lechner A, Broessner G, Lampl C, Luthringshausen G, et al. Prevalence, management and burden of episodic and chronic headaches—a cross-sectional multicentre study in eight Austrian headache centres. J Headache Pain. 2015;16:46.
7. Lanteri-Minet M. Economic burden and costs of chronic migraine. Curr Pain Headache Rep. 2014;18:385.
8. Yu S, Han X. Update of chronic tension-type headache. Curr Pain Headache Rep. 2014;19:469.
9. WHO Lifting the Burden [http://www.who.int/mental_health/management/ who_atlas_headache_disorders.pdf?ua=1]. Accessed 1 Sept 2018.
10. Zhang Y, Dennis JA, Leach MJ, Bishop FL, Cramer H, Chung VC, et al. Complementary and alternative medicine use among US adults with headache or migraine: results from the 2012 National Health Interview Survey. Headache. 2017;57:1228–42.
11. Bigal ME, Serrano D, Reed M, Lipton RB. Chronic migraine in the population burden, diagnosis, and satisfaction with treatment. Neurology. 2008;71:559–66.
12. Xue C, Zhang A, Lin V, Myers R, Polus B, Story D. Acupuncture, chiropractic and osteopathy use in Australia: a national population survey. BMC Public Health. 2008;8:105.
13. Sanderson JC, Devine EB, Lipton RB, Bloudek LM, Varon SF, Blumenfeld AM, et al. Headache-related health resource utilisation in chronic and episodic migraine across six countries. J Neurol Neurosurg Psychiatry. 2013;84:1309–17.
14. Nicol AL, Hammond N, Doran SV. Interdisciplinary management of headache disorders. Tech Reg Anesth Pain Manag. 2013;17:174–87.
15. Gaul C, Liesering-Latta E, Schäfer B, Fritsche G, Holle D. Integrated multidisciplinary care of headache disorders: a narrative review. Cephalalgia 2016; 36: 1181–91.
16. Adams J, Steel A, Moore C, Amorin-Woods L, Sibbritt D. Establishing the ACORN National Practitioner Database: strategies to recruit practitioners to a National Practice-Based Research Network. J Manip Physiol Ther. 2016;39:594 602.

17. Adams J, Peng W, Steel A, Lauche R, Moore C, Amorin-Woods L, et al. A cross-sectional examination of the profile of chiropractors recruited to the Australian chiropractic research network (ACORN): a sustainable resource for future chiropractic research. BMJ Open. 2017;7:1–8.

18. Kernick D, Stapley S, Hamilton W. GPs' classification of headache: is primary headache underdiagnosed? Br J Gen Pract. 2008;58:102–4.

19. Vuillaume De Diego E, Lanteri-Minet M. Recognition and management of migraine in primary care: influence of functional impact measured by the headache impact test (HIT). Cephalalgia. 2005;25:184–90.

20. Adams J, Barbery G, Lui C-W. Complementary and alternative medicine use for headache and migraine: a critical review of the literature. Headache. 2013;53:459–73.

21. Moore CS, Sibbritt DW, Adams J. A critical review of manual therapy use for headache disorders: prevalence, profiles, motivations, communication and self-reported effectiveness. BMC Neurol. 2017;17:1–11.

22. Kristoffersen ES, Grande RB, Aaseth K, Lundqvist C, Russell MB. Management of primary chronic headache in the general population: the Akershus study of chronic headache. J Headache Pain. 2012;13:113–20.

23. Headache Classification Committee of the International Headache S. The international classification of headache disorders, 3rd edition (beta version). Cephalalgia. 2013;33:629–808.

24. Stewart WF, Lipton RB, Kolodner KB, Sawyer J, Lee C, Liberman JN. Validity of the migraine disability assessment (MIDAS) score in comparison to a diary-based measure in a population sample of migraine sufferers. Pain 2000;88:41–52.

25. Jacobson GP, Ramadan NM, Aggarwal SK, Newman CW. The Henry ford hospital headache disability inventory (HDI). Neurology. 1994;44:837.

26. Phillip D, Lyngberg A, Jensen R. Assessment of headache diagnosis. A comparative population study of a clinical interview with a diagnostic headache diary. Cephalalgia. 2007;27:1–8.

27. Chiropractic Board of Australia. Chiropractic registrant data [http://www.chiropracticboard.gov.au/About-the-Board/Statistics.aspx]. Accessed 1 Oct 2018.

28. Chaibi A, Tuchin PJ, Russell MB. Manual therapies for migraine: a systematic review. J Headache Pain. 2011;12:127–33.

29. Posadzki P, Ernst E. Spinal manipulations for the treatment of migraine: a systematic review of randomized clinical trials. Cephalalgia. 2011;31:964–70.

30. Lozano López C, Mesa Jiménez J, de la Hoz Aizpurúa JL, Pareja Grande J, Fernández de las Peñas C. Efficacy of manual therapy in the treatment of tension-type headache. A systematic review from 2000 to 2013. Neurología (English Edition). 2016;31:357–69.

31. Mesa-Jiménez JA, Lozano-López C, Angulo-Díaz-Parreño S, Rodríguez-Fernández ÁL, De-la-Hoz-Aizpurua JL, Fernández-de-las-Peñas C. Multimodal manual therapy vs pharmacological care for management of tension type headache: a meta-analysis of randomized trials. Cephalalgia. 2015;35:1323–32.

32. Racicki S, Gerwin S, DiClaudio S, Reinmann S, Donaldson M. Conservative physical therapy management for the treatment of cervicogenic headache: a systematic review. J Man Manip Ther. 2013;21:113–24.

33. Chaibi A, Russell MB. Manual therapies for cervicogenic headache: a systematic review. J Headache Pain. 2012;13:351–9.

34. Kingston WS, Halker R. Determinants of suboptimal migraine diagnosis and treatment in the primary care setting. JCOM. 2017;24:319–24.

35. Sarah N, TL P. Headaches in brain tumor patients: primary or secondary? Headache. 2014;54:776–85.

36. Obermann M, Katsarava Z. Management of medication-overuse headache. Expert Rev Neurother. 2007;7:1145–55.

37. Fredriksen T, Antonaci F, Sjaastad O. Cervicogenic headache: too important to be left un-diagnosed. J Headache Pain. 2015;16:1–3.

38. Antonaci F, Bono G, Chimento P. Diagnosing cervicogenic headache. J Headache Pain. 2006;7:145–8.

39. Pohlman KA, Hondras MA, Long CR, Haan AG. Practice patterns of doctors of chiropractic with a pediatric diplomate: a cross-sectional survey. BMC Complement Altern Med. 2010;10:26.

40. Adams J, Lauche R, Peng W, Steel A, Moore C, Amorin-Woods LG, et al. A workforce survey of Australian chiropractic: the profile and practice features of a nationally representative sample of 2,005 chiropractors. BMC Complement Altern Med. 2017;17:14.

41. Chiropractic and you. https://chiropractors.asn.au/about-chiropractic/chiropractic-and-you. Accessed 1 Oct 2018.

42. World Federation of Chiropractic Identity Task Report [https://www.wfc.org/website/images/wfc/docs/as_tf_final_rept-Am_04-29-05_001.pdf]. Accessed 3 Jan 2017.

43. Engel RM, Beirman R, Grace S. An indication of current views of Australian general practitioners towards chiropractic and osteopathy: a cross-sectional study. Chiropr Man Therap. 2016;24:37.

44. Chaibi A, Russell MB. Manual therapies for primary chronic headaches: a systematic review of randomized controlled trials. J Headache Pain. 2014;15:67.

45. Rossi P, Di Lorenzo G, Faroni J, Malpezzi MG, Cesarino F, Nappi G. Use of complementary and alternative medicine by patients with chronic tension-type headache: results of a headache clinic survey. Headache. 2006;46:622–31.

46. Gaul C, Eismann R, Schmidt T, May A, Leinisch E, Wieser T, et al. Use of complementary and alternative medicine in patients suffering from primary headache disorders. Cephalalgia. 2009;29:1069–78.

47. Malone CD, Bhowmick A, Wachholtz AB. Migraine: treatments, comorbidities, and quality of life, in the USA. J Pain Res. 2015;8:537–47.

48. Starling AJ, Dodick DW. Best practices for patients with chronic migraine: burden, diagnosis, and management in primary care. Mayo Clin Proc. 2015; 90:408–14.

49. Grant T, Niere K. Techniques used by manipulative physiotherapists in the management of headaches. Aust J Physiother. 2000;46:215–22.

50. Schabert E, Crow WT. Impact of osteopathic manipulative treatment on cost of care for patients with migraine headache: a retrospective review of patient records. J Am Osteopath Assoc. 2009;109:403–7.

51. Bendtsen L, Evers S, Linde M, Mitsikostas DD, Sandrini G, Schoenen J. EFNS guideline on the treatment of tension-type headache – report of an EFNS task force. Eur J Neurol. 2010;17:1318–25.

52. Pringsheim T, Davenport WJ, Mackie G, Worthington I, Aubé M, Christie SN, et al. Canadian headache society guideline for migraine prophylaxis. Can J Neurol Sci. 2012;39:S1–S59.

53. Seng EK, Mayson SJ, Sonty N, Stein T, Tsui P, Qian S, et al. Psychological considerations in the migraine patient. In: Migraine Surgery edn; 2014. p. 59–90.

54. Jensen R, Zeeberg P, Dehlendorff C, Olesen J. Predictors of outcome of the treatment programme in a multidisciplinary headache centre. Cephalalgia. 2010;30:1214–24.

55. Hoque B, Rahman KM, Hasan ATMH, Chowdhury RN, Khan SU, Alam MB, et al. Precipitating and relieving factors of migraine versus tension type headache. BMC Neurol. 2012;12:1–4.

56. Haas M, Spegman A, Peterson D, Aickin M, Vavrek D. Dose-response and efficacy of spinal manipulation for chronic Cervicogenic headache: a pilot randomized controlled trial. Spine J. 2010;10:117–28.

57. Castien RF, Windt DA, Grooten A, Dekker J. Effectiveness of manual therapy for chronic tension-type headache: a pragmatic, randomised, clinical trial. Cephalalgia. 2011;31:133–43.

58. Hurwitz EL, Vassilaki M, Li D, Schneider MJ, Stevans JM, Phillips RB, et al. Variations in patterns of utilization and charges for the Care of Headache in North Carolina, 2000-2009: a statewide claims data analysis. J Manip Physiol Ther. 2016;39:229–39.

59. Jensen R, Tassorelli C, Rossi P, Allena M, Osipova V, Steiner T, et al. A basic diagnostic headache diary (BDHD) is well accepted and useful in the diagnosis of headache. A multicentre European and Latin American study. Cephalalgia. 2011;31:1549–60.

60. Minen MT, Loder E, Tishler L, Silbersweig D. Migraine diagnosis and treatment: a knowledge and needs assessment among primary care providers. Cephalalgia. 2016;36:358–70.

61. Stewart WF, Lipton RB, Kolodner K. Migraine disability assessment (MIDAS) score: relation to headache frequency, pain intensity, and headache symptoms. Headache. 2003;43:258–65.

62. Lipton RB, Stewart WF, Sawyer J, Edmeads JG. Clinical utility of an instrument assessing migraine disability: the migraine disability assessment (MIDAS) questionnaire. Headache. 2001;41:854–61.

19

Atypical sensory processing pattern following median or ulnar nerve injury

Pernilla Vikström[1], Anders Björkman[1], Ingela K. Carlsson[1], Anna-Karin Olsson[2] and Birgitta Rosén[1*]

Abstract

Background: Due to brain plasticity a transection of a median or ulnar nerve results in profound changes in the somatosensory areas in the brain. The permanent sensory deprivation after a peripheral nerve injury might influence the interaction between all senses.

The aim of the study was to investigate if a median and/or ulnar nerve injury gives rise to a changed sensory processing pattern. In addition we examined if age at injury, injured nerve or time since injury influence the sensory processing pattern.

Methods: Fifty patients (40 men and 10 women, median age 43) operated due to a median and/or ulnar nerve injury were included. The patients completed the Adolescent/Adult Sensory Profile questionnaire, which includes a comprehensive characterization on how sensory information is processed and how an individual responds to multiple sensory modalities. AASP categorizes the results into four possible Quadrants of behavioral profiles (Q1-low registration, Q2-sensory seeking, Q3-sensory sensitivity and Q4-sensory avoiding). The results were compared to 209 healthy age and gender matched controls. Anova Matched Design was used for evaluation of differences between the patient group and the control group. Atypical sensory processing behavior was determined in relation to the normative distribution of the control group.

Results: Significant difference was seen in Q1, low registration. 40% in the patient group scored atypically in this Quadrant compared to 16% of the controls. No correlation between atypical sensory processing pattern and age or time since injury was seen.

Conclusion: A peripheral nerve injury entails altered sensory processing pattern with increased proportion of patients with low registration to sensory stimulus overall. Our results can guide us into more client centered rehabilitation strategies.

Keywords: Sensory, Median nerve, Ulnar nerve, Injury, Sensory profile

Background

An injury to a major nerve in the upper extremity in adults causes long-lasting disability due to loss of fine sensory and motor function [1, 2]. In addition, such injuries often cause psychological stress and may have devastating long-term effects on ADL and quality of life [3–9].

Sensibility is the function most seriously affected by a nerve injury [4, 10]. However, "sensibility" is much more than just touch sensation. Touch is one aspect of perception where perception is a range of processes involved in turning sensations from all sense organs into meaningful information [11]. These perceptual processes are necessary to help us, among other things, orient in the environment and sort out the importance from all stimulus we are exposed to continuously, including touch stimulus.

The interaction between all senses are crucial for our understanding of, and interaction with, the surrounding world, where cross-modal association areas of the brain merge stimulus from all senses [12, 13].

* Correspondence: birgitta.rosen@med.lu.se
[1]Department of Translational Medicine – Hand Surgery, Skåne University Hospital and Lund University, Jan Waldenströms gata 5, SE-205 03 Malmö, Sweden
Full list of author information is available at the end of the article

A person's *"sensory profile"* describes how an individual processes information from all senses and the sensory profile is thus highly individual. The Adolescent/Adult Sensory Profile (AASP) is a standardized self-reported questionnaire that classifies sensory experiences and behavioral responses [14]. It includes a comprehensive characterization on how sensory information is processed and how an individual responds to multiple sensory modalities (Touch, Taste/Smell, Visual, Auditory, Movement and Activity). Based on the results from the questionnaire, a sensory profile is created [15, 16]. The concept was developed from Dunn's model of Sensory Processing. Dunn proposes that four sensory processing patterns characterize the perceptual process. These patterns are thought to arise from both individual differences in neurological thresholds to notice or react to stimuli, but also from self-regulation strategies, the so-called response behavior. The neurological thresholds refers to how readily the nervous system detects and reacts to stimuli, a lower threshold, the greater the probability of nervous system will be to detect and react to stimuli. The self-regulatory behavioral responses depicts how people behave in responses to stimuli according to their neurological thresholds. A person can respond in accordance to the neurological threshold (passive behavior response) or by counteract their neurological threshold (active behavior response). Combinations of these dimensions gives us four sensory processing styles [17]. AASP has primarily been used in rehabilitation of neuropsychiatric disorders and is suggested to be useful in planning clinical interventions [14]. In addition, AASP has also been shown to facilitate planning of clinical interventions in a few studies of patients with physical disorders such as atopic dermatitis, stroke and asthma [18–22].

A transection of a median or ulnar nerve results in rapid and profound changes in the somatosensory areas in the brain due to brain plasticity [23–28], and there are changes in the peripheral nerve as well [29]. Therefore, there are reasons to believe that the permanent sensory deprivation after a peripheral nerve transection might interact and influence the cross-modality between all senses as well as the higher cognitive functions in the brain. The proportionally large representation of the hand in the somatosensory cortex [30] is another reason to believe that a person's sensory profile may change. This depends on whether the extensive changes in this area can contribute to changes in other areas after median and/or ulnar nerve injury. Hypothetically, the changes in the somatosensory cortex may also affect processing of information from other senses.

If sensory processing changes could be demonstrated, it would teach us more about the plasticity of the brain following a peripheral nerve transection. In addition, knowledge about the patient's sensory profile might improve the possibility to individualize rehabilitation following nerve transection. Hence, given that an adult person with a severe nerve injury has a permanent limited perception of touch we hypothesized that patients with such injuries have an atypical experience and behavior in sensory processing overall.

Age at injury is a well-known influencing factor for sensory outcome after a nerve injury [31, 32] and improvement of sensory function following a major nerve trauma continues for years [33–35].

The aim of the present study was to investigate if a median and/or ulnar nerve transection gives rise to a changed sensory profile. An additional aim was to investigate how age at injury and time since injury influence the sensory profile.

Methods

Participants

Fifty adult (> 18 years) patients with at least 50% repair of the median and/or ulnar nerve were included in the study. All available patients from two earlier studies were asked to participate in the present study. The inclusion criteria were described in detail in those reports [36, 37]. Exclusion criteria were severe psychiatric or neurological disorder and communication problems due to language difficulties. Each patient was matched with four to six individual age (± 2 years) and gender matched controls from a healthy control group. The matched controls were extracted from the normative population from validation of the Sensory Profile into Swedish [38]. Depending on the varying amount of available matched controls in the normative population the number of controls vary between four and six.

Measures

The adolescent/Adult Sensory Profile [14] is a self-reported 60 item questionnaire based on Dunn's Model of Sensory Processing [17].

The 60 items are divided into four quadrants, based on a combination of behavioral response and neurological threshold. The four Quadrants are Low registration, Sensation Seeking, Sensory Sensitivity, and Sensory Avoiding. The questions concern experiences of sensory processing in everyday sensory experiences across different sensory processing domains (Taste/Smell, Movement, Visual, Touch, Activity and Auditory). Every item is scored on a 5-point scale where 1 = almost never, to 5 = almost always. The sum of the scores for each Quadrant and the six Domains are calculated from the answers.

Data analysis

To investigate whether a median and/or ulnar nerve injury gives rise to a changed sensory profile, Anova Matched Design was used for calculation of differences between the patient group and the age and gender matched control group. This was done for each of the four Quadrants (Q1-low registration, Q2-sensory seeking, Q3-sensory sensitivity and Q4-sensory avoiding) and the six Domains (Taste/Smell, Movement, Visual, Touch, Activity and Auditory). Level of significance was ≤0.05.

For the Quadrants/Domains with a significant difference between the groups, the percentage of patients who scored Atypically High and Atypically Low was calculated. A patient score ± 1 SD of the control group mean was categorized as "Atypically High" or "Atypically Low" respectively. We compared this percentage against a test value of 16%, indicating ± ≥ 1 SD, from the control group mean, which is interpreted as "more/less than most people".

The same calculation was then made for the scores of Definitely High/Low. A patient score ± 2 SD of the control group mean was categorized as "Definitely High" or "Definitely Low" respectively. We compared this percentage against a test value of 2.5%, indicating ± ≥ 2 SD from the control group mean, which is interpreted as "much more/much less than most people" [39]. Deviations from the mean were analyzed separately for each direction and confidence interval was calculated according to Binomial distribution.

Spearman correlation was used to examine the relationship between the Sensory Profile™ score and the possible influencing factors age and time since injury.

Ethics

The study was approved by the Ethical Committee of Lund University and it was conducted.

according to the declaration of Helsinki. All participants gave written consent.

Results

Participants

Fifty patients were included in the study. One patient was lost due to incomplete filling of the AASP questionnaire (Table 1).

Table 1 Demographics

	Patient group n = 49	Control group n = 209
Gender Men/Women	39/10	164/45
Age[a]	43 (19–75)	44 (18–76)
Months since injury[a]	24 (7–108)	–
Injured nerve median /ulnar/both	18/27/4	–
Complete/Partial nerve transection	45/4	–

[a]Presented with median (range)

Sensory profile quadrants comparison

When comparing patients with controls, the results in the Low Registration Quadrant differed significantly (Table 2). An increased amount of the patients scored Atypically/Definitely High in the Low Registration Quadrant and an increased amount of patients scored Atypically/Definitely Low in the Low Registration Quadrant compared to their controls (Table 3 and Fig. 1). No significant differences were seen for the other three Quadrants.

Sensory profile domains comparison

No differences between the patients and the controls were seen in any of the six specific Domains (Taste/Smell, Movement, Vision, Touch, Activity and Auditory).

Influencing factors

No statistical correlations were seen between Sensory Profile™ score and age or time since injury.

Discussion

This study shows that patients with median or ulnar nerve injuries have an altered sensory processing pattern with increased incidence of low registration of impressions from all senses.

Low registration means high neurological thresholds, which in turn means that these persons fail to detect stimuli that others notice and more intense stimuli are needed for the nervous system to respond and enable the patients to sustain attention [39]. Atypical sensory processing patterns have also been seen in adults with atopic dermatitis and following a stroke, but in contrast to nerve injured patients, the patients with atopic dermatitis and post stroke showed decreased neurological thresholds, which in turn means that they respond to a low amount of stimulus [19, 22]. The present study supports the idea that the sensory profile also changes in physical disorders. It is important to remember that a multitude of combinations in scores in the four Quadrants are possible, which gives the individual a unique sensory processing pattern. The score does not tell when a pattern is problematic for the individual in daily life, instead it shows how the person compares to a larger matched control group [39] and gives insight into personal behavior and responses to different environments [14]. Problems arise only when there is a conflict between the patient's will or

Table 2 Significance of differences between patients and controls

	p-value
Low registration, Q 1	0.029
Sensory seeking, Q 2	0.956
Sensory sensitivity, Q 3	0.206
Sensory avoiding, Q 4	0.268

Level of significance = p-value ≤0.05

Table 3 Percentage distribution of scoring in the Low Registration Quadrant

	Patient group	95% CI	Control group
Atypically High	40%	32–48	16%
Definitely High	13%	8–19	2.5%
Atypically Low	8%	4–14	16%
Definitely Low	0%	0–4	2.5%

Percentage distribution of scoring Atypically High/Low (± 1 SD compared with the control group mean) and Definitely High/Low in Q1-Low Registration Quadrant (± 2 SD compared with the control group mean)

wishes and the current performance [39], meaning that there are no definitive cut-off scores when the profile is problematic. We have not investigated the relationship between divergent sensory processing pattern and quality of life. This, on the other hand, has been investigated in a very recent study on patients with multiple sclerosis where a significant correlation was found between high scores in Low Registration Quadrant and reduced quality of life [40]. In addition, Kinnealy [41] also demonstrated a correlation between Low Registration Quadrant and reduced quality of life including all four areas encompassing emotional health in Short Form-36 Health Survey.

Sensory relearning is a vital part of the rehabilitation following peripheral nerve repair and it is the training technique used to prepare and "teach" the somatosensory cortex to interpret the new afferent signaling at touch [1].This training is a process of stimulating the brain through the use of cognitive learning techniques. Sensory relearning is designed to stimulate sensory areas in order to improve the cortical processing of the changed afferent input [35] and starts immediately after the nerve repair [1]. Sensory relearning uses the plastic capacity of the brain for therapeutic purpose, i.e. guided plasticity [42] and also the cross-modal capacity of the

brain [13]. By using different techniques for guided plasticity, such as motor or sensory observation [43, 44] and motor or sensory imagery exercises [45, 46], activation of the somatosensory cortex is achieved. These techniques are used in rehabilitation during the sensory deprivation after the nerve injury to stimulate the somatosensory cortex in in the initial phase after the nerve transection, before the axons have reinnervated their targets in the hand. Furthermore, to replace one sensory modality with another, cross-modal plasticity, is a concept that in previous studies has been proved beneficial for sensory re-learning after peripheral nerve injuries [9, 36, 47–50].

The results from the current study may support that cross-modal rehabilitation techniques, with multiple simultaneous sensory stimulus, would be beneficial in sensory relearning since it is suggested for people scoring atypically high in the Low Registration Quadrant, to increase the intensity of stimuli [39]. The literature about sensory profile also advocates for such "low registrators" to vary the kind of stimulus and to slow down the pace of presentation of stimuli, with purpose to let the patient get enough time to detect and process the information.

In addition, knowledge about sensory profile can help to individualize components in the rehab design such as the amount and frequency of training sessions and visits to the hospital. The individual patient can then practice, understand and exercise at his/her own pace. This is in line with what was reported in a qualitative report of patients' experiences of early sensory relearning where it was found that there is a great variation in the need of guidance in the specific training –sensory relearning – following a nerve injury [37]. An advantage for people who score high in the Low Registration Quadrant in the Sensory Profile questionnaire is that they find it easier to focus on tasks that they find interesting, even in distracting environments [39]. Ideally this

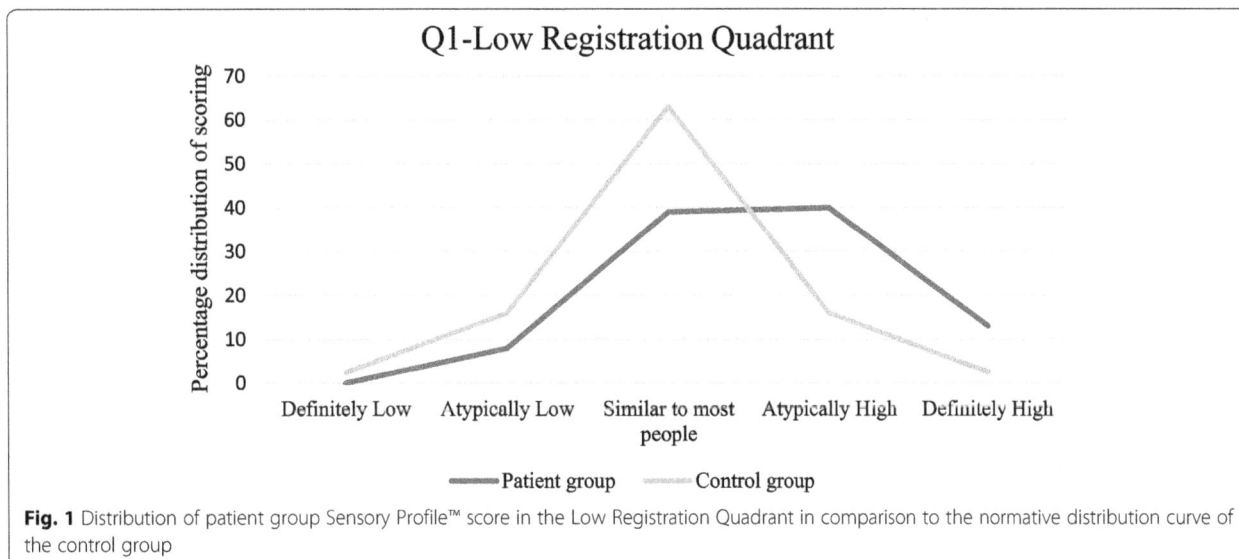

Fig. 1 Distribution of patient group Sensory Profile™ score in the Low Registration Quadrant in comparison to the normative distribution curve of the control group

should be used in sensory relearning however, the challenge is to make the relearning interesting and meaningful for the patient.

There are limitations in this study. The number of individuals is limited, but a strength is that we had access to a large control group where every patient could be matched to four to six individual controls. A confounding factor in this study is the possibility of influencing neuropsychological factors that are not investigated here, but which contribute to the result in the Sensory Profile. The AASP questionnaire was developed for use in neuropsychiatric disorders. However, several studies including patients with more somatic disorders such as atopic dermatitis, stroke and multiple sclerosis [19, 22, 40] have revealed interesting findings in sensory processing when using the AASP. Our findings can also guide the rehabilitation strategies. This exploratory study also gives us an idea of the deviation and atypical sensory processing patterns that exist in patients with median/ulnar nerve transection.

Surprisingly, neither age nor time since injury influenced the sensory processing patterns. An addition of direct measures of the patient's sensory function [51] maybe had gained knowledge of if there is a relationship between abnormal sensory processing patterns and sensory outcome following peripheral nerve injury.

Previous research on patients with severe peripheral nerve injuries [37] showed that a majority of patients expressed a need for strong support from the therapist. Furthermore, at least 14% of the patients expressed a need for creating routines for their sensory relearning program. The present study show that the patients with severe peripheral nerve injuries have an atypically sensory processing pattern. Proposed interventions for these individuals with atypical high scoring in the Low Registration Quadrant [39] e.g. intense, ideally multisensory, stimuli and to give the person enough time to perceive the stimuli. Multisensory stimulations in sensory re-learning have also been suggested previously [52] and that is also in line with our results here. In order to meet the needs found in this study, an example of a multisensory technique that can be used more in client centered rehabilitation is in a familiar self-chosen meal situation. In the meal situation the patient should be encouraged to use all senses. For example, when handling an orange, "sense not only the texture and shape but also the scent, color and taste". In such an everyday situation the amount of sensory input is increased, which may be useful in rehabilitation for these "low registrators".

Among proposed interventions for patients scoring high in Low Registration Quadrant [39] are also repeated oral and written information, as well as individually structured time and environments with varying and contrasting stimulus.

Future studies should focus on the development of multisensory rehabilitation applications with enhanced opportunity for repeated information, a motivational client centered approach in training and variation of the intensity and complexity of stimuli/objects in sensory relearning.

Conclusion

We have here showed that a peripheral nerve injury causes altered sensory processing pattern with an increased proportion of patients with low registration to sensory stimulus overall, and the results can guide us into more client centered rehabilitation strategies.

Abbreviations
AASP: Adolescent/Adult Sensory Profile; ADL: Activities of Daily Life

Funding
This work was supported by grants from the County Council of Skåne; and the Healthcare Academy at Skåne University Hospital.

Authors' contributions
PV made substantial contributions to conception and design, collected the data, analyzed and interpreted the data and was a major contributor in writing the manuscript. AB contributed to the design, manuscript and critically reviewed important content on neuroscience. IC contributed to the concept and design, interpretation of the data and contributed to the manuscript. A-KO contributed with her collected data of the normal population, supervision and expertise regarding sensory profile and contributed to the manuscript. BR made substantial contributions to conception and design, analyzed and interpreted the data and was a contributor in writing the manuscript. All authors read and approved the final manuscript.

Competing interests
The authors declare that they have no competing interests.

Author details
[1]Department of Translational Medicine – Hand Surgery, Skåne University Hospital and Lund University, Jan Waldenströms gata 5, SE-205 03 Malmö, Sweden. [2]Department of Psychiatry, NU Health Care, Trollhättan and Department of Psychology, Karlstad University, Karlstad, Sweden.

References
1. Lundborg G, Rosen B. Hand function after nerve repair. Acta Physiol (Oxf). 2007;189(2):207–17.
2. Jaquet JB, Luijsterburg AJ, Kalmijn S, Kuypers PD, Hofman A, Hovius SE. Median, ulnar, and combined median-ulnar nerve injuries: functional outcome and return to productivity. J Trauma. 2001;51(4):687–92.
3. Novak CB, Anastakis DJ, Beaton DE, Katz J. Patient-reported outcome after peripheral nerve injury. J Hand Surg Am. 2009;34(2):281–7.
4. Chemnitz A, Dahlin LB, Carlsson IK. Consequences and adaptation in daily life -- patients' experiences three decades after a nerve injury sustained in adolescence. BMC Musculoskelet Disord. 2013;14(1):252.
5. Bailey R, Kaskutas V, Fox I, Baum CM, Mackinnon SE. Effect of upper extremity nerve damage on activity participation, pain, depression, and quality of life. J Hand Surg Am. 2009;34(9):1682–8.
6. Jaquet JB, Kalmijn S, Kuypers PD, Hofman A, Passchier J, Hovius SE. Early psychological stress after forearm nerve injuries: a predictor for long-term functional outcome and return to productivity. Ann Plast Surg. 2002;49(1): 82–90.
7. Ultee J, Hundepool CA, Nijhuis TH, van Baar AL, Hovius SE. Early posttraumatic psychological stress following peripheral nerve injury: a prospective study. J Plast Reconstr Aesthet Surg. 2013;66(10):1316–21.
8. Stonner MM, Mackinnon SE, Kaskutas V. Predictors of disability and quality of life with an upper-extremity peripheral nerve disorder. Am J Occup Ther. 2017;71(1):7101190050p1–8.

9. Vikström P, Rosén B, Carlsson I, Björkman A. The effect of early relearning on sensory recovery 4 to 9 years after nerve repair: a report of a randomized controlled study. J Hand Surg Eur Vol. 2018;0(0):1–5.

10. Lundborg G. Nerve injury and repair-regeneration, reconstruction and cortical remodeling. 2nd ed. Philadelphia: Churchill Livingstone; 2004.

11. Goldstein EB, Brockmole JR. Sensation & Perception. 10th edition ed. In: Boston Cengage learning; 2017.

12. Pascual-Leone A, Hamilton R. Chapter 27 the metamodal organization of the brain. Prog Brain Res. 2001;134:427–45.

13. Merabet LB, Pascual-Leone A. Neural reorganization following sensory loss: the opportunity of change. Nat Rev Neurosci. 2010;11(1):44–52.

14. Brown C, Filion D, Tollefson N, Dunn W, Cromwell R. The adult sensory profile: measuring patterns of sensory processing. Am J Occup Ther. 2001; 55(1):75–82.

15. Dunn W. The sensory profile. San Antonio: Psychological Corporation; 1999.

16. Dunn W. The sensations of everyday life: empirical, theoretical, and pragmatic considerations. Am J Occup Ther. 2001;55(6):608–20.

17. Dunn W. The impact of sensory processing abilities on the daily lives of young children and their families: a conceptual model. Infants Young Child. 1997;9(4):23–35.

18. Engel-Yeger B, Habib-Mazawi S, Parush S, Rozenman D, Kessel A, Shani-Adir A. The sensory profile of children with atopic dermatitis as determined by the sensory profile questionnaire. J Am Acad Dermatol. 2007;57(4):610–5.

19. Engel-Yeger B, Mimouni D, Rozenman D, Shani-Adir A. Sensory processing patterns of adults with atopic dermatitis. J Eur Acad Dermatol. 2011;25(2): 152–6.

20. Demopoulos C, Arroyo MS, Dunn W, Strominger Z, Sherr EH, Marco E. Individuals with agenesis of the Corpus callosum show sensory processing differences as measured by the sensory profile. Neuropsychology. 2015; 29(5):751–8.

21. Engel-Yeger B, Almog M, Kessel A. The sensory profile of children with asthma. Acta Paediatr. 2014;103(11):e490–e4.

22. Chung SM, Song BK. Evaluation of sensory processing abilities following stroke using the adolescent/adult sensory profile: implications for individualized intervention. J Phys Ther Sci. 2016;28(10):2852–6.

23. Taylor KS, Anastakis DJ, Davis KD. Cutting your nerve changes your brain. Brain. 2009;132:3122–33.

24. Chemnitz A, Weibull A, Rosen B, Andersson G, Dahlin LB, Bjorkman A. Normalized activation in the somatosensory cortex 30years following nerve repair in children: an fMRI study. Eur J Neurosci. 2015;42(4):2022–7.

25. Liss AG, afEkenstam FW, Wiberg M. Loss of neurons in the dorsal root ganglia after transection of a peripheral sensory nerve - an anatomical study in monkeys. Scand J Plast Reconstr Surg Hand Surg. 1996;30(1):1–6.

26. Witzel C, Rohde C, Brushart TM. Pathway sampling by regenerating peripheral axons. J Comp Neurol. 2005;485(3):183–90.

27. Silva AC, Rasey SK, Wu X, Wall JT. Initial cortical reactions to injury of the median and radial nerves to the hands of adult primates. J Comp Neurol. 1996;366(4):700–16.

28. Kandel ER, Schwartz JH, Jessell TM, Siegelbaum SA, Hudspeth AJ. Principles of neural science. 5th ed. New York: McGraw-Hill; 2013.

29. Dahlin LB, Wiberg M. Nerve injuries of the upper extremity and hand. EFORT Open Rev. 2017;2(5):158–70.

30. Purves D, Cabeza R, Huettel S, LaBar K, Platt M, Waldorff M. Principles of cognitive neuroscience. 2nd ed. Sunderland: Sinauer Associates Inc; 2013.

31. Rosen B. Recovery of sensory and motor function after nerve repair. A rationale for evaluation. J Hand Ther. 1996;9(4):315–27.

32. Chemnitz A, Bjorkman A, Dahlin LB, Rosen B. Functional outcome thirty years after median and ulnar nerve repair in childhood and adolescence. J Bone Joint Surg Am. 2013;95(4):329–37.

33. Rosen B, Lundborg G. The long term recovery curve in adults after median or ulnar nerve repair: a reference interval. J Hand Surg Br. 2001;26(3):196–200.

34. Vordemvenne T, Langer M, Ochman S, Raschke M, Schult M. Long-term results after primary microsurgical repair of ulnar and median nerve injuries. A comparison of common score systems. Clin Neurol Neurosurg. 2007; 109(3):263–71.

35. Miller LK, Chester R, Jerosch-Herold C. Effects of sensory reeducation programs on functional hand sensibility after median and ulnar repair: a systematic review. J Hand Ther. 2012;25(3):297–307.

36. Rosen B, Vikstrom P, Turner S, McGrouther DA, Selles RW, Schreuders TA, et al. Enhanced early sensory outcome after nerve repair as a result of immediate post-operative re-learning: a randomized controlled trial. J Hand Surg Eur Vol. 2015;40(6):598–606.

37. Vikström P, Carlsson I, Rosén B, Björkman A. Scientific/clinical article: Patients' views on early sensory relearning following nerve repair—a Q-methodology study. J hand Ther. 2017. Published online. https://doi.org/10.1016/j.jht.2017.07.003.

38. Brown CE, Dunn W. Adolecent/adult sensory profile Manualsupplement, Swedish version. Sweden: Pearson AB; 2014.

39. Brown CE, Dunn W. Adolecent/adult sensory profile User's manual. Bloomington: Pearson; 2002.

40. Colbeck M. Sensory processing, cognitive fatigue, and quality of life in multiple sclerosis: Traitement de l'information sensorielle, fatigue cognitive et qualite de vie des personnes atteintes de sclerose en plaques. Can J Occup Ther. 2018;85(2):169–75.

41. Kinnealey M, Koenig KP, Smith S. Relationships between sensory modulation and social supports and health-related quality of life. Am J Occup Ther. 2011;65(3):320–7.

42. Duffau H. Brain plasticity: from pathophysiological mechanisms to therapeutic applications. J Clin Neurosci. 2006;13(9):885–97.

43. Pihko E, Nangini C, Jousmaki V, Hari R. Observing touch activates human primary somatosensory cortex. Eur J Neurosci. 2010;31(10):1836–43.

44. Bassolino M, Campanella M, Bove M, Pozzo T, Fadiga L. Training the motor cortex by observing the actions of others during immobilization. Cereb Cortex. 2014;24(12):3268–76.

45. Ehrsson HH, Geyer S, Naito E. Imagery of voluntary movement of fingers, toes, and tongue activates corresponding body-part-specific motor representations. J Neurophysiol. 2003;90(5):3304–16.

46. Yoo SC, Freeman DK, McCarthy JJ, Jolesz FA. Neural substrates of tactile imagery: a functional MRI study. Neuroreport. 2003;14(4):581–5.

47. Rosen B, Lundborg G. Enhanced sensory recovery after median nerve repair using cortical audio-tactile interaction. A randomised multicentre study. J Hand Surg Eur Vol. 2007;32(1):31–7.

48. Lanzetta M, Perani D, Anchisi D, Rosen B, Danna M, Scifo P, et al. Early use of artificial sensibility in hand transplantation. Scand J Plast Reconstr Surg Hand Surg. 2004;38(2):106–11.

49. Svens B, Rosén B. Early sensory re-learning after nerve repair using mirror-training and sense-substitution - a case report. Hand Ther. 2009;14:75–82.

50. Lundborg G, Björkman A, Hansson T, Nylander L, Nyman T, Rosén B. Artificial sensibility of the hand based on cortical audiotactile interaction: a study using functional magnetic resonance imaging. Scand J Plast Reconstr Surg Hand Surg. 2005;39(6):370–2.

51. Rosén B, Lundborg G. A model instrument for the documentation of outcome after nerve repair. J Hand Surg Am. 2000;25(3):535–43.

52. Rosén B, Lundborg G. Sensory reeducation. In: Skirven O, Fedorczyk A, editors. Rehabilitation of the hand and upper extremity. 1. 6 ed. Philadelphia: Mosby Inc; 2011.

20

Long-term, telephone-based follow-up after stroke and TIA improves risk factors: 36-month results from the randomized controlled NAILED stroke risk factor trial

Joachim Ögren[1]*[iD], Anna-Lotta Irewall[1], Lars Söderström[2] and Thomas Mooe[1]

Abstract

Background: Strategies are needed to improve adherence to the blood pressure (BP) and low-density lipoprotein cholesterol (LDL-C) level recommendations after stroke and transient ischemic attack (TIA). We investigated whether nurse-led, telephone-based follow-up that included medication titration was more efficient than usual care in improving BP and LDL-C levels 36 months after discharge following stroke or TIA.

Methods: All patients admitted for stroke or TIA at Östersund hospital that could participate in the telephone-based follow-up were considered eligible. Participants were randomized to either nurse-led, telephone-based follow-up (intervention) or usual care (control). BP and LDL-C were measured one month after discharge and yearly thereafter. Intervention group patients who did not meet the target values received additional follow-up, including lifestyle counselling and medication titration, to reach their treatment goals (BP < 140/90 mmHg, LDL-C < 2.5 mmol/L). The primary outcome was the systolic BP level 36 months after discharge.

Results: Out of 871 randomized patients, 660 completed the 36-month follow-up. The mean systolic and diastolic BP values in the intervention group were 128.1 mmHg (95% CI 125.8–130.5) and 75.3 mmHg (95% CI 73.8–76.9), respectively. This was 6.1 mmHg (95% CI 3.6–8.6, $p < 0.001$) and 3.4 mmHg (95% CI 1.8–5.1, $p < 0.001$) lower than in the control group. The mean LDL-C level was 2.2 mmol/L in the intervention group, which was 0.3 mmol/L (95% CI 0.2–0.5, $p < 0.001$) lower than in controls. A larger proportion of the intervention group reached the treatment goal for BP (systolic: 79.4% vs. 55.3%, $p < 0.001$; diastolic: 90.3% vs. 77.9%, $p < 0.001$) as well as for LDL-C (69.3% vs. 48.9%, $p < 0.001$).

Conclusions: Compared with usual care, a nurse-led telephone-based intervention that included medication titration after stroke or TIA improved BP and LDL-C levels and increased the proportion of patients that reached the treatment target 36 months after discharge.

Keywords: Stroke, TIA, Secondary prevention, Modifiable risk factors, Blood pressure, Cholesterol, Randomized controlled study, Telemedicine, Nurses

* Correspondence: joachim.ogren@regionjh.se
[1]Department of Public Health and Clinical Medicine, Umeå University, Östersund, Sweden
Full list of author information is available at the end of the article

Background

Stroke is a major cause of mortality and morbidity worldwide. Today, more patients than ever survive strokes, thereby increasing the prevalence of stroke survivors [1]. These patients have an increased risk of new vascular events [2–4], but this risk can be reduced by hypertension treatment as well as by statin treatment [5, 6]. Current guidelines therefore recommend both [7, 8].

Notably, observational studies show that after stroke, only 25 to 49% of all patients reach treatment targets for blood pressure (BP) and only 14 to 77% reach treatment targets for low-density lipoprotein cholesterol (LDL-C) [9–13]. Strategies to improve patient control of modifiable risk factors have been tested in randomized controlled trials (RCTs) with heterogeneous results [13–18]. Considering the high prevalence of stroke survivors and the limited available resources for public health care, involving health care professionals other than physicians as well as telemedicine-based strategies might offer alternative cost-effective solutions to improve secondary prevention.

The RCTs of risk factor interventions delivered mainly by nurses or pharmacists have a variety of designs and have shown variable results [13, 14, 17, 19]. Most programs that improve risk factor control after stroke or transient ischemic attack (TIA) include medical treatments that can be adjusted by a physician or by a nurse or pharmacist [15, 17, 20, 21]. In a recent systematic review of telemedicine strategies in patients after a stroke or TIA, a meta-analysis including four studies showed significant improvements in BP [22] using telemedicine compared to usual care. The studies were heterogeneous in terms of their methods and results, and the components, duration, and intensity of the follow-up programs also varied in the studies. However, in two of the four studies, the intervention program included follow-up and adjustment of medical treatment.

The nurse-based age independent intervention to limit evolution of disease after stroke or TIA (NAILED) trial combined a nurse-based, telemedicine strategy with systematic review of medical treatment, including titration of medicine. This approach decreased BP and LDL-C compared significantly better than in a control group at 12 months [20]. However, the secondary preventive perspective is generally considerably longer in terms of treatment duration, and there is currently insufficient knowledge of how to perform cost-effective follow-up to ensure long-term adherence to risk factor treatment goals. Currently, the only available study with an intervention that continued beyond 12 months after stroke or TIA did not show significant improvements in BP or LDL-C [23], but it did not use medication titration

Objectives

The primary aim of the present study was to investigate whether the NAILED trial intervention improved BP values and LDL-C levels 36 months after stroke or TIA compared to usual care. The secondary aim was to evaluate whether a larger proportion of the intervention group reached set treatment targets. Finally, we aimed to investigate whether there were any trends in the effects of the intervention during the study period. An abstract of the current study has been previously published [24].

Methods

Trial design

The NAILED stroke risk factor trial was a population-based RCT with two parallel groups and an allocation ratio of 1:1. The design of the study was described previously in the published study protocol [25] and has been used and described in the published analysis of the 12 months follow-up of the NAILED-stroke trial [20]. It is described briefly below.

Participants

All patients treated with an intracerebral hematoma (ICH), ischemic stroke (IS) or TIA at Östersund hospital, the only hospital in the county of Jämtland Sweden between January 1, 2010 and December 31, 2013 were considered for participation in the study. To be considered eligible the participants also had to be able to participate in a telephone-based follow-up and sign an informed, written consent. Patients with aphasia, impaired hearing, cognitive impairment, or severe, often terminal disease, were excluded..

Randomization and blinding

Eligible patients were randomly assigned to the intervention group or the control group. The randomized allocation sequence was computer-generated in blocks of four and stratified for sex and for degree of disability (modified Rankin Scale < 3 or ≥ 3). The resulting group allocation was not blinded to participants, the study team, or other caregivers.

Data collection and follow-up

Measurments of BP and blood lipids were performed at the patients' closest healthcare facility at 1, 12, 24, and 36 months post-discharge. A study nurse then interviewed participants in both the intervention and control groups about their compliance with recommended treatment, sense of well-being, use of tobacco, and physical activity level. The information was collected systematically according to the variables in the study protocol. To perform the follow-up a nurse working 0.5–0.75 of a full time was required. The study nurse was experienced in stroke care and had participated in courses in motivational interviewing (MI) and good clinical practice (GCP).

Intervention

The intervention group received telephone-based counselling and an assessment of their pharmacological treatment [25]. A study physician was consulted to assess and adjust the medical treatment when the participants did not achieve the set target for LDL-C and/or BP. There were no pre-specified algorithm to the pharmacological adjustments; rather, individualized for each participant. The process was repeated after approximately 4 weeks, when necessary (see flow chart in Fig. 1). Lipid-lowering therapy was restricted to patients with ischemic events.

In the control group, treatment was generally initiated in-hospital and after discharge they received secondary preventive care according to local standards, most often by each patient's general practitioner.

Outcomes

Outcome variables were measured at 1, 12, 24 and 36 moths and included sitting systolic blood pressure (SBP) and diastolic blood pressure (DBP), LDL-C, and the proportion of patients reaching set targets for these variables. Sitting SBP at 36 months was analyzed as the primary outcome, and the other variables were analyzed as secondary outcomes. SBP < 140 mmHg, DBP < 90 mmHg, and an LDL-C value < 2.5 mmol/L (or < 1.8 mmol/L in patients with diabetes) were considered to be within the target range according to local guidelines at the time of the assessments.

BP was measured once in the seated position after 5 min of rest. LDL-C values were calculated using the Friedewald formula. Cause of death data were obtained from the national cause of death register.

Sample size

To reliably detect a difference of 5 mmHg between the groups for the mean SBP, we needed study groups of 180 participants (standard deviation 19, mean SBP 140 versus 135, alpha 0.05 two-tailed, power 80%). Study groups of at least 200 participants were planned to allow for drop-outs. This sample size was also adequate for detection of a group difference of 0.3 mmol/L in LDL values.

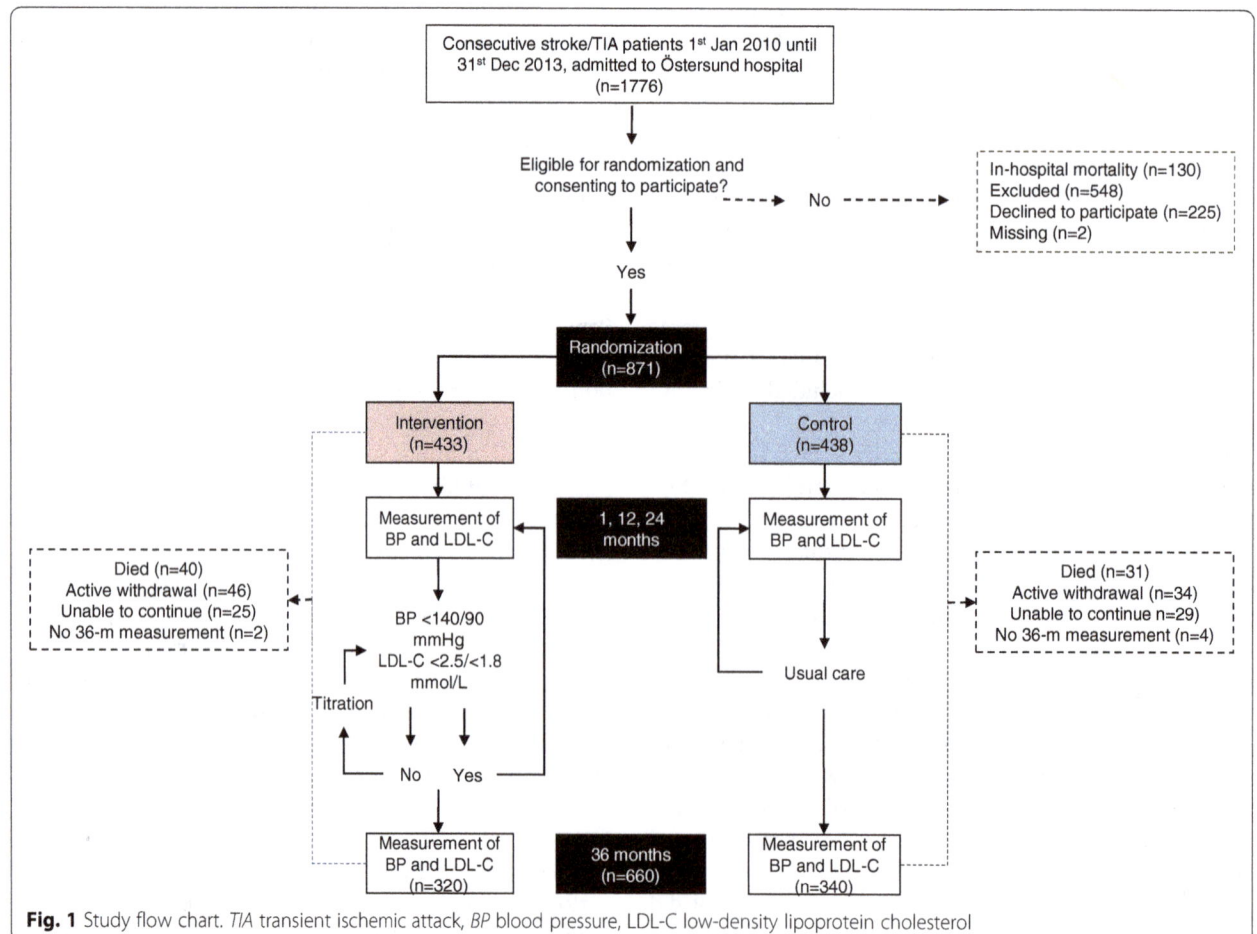

Fig. 1 Study flow chart. *TIA* transient ischemic attack, *BP* blood pressure, LDL-C low-density lipoprotein cholesterol

Statistical methods

The analyses were performed according to the intention to treat principle. Baseline characteristics comparisons between groups were performed using an independent sample t-test or a chi-square test as appropriate.

We calculated the adjusted mean differences between groups (intervention vs. control) in BP and LDL-C levels at 36 months using a general linear model adjusted for sex and degree of disability in order to reflect the stratified randomization. We used paired sample t-tests to evaluate changes in mean BP and LDL-C values between 1 and 36 months within a single group.

All analyses were performed using SPSS software, version 24.0, and we defined the significance threshold at the level of $p = 0.05$.

Trial registration

The NAILED stroke risk factor trial is registered in the ISRCTN registry (ISRCTN23868518). The ICMJE strict requirement of prospective registration of clinical trials came to our attention when the recruitment had already begun. The study was therefore retrospectively registered on June 19, 2012. The authors confirm that all ongoing and related trials for this intervention are now registered.

Results

Out of the 871 randomized patients, 660 participants completed the 36-month follow-up and were included in the analysis (mean age: 69.6 years, 40.8% women, 58.6% with IS, 3.5% with ICH, and 37.9% with TIA). Figure 1 shows the flow chart of the participants. The baseline characteristics of the participants that are included in the final analysis were well balanced, except for diabetes, which was more common in the control group. Table 1 shows the baseline data of the participants in the final analysis, and Additional file 1: Table S1 shows the baseline characteristics of all of the participants who were randomized in the study.

Of the 211 participants that did not complete the 36-month follow-up, 80 patients chose to discontinue follow-up, 54 were not able to continue due to severe disease, and 71 died. Six participants wanted to continue to participate in the study but were unable to complete the 36-month follow-up. The participants who did not complete the 36-month follow-up were older and had more co-morbidities. A total of 99 patients died between randomization and the 36-month follow-up; of these, 21 of 55 deaths in the intervention group and 17 of 44 deaths in the control group were classified as cardiovascular-related deaths. The intervention group and the control group did not differ significantly in terms of the proportions of cardiovascular or all-cause mortality ($p = 0.51$ and $p = 0.24$).

SBP at the 36-month follow-up

At 36 months, the mean adjusted SBP was 128.1 mmHg (95% CI 125.8–130.5) in the intervention group and 134.2 mmHg (95% CI 131.8–136.6) in the control group, with a difference of 6.1 mmHg (95% CI 3.6–8.6, $p < 0.001$) between the groups. The decreases in BP compared to the 1 month measurements were 8.1 mmHg (95% CI 5.8–10.3) and 2.3 mmHg (95% CI 0.1–4.4) in the intervention and control groups, respectively.

DBP at the 36-month follow-up

The mean adjusted DBP values in the intervention and control groups were 75.3 mmHg (95% CI 73.8–76.9) and 78.8 mmHg (95% CI 77.2–80.3), respectively, with a difference of 3.4 mmHg (95% CI 1.8–5.1, $p < 0.001$) between the groups. The mean DBP decreased between 1 and 36 months by 4.4 mmHg (95% CI 2.9–5.8) and 0.2 mmHg (95% CI -1.0–1.5), respectively.

LDL-C at the 36-month follow-up

The mean adjusted LDL-C values in the intervention and control groups were 2.2 mmol/L (95% CI 2.1–2.4, 86.5 mg/dL) and 2.5 mmol/L (95% CI 2.4–2.7, 98.1 mg/dL), respectively, a mean difference of 0.3 mmol/L (95% CI 0.2–0.5, $p < 0.001$). The decrease in the intervention group was 0.2 mmol/L (95% CI 0.1–0.3), while there was a significant increase of 0.1 mmol/L (95% CI 0.0–0.2) in the control group.

Proportion of patients reaching the treatment targets

At 36 months, 79.4% and 55.3% of participants reached the treatment target for SBP in the intervention and control groups, respectively ($p < 0.001$). The corresponding proportion were 90.3% vs. 77.9% ($p < 0.001$) for DBP and 69.3% vs. 48.9% ($p < 0.001$) for LDL-C. Figure 2 shows the results for 36 months as well as for 1, 12, and 24 months before and after titration of medication.

Trends over time

At 1 month, 71.9% and 73.2% ($p = 0.727$) of the participants in the intervention and the control groups, respectively, had at least one LDL-C, SBP, or DBP measurement that did not reach the treatment target. At 36 months, the corresponding percentages were 44.1% and 72.9% ($p < 0.001$). Only 5.9% and 4.7% ($p = 0.493$) of the participants were below the treatment target values at all measurements during the study period (Fig. 3). The difference in the mean SBP and DBP values between the two groups increased during the study period, while the difference at 12 months remained unchanged at 36 months for LDL-C (Fig. 2).

Table 1 Baseline characteristics of the study participants

	Intervention group (n = 320)	Control group (n = 340)	P value
Mean age, years	69.9	69.3	ns
Women no. (%)	130 (40.6)	139 (40.9)	ns
Qualifying event no. (%)			
Ischemic stroke	181 (56.6)	206 (60.6)	ns
Intracerebral hematoma	11 (3.4)	12 (3.5)	ns
TIA	128 (40.0)	122 (35.9)	ns
mRS 3–5 no. (%)	37 (11.6)	31 (9.1)	ns
Medical history no. (%)			
Stroke	41 (12.9)	37 (10.9)	ns
Myocardial infarction	22 (6.9)	30 (8.8)	ns
Heart failure	8 (2.5)	9 (2.6)	ns
Atrial fibrillation	47 (15.2)	52 (15.4)	ns
Diabetes	45 (14.1)	68 (20.1)	0.049
Smoker no. (%)	42 (13.1)	48 (14.1)	ns
Medications at 1 month no. (%)			
Antihypertensive drug	231 (72.2)	264 (77.6)	ns
Statin	253 (79.8)	276 (81.7)	ns
Antiplatelet drug	253 (79.1)	276 (81.2)	ns
Anticoagulant drug	48 (15.1)	45 (13.3)	ns
Baseline values ± SD			
SBP (mmHg)	136.9 ± 16.7	137.2 ± 18.5	ns
DBP (mmHg)	80.8 ± 11.6	80.2 ± 10.4	ns
LDL-C (mmol/L)	2.5 ± 0.8	2.4 ± 0.8	ns

mRS modified Rankin scale, *TIA* transient ischemic attack, *SBP* systoilc blood pressure, *DBP* diastolic blood pressure, *LDL-C* low-density lipoprotein cholesterol

Discussion

The present study analyzed 660 participants at the end of 36-month follow-up. The results showed that nurse-led, telephone-based, secondary preventive follow-up that included medication titration improved SBP, DBP, and LDL-C 36 months after a stroke or TIA compared to the usual-care control group. Furthermore, a significantly larger proportion of participants in the intervention group reached the treatment targets for SBP and DBP as well as for LDL-C. The BP levels and the proportion of participants who reached the BP targets improved each year in the intervention group, but the proportion remained almost unchanged in the control group.

The final SBP and DBP levels were 6.1 mmHg and 3.4 mmHg lower in the intervention group than in the control group. These differences were comparable to the reductions seen in RCTs of antihypertensive treatment after stroke or TIA, which showed a 22 to 34% relative risk reduction of recurrent stroke [5, 26]. The LDL-C was reduced by 0.3 mmol/L in the intervention group, less than in the Stroke Prevention by Aggressive Reduction in Cholesterol Levels (SPARCL) study [6]. The clinical relevance of this reduction is uncertain.

Previous studies of interventions that aimed to improve the control of modifiable risk factors in the secondary prevention of stroke and TIA have had different designs and variable results [14–19, 21]. This makes it hard to distinguish which factors are responsible for observed benefits. A Cochrane meta-analysis from 2014 found a non-significant decrease in SBP and a non-significant increase in the proportion of patients who reached the treatment target for BP [14], but it did not identify any trends towards improvement in the LDL-C levels or in the proportion of participants reaching LDL-C treatment targets. Some studies have shown promising results for the improvement of modifiable risk factors after stroke or TIA and also in patients at risk of other cardiovascular diseases. These studies [15, 17, 19, 21, 27], as well as the present trial, all involved adjustment of pharmacological treatment by a nurse, a pharmacist, or a physician.

At discharge, 73% to 78% of the participants were on antihypertensive medication, and 80% were being treated with statins (Table 1). These proportions are comparable with the treatment data found in Riksstroke, the Swedish national stroke register [28]. Despite the high proportion

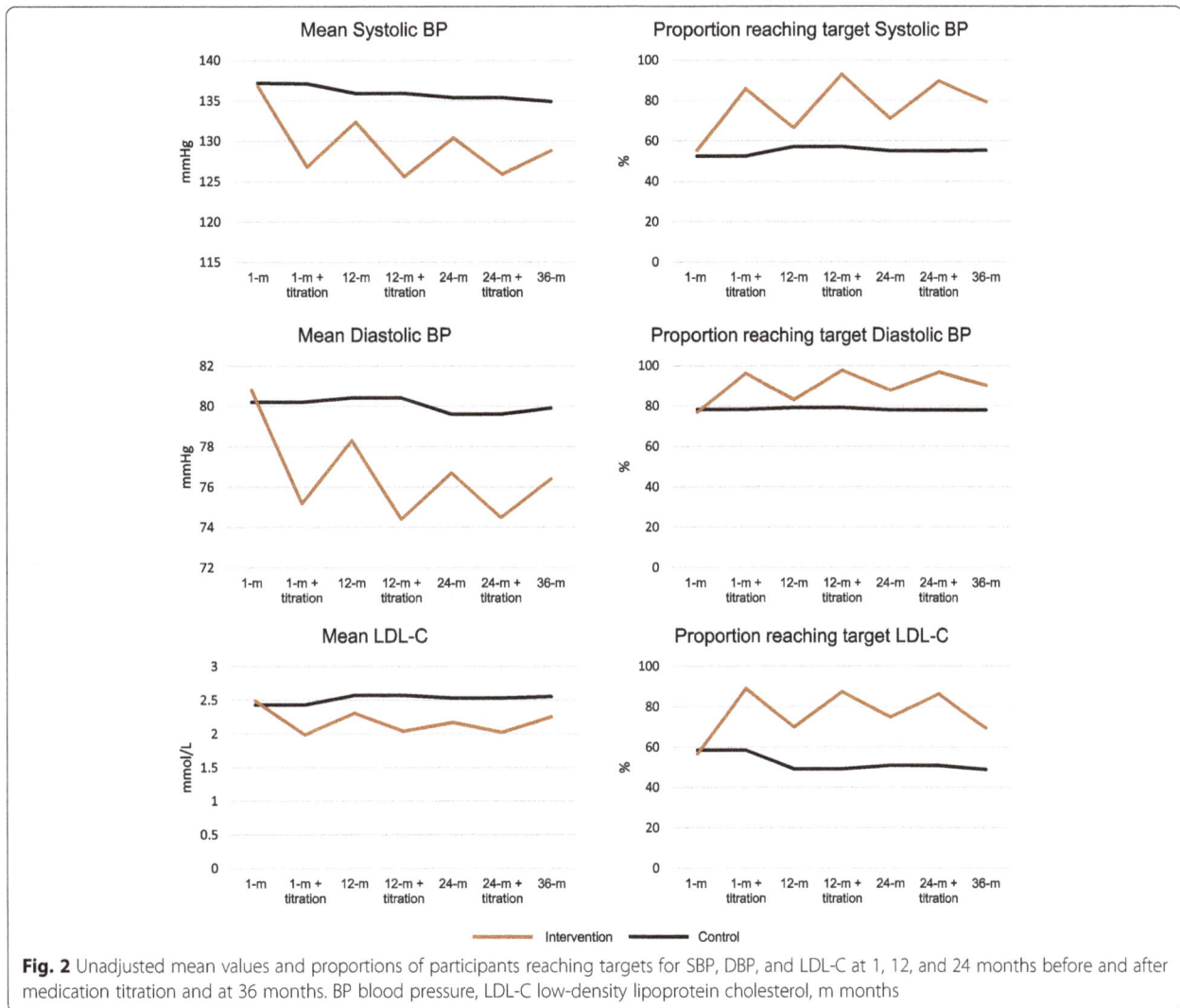

Fig. 2 Unadjusted mean values and proportions of participants reaching targets for SBP, DBP, and LDL-C at 1, 12, and 24 months before and after medication titration and at 36 months. BP blood pressure, LDL-C low-density lipoprotein cholesterol, m months

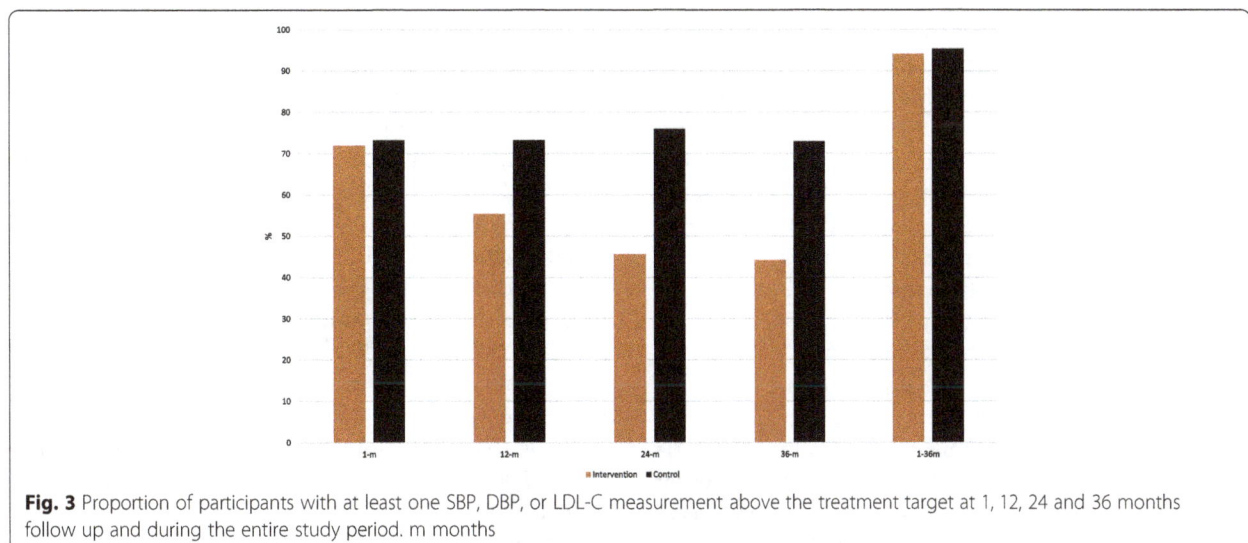

Fig. 3 Proportion of participants with at least one SBP, DBP, or LDL-C measurement above the treatment target at 1, 12, 24 and 36 months follow up and during the entire study period. m months

of treated participants, only about half of the study participants reached the treatment target for SBP and LDL-C at the baseline assessment one month after discharge (Fig. 2). It is possible that the medication initiated during the hospital stay had not yet reached its full effect because there were plans to titrate it during follow-up or because the doses were inadequate.

During the follow-up of high-risk cardiovascular patients, failure to reach the treatment target should prompt a review of the medical treatment, an inquiry about adherence, and in most cases, reinforcement of medication to improve risk factor levels. In addition, the patient needs to be motivated and capable of following treatment recommendations to ensure adherence. In this study, the proportion of participants in the control group who reached treatment targets remained unchanged for BP and decreased for LDL-C over time, whereas the proportions increased in the intervention group. The lack of improvement was seen in the control group despite sending the follow-up measurements to each patient's general practitioner. Plus, as a consequence of study participation, there was probably a higher-than-usual awareness of cardiovascular risk factors among the control group participants. The interference of the study with normal clinical practice in the control group was unavoidable. However, it might have been expected to contribute to an underestimation of the effect of the NAILED intervention. In addition, the control group achieved less than the intervention group despite a fairly equal number of healthcare contacts and risk factor assessments, at least during the first year, according to previously published results from the NAILED stroke risk factor trial [20]. We cannot know for sure why these contacts resulted in improved risk factor levels in the intervention group, but it is likely that the NAILED trial intervention, with systematic medication titration, decreased the risk that the physician would not respond to a value above the treatment target (i.e. therapeutic inertia), a problem that has been described in the follow-up after stroke or TIA [29]. Moreover, contact with the study nurse gave participants the chance to discuss their treatment and possible side effects, and this may have increased the participants' adherence to medication. The combination of decreased therapeutic inertia and increased adherence might explain the positive results of the intervention.

Time trends and the duration of follow-up

Stroke survivors have a life-long increased risk of recurrent stroke [3]. The effect of antihypertensive or lipid-lowering treatment on new vascular events in RCTs remains during follow-up periods of at least 36 months [5, 6, 30]. However, only two studies on interventions to improve secondary prevention after stroke or TIA had follow-up of more than 12 months [23, 31], and only one implemented interventions after 12 months [23]. None of the studies showed any significant improvements in BP or LDL-C levels. In the present study, we found a clinically relevant effect of the intervention on BP levels at 36 months. Furthermore, we found that the difference in BP between the study groups increased continuously during follow-up (Fig. 2). During the study period, the proportion of participants with at least one SBP, DBP, or LDL-C measurement that did not reach the target was nearly 95% in both the intervention and control groups (Fig. 3). However, the proportion of participants that needed treatment adjustment decreased continuously in the intervention group but not in the control group. In the intervention group, the proportion of participants that needed adjustment markedly increased between the end of each titration and the next follow-up (Fig. 2), and at 36 months, more than 40% of the participants in the intervention group had at least one SBP, DBP, or LDL-C value above the treatment target. Furthermore, almost all of the participants who did not need any medication adjustments at 1 month had at least one value above the treatment target during the follow-up period. Thus, regardless of the initial risk factor levels, life-long follow-up, similar to the routines for diabetic patients, seems necessary for an acceptable level of secondary prevention after stroke or TIA.

Continuous improvement was not seen for LDL-C, and the underlying reasons for this are unclear. This may be attributable to side effects and decreasing adherence to statin treatment. Further analyses are planned to explore this finding.

Treatment target and endpoints

The present study focused on risk factor levels and on reaching treatment targets to decrease the risk of new vascular events [5, 6]. There are presently insufficient data about the optimal treatment target for BP after stroke or TIA, but guidelines recommend BP levels < 140/< 90 mmHg [7, 8]. Moreover, no trials have compared the use of different treatment targets for LDL-C after stroke or TIA. In this study, we chose BP levels < 140/< 90 mmHg and an LDL-C level < 2.5 mmol/L (< 1.8 in participants with diabetes) to be consistent with the treatment goals used in primary care during the study period, since the control group participants were treated in primary care.

At 36 months of follow-up, there were more deaths in the intervention group than in the control group ($n = 55$ vs. $n = 44$; $p = 0.24$). However, the present study was not designed and powered to investigate mortality or new vascular events. These analyses will be performed based on the entire follow-up period for the NAILED cohort.

Strengths and limitations

With 871 participants randomized and 660 in the final analysis, this study is one of the largest in the field. We used a population-based approach and a simple follow-up routine in order to include a large proportion of the targeted population. Furthermore, the baseline treatments corresponded well with national level data in the Riksstroke registry. This should give the study high external validity. However, 35.7% of the patients could not participate in the study due to physical or cognitive impairment [32]. Moreover, 211 out of the 871 randomized participants did not reach the 3-year follow-up. This could be considered a weakness of the study, but it also reflects the reality of the characteristics of this study population. Severe co-morbidities and a high mortality rate in this population unavoidably increase the proportion of patients who cannot participate or who discontinue participation during follow-up. This limits the potential for secondary prevention.

Conclusion

A nurse-led telephone-based intervention that included medication titration after stroke or TIA improved BP and LDL-C levels and increased the proportion of patients that reached treatment targets 36 months after discharge. The effect of the intervention on BP increased over time. If implemented, the NAILED strategy could improve BP and LDL-C levels in many stroke survivors.

Abbreviations

BP: Blood pressure; DBP: Diastolic blood pressure; ICH: Intracerebral hematoma; IS: Ischemic stroke; LDL-C: Low-density lipoprotein cholesterol; NAILED: Nurse based Age-independent Intervention to Limit Evolution of Disease after stroke or TIA; RCT: Randomized controlled trial; SBP: Systolic blood pressure; TIA: Transient ischemic attack

Acknowledgements
The authors would like to thank the study nurses for their indispensable contributions to the study.

Funding
The study received funding from the Research Development and Education Unit, Region Jämtland Härjedalen (grant numbers: JLL-376981, JLL-377161) and the Swedish Heart-Lung Foundation (grant number 20140541). The funders had no role in study design, data collection and analysis, decision to publish, or preparation of the manuscript.

Authors' contributions
TM conceived the general trial design with input from ALI, LS and JÖ. TM, ALI, and JÖ were consulted as study doctors during the trial. JÖ performed all analyses after discussions and statistical input from LS. JÖ led the writing of the manuscript with input from ALI, LS and TM. All authors approved the final version of the manuscript and agreed to be accountable for all aspects or the work.

Competing interests
The authors declare that they have no competing interests.

Author details
[1]Department of Public Health and Clinical Medicine, Umeå University, Östersund, Sweden. [2]Unit of Research, Development and Education, Östersund, Sweden.

References
1. Feigin VL, Forouzanfar MH, Krishnamurthi R, Mensah GA, Connor M, Bennett DA, Moran AE, Sacco RL, Anderson L, Truelsen T, et al. Global and regional burden of stroke during 1990-2010: findings from the global burden of disease study 2010. Lancet. 2014;383:245–55.
2. Feng WHR, Adams RJ. Risk of recurrent stroke, myocardial infarction, or death in hospitalized stroke patients. Neurology. 2010;74:588–93.
3. Mohan KMWC, Rudd AG, Heuschmann PU, Kolominsky-Rabas PL, Grieve AP. Risk and cumulative risk of stroke recurrence: a systematic review and meta-analysis. Stroke. 2011;42:1489–94.
4. Touzé EVO, Chatellier G, Peyrard S, Rothwell PM, Mas JL. Risk of myocardial infarction and vascular death after transient ischemic attack and ischemic stroke: a systematic review and meta-analysis. Stroke. 2005;36:2748–55.
5. Liu L, Wang Z, Gong L, Zhang Y, Thijs L, Staessen JA, et al. Blood pressure reduction for the secondary prevention of stroke: a chinese trial and a systematic review of the literature. Hypertens Res. 2009;32:1032–40.
6. Amarenco PBJ, Callahan A 3rd, Goldstein LB, Hennerici M, Rudolph AE, Sillesen H, Simunovic L, Szarek M, Welch KM, Zivin JA. Stroke prevention by aggressive reduction in cholesterol levels (SPARCL) investigators. High-dose atorvastatin after stroke or transient ischemic attack NEJM. 2006;355:549–59.
7. Kernan WN, Ovbiagele B, Black HR, Bravata DM, Chimowitz MI, Ezekowitz MD, Fang MC, Fisher M, Furie KL, Heck DV, et al. Guidelines for the prevention of stroke in patients with stroke and transient ischemic attack: a guideline for healthcare professionals from the american heart association/ american stroke association. Stroke. 2014;45:2160–236.
8. Piepoli MF, Hoes AW, Agewall S, Albus C, Brotons C, Catapano AL, Cooney MT, Corra U, Cosyns B, Deaton C, et al. 2016 european guidelines on cardiovascular disease prevention in clinical practice: the sixth joint task force of the european society of cardiology and other societies on cardiovascular disease prevention in clinical practice (constituted by representatives of 10 societies and by invited experts)developed with the special contribution of the european association for cardiovascular prevention & rehabilitation (eacpr). Eur Heart J. 2016;37:2315–81.
9. Amar JCJ, Touzé E, Bongard V, Jullien G, Vahanian A, Coppé G, Mas JL. ECLAT1 study investigators. Comparison of hypertension management after stroke and myocardial infarction: results from eclat1--a french nationwide study. Stroke. 2004;35:1579–83.
10. Brewer L, Mellon L, Hall P, Dolan E, Horgan F, Shelley E, Hickey A, Williams D. Secondary prevention after ischaemic stroke: the aspire-s study. BMC Neurol. 2015;15:216.
11. Heuschmann PUKJ, Nowe T, Dittrich R, Reiner Z, Cifkova R, Malojcic B, Mayer O, Bruthans J, Wloch-Kopec D, Prugger C, et al. Control of main risk factors after ischaemic stroke across europe: data from the stroke-specific module of the EUROASPIRE III survey. Eur J Prev Cardiol. 2015;22:1354–62.
12. Alvarez-Sabin JQM, Hernandez-Presa MA, Alvarez C, Chaves J, Ribo M. Therapeutic interventions and success in risk factor control for secondary prevention of stroke. J Stroke Cerebrovas Dis. 2009;18:460–5.
13. Jonsson AC, Hoglund P, Brizzi M, Pessah-Rasmussen H. Secondary prevention and health promotion after stroke: can it be enhanced? J Stroke Cerebrovas Dis. 2014;23:2287–95.
14. Lager KE, Mistri AK, Khunti K, Haunton VJ, Sett AK, Wilson AD. Interventions for improving modifiable risk factor control in the secondary prevention of stroke. The Cochrane database Syst Rev. 2014:Cd009103.
15. Ihle-Hansen H, Thommessen B, Fagerland MW, Oksengard AR, Wyller TB, Engedal K, Fure B. Multifactorial vascular risk factor intervention to prevent cognitive impairment after stroke and tia: a 12-month randomized controlled trial. Int J Stroke. 2014;9:932–8.
16. Kronish IM, Goldfinger JZ, Negron R, Fei K, Tuhrim S, Arniella G, Horowitz CR. Effect of peer education on stroke prevention: the prevent recurrence of all inner-city strokes through education randomized controlled trial. Stroke. 2014;45:3330–6.
17. McAlister FA, Majumdar SR, Padwal RS, Fradette M, Thompson A, Buck B, Dean A, Bakal JA, Tsuyuki R, Grover S, et al. Case management for blood pressure and lipid level control after minor stroke: prevention randomized controlled trial. CMAJ. 2014;186:577–84.

18. O'Carroll RE, Chambers JA, Dennis M, Sudlow C, Johnston M. Improving medication adherence in stroke survivors: mediators and moderators of treatment effects. Health Psychol. 2014;33:1241–50.

19. Glynn LG, Murphy AW, Smith SM, Schroeder K, Fahey T. Interventions used to improve control of blood pressure in patients with hypertension. Cochrane database Syst Rev. 2010:Cd005182.

20. Irewall ALÖJ, Bergström L, Laurell K, Söderström L, Mooe T. Nurse-led, telephone-based, secondary preventive follow-up after stroke or transient ischemic attack improves blood pressure and ldl cholesterol: results from the first 12 months of the randomized, controlled nailed stroke risk factor trial. PLoS One. 2015;10:e0139997.

21. Joubert J, Reid C, Barton D, Cumming T, McLean A, Joubert L, Barlow J, Ames D, Davis S. Integrated care improves risk-factor modification after stroke: initial results of the integrated care for the reduction of secondary stroke model. J Neurol Neurosurg Psychiatry. 2009;80:279–84.

22. Kraft P, Hillmann S, Rucker V, Heuschmann PU. Telemedical strategies for the improvement of secondary prevention in patients with cerebrovascular events-a systematic review and meta-analysis. Int J Stroke. 2017;12:597–605.

23. Brotons C, Soriano N, Moral I, Rodrigo MP, Kloppe P, Rodriguez AI, Gonzalez ML, Arino D, Orozco D, Buitrago F, et al. Randomized clinical trial to assess the efficacy of a comprehensive programme of secondary prevention of cardiovascular disease in general practice: the preseap study. Revista espanola de cardiologia. 2011;64:13–20.

24. Oral Abstracts. European Stroke Journal. 2017;2(IS)3–97 https://doi.org/10.1177/2396987317705236

25. Mooe TBL, Irewall A-L, Ögren J. The nailed stroke risk factor trial (nurse based age independent intervention to limit evolution of disease after stroke): Study protocol for a randomized controlled trial. Trials. 2013;14:5.

26. Law MR, Morris JK, Wald NJ. Use of blood pressure lowering drugs in the prevention of cardiovascular disease: meta-analysis of 147 randomised trials in the context of expectations from prospective epidemiological studies. BMJ. 2009;338:b1665.

27. Snaterse M, Dobber J, Jepma P, Peters RJ, Ter Riet G, Boekholdt SM, et al. Effective components of nurse-coordinated care to prevent recurrent coronary events: a systematic review and meta-analysis. Heart. 2016;102:50–6.

28. collaboration TR. Riksstroke annual report 2014; stroke and tia. 2015.

29. Roumie CL, Zillich AJ, Bravata DM, Jaynes HA, Myers LJ, Yoder J, Cheng EM. Hypertension treatment intensification among stroke survivors with uncontrolled blood pressure. Stroke. 2015;46:465–70.

30. Group. PC. Randomised trial of a perindopril-based blood-pressure-lowering regimen among 6,105 individuals with previous stroke or transient ischaemic attack. Lancet. 2001;358:1033–41.

31. Welin L, Bjalkefur K, Roland I. Open, randomized pilot study after first stroke: a 3.5-year follow-up. Stroke. 2010;41:1555–7.

32. Irewall AL, Bergstrom L, Ogren J, Laurell K, Soderstrom L, Mooe T. Implementation of telephone-based secondary preventive intervention after stroke and transient ischemic attack - participation rate, reasons for nonparticipation and one-year mortality. Cerebrovasc Dis extra. 2014;4:28–39.

Visual outcome is similar in optic neuritis patients treated with oral and i.v. high-dose methylprednisolone: a retrospective study on 56 patients

Magdalena Naumovska[1], Rafi Sheikh[1], Boel Bengtsson[2], Malin Malmsjö[1] and Björn Hammar[1]*

Abstract

Background: To investigate visual recovery after treatment of acute optic neuritis (ON) with either oral or intravenous high-dose methylprednisolone, in order to establish the best route of administration.

Methods: Retrospective analysis of patients treated with oral or intravenous high-dose (≥ 500 mg per day) methylprednisolone for acute ON of unknown or demyelinating etiology. Twenty-eight patients were included in each treatment group. Visual acuity was measured with the Snellen letter chart, color vision with Boström-Kugelberg pseudo-isochromatic plates, and visual field with a Humphrey Field Analyzer.

Results: The treatment results were similar in the two groups at follow-up, with no significant difference in visual acuity ($p = 0.54$), color vision ($p = 0.18$), visual field mean deviation ($p = 0.39$) or the number of highly significantly depressed test points ($p = 0.46$).

Conclusions: The results show no clinical disadvantage of using oral high-dose corticosteroids compared to intravenous administration in the treatment of acute ON, which would facilitate the clinical management of these patients.

Keywords: Optic neuritis, Methylprednisolone, Corticosteroids, Multiple sclerosis

Background

Optic neuritis (ON) is an inflammatory disease of the optic nerve. It typically manifests as subacute visual loss with pain that is often exacerbated by eye movement. ON is closely linked to multiple sclerosis (MS) and, in most cases, the pathogenesis is similar [1]. Approximately half the patients with ON will develop MS [1, 2].

Corticosteroids have been widely used for the treatment of MS relapse and optic neuritis, and the effect on short-term recovery of visual function has been well documented, while there are no long-term effects on visual outcome [3–8]. However, the best dosage, length of treatment and route of administration have not yet been established. Previous studies on the treatment of ON have compared the effect of a single route of administration of corticosteroids, either intravenous (i.v.) or oral, with a placebo [5–8], or unequally high doses have been compared [3, 9]. In the Optic Neuritis Treatment Trial (ONTT), a lower dose of oral prednisone was compared with a high i.v. dose of methylprednisolone (MP) [3]. The results suggested that high-dose i.v. MP increased the rate of recovery and visual function at six months, however, equally high doses of corticosteroids were not evaluated. The bioavailability of orally administered MP has been estimated to be 82% of that when MP is administered intravenously [10, 11]. Oral administration should therefore be of no disadvantage. Indeed, oral administration would facilitate the clinical management of these patients and is also safe, well-tolerated and less expensive than intravenously administered corticosteroids.

* Correspondence: bjorn.hammar@med.lu.se
[1]Department of Clinical Sciences Lund, Ophthalmology, Lund University, Skane University Hospital, Ögonklinik A Kioskgatan 1, SE-221 85 Lund, Sweden
Full list of author information is available at the end of the article

The aim of the present study was to compare the effects of oral and i.v. corticosteroids, both at high dose (≥500 mg MP per day), with regard to visual outcome in patients with acute ON. Twenty-eight patients were included in each treatment group. Visual acuity, color vision and visual fields were compared in the groups at follow-up.

Methods
Procedure
Patient records of subjects who were treated at the Department of Neurology and the Department of Ophthalmology at Skane University Hospital in Lund and Malmo, Sweden, between the years 2006 and 2017, were reviewed to identify patients with acute ON. According to local practice, all patients were first diagnosed with optic neuritis at the Department of Opthalmology and then treated at the Department of Neurology. Visual function was followed by an ophthalmologist. Patients were identified by searching the medical records for the diagnosis "optic neuritis", "multiple sclerosis" and/or "retrobulbar neuritis". By tradition, patients at the Lund clinic are more often treated with i.v. MP, whereas patients at the Malmo clinic more frequently receive oral MP regardless of the severity of symptoms. This is due to regional differences, in which the route of administration of corticosteroids is different but the treatment and follow-up is otherwise the same. In case of oral treatment, patients received methylprednisolone in tablet form for treatment at home, whereas those who were treated with intravenous corticosteroids were either hospitalized or had to visit the neurological department once daily to receive the treatment.

Inclusion and exclusion criteria
Inclusion criteria were acute ON of unknown or demyelinating etiology in patients aged 18 years or older and treatment with high-dose MP (≥500 mg per day) orally or intravenously, without oral tapering. Exclusion criteria were previous ON in the same eye, repeated treatment with corticosteroids during the follow-up period, recent treatment (< 6 months) with corticosteroids for other complaints, neuromyelitis optica or systemic disease other than MS that might be the cause of the ON, initiated treatment with disease-modifying drugs in patients recently diagnosed with MS, and follow-up period less than 1 month or more than 6 months after the commencement of treatment. Patients were also excluded in cases when neuromyelitis optica was suspected, and aquaporin-4-antibodies were detected. Patients with MS who were already being treated with disease-modifying drugs prior to the advent of ON, and in whom this therapy was not changed, were not excluded. Patients with

previous ON in the other eye were not excluded. In cases where data were available from several occasions during the follow-up period, the data closest to the six-month endpoint were chosen. Note that magnetic resonance imaging (MRI) pattern and cerebrospinal fluid oligoclonal band are not included in the current study as these tests were not reliably obtained in all subjects.

Sample size
Electronic patient records between the years 2006 and 2017 were reviewed in order to find patients with acute ON. Four hundred and sixty patients with suspected acute ON were assessed for eligibility and of these, 404 patients were excluded as a result of the inclusion and exclusion criteria. A total of 56 patients were included, with 28 subjects per treatment group. For participant enrollment, see Fig. 1.

Patient characteristics
The two groups had similar durations of symptoms before the commencement of treatment and similar median follow-up times. They did not differ in total dose of MP or in treatment duration. Fewer patients had MS and were undergoing disease-modifying therapy for MS in the oral group than in the i.v. group before treatment for ON. There were no statistical differences in patient characteristics between groups. Data was not sufficient to explore side effects by treatment group. The detailed characteristics are given in Table 1.

Visual function measurements and calculations
The primary efficacy measures used were visual acuity, color vision and visual field outcome. Visual acuity was measured with the Snellen letter chart (Ortho-KM, Lund, Sweden), color vision with Boström-Kugelberg pseudo-isochromatic plates (BK) (KIFA, Stockholm, Sweden) [12], and visual field with a Humphrey Field Analyzer (HFA), SITA Standard program 30–2 or 24–2 (Carl Zeiss Meditec, Dublin, Calif, USA).

Decimal visual acuities were converted to logMAR units for statistical analysis. In cases where patients had poor visual acuity, hand movements were converted into a decimal visual acuity of 0.005, and finger counting was converted to 0.01 [13]. Color vision was described as the percentage of correct pseudo-isochromatic plates.

The results obtained with the HFA were expressed in two ways: the mean deviation (MD) in decibels, and the number of highly significantly depressed test points (DP) at the $p < 0.005$ level in the total deviation probability map. The total deviation probability map identifies and highlights test locations where the age-corrected threshold sensitivity is outside normal limits compared to healthy subjects. A highly significantly depressed test

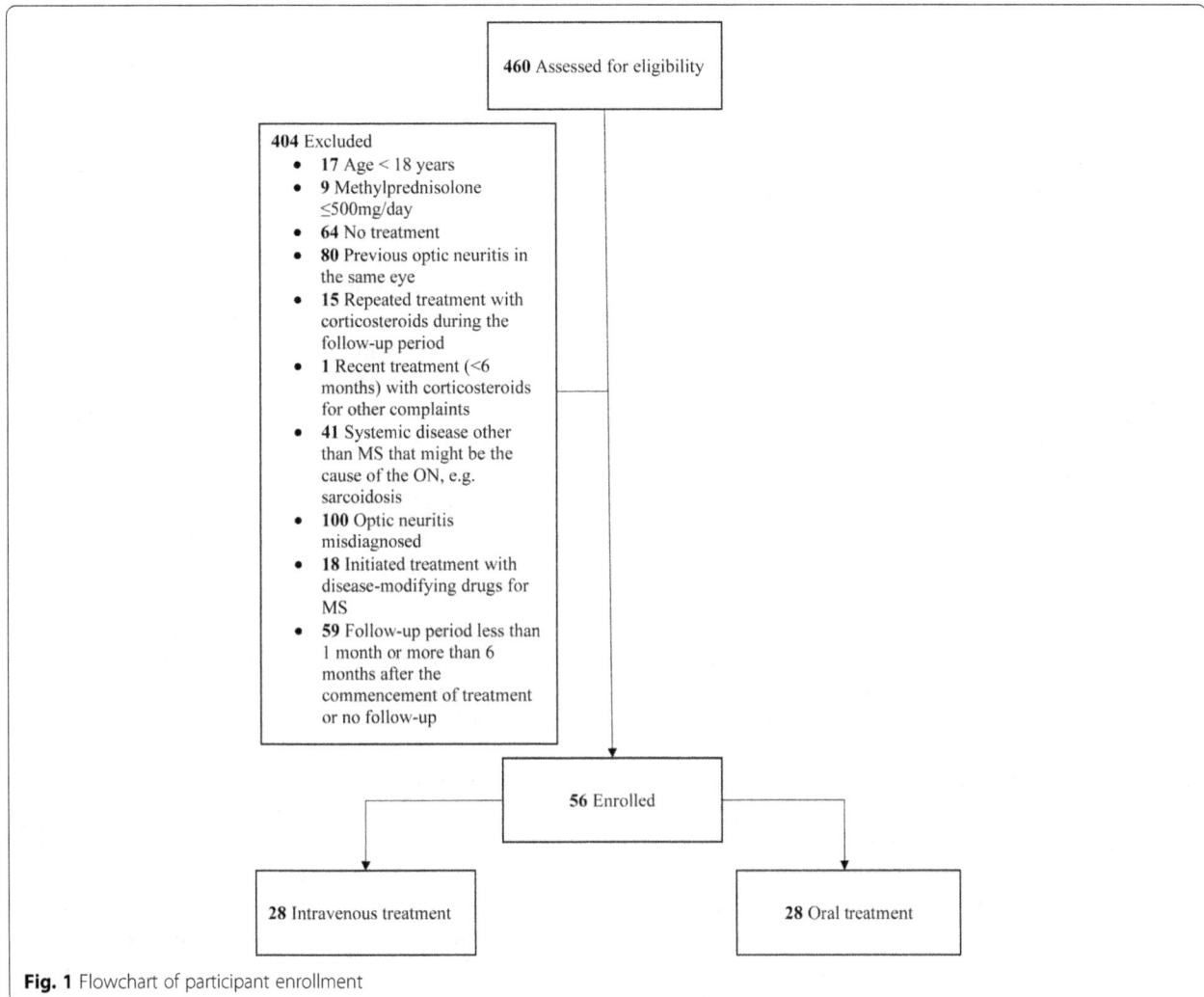

Fig. 1 Flowchart of participant enrollment

point indicates that 99.5% of normal subjects of the same age would be expected to have a sensitivity that is higher than the recorded value. This is considered to provide a more sensitive measure of visual field defects than the MD, as the MD is the weighted average measure of the deviations from the normal age-corrected threshold values of all test points in the visual field. To obtain the value of DP, HFA 24–2 was analyzed by counting and summing the number of highly significantly depressed test points. In subjects

Table 1 Patient characteristics

	All patients ($n = 56$)	Oral ($n = 28$)	i.v. ($n = 28$)
Gender (female/male)	42/14	20/8	22/6
Median age (range) (years)		33 (23 to 60)	35 (18 to 60)
Median duration of symptoms before treatment (range) (days)		7 (1 to 35)	7 (1 to 30)
Median total dose MP (range) (grams)		3.0 (1.5 to 5)	3.0 (2.8 to 6)
Median treatment duration (range) (days)		3 (3 to 5)	3 (3 to 6)
Median follow-up time (range) (weeks)		9 (4 to 24)	9 (4 to 24)
Multiple sclerosis before treatment (number of patients)	13	5	8
Undergoing disease-modifying therapy for MS (number of patients)	8	2	6
Previous ON in other eye (number of patients)	8	5	3

where HFA 30–2 was performed, only the test points corresponding to the HFA 24–2 program were included.

Statistics

Results are presented as median values (range). Calculations and statistical analysis were performed using GraphPad Prism 7.0c and the Mann–Whitney test for comparisons (GraphPad Software Inc., San Diego, CA, USA). Significance was defined as $p < 0.05$.

Results

The results of treatment at follow-up were similar in the two groups treated with oral and i.v. corticosteroids, showing no differences in visual acuity, color vision, visual field MD, or the number of highly significantly depressed test points. There was no difference in visual recovery between younger patients (age < 40 years) or older patients (age ≥ 40 years). See Table 2, Figs. 2 and 3 for detailed results.

Discussion

The results of this study show that there is no difference in visual outcome in patients with acute ON, treated with high-dose MP (≥500 mg per day) given orally or intravenously. Interestingly, in analogy with the present study on ON, others have studied the effect on MS relapses following high-dose oral corticosteroids, showing no inferiority of oral administration compared to i.v. administration, regarding MS disability outcome [14–16]. Furthermore, the results of our study are supported by a recently published prospective study on bioequivalent doses of corticosteroids in the treatment of acute ON, showing that oral administration of corticosteroids is not inferior to i.v. administration in terms of visual acuity and visual evoked potentials at follow-up [17]. It could be expected that the effects of oral and i.v. treatment would be similar as the bioavailability of oral MP has been reported to be as high as 82% of that given intravenously [11]. Interestingly, we found no difference in visual outcome, even though the oral group did not receive bioequivalent doses. Replacing high-dose i.v. administration of corticosteroids with oral administration

would be of benefit to both the patient and the health care system. Indeed, the tolerability has been reported to be similar for both oral and i.v. administration of corticosteroids [15, 16].

In previous studies of oral versus i.v. administration of corticosteroids for the treatment of ON, equally high doses have not been tested, i.e. low-dose oral corticosteroids have been compared to high-dose i.v. corticosteroids. This is the case in the ONTT, in which the patients treated with oral corticosteroids received much lower doses of corticosteroids than those receiving i.v. treatment [3]. The rate of return of visual function was found to be higher following i.v. MP than with placebo, and the i.v. group exhibited slightly better visual field, contrast sensitivity, and color vision, but not better visual acuity, at 6 months. This was not found to be the case when oral administration of prednisone was compared to placebo. At 1 year, no difference was found between the groups, regardless of the route of administration [18].

In other studies, only a single route of administration of corticosteroids has been assessed, i.e. either i.v. or oral, and compared to the effect of a placebo. It has been reported that i.v. administration of corticosteroids increased the rate of recovery compared to placebo, but did not influence the final visual outcome [5–7], or the length of the lesion in the optic nerve [5]. Interestingly, in a study by Sellebjerg et al., the rate of recovery of visual function was improved in patients receiving high-dose MP orally compared to those given the placebo [8], showing the beneficial effects of high-dose oral steroids in the treatment of ON, supporting the findings in the present study.

As disease-modifying therapy may alter the course of recovery in acute demyelinating events [19, 20], such cases were excluded from the present study. However, patients undergoing therapy prior to the incident of ON were not excluded. The number of patients undergoing disease-modifying therapy was higher in the group receiving i.v. MP. The contributing effect of these agents on the course of recovery in acute demyelinating events has rarely been evaluated [21], and an additional effect

Table 2 Results of treatment with oral versus i.v. high-dose methylprednisolone, expressed as median values (range)

	Before treatment			After treatment		
	Oral (N = 28)	i.v. (N = 28)	p-value	Oral (N = 28)	i.v. (N = 28)	p-value
Visual acuity, logMAR (units)	0.30 (0 to 2)	0.35 (0 to 2)	0.98	0.05 (0 to 0.60)	0.05 (0 to 1.22)	0.54
Color vision (percentage correct plates)	22.22 (0 to 100)	6.67 (0 to 100)	0.049	76.67 (0 to 100)	93.33 (13.33 to 100)	0.18
Visual field, MD (decibels)	−18.47 (−33.48 to −1.59)	−12.80 (−27.71 to −3.06)	0.58	−2.56 (−31.75 to −0.26)	−1.80 (−11.4 to 0.48)	0.39
Number of highly significantly depressed test points in visual field	31 (0 to 52)	34 (2 to 52)	0.88	0 (0 to 52)	0 (0 to 45)	0.46

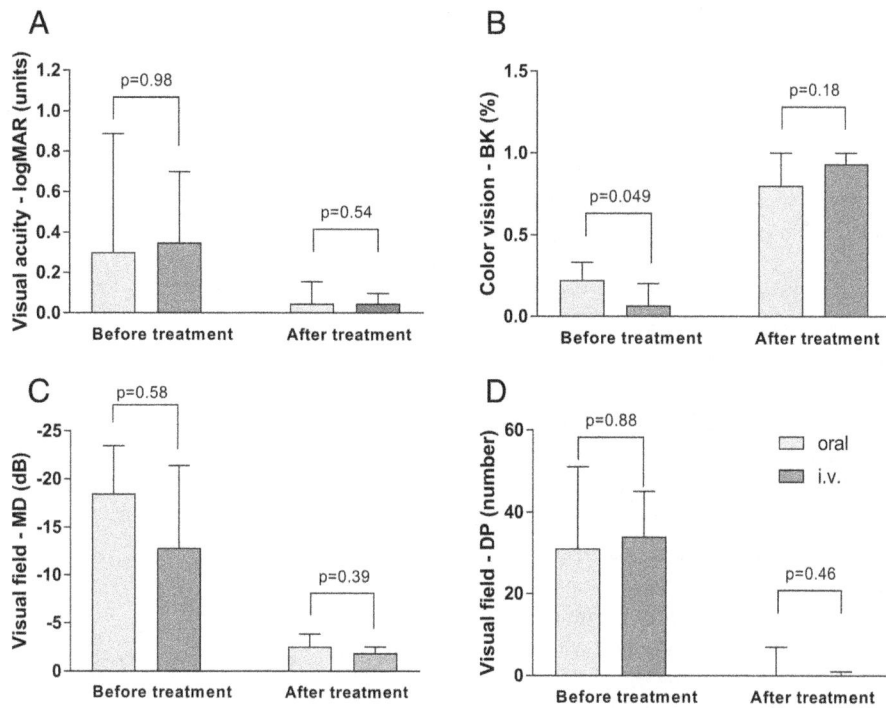

Fig. 2 Results before and after treatment with oral or i.v. high-dose methylprednisolone. **a** Visual acuity expressed in logMAR units. **b** Color vision expressed as the percentage correct plates. **c** Visual field expressed as the mean deviation (MD) in decibels. **d** Visual field expressed as the number of highly significantly depressed test points (DP) in the total deviation probability map. Note that the visual outcome is similar in the two groups

can therefore not be ruled out. Prospective studies evaluating the effect of corticosteroids without disease-modifying therapy in the acute phase might be difficult in patients with demyelinating acute ON, as the criteria for the diagnosis of MS have changed during the past decade, and treatment with disease-modifying agents is now initiated early.

The test methods chosen to measure visual function were visual acuity, visual field and color vision, as these together provide a comprehensive picture of visual function. Regarding the visual field, a strength of our study is that we measured visual field defects by counting the number of highly significantly depressed test points in the total deviation probability map. This is likely to

provide a more sensitive measure of visual field defects than the MD, since the latter is the average value of all deviations from the age-corrected normal threshold values of all test points in the visual field. We included the MD in our analysis to enable comparison with previous studies using MD as a measure of the visual field.

One limitation of the present study is the small number of subjects, which makes it difficult to draw definitive statistically supported conclusions. As this was a retrospective study, the data available in the patient records were also limited. For example, there was no information on visual evoked potentials (VEP) or Optical Coherence Tomography (OCT), as these are not

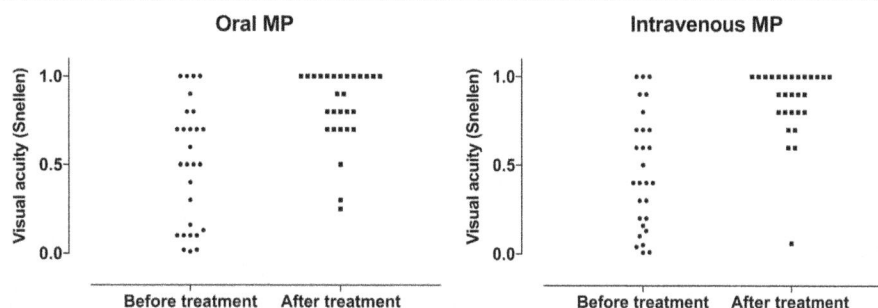

Fig. 3 Visual acuity before and after treatment with oral or i.v. high-dose methylprednisolone, expressed in decimal visual acuity

standard tools for evaluating recovery after optic neuritis in a clinical setting at the departments included in the current study. For future prospective studies, this information would be of interest to analyze. Furthermore, the test used for color vision measurement is a non-specific test that is not optimized for the detection of acquired color vision deficiencies. A more suitable test should be used in future trials evaluating acquired color vision deficiency.

Regardless of whether ON is treated or not, the visual function starts to recover within 1 month [3, 22]. As ON improves spontaneously, treatment with corticosteroids has been questioned. A Cochrane review found that there was no evidence of any beneficial effect of oral or i.v. corticosteroids compared to placebo regarding visual acuity, visual field or contrast sensitivity outcomes [23]. However, even when visual acuity returns to normal, many patients have lasting symptoms of visual disability [24]. Optimal treatment should include the rapid relief of symptoms, as well as the prevention of tissue damage. Previous studies have shown that treatment with corticosteroids in ON has an effect on the rate of recovery and that the short-term risk of development of MS is reduced [25]. The effects of corticosteroid treatment have also been evaluated on brain MRI-derived quantities in MS, including gadolinium-enhancing lesions, showing a decrease in the number of lesions after treatment, also indicating the positive effect of corticosteroids [26, 27].

Conclusions
The results of this study show no clinical disadvantage of using oral high-dose (≥500 mg MP per day) corticosteroids compared to intravenous administration in the treatment of acute ON. Oral corticosteroids are safe, well-tolerated, easy to administer and less expensive than i.v. corticosteroids. However, more prospective randomized trials must be carried out to evaluate the role of high-dose oral corticosteroids as a treatment option in ON before any clinical recommendations can be made.

Abbreviations
BK: Boström-Kugelberg pseudo-isochromatic plates; DP: Number of highly significantly depressed test points; HFA: Humphrey field analyzer; i.v: Intravenous; MD: Mean deviation; MP: Methylprednisolone; MRI: Magnetic resonance imaging; MS: Multiple sclerosis; ON: Optic neuritis; ONTT: Optic Neuritis Treatment Trial

Funding
This study was supported by the Swedish Government Grant for Clinical Research (ALF), the Skåne University Hospital (SUS) Research Grants, the Region Skåne County Council Research Grants, the Foundation for the Visually Impaired in the County of Malmöhus, The Nordmark Foundation for Eye Diseases at Skåne University Hospital, the Swedish Eye Foundation.

Authors' contributions
Study concept and design: BJH, MN, RS, MM, BB. Reviews of patient records and data collection: MN. Analysis and interpretation of data: MN, RS, BJH. Statistical analysis: MN, RS, MM. Drafting of the manuscript: MN, RS, BJH, BB, MM. All authors read and improved the final manuscript.

Competing interests
The authors declare that they have no competing interests.

Author details
[1]Department of Clinical Sciences Lund, Ophthalmology, Lund University, Skane University Hospital, Ögonklinik A Kioskgatan 1, SE-221 85 Lund, Sweden. [2]Department of Clinical Sciences Malmo, Ophthalmology, Lund University, Lund, Sweden.

References
1. Lightman S, McDonald WI, Bird AC, Francis DA, Hoskins A, Batchelor JR, Halliday AM. Retinal venous sheathing in optic neuritis. Its significance for the pathogenesis of multiple sclerosis. Brain. 1987;110(Pt 2):405–14.
2. Optic Neuritis Study G. Multiple sclerosis risk after optic neuritis: final optic neuritis treatment trial follow-up. Arch Neurol. 2008;65:727–32.
3. Beck RW, Cleary PA, Anderson MM, Jr., Keltner JL, Shults WT, Kaufman DI, Buckley EG, Corbett JJ, Kupersmith MJ, Miller NR, et al.: A randomized, controlled trial of corticosteroids in the treatment of acute optic neuritis. The optic neuritis study group. N Engl J Med 1992, 326:581–588.
4. Brusaferri F, Candelise L. Steroids for multiple sclerosis and optic neuritis: a meta-analysis of randomized controlled clinical trials. J Neurol. 2000;247: 435–42.
5. Kapoor R, Miller DH, Jones SJ, Plant GT, Brusa A, Gass A, Hawkins CP, Page R, Wood NW, Compston DA, et al. Effects of intravenous methylprednisolone on outcome in MRI-based prognostic subgroups in acute optic neuritis. Neurology. 1998;50:230–7.
6. Spoor TC, Rockwell DL. Treatment of optic neuritis with intravenous megadose corticosteroids. A consecutive series. Ophthalmology. 1988;95: 131–4.
7. Wakakura M, Mashimo K, Oono S, Matsui Y, Tabuchi A, Kani K, Shikishima K, Kawai K, Nakao Y, Tazawa Y, et al. Multicenter clinical trial for evaluating methylprednisolone pulse treatment of idiopathic optic neuritis in Japan. Optic Neuritis Treatment Trial Multicenter Cooperative Research Group (ONMRG). Jpn J Ophthalmol. 1999;43:133–8.
8. Sellebjerg F, Nielsen HS, Frederiksen JL, Olesen J. A randomized, controlled trial of oral high-dose methylprednisolone in acute optic neuritis. Neurology. 1999;52:1479–84.
9. Alejandro PM, Castanon Gonzalez JA, Miranda Ruiz R, Edgar Echeverria R, Adriana Montano M: [comparative treatment of acute optic neuritis with "boluses" of intravenous methylprednisolone or oral prednisone]. Gac Med Mex 1994, 130:227–230.
10. Morrow SA, Stoian CA, Dmitrovic J, Chan SC, Metz LM. The bioavailability of IV methylprednisolone and oral prednisone in multiple sclerosis. Neurology. 2004;63:1079–80.
11. Groenewoud G, Hundt HK, Luus HG, Muller FO, Schall R. Absolute bioavailability of a new high dose methylprednisolone tablet formulation. Int J Clin Pharmacol Ther. 1994;32:652–4.
12. Hedin A, Tallstedt L. The Bostrom-Kugelberg pseudo-isochromatic plates. How efficient is the third edition? Acta Ophthalmol (Copenh). 1985;63:701–5.
13. Schulze-Bonsel K, Feltgen N, Burau H, Hansen L, Bach M. Visual acuities "hand motion" and "counting fingers" can be quantified with the freiburg visual acuity test. Invest Ophthalmol Vis Sci. 2006;47:1236–40.
14. Le Page E, Veillard D, Laplaud DA, Hamonic S, Wardi R, Lebrun C, Zagnoli F, Wiertlewski S, Deburghgraeve V, Coustans M, et al. Oral versus intravenous high-dose methylprednisolone for treatment of relapses in patients with multiple sclerosis (COPOUSEP): a randomised, controlled, double-blind, non-inferiority trial. Lancet. 2015;386:974–81.
15. Ramo-Tello C, Grau-Lopez L, Tintore M, Rovira A, Ramio i Torrenta L, Brieva L, Cano A, Carmona O, Saiz A, Torres F, et al. A randomized clinical trial of oral versus intravenous methylprednisolone for relapse of MS. Mult Scler. 2014;20:717 25.

16. Alam SM, Kyriakides T, Lawden M, Newman PK. Methylprednisolone in multiple sclerosis: a comparison of oral with intravenous therapy at equivalent high dose. J Neurol Neurosurg Psychiatry. 1993;56:1219–20.

17. Morrow SA, Fraser JA, Day C, Bowman D, Rosehart H, Kremenchutzky M, Nicolle M. Effect of treating acute optic neuritis with bioequivalent Oral vs intravenous corticosteroids a randomized clinical trial. Jama Neurol. 2018;75:690–6.

18. Beck RW, Cleary PA. Optic neuritis treatment trial. One-year follow-up results. Arch Ophthalmol. 1993;111:773–5.

19. O'Connor PW, Goodman A, Willmer-Hulme AJ, Libonati MA, Metz L, Murray RS, Sheremata WA, Vollmer TL, Stone LA. Natalizumab multiple sclerosis trial G: randomized multicenter trial of natalizumab in acute MS relapses: clinical and MRI effects. Neurology. 2004;62:2038–43.

20. An X, Kezuka T, Usui Y, Matsunaga Y, Matsuda R, Yamakawa N, Goto H. Suppression of experimental autoimmune optic neuritis by the novel agent fingolimod. J Neuroophthalmol. 2013;33:143–8.

21. Bennett JL, Nickerson M, Costello F, Sergott RC, Calkwood JC, Galetta SL, Balcer LJ, Markowitz CE, Vartanian T, Morrow M, et al. Re-evaluating the treatment of acute optic neuritis. J Neurol Neurosurg Psychiatry. 2015;86:799–808.

22. Beck RW, Cleary PA, Backlund JC. The course of visual recovery after optic neuritis. Experience of the optic neuritis treatment trial. Ophthalmology. 1994;101:1771–8.

23. Gal RL, Vedula SS, Beck R. Corticosteroids for treating optic neuritis. Cochrane Database Syst Rev. 2015:CD001430.

24. Optic Neuritis Study G. Visual function 15 years after optic neuritis: a final follow-up report from the optic neuritis treatment trial. Ophthalmology. 2008;115:1079–82 e1075.

25. Beck RW, Trobe JD. What we have learned from the optic neuritis treatment trial. Ophthalmology. 1995;102:1504–8.

26. Martinelli V, Rocca MA, Annovazzi P, Pulizzi A, Rodegher M, Martinelli Boneschi F, Scotti R, Falini A, Sormani MP, Comi G, Filippi M. A short-term randomized MRI study of high-dose oral vs intravenous methylprednisolone in MS. Neurology. 2009;73:1842–8.

27. Barkhof F, Hommes OR, Scheltens P, Valk J. Quantitative MRI changes in gadolinium-DTPA enhancement after high-dose intravenous methylprednisolone in multiple sclerosis. Neurology. 1991;41:1219–22.

Comorbidity of migraine with ADHD in adults

Thomas Folkmann Hansen[1,2,13]*, Louise K. Hoeffding[3], Lisette Kogelman[1], Thilde Marie Haspang[1], Henrik Ullum[3], Erik Sørensen[3], Christian Erikstrup[4], Ole Birger Pedersen[5], Kaspar René Nielsen[6], Henrik Hjalgrim[7,8], Helene M. Paarup[9], Thomas Werge[10,11,12] ⓘD and Kristoffer Burgdorf[3]

Abstract

Background: Migraine and Attention Deficit and Hyperactivity Disorder (ADHD) have been found to be associated in child and adolescent cohorts; however, the association has not been assessed in adults or otherwise healthy population. Assessing the comorbidity between ADHD and migraine may clarify the etiopathology of both diseases. Thus, the objective is to assess whether migraine (with and without visual disturbances) and ADHD are comorbid disorders.

Methods: Participants from the Danish Blood Donor Study (N = 26,456, age 18–65, 46% female) were assessed for migraine and ADHD using the ASRS ver 1.1 clinically validated questionnaire and self-reported migraine in a cross-sectional study. Logistic regression was used to examine the comorbidity between migraine and ADHD, and their associated endophenotypes.

Results: Migraine was strongly associated with ADHD (OR = 1.8, 95% CI = 1.5–2.1), (238/6152 vs 690/19,376). There was a significant interaction between age and gender, with comorbidity increasing with age and female sex. Post-hoc analysis showed that migraine with visual disturbance was generally associated with a marginally higher risk of ADHD and this was independent of ADHD endophenotypes.

Conclusion: Migraine and ADHD were demonstrated to be comorbid disorders; the association with ADHD was most prominent for participants with migraine with visual disturbances. Future studies will elucidate which genetic and environmental factors contribute to migraine-ADHD comorbidity.

Keywords: Migraine, Attention deficiency and hyperactivity disorder, Comorbidity

Background

Migraine is a complex and multifactorial headache disorder with a lifetime prevalence of 16–18% [1–3]. Migraine is twice as prevalent in females, and onset is typically between adolescence and the late 50s [1–3]. According to the World Health Organization (WHO), migraine is the sixth most disabling disease in the world with high financial costs to society [4]. Response to acute treatment varies considerably and approximately 20% of the pharmacologically treated patients experience no symptom relief after medication [5]. There are two major endophenotypes in migraine: migraine

with or without aura. Aura is a sensory disturbance, which is predominantly seen as visual disturbances (99%) with a subsequent headache or migraine [6, 7].

Attention deficit and hyperactivity disorder (ADHD) is characterized by inappropriate levels of inattention, e.g., difficulty keeping attention, keeping track of details, and difficulty structuring trivial duties or following instructions, hyperactivity, e.g., speaks a lot, difficulty relaxing or sitting still, and impulsivity, e.g., often interrupts other people during conversations or answers a question before the question is finished [8]. In contrast to migraine, ADHD has an early onset and a pooled worldwide prevalence of 5.3% in child and adolescent populations [9]. The current treatment strategies do not completely remove the symptoms in both children and adults and approximately 30% of all patients

* Correspondence: Thomas.hansen@regionh.dk
[1]Danish Headache Center, Department of Neurology, Rigshospitalet Glostrup, University Hospital of Copenhagen, Copenhagen, Denmark
[2]Novo Nordisk Foundation Center for Protein Research, Faculty of Health and Medical Sciences, University of Copenhagen, Copenhagen, Denmark
Full list of author information is available at the end of the article

do not respond to medical treatment or develop serious adverse reactions [10, 11].

It is well established that migraine is comorbid with psychiatric traits, in particular depressive and bipolar disorder [12, 13], and that the comorbidity is partly explained by shared genetics [14]. More recently, the comorbidity between migraine and ADHD has also been assessed [15–18]. In adults, a clinical case-control study of ADHD ($n = 572/675$) found an increased prevalence of migraine when compared to community controls [16], and subsequently the same investigators showed a positive association between prescription of anti-migraine and anti-ADHD drugs to adults in the total Norwegian population($n > 4$mill) [17]. In line with this, Arruda et al. reported a higher prevalence of ADHD among children with migraine (5–12 years) than for non-headache individuals in a pediatric population cohort ($n = 5671$) [19]. According to the recently published meta-analysis including child and adolescence studies and the Fasmer et al. adult study, there is a positive association between migraine and ADHD with odds-ratio of 1.3 [16, 20].

Using a cross-sectional study of adults (age 18–65 years), we test the hypothesis that migraine is comorbid with ADHD in 26,456 participants using clinically validated questionnaires.

Methods

Participants

From November 2015 to September 2017 voluntary blood donors were recruited as part of the Danish Blood Donor Study (DBDS) (www.DBDS.dk). In brief, the DBDS was initiated in 2010 and is an ongoing prospective research cohort and biobank that recruits participants between 17 and 67 years of age from blood banks across Denmark [21, 22]. Individuals in chronic medical treatment or frequent travelers to countries considered resulting in high-risk of blood disease are not allowed to participate. Approximately 95% of all invited individuals are consented to participate in DBDS [22]. At enrolment, each individual gives oral and written informed consent to participate in DBDS and subsequently answers a digital tablet-based questionnaire including a migraine (two questions) and an ADHD (18 questions) module. In total, 29,489 participants were recruited to the study. The study is approved by the Danish Data Protection Agency (2007-58-0015) and the Ethical Committee of Central Denmark (M-20090237). For further details about the DBDS platform and questionnaire, see Pedersen et al. [22] or Burgdorf et al. [21]

In total, 29,489 participants were given a questionnaire. We excluded 3033 individuals due to missing answers on either the SQM ($n = 2057$) or the ASRS items ($n = 1108$) of which $n = 132$ were missing both. The excluded individuals did not differ significantly with respect to age (chi-square

test, P-value = 0.24) compared to the study population. The excluded individuals were slightly older (median age: 44 years, IQR = 31–54 years) when compared to the study population (median age: 42 years, IQR = 30–52 years) (Wilcoxon test, P-value = 3.7e-8). Importantly, the frequency of migraine in individuals excluded because of missing information in the ASRS questionnaire was similar to that of the study population (24.1%). Further, the frequency of ADHD in individuals excluded because of missing items in the SQM questionnaire was similar to that of the study population 4.2%.

The migraine module

The presence of migraine was evaluated by two questions from the population screening questionnaire for migraine (SQM). The participants were asked two questions ("Have you ever had migraine?" and "Have you ever had visual disturbances lasting 5-60 min followed by headache?") of the original SQM. Participants who had a positive response to either of the two questions were considered to have migraine and are referred as migraine cases in this study. Individuals with missing information or who answered "I don't know" were excluded. A detailed description of the SQM questionnaire can be found elsewhere [23]. In short, the SQM has previously been shown to identify 93% of those with migraine with aura and 75% of those with migraine without aura in a Danish setting [23]. Using the national prescription register, we found that 89.5% of those prescribed migraine-specific treatment, i.e. triptans ATC-codes N02CC01–7, are captured using these two questions.

The ADHD module

Current self-reported ADHD symptoms were assessed using the current national recommendation for clinical assessment of adults by using the ADHD Self-Report Scale v1.1 (ASRS) [24, 25] translated to Danish Dalsgaard et al. [26]. The ASRS consists of 18 items based on the *Diagnostic and Statistical Manual of Mental Disorders fourth edition* (DSM-IV) diagnostic criteria for ADHD and is the recommended version for clinical use in Denmark. Each of the 18 questions was scored on a five-point Likert scale ranging from never = 0 to very often = 4. In this study we use the optimal Kessler et al. 18-item ASRS scale score obtained by summarizing all items (total range of 0–72) as the primary outcome. The ASRS has been validated in multiple countries using different populations [27–30]. The scale dichotomizes ADHD based upon all items for ADHD (having a score > 36), inattentive subtype (items 1–4 + 7–11, having a score > 23), the hyperactivity-impulsivity subtype (items 5–6 + 12–18, having a score > 23), and the 6-item screening score (having a score > 13) [28]. A more detailed description of the ASRS questionnaire can be found elsewhere [24].

Statistical analysis

The study population was described by numbers and percentages for categorical variables and as median and interquartile range (IQR) for continuous variables. Differences in distributions between participants with and without migraine and ADHD symptoms were analyzed using Fisher's exact test or Mann-Whitney/Wilcoxon test (age does not follow a normal distribution, thus non-parametric analysis is used).

Logistic regression was used to analyze the association between migraine and ADHD (dichotomous variables) in the study population, adjusting for age, sex, and the interaction between sex and age, with migraine as the dependent variable. We used a logistic regression model with a binary outcome of either migraine, migraine with visual disturbance, or migraine without visual disturbances. We did not include sampling weights, as these are not available for DBDS. We calculatedthe regression in two ways including age as a quantitative trait or as a categorical trait (10 year interval). We report the derived odds ratios (OR) and 95% confidence intervals (CIs). A P-value< 0.05 was considered statistically significant. Post-hoc analyses were performed using different thresholds of the ASRS score (from 0 and 52), and single ASRS items (data not shown). To check if the specified model is appropriate for the data, the predicted and observed residuals were inspected for each analysis and no issues were observed.

All statistical analyses were performed using the statistical package for R version 3.3.3: stat, basic, ggplot2, eeptools, cowplot, and GirdExtra.

Results

Study population

The population consisted of 26,456 participants (median age: 42 years, IQR = 30–52 years) from the DBDS, of whom 24.2% screened positive for migraine (median age: 42 years, IQR = 31–51 years, female-to-male ratio: 1:0.6), 2.61% screened positive for ADHD (median age: 29 years, IQR = 25–40 years, female-to-male ratio: 1:1.4), and 0.90% reported having both migraine and ADHD (median age: 31 years, IQR = 24–41 years, male-to-female ratio: 1:0.74), see Table 1 for the prevalence. There was a significant difference in the age and sex distributions for participants with either migraine or ADHD (Wilcoxon test and chi-square exact, $P < 1e$-15 and $P < 1e$-15, respectively) (Fig. 1), thus we included a correction for age, sex and interaction of age and sex in the model.

There was an association between migraine and ADHD symptoms with OR = 1.81 (95CI%: 1.53–2.12, $P = 1.4e$-14) including corrections for age, sex and the interaction of age and sex as covariates (Table 2a). As expected, male sex is protective (OR = 0.57), and increased age further increased protection with OR = 9.99 per year (Table 2a). To ease literature comparison, we present the sex-stratified results (Table 2b + c) and repeated the regression analysis using age bins (10 years), see Table 3. The association was not explained by one specific item in the ASRS questionnaire (data not shown). The highest risk was found for migraine with visual disturbances and ADHD symptoms (OR = 2.05, 95CI%: 1.55–2.68, $P = 3.3e$-11). Using the national prescription register we did not find any difference in frequency of triptan purchases with and without ADHD symptoms (at least one purchase: 22.1% vs 23.2%, $p = 0.80$, at least 2 purchases: 13.7% vs 14.4%, and at least 10 purchases: 3.2% vs 4.9%, $p = 0.39$).

The association between migraine and ADHD symptoms was statistically significant irrespective of the employed ASRS score threshold (Fig. 2a), with a tendency to increase with the ASRS score. The same results were observed for ADHD symptoms and migraine with visual disturbances (Fig. 2b), however; no association was detected for migraine without visual disturbances with ASRS scores below 10 and above 51 (Fig. 2c).

Migraine was associated with both ADHD endophenotypes (inattention and hyperactivity-impulsivity), with migraine with visual disturbances showing a marginally

Table 1 Characteristics of the study population ($N = 26,456$) with respect to migraine and ADHD symptoms

Description	N Female	(%[e])	Male	Total	(%[f])	P-value[d]
The total study population	12,247	(46.3)	14,209	26,456	(100)	
Migraine[a]	4024	(63.0)	2366	6390	(24.2)	< 0.001
- Without visual disturbances	2187	(62.0)	1343	3530	(13.3)	< 0.001
- With visual disturbances	1832	(64.2)	1019	2851	(10.8)	< 0.001
ADHD[b]	285	(41.3)	405	690	(2.6)	0.0085
- Inattention	83	(39.7)	126	209	(0.79)	0.06
- Hyperactivity-impulsivity	67	(43.0)	89	156	(0.59)	0.42
- Screening items[c]	182	(26.7)	400	682	(2.58)	< 0.001
Migraine and ADHD	137	(57.6)	101	238	(0.90)	< 0.001

[a]Symptoms of migraine was assessed by the SQM [19], [b] ADHD symptoms were assessed by the ASRS [20], [c] Screening as described by Kessing et al. [23], [d] Test of gender differences of total population and subgroup by chi-square test, [e] percentage females of the subgrup, [f] percentage of the total sample

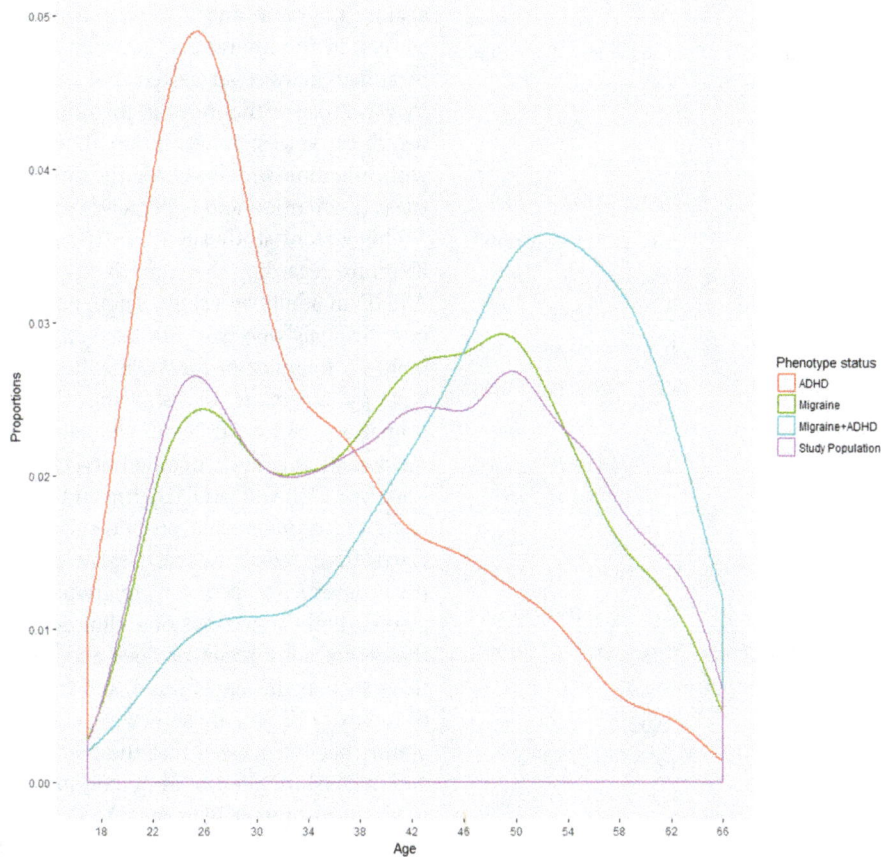

Fig. 1 Age distribution. The X-axis shows age from 17 to 66 years, the Y-axis shows the proportional distribution by age of the study population, colored according to phenotype status on the right

Table 2 Multivariable Logistic regression analysis

Model		a) All genders			b) Females only			c) Males only		
Outcome	Variable	OR	CI 95%	P-value	OR	CI 95%	P-value	OR	CI 95%	P-value
Migraine	ADHD	1.81	1.53–2.12	< 0.001	2.01	1.58–2.54	< 0.001	1.64	1.30–2.06	< 0.001
	Age	1.00	1.00–1.01	0.001	1.01	1.00–1.01	< 0.001	1.00	0.99–1.00	0.051
	Gender (Male)	0.57	0.47–0.69	< 0.001						
	Age:Gender (Male)	0.99	0.99–0.99	< 0.001						
With Visual Disturbances	ADHD	1.98	1.61–2.41	< 0.001	2.05	1.55–2.68	< 0.001	1.89	1.38–2.53	< 0.001
	Age	1.00	1.00–1.00	0.84	1.00	1.00–1.00	0.11	1.00	0.99–1.00	0.11
	Gender (Male)	0.53	0.40–0.69	< 0.001						
	Age:Gender (Male)	1.00	0.99–1.00	0.16						
Without Visual Disturbances	ADHD	1.52	1.22–1.88	< 0.001	1.69	1.24–2.27	< 0.001	1.37	0.99–1.86	0.047
	Age	1.01	1.00–1.01	< 0.001	1.01	1.00–1.01	< 0.001	1.00	0.99–1.00	0.23
	Gender (Male)	0.63	0.49–0.82	< 0.001						
	Age:Gender (Male)	0.99	0.98–1.00	< 0.001						

Multivariable Logistic regression analysis of migraine and migraine with and without visual disturbances, subsequent stratified on gender.
Reference of the regression model is given in ()

Table 3 Multivariable logistic regression analysis

Outcome	Variable	OR	CI 95%	P-value
Migraine	ADHD	1,86	1,58-2,19	< 0.001
	Age 3X[a]	1,34	1,20-1,51	< 0.001
	Age 4X[a]	1,59	1,43-1,76	< 0.001
	Age 5X[a]	1,27	1,14-1,42	< 0.001
	Age 60+[a]	0,98	0,84-1,15	0.80
	Gender (Male)	0,49	0,44-0,56	< 0.001
	Gender (Male) interaction with:			
	Age 3X[a]	0,78	0,66-0,93	0.007
	Age 4X[a]	0,75	0,63-0,88	< 0.001
	Age 5X[a]	0,75	0,63-0,89	0.0013
	Age 60+[a]	0,84	0,66-1,07	0.16
With Visual Disturbances	ADHD	2,01	1,63-2,45	< 0.001
	Age 3X[a]	1,13	0,97-1,31	0.110
	Age 4X[a]	1,20	1,05-1,38	0.0095
	Age 5X[a]	1,13	0,98-1,31	0.090
	Age 60+[a]	0,78	0,63-0,97	0.028
	Gender (Male)	0,49	0,41-0,57	< 0.001
	Gender (Male) interaction with:			
	Age 3X[a]	0,90	0,71-1,15	0.41
	Age 4X[a]	0,83	0,66-1,05	0.13
	Age 5X[a]	0,79	0,62-1,01	0.06
	Age 60+[a]	1,12	0,80-1,57	0.5
Without Visual Disturbances	ADHD	1,59	1,28-1,97	< 0.001
	Age 3X[a]	1,47	1,27-1,70	< 0.001
	Age 4X[a]	1,81	1,59-2,07	< 0.001
	Age 5X[a]	1,34	1,16-1,54	< 0.001
	Age 60+[a]	1,15	0,94-1,39	0.16
	Gender (Male)	0,53	0,46-0,63	< 0.001
	Gender (Male) interaction with:			
	Age 3X[a]	0,73	0,58-0,92	0.0069
	Age 4X[a]	0,72	0,59-0,89	0.0026
	Age 5X[a]	0,75	0,60-0,93	0.011
	Age 60+[a]	0,69	0,50-0,94	0.021

[a] Reference is age < 30

larger effect than migraine without visual disturbances, notably with overlapping confidence intervals (Fig. 3).

Discussion

We address the comorbidity of migraine and ADHD symptoms in a healthy population of 29,489 adults using two clinically validated questionnaires (SQM and ASRS). Our results show a strong and statistically significant comorbidity between the two disorders which was irrespective of the threshold (i.e., not restricted to the commonly used ASRS score threshold of 37 (Fig. 2). The

regression model clearly shows that being male protects against migraine and increased age is further protective as seen in the interaction between age and sex (Table 2). Stratified analyses suggested that the observed comorbidity was more pronounced in migraineurs experiencing visual disturbances; however, no differences in association with migraine were seen for the two ADHD endophenotypes (inattention and hyperactivity-impulsivity).

The current study significantly supplements the sparse literature regarding the comorbidity between migraine and ADHD in adults by using a large, healthy study population of individuals who have not been exposed to chronic treatment for migraine or for ADHD. It supports the meta-analysis by Salem et al., showing OR of 1.3, consisting primarily of child and adolescence studies. This meta-analysis cohort consisted of a clinical case-control cohort, (n = 572) with ADHD [16], and a cross-sectional study using prescription data on anti-migraine and anti-ADHD drugs from the entire Norwegian population [17]. Thus, the comorbidity between migraine and ADHD seems present both in and out of a clinical setting. The origin of the comorbidity is not obvious and typical prognostic features such as the age of onset, and the female-to-male ratio of the two diseases are somewhat contradicting. It has previously been suggested that the co-occurrence of migraine and ADHD originates from common pathophysiological mechanisms potentially related to dysfunctions in the dopaminergic system [16, 17, 31]. This arises because many of the migraine symptoms, including prodromal symptoms, can be provoked with dopamine receptor stimulation, and some can even be quantified in rat models with dopaminergic activiation [31]. Dopamine has long been thought to be involved in ADHD pathology, and the effective ADHD drug, methylphenidate, acts by inhibiting dopamine reuptake. However, the comorbidity could also be more complex because of common co-morbidities of other psychiatric disorders such as anxiety and mood disorders [13, 32–36]. Their etiological comorbidity may arise because of pleiotropic factors. This has recently been supported by Antilla et al., showing a significant genetic correlation between migraine and ADHD [37]. Interestingly, major depressive disorder was also found to significantly correlate with both migraine and ADHD suggesting that common pleiotropic factors exist.

The observed prevalence of migraine and ADHD (34.7%) was higher than reported by Fasmer et al. (28.3%) in a sample of ADHD patients with similar age and sex distribution [16]. However, there is an anecdote among headache individuals with headache that donating blood gives symptom relief, which could explain the frequency of migraine, i.e. bloodletting by phlebotomy. Furthermore, we used self-reported ADHD rather than formal clinical diagnoses in our analysis, which may influence the results with false positive and negative cases. Despite these methodological

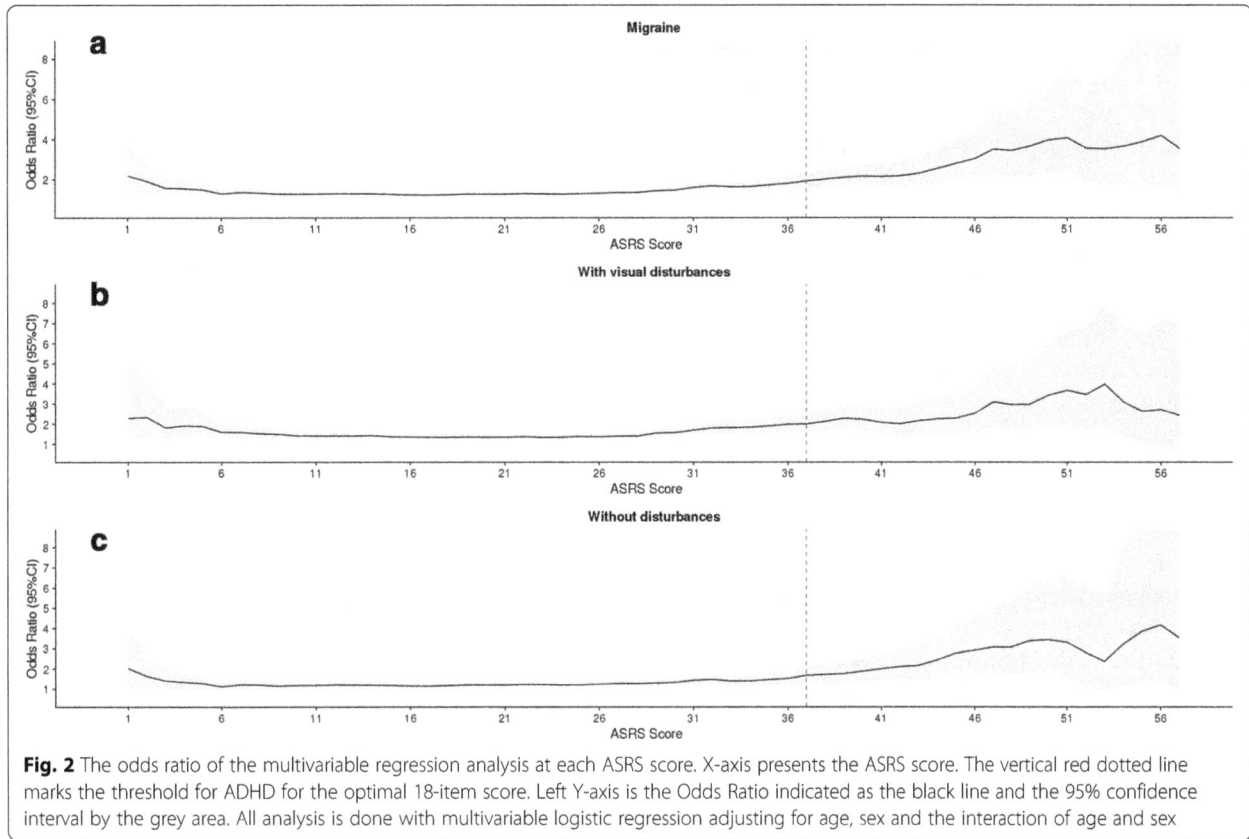

Fig. 2 The odds ratio of the multivariable regression analysis at each ASRS score. X-axis presents the ASRS score. The vertical red dotted line marks the threshold for ADHD for the optimal 18-item score. Left Y-axis is the Odds Ratio indicated as the black line and the 95% confidence interval by the grey area. All analysis is done with multivariable logistic regression adjusting for age, sex and the interaction of age and sex

differences, we found the prevalence of self-reported migraine and ADHD symptoms in males (24% vs. 23%) to be like that reported by Fasmer et al. [16].

We found that the comorbidity between migraine and ADHD was most prevalent among participants peaking at 52 to 53 years of age, and in the 40 decade compared to the 17–29 age group, which is somewhat inversely correlated with the age distribution of ADHD symptoms in the study population (Fig. 1). This could imply that the manifestations of comorbid migraine and ADHD occur rather late in life when compared to ADHD in general, or that ADHD symptoms mask the presence of migraine in the younger participants. Similar results have been reported by Fasmer et al. [17] using simultaneous

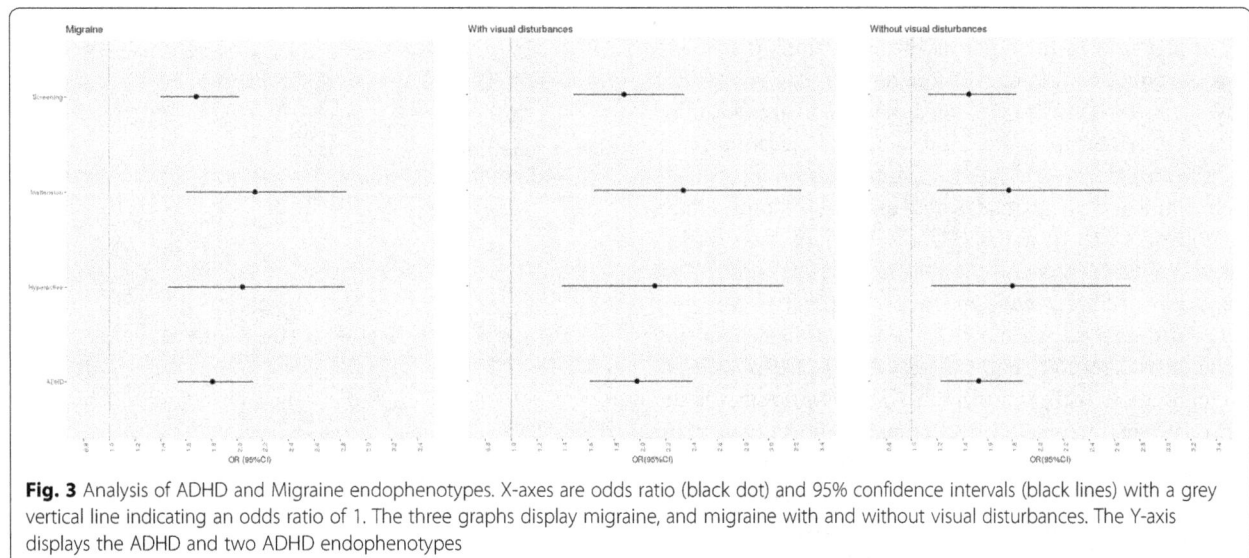

Fig. 3 Analysis of ADHD and Migraine endophenotypes. X-axes are odds ratio (black dot) and 95% confidence intervals (black lines) with a grey vertical line indicating an odds ratio of 1. The three graphs display migraine, and migraine with and without visual disturbances. The Y-axis displays the ADHD and two ADHD endophenotypes

prescriptions of anti-migraine and anti-ADHD medication as a proxy for comorbidity. However, this was not true for the 10–19 years age group, suggesting that ADHD among adolescents may have no comorbidity with migraine and thus having a distinct etiopathology or, as previously mentioned, there is a masking of migraine symptoms in young individuals with ADHD. The notion of a different etiopathology among ADHD patients is suggested by Johansson et al. (Johansson et al. 2008), showing that susceptibility genes differ between persistent and juvenile ADHD [38]. Furthermore, the transition of ADHD symptoms from childhood to adulthood is well recognized where the hyperactivity-impulsivity often becomes less prominent.

We did not detect a specific association between any ADHD endophenotypes and migraine which is congruent with previous reports for children, e.g., Pakainis et al. and Arruda et al [19, 39] It is noteworthy that we do not see a large difference between ADHD inattention and hyperactive endophenotype. Although speculative, the smaller difference between hyperactive and inattention endophenotype in the study cohort could reflect that the inattention is more often referred to treatment and thus are not permitted to donate blood [40].

Participants reporting migraine preceded by visual disturbances (migraine with visual aura symptoms) were more often affected by co-occurring ADHD symptoms when compared to participants reporting no visual disturbances and combined (Table 2, Fig. 2). No obvious shared mechanism between visual disturbances and ADHD symptoms is known. The neurovascular phenomenon cortical depression spreading is suggested as the pathophysiology of aura symptoms in migraine patients [41], however, there are no published studies on ADHD patients. Ophthalmologic disturbances appear to be more frequent in patients diagnosed with ADHD [42], however, it is very speculative whether this could explain the observed comorbidity and further studies are needed.

The strength of the study is the large sample size and that chronic treatment of migraine and ADHD do not influence the results, e.g., treatment-induced migraine attacks. Furthermore, we used validated questionnaires to assess migraine and ADHD symptoms. In accordance with Danish clinical guides we use the recommended version of ASRS to assess ADHD. While a new version based on DSM V exists, a recent study found almost identical specificity and sensitivity of the two versions [43]. Furthermore, we show that 89% of individuals using triptans are captured, and the prevalence of triptan users in migraineurs with and without ADHD symptoms is the same. When interpreting the results, it is important to take into consideration that the study population is a healthy donor population, presumably producing a conservative estimate of the association as individuals exposed to chronic medication or chronic illness are excluded as

donors. Further, we suggest carrying out longitudinal cohort and twin studies to assess causality.

Conclusion

We demonstrate a significant corbobidity between migraine and ADHD in adults, and this is most prominent for participants with migraine with visual disturbances. These results contribute to the understanding of genetic correlation seen between ADHD and migraine and seeds future studies that will elucidate which genetic and environmental factors contribute to migraine-ADHD comorbidity.

Article highlights

- This study examined the association between migraine and ADHD in a large adult population
- There is a strong association between migraine and ADHD (odds ratio = 1.8, 95% CI = 1.5–2.1)
- The association between migraine and ADHD seems strongest for individuals with visual disturbances

Abbreviations
95%CI95: Confidence interval; ADHD : Attention Deficit and Hyperactivity Disorder; ASRS: ADHD Self-Report Scale; IQR: Interquartile range; OR: Odss Ratio; SQM: Screening questionnaire for migraine; WHO: World Health Organization

Acknowledgments
We acknowledge the Danish blood donors and the staff at the Danish blood banks involved in the present study. We thank Shantel Weinsheimer for reviewing the final manuscript.

Funding
This work was supported by RegionH research foundation (R129-A3973 to Dr. Hansen); Candy foundation CEHEAD (Prof Jes Olesen, Co-PI Dr. Hansen); the Lundbeck Foundation, Denmark under Grant (R219–2016–1030 to Dr. Hoeffding); The Danish Council for Independent Research - Medical Sciences under Grant (1333-00275A to Dr. Burgdorf and 09–069412); The Danish Administrative Regions; The Danish Administrative Regions' Bio- and Genome Bank; and The Danish Blood Donor Research Foundation (Bloddonorernes Forskningsfond). The funders had no role in study design, data collection, and analysis, decision to publish, or preparation of the manuscript.

Authors contributions
TFH, LKH, study design and analysis. LK and TMH statistical design and analysis. HU, ES, CE, OBP, KRN, HH, HMP, TW, and KB study design. All authors contributed to creating this manuscript and approved the final version.

Competing interests
TW: has served as a lecturer for and consultant to H. Lundbeck A/S. TFH, LKH,KB,LK,TMH,HH,HMP,KRN,OBP,CE,ES,HU and TW reports no competing interest.

Author details
[1]Danish Headache Center, Department of Neurology, Rigshospitalet Glostrup, University Hospital of Copenhagen, Copenhagen, Denmark. [2]Novo Nordisk Foundation Center for Protein Research, Faculty of Health and Medical Sciences, University of Copenhagen, Copenhagen, Denmark. [3]Department of Clinical Immunology, the Blood Bank, Rigshospitalet, University Hospital of

Copenhagen, Copenhagen, Denmark. [4]Department of Clinical Immunology, Aarhus University Hospital, Aarhus, Denmark. [5]Department of Clinical Immunology, Naestved Hospital, Naestved, Denmark. [6]Department of Clinical Immunology, Aalborg University Hospital, Aalborg, Denmark. [7]Department of Epidemiology Research, Statens Serum Institut, Copenhagen, Denmark. [8]Department of Hematology, Copenhagen University Hospital, Rigshospitalet, Copenhagen, Denmark. [9]Department of Clinical Immunology, Odense University Hospital, Odense, Denmark. [10]Institute of Biological Psychiatry, Mental Health Centre Sct. Hans, Copenhagen University Hospital, Roskilde, Denmark. [11]Department of Clinical Medicine, University of Copenhagen, Copenhagen, Denmark. [12]The Lundbeck Foundation Initiative for Integrative Psychiatric Research, iPSYCH, Copenhagen, Denmark. [13]Danish Headache Center, Neurological department, Copenhagen University Hospital, Nordre Ringevej 69, DK-2600 Glostrup, Denmark.

References

1. Dahlof C, Linde M. One-year prevalence of migraine in Sweden: a population-based study in adults. Cephalalgia. 2001;21:664–71.
2. Hagen K, Zwart JA, Vatten L, Stovner LJ, Bovim G. Prevalence of migraine and non-migrainous headache--head-HUNT, a large population-based study. Cephalalgia. 2000;20:900–6.
3. Russell MB, Rasmussen BK, Thorvaldsen P, Olesen J. Prevalence and sex-ratio of the subtypes of migraine. Int J Epidemiol. 1995;24:612–8.
4. Gustavsson A, Svensson M, Jacobi F, et al. Cost of disorders of the brain in Europe 2010. Eur Neuropsychopharmacol. 2011;21:718–79.
5. Oldman AD, Smith LA, McQuay HJ, Moore RA. Pharmacological treatments for acute migraine: quantitative systematic review. Pain. 2002;97:247–57.
6. Headache Classification Committee of the International Headache Society (IHS) The International Classification of Headache Disorders, 3rd edition. Cephalalgia 2018;38:1–211.
7. Russell MB, Olesen J. A nosographic analysis of the migraine aura in a general population. Brain. 1996;119:355–61.
8. Organization WH. International Statistical Classification of Diseases and Related Health Problems: tenth revision-Version for 2007. http://www.who.int/classifications/icd/en/. Accessed 1 Dec 2017.
9. Polanczyk G, de Lima MS, Horta BL, Biederman J, Rohde LA. The worldwide prevalence of ADHD: a systematic review and metaregression analysis. Am J Psychiatry. 2007;164:942–8.
10. Maia CR, Cortese S, Caye A, et al. Long-term efficacy of methylphenidate immediate-release for the treatment of childhood ADHD. J Atten Disord. 2017;21:3–13.
11. Spencer T, Biederman J, Wilens T, et al. A large, double-blind, randomized clinical trial of methylphenidate in the treatment of adults with attention-deficit/hyperactivity disorder. Biol Psychiatry. 2005;57:456–63.
12. Antonaci F, Nappi G, Galli F, Manzoni GC, Calabresi P, Costa A. Migraine and psychiatric comorbidity: a review of clinical findings. J Headache Pain. 2011;12:115–25.
13. Jette N, Patten S, Williams J, Becker W, Wiebe S. Comorbidity of migraine and psychiatric disorders--a national population-based study. Headache. 2008;48:501–16.
14. Yang Y, Zhao H, Heath AC, Madden PA, Martin NG, Nyholt DR. Shared genetic factors underlie migraine and depression. Twin Res Hum Genet. 2016;19:341–50.
15. Arruda MA, Guidetti V, Galli F, Albuquerque RC, Bigal ME. Migraine, tension-type headache, and attention-deficit/hyperactivity disorder in childhood: a population-based study. Postgrad Med. 2010;122:18–26.
16. Fasmer OB, Halmoy A, Oedegaard KJ, Haavik J. Adult attention deficit hyperactivity disorder is associated with migraine headaches. Eur Arch Psychiatry Clin Neurosci. 2011;261:595–602.
17. Fasmer OB, Riise T, Lund A, Dilsaver SC, Hundal O, Oedegaard KJ. Comorbidity of migraine with ADHD. J Atten Disord. 2012;16:339–45.
18. Instanes JT, Klungsoyr K, Halmoy A, Fasmer OB, Haavik J. Adult ADHD and comorbid somatic disease: a systematic literature review. J Atten Disord. 2016.
19. Arruda MA, Arruda R, Guidetti V, Bigal ME. ADHD is comorbid to migraine in childhood: a population-based study. J Atten Disord. 2017: 1087054717710767. https://www.ncbi.nlm.nih.gov/pubmed/28587507.
20. Salem H, Vivas D, Cao F, Kazimi IF, Teixeira AL, Zeni CP. ADHD is associated with migraine: a systematic review and meta-analysis. Eur Child Adolesc Psychiatry. 2018;27(3):267–77.
21. Burgdorf KS, Felsted N, Mikkelsen S, et al. Digital questionnaire platform in the Danish blood donor study. Comput Methods Prog Biomed. 2016;135:101–4.
22. Pedersen OB, Erikstrup C, Kotze SR, et al. The Danish blood donor study: a large, prospective cohort and biobank for medical research. Vox Sang. 2012;102:271.
23. Gervil M, Ulrich V, Olesen J, Russell MB. Screening for migraine in the general population: validation of a simple questionnaire. Cephalalgia. 1998;18:342–8.
24. Kessler RC, Adler L, Ames M, et al. The World Health Organization adult ADHD self-report scale (ASRS): a short screening scale for use in the general population. Psychol Med. 2005;35:245–56.
25. NKR: Udredning og behandling af ADHD hos voksne. at https://www.sst.dk/da/udgivelser/2015/nkr-adhd-hos-voksne. Accessed 1 Dec 2017.
26. Poulsen L, Jorgensen SL, Dalsgaard S, Bilenberg N. Danish standardization of the attention deficit hyperactivity disorder rating scale. Ugeskr Laeger. 2009;171:1500–4.
27. Adler LA, Spencer T, Faraone SV, et al. Validity of pilot adult ADHD self-report scale (ASRS) to rate adult ADHD symptoms. Ann Clin Psychiatry. 2006;18:145–8.
28. Kessler RC, Adler LA, Gruber MJ, Sarawate CA, Spencer T, Van Brunt DL. Validity of the World Health Organization adult ADHD self-report scale (ASRS) screener in a representative sample of health plan members. Int J Methods Psychiatr Res. 2007;16:52–65.
29. Kim JH, Lee EH, Joung YS. The WHO adult ADHD self-report scale: reliability and validity of the Korean version. Psychiatry Investig. 2013;10:41–6.
30. Sonnby K, Skordas K, Olofsdotter S, Vadlin S, Nilsson KW, Ramklint M. Validation of the World Health Organization adult ADHD self-report scale for adolescents. Nord J Psychiatry. 2015;69:216–23.
31. Emilien G, Maloteaux JM, Geurts M, Hoogenberg K, Cragg S. Dopamine receptors--physiological understanding to therapeutic intervention potential. Pharmacol Ther. 1999;84:133–56.
32. Fasmer OB. The prevalence of migraine in patients with bipolar and unipolar affective disorders. Cephalalgia. 2001;21:894–9.
33. Fasmer OB, Oedegaard KJ. Clinical characteristics of patients with major affective disorders and comorbid migraine. World J Biol Psychiatry. 2001;2:149–55.
34. Low NC, Du Fort GG, Cervantes P. Prevalence, clinical correlates, and treatment of migraine in bipolar disorder. Headache. 2003;43:940–9.
35. Breslau N, Merikangas K, Bowden CL. Comorbidity of migraine and major affective disorders. Neurology. 1994;44:S17–22.
36. d'Onofrio F, Barbanti P, Petretta V, et al. Migraine and movement disorders. Neurol Sci. 2012;33(Suppl 1):S55–9.
37. Brainstorm C, Anttila V, Bulik-Sullivan B, et al. Analysis of shared heritability in common disorders of the brain. Science. 2018:360.
38. Johansson S, Halleland H, Halmoy A, et al. Genetic analyses of dopamine related genes in adult ADHD patients suggest an association with the DRD5-microsatellite repeat, but not with DRD4 or SLC6A3 VNTRs. Am J Med Genet B Neuropsychiatr Genet. 2008;147B:1470–5.
39. Pakalnis A, Gibson J, Colvin A. Comorbidity of psychiatric and behavioral disorders in pediatric migraine. Headache. 2005;45:590–6.
40. Millstein RB, Wilens TE, Biederman J, Spencer TJ. Presenting ADHD symptoms and subtypes in clinically referred adults with ADHD. J Atten Disord. 1997;2:159–66.
41. Lauritzen M. Pathophysiology of the migraine aura. The spreading depression theory. Brain. 1994;117(Pt 1):199–210.
42. Gronlund MA, Aring E, Landgren M, Hellstrom A. Visual function and ocular features in children and adolescents with attention deficit hyperactivity disorder, with and without treatment with stimulants. Eye (Lond). 2007;21: 494–502.
43. Bastiaens L, Galus J. Comparison of the adult ADHD self report scale screener for DSM-IV and DSM-5 in a dually diagnosed correctional population. Psychiatr Q. 2018;89:505–10.

Study protocol: Care of Late-Stage Parkinsonism (CLaSP)

Monika Balzer-Geldsetzer[1,10], Joaquim Ferreira[2], Per Odin[3], Bastiaan R. Bloem[4], Wassilios G. Meissner[5,6], Stefan Lorenzl[7,8], Michael Wittenberg[9], Richard Dodel[1,10] and Anette Schrag[11]* [ID]

Abstract

Background: Parkinson's disease (PD) is a chronic progressive disorder leading to increasing disability. While the symptoms and needs of patients in the early stages of their disease are well characterized, little information is available on patients in the late stage of the disease.

Methods/design: The Care of Late-Stage Parkinsonism (CLaSP) study is a longitudinal, multicenter, prospective cohort study to assess the needs and provision of care for patients with late stage Parkinsonism and their carers in six European countries (UK, France, Germany, Netherlands, Portugal, Sweden). In addition, it will compare the effectiveness of different health and social care systems. Patients with Parkinsonism with Hoehn and Yahr stage ≥IV in the "On"-state or Schwab and England stage 50% or less are evaluated at baseline and three follow-up time-points. Standardised questionnaires and tests are applied for detailed clinical, neuropsychological, behavioural and health-economic assessments. A qualitative study explores the health care needs and experiences of patients and carers, and an interventional sub-study evaluates the impact of specialist recommendations on their outcomes.

Discussion: Through the combined assessment of a range of quantitative measures and qualitative assessments of patients with late stage parkinsonism, this study will provide for the first time comprehensive and in-depth information on the clinical presentation, needs and health care provision in this population in Europe, and lay the foundation for improved outcomes in these patients.

Keywords: Late stage parkinsonism, Care provision, Non-motor complications, Quality of care, Health-related quality of life, Health-economic evaluation, Patient-reported outcomes

Introduction

Parkinson's disease (PD) is the second most common neurodegenerative disorder, affecting approximately 1.2 million people in Europe [1]. There is increasing disability with disease progression, but whilst there is an abundant number of studies on the health and social care needs of patients in the early stages of PD, there is surprisingly little information on the medical and care needs of the late stage population, and how these needs are currently met. In addition, there is little information on the use and effectiveness of the pharmacological and non-pharmacological interventions for PD in these late stages, when there may be multiple features and comorbidities. These include motor complications and non-motor symptoms such as behavioral and psychological symptoms, autonomic disturbances and sleep disorders, which can contribute to the burden of the disease to patients and their carers [2, 3] and may lead to nursing home placement and higher mortality [3–5]. Most studies on the management and care needs of patients with PD include only small subgroups in the late stages of the disease [6, 7] and patients in Hoehn and Yahr stages IV

* Correspondence: a.schrag@ucl.ac.uk
[11]UCL Institute of Neurology, University College London, Royal Free Campus, Rowland Hill street, NW3 2PF, London, UK
Full list of author information is available at the end of the article

and V [8] are usually excluded from clinical trials [9]. In specialist practice, the proportion of patients in the late stages is also underrepresented as they are often too disabled to attend hospital or office-based appointments and do not receive adequate care [10]. It is therefore currently relatively unknown what the exact health care needs are in patients with late stage Parkinsonism, and no large study has evaluated the provision of health care for these patients and associated costs across different European health care systems. Small studies point to an increased use of health as well as social care resources (hospitalization and institutionalization) in late PD stages [11–14] and a high need for informal care with increased caregiver burden [12, 14].

The Care of Late-Stage Parkinsonism (CLaSP) study aims to establish a large European cohort of patients with parkinsonism in the late stage of the disease (i.e. HY stages IV/V in the "On"-stage or Schwab and England stage 50% or less) in six European countries to examine the health and social care needs of this patient group and their carers, available health care provision and costs to society. Alongside the cohort study, eligible patients are randomised in an interventional trial evaluating the impact of specialist recommendations in patients in late stages of Parkinsonism, and a qualitative study explores the health care needs and experiences of patients and carers. This article describes in detail the methodology of the study and the assessments used in this large and unique cohort. An abstract on the study design has been previously published [15].

Methods
Study design
The CLaSP study is a longitudinal multicenter cohort study of patients with late stage Parkinsonism and their carers. In the six European health care systems (London and Luton, UK; Marburg-Giessen, Essen, and Munich, Germany; Nijmegen, The Netherlands; Bordeaux, France; Lisbon, Portugal; and Lund, Sweden) patients with late-stage Parkinsonism and their informal carers are identified from neurology, care of the elderly, palliative care, and primary care settings. Patients for the qualitative interviews and for the intervention trial are recruited from the participants in the cohort study.

Cohort study
Inclusion criteria
Patients are eligible for enrolment in the CLaSP study, if they had been diagnosed for at least seven years with Parkinsonism and are classified as Hoehn and Yahr stage (HY) IV or V in the "On"-state OR have developed significant disability (Schwab and England stage ≤50%) in the "On"-state [16]. Established clinical criteria (UK Parkinson's Disease Society Brain Bank Diagnostic Criteria

[17]) are applied to distinguish subjects with PD from those with different atypical parkinsonian syndromes. However, since distinction in late stages of the disease can be difficult and patient needs are likely to be similar despite different underlying pathology, patients with atypical parkinsonian disorders are not excluded.

Exclusion criteria
Patients with PD in HY stages I-III are excluded as well as patients with a diagnosis of "symptomatic PD" such as normal pressure hydrocephalus or drug-induced Parkinsonism, except if persisting following discontinuation of the causative drug.

Assessments (see Table 1) are conducted in person at baseline and at 12 months, with optional telephone follow-up at 6 and 18 months.

Interventional trial
Inclusion criteria
For the interventional trial, patients are eligible if they experience at least one of the following insufficiently treated symptoms/problems (based on clinical judgment): motor parkinsonism according to Unified Parkinson's Disease Rating Scale (UPDRS; including nocturnal motor problems), levodopa-induced motor complications, including Off-time > 50% of waking day (assessed on UPDRS part IV), moderately disabling dyskinesias (item 33 ≥ 2) or Off time dystonia, PD dementia (defined according to MDS Task Force definition [18], depression (GDS > 4 points) not receiving adequate treatment, psychotic symptoms, agitation/ aggression; anxiety and irritability/ liability (all NPI items > 4 points), symptomatic orthostatic hypotension, pain, constipation, urinary symptoms, insomnia or daytime sleepiness, falls OR are treated medications potentially associated with exacerbation of PD-related problems: (a) typical antipsychotics other than quetiapine or clozapine, anticholinergics, benzodiazepines, pills with protein rich meal, antihypertensives in symptomatic hypotensive patients, valproate, calcium antagonists, other medications with side effect exacerbating PD motor or non-motor symptoms OR are at risk of contractures and skin ulceration OR inadequate management of dysphagia with risk of choking, of dysarthria or of hypersalivation OR live in an inadequate home environment.

Exclusion criteria
Patients with parkinsonism seen by a movement disorders specialist in the four months prior to inclusion, and patients unable to comply with management plans (such as attending physiotherapy or change of medication) are excluded from the intervention trial.

Participants fulfilling the inclusion criteria are randomised in an open-label trial to two-arms in 3:1 allocation:

Table 1 Assessment instruments and time points of application

Scales/Domains	Instruments	Reference	Application at			
			T1	T2	T3	T4
Patient-completed						
Quality of life and health status	EuroQol instrument	[20]	x	x	(x)	(x)
	PDQ-8[a]	[21]	x	x	x	x
Meaning in Life	SMiLE	[22]	x	x	(x)	(x)
Satisfaction with Care	Likert scale		x	x	(x)	(x)
Carer-completed						
Quality of life and health status	EuroQol instrument	[20]	x	x	(x)	(x)
Patient Quality of Life	DEMQOL-Proxy[b]	[23]	x	x	x	x
Satisfaction with Support	Likert Scale		x	x	(x)	(x)
Caregiver burden	Zarit burden scale	[24]	x	x	(x)	(x)
Clinician-completed						
Activities of daily living	UPDRS (pt. II)	[25]	x	x	x	x
	Schwab&England	[16]	x	x	x	x
Demographic/social data			x			
Checklist of symptoms, treatments, tests						
Comorbidities	Charlson-Index	[34]	x	x	(x)	(x)
Resource Utilisation questionnaire		[19]	x	x	x	
Clinical rating/judgement	CGI	[26]	x	x	x	x
	Hoehn and Yahr	[8]	x	x	(x)	(x)
	UPDRS (pts. I, III, IV)	[25]	x	x	(x)	(x)
Cognitive assessment	MMSE+clock drawing+fluency	[27–29]	x	x	(x)	(x)
	Pill questionnaire	[18]	x	x	(x)	(x)
Neuropsychiatric and other non-motor symptoms	Neuropsychiatric Inventory (NPI-12)	[30]	x	x	(x)	(x)
	Non-motor symptom scale	[31]	x	x	x	x
	Geriatric Depression Scale (GDS)	[32]	x	x	(x)	(x)
Basic palliative assessment	ESAS-(PD)	[33]	x	x	(x)	(x)
Supine and standing blood pressure			x			
Evaluation of Implementation				x		

[a]in patients with a diagnosis Parkinson's disease only; [b]in patients with dementia instead of PDQ8 and EQ-5D; (x) optional; T1 = Baseline with randomisation, T2: 6 months after baseline (in-person for intervention participants only), T3: 12 months after baseline (telephone with patient and/or carer or optional in-person assessment), and T4: 18 months after baseline (telephone with patient and/or carer or optional in-person assessment). Abbreviations used: PDQ-8 The Parkinson's Disease Questionnaire, short form, SMiLE Schedule for Meaning in Life Evaluation. Euroqol-Instrument (EQ-5D Index and visual analogue scale), DEMQOL-Proxy health-related quality of life for people with dementia - proxy version. CGI Clinical Global Impression, UPDRS Unified Parkinson's Disease Rating Scale, UPDRS Unified Parkinson's Disease Rating Scale, MMSE Mini Mental State Examination, ESAS-PD Edmonton Symptom Assessment System – Parkinson's Disease

to an intervention or care as usual, and assessed at 6 months (in-person; primary outcome) and optionally at 12 and 18 months (telephone review, secondary outcome). The intervention consists of individually tailored treatment strategies suggested by specialists after review of the baseline assessment and treatment regime.

Qualitative study
Inclusion criteria
For the qualitative study, approximately 10 PD patients and an informal carer in each participating center (London, UK, Lund, Sweden, and Lisbon, Portugal) are being recruited

consecutively. For inclusion, the same criteria apply as for the cohort study.

Exclusion criteria
In addition to the exclusion criteria of the cohort study, patients unable to communicate in words (because of either dysarthria or language problems) are excluded from the qualitative study.

Semi-structured interviews with patients and informal carers are conducted on the needs of patients with late stage Parkinsonism. The questions addressed are: perceived met and unmet needs, including palliative care needs, the experience and perceived impact of receipt of services, formal and informal support, exploration of deficits and barriers to adequate care provision, identification of factors influencing the decision as to whether patients are cared for at home or in residential care/institution, and advanced care planning (attitudes of patients towards advance directives and preferred place of death). These interviews are audio-recorded and transcribed; and then subject to thematic analysis aided by the N-VIVO computer program to identify the range of experiences and perceived needs and outcomes of different services provisions and treatments.

Recruitment strategies

The major challenge in the CLaSP project is the identification, recruitment, and assessment of patients in late stages. We particularly aim to include patients who are not under regular specialist follow-up. Therefore, several methods to reach this target group are employed, particularly aiming to recruit individuals not currently attending routine specialist clinics: The centers contacted general practitioners, hospitals, nursing homes, patient advocate groups as well as self-help groups to draw attention to the CLaSP project and identify and recruit eligible patients.

Clinical assessment

Cohort study

The assessment of patients and carer comprise of standardised questionnaires to evaluate disease severity, comorbidities, depression, cognition, non-motor symptoms, quality of life in patients and carers as well as caregiver burden (for an overview of timepoints and instruments/questionnaires applied, see Table 1). The patients of the cohort study are followed up in person at 12 months and optionally via telephone at 6-month and 18 months. A special resource use questionnaire for patients with Parkinson's disease and their carers was developed and used in a previous health economic cost of illness study [19] was applied. The questionnaire was adapted to the requirements of the respective country-specific health care system.

Intervention study

Baseline assessments are repeated at 6 months (T2) in person and on the telephone at 12 months. In addition, at T2, information is collected whether the individual intervention has been implemented into the patient's treatment schedule.

Outcome measures

The following instruments are used to collect data on the patients and their caregivers at different time points during the study (see also Table 1):

Health-related quality of life in PD patients and their caregivers is evaluated using the self-completed, generic EuroQol instrument, which comprises a questionnaire (EQ-5D) and a visual analogue scale (EQ VAS) [20]. The questionnaire consists of five questions with three levels of possible answers, representing the dimensions Mobility, Self-Care, Usual Activities, Pain/Discomfort, and Anxiety/Depression. In the EQ VAS, the participants rate their subjective health status on a scale with a range of 0 to 100 with higher scores indicating a better quality of life. Additionally, the self-administered, disease-specific PDQ-8 instrument is used in patients [21]. It is derived from the PDQ-39 and assesses eight domains: Activities of Daily Living, Attention and Working Memory, Communication, Depression, Quality of Life, and Social Relationships. Higher scores in the PDQ-8 indicate more problems and a worse quality of life. Satisfaction with Care is assessed in the patient via a 5-point Likert scale, with higher rating reflecting less satisfaction. The Schedule for Meaning in Life Evaluation (SMiLE) is an instrument to assess individual meaning in life [22]. First, the patients list one to seven areas that provide meaning to their lives and subsequently rate the current level of importance and satisfaction of each area. From these answers, a sum score can be calculated where higher scores indicate higher satisfaction in life. The DEMQOL proxy is used to obtain caregiver reports on the patient's quality of life [23]. In our study, it is applied in patients with dementia instead of the PDQ-8 and the Euroqol instrument. Satisfaction with Support is assessed in the caregiver via a 5-point Likert scale, with higher rating indicating less satisfaction. The caregiver burden is assessed via the revised 22-items version of the Zarit Burden Scale [24]. Each item on the interview is answered by the caregiver on a 5-point scale with higher sum scores reflecting higher burden on the caregiver. The clinician completes the following assessments on the patient: For the clinical evaluation of Parkinson's disease, the Unified Parkinson's disease Rating Scale (UPDRS) is used to assess patients in four sections: Mentation, Behavior and Mood, Activities of Daily Living, Motor Examination, and Complications of Therapy [25]. In addition, the Hoehn and Yahr scale (HY) is used to describe the stage of PD severity [8]. The patient's ability to perform activities of daily living is assessed with the Schwab & England Scale [16]. The score reflects the patient's situation on a 0 (= complete dependence/bedridden) to 100% (= complete independence) scale. The Clinical Global Impression (CGI) rating scale is used to evaluate the patients' symptom severity and change of symptoms over time [26]. The Mini-Mental State Examination (MMSE) is an assessment tool for general cognitive impairment, with higher overall total scores (range 0–30) indicating better performance [27]. The clock-drawing test is used for screening for cognitive impairment and dementia [28], which is sensitive to visuo-spatial impairment. The verbal fluency test (letter s) is used as a short test of executive function [29]. The Pill Questionnaire is a screening tool for mild cognitive impairment in nondemented Parkinson's disease patients, using the ability to remember Parkinson's disease-specific medications as an indicator of cognitive function [18]. The Neuropsychiatric Inventory (NPI-12) is an informant-based instrument to assess the presence and severity of twelve neuropsychiatric symptoms (i.e. delusions, hallucinations, agitation/aggression, dysphoria/depression, anxiety, euphoria/elation, apathy/indifference, disinhibition, irritability/lability, aberrant motor behaviors, night-time behavioral disturbances, appetite/eating disturbances) in patients with dementia, as well as informant distress [30]. To assess the occurrence and severity of non-motor symptoms, the Non-Motor Symptom Scale (NMSS) is used [31]. The Geriatric Depression Scale (GDS) is a 15-item screening tool with higher overall total scores (range 0–15) indicating higher depression levels [32]. The modified Edmonton Symptom Assessment System Scale for PD (ESAS-PD) was modified from symptom assessment in palliative care for patients with PD [33]. Comorbidities are assessed with the Charlson Comorbidity Index (CCI) [34].

Primary endpoint

The primary endpoint is the absolute change in UPDRS-ADL score from baseline to month 6 (intervention study) and to month 12 (cohort study). The UPDRS is administered by a researcher blinded to the treatment group.

Secondary endpoints

Secondary endpoints are the patients' quality of life, mental health, disease severity and disability, non-motor symptoms scale score, occurrence of disease severity milestones (psychosis, dementia, falls, wheelchair-bound, institutionalization, and death), satisfaction with care as well as caregiver burden.

Ethical approval

The CLaSP study is being conducted in compliance with the Helsinki Declaration [35], i.e. detailed oral and written information is given to the patients and their informant to ensure that the patient fully understands potential risks and benefits of the study. The study protocol was approved by the local ethics committees of all participating study sites (London:Camden and Islington NRES Committee 14/LO/0612, Bordeaux: South West and Overseas Protection Committee III (South West and Overseas Protection Committee). 2014-A01501–46, Lisbon:Centro Hospitalar Lisboa Norte, DIRCLN-19SET2014–275, Lund: EPN Regionala etikprovningsnamnden: Lund (EPN Regional Ethics Name: Lund). *JPND NC 559–002*, Marburg: Ethik-Kommission bei der Landesarztekammer Hessen

(Ethics Commission at the State Medical Association Hesse). MC 309/2014, Munich: Ethikkommission bei der LMU Munchen (Ethics committee at the LMU Munchen). 193–14, Nijmegen: Radboud universitair medisch centrum, Concernstaf Kwaliteit en Veiligheid, Commissie Mensgebonden Onderzoek Regio Arnhem-Nijmegen (Radboud university medical center,Group staff Quality and Safety Human Research Committee, Arnhem-Nijmegen region). DJ/CMO300).

Informed consent

Participants (patients and their caregivers) are included in the study after giving their written informed consent. In case the patient lacks capacity to give consent to the study due to severe cognitive impairment, the decision on study participation is made by a legal guardian or consultee, depending on the ethical and legal requirements at each site. All participants (patients and caregivers) can withdraw from the study at any point in time without any negative implications.

Sample size

For the baseline evaluation of the **Cohort study**, at least 70 patients will be recruited per country. Out of this sample, 48 patients per country will be randomised for the intervention study. Permuted block randomization is used, stratified by country, dementia (yes/ no) and residence (nursing home or similar/ home). Applying a one-way ANOVA at a significance level of 5% and power of 80%, a sample size of 70 per country allows to detect differences in UPDRS-ADL scores between health care systems with a standard deviation of means of 1.76. The common standard deviation within each county is assumed to be 10.

For the **Intervention study**, the power calculations were based on the analysis of the primary efficacy endpoint: absolute change in UPDRS-ADL (Unified Parkinson's Disease Rating Scale – part II, activities of daily living) score from baseline to month 6 (time to complete the intervention). Assumptions for mean and standard deviation of change in UPDRS-ADL scores of the intervention group are based on results of a previous study using the UPDRS-ADL [36]. An independent sample t-test was used to determine the sample size needed for detecting a difference in change of 4.8 between the two treatment groups. Assuming a standard deviation of 10 for difference in change, a two-sided significance level of 5%, a power of 80%, and non-participating and dropout rates of 20% each, 216 patients were calculated to be needed for the intervention group and 72 patients to the standard group (3:1 allocation).

Statistical analysis

Categorical variables will be analysed by absolute and relative frequency, continuous variables by median, mean, standard deviation, 95% confidence interval, minimum, and maximum. Differences in continuous variables between groups (e.g. countries) at time points will be tested by analysis of variance (ANOVA) and analysis of covariance (ANCOVA) or their nonparametric analogues, respectively. Differences between groups at time points assessed by proportions will be analysed by the Chi-square or Fisher's exact test, if applicable, and logistic regression.

Changes in continuous variables between two time points will be evaluated by the paired t-test or Wilcoxon signed rank test, respectively. Changes in proportions between two time points will be analysed by the McNemar test. Longitudinal analyses will be performed by applying linear and generalized linear mixed models with patient or carer as random effect, main effects for country and time, as well as a country-by-time interaction term and possible confounders.

In the intervention study, all analyses of outcome parameters will be done in the intent-to-treat population. The primary efficacy analysis will be to investigate the treatment effect on absolute change in UPDRS-ADL score from baseline to month 6 in the intervention and standard care group. Data will be analyzed using ANCOVA with categorical factors (treatment, country, dementia, residence) and baseline UPDRS-ADL score as a covariate. The null hypothesis "no difference in the primary endpoint between the intervention group and standard care group" will be tested against the alternative hypothesis "difference in the primary endpoint between both groups". The primary efficacy analysis will be repeated using the per-protocol population to confirm the overall study results. Safety data will be analyzed in the as-treated population.

All tests will be performed two-sided, p values < 0.05 will be considered statistically significant.

Discussion

Despite a large variety of symptomatic and supportive treatment options, PD remains a progressive and ultimately very disabling disorder, for which as yet no disease-modifying drugs exist. With the increasing population age and rising prevalence of PD expected over the next decades there is a growing challenge in the appropriate care for patients who reach the late stages of this disorder [37]. Improvements in care of late stage Parkinsonism are likely not only to improve patients' health-related quality of life and caregiver burden, but also to reduce health care costs substantially by reducing the rate of institutionalization, hospital admissions, and polypharmacy. The CLaSP study is the first study that specifically characterises the clinical features, comorbidities, health care and social care needs, current treatment strategies and outcomes of patients with late stage parkinsonism across several European countries. It will

evaluate the impact on patients as well as their carers, identify the current provision of health care and how it meets these needs, evaluate the adequacy of standard assessment methods and examine whether specialised, tailored review improves outcomes in patients with parkinsonism. It will also provide essential information on health economic data on the costs of providing health and social care for patients with this condition. Combining the cohorts' detailed assessments, using quantitative and qualitative data, in six different countries and across neurology, geriatric and palliative care settings, and studying this cohort longitudinally, will provide multifaceted, in-depth knowledge on this little studied population. This information can then inform how best to provide effective and cost-effective health and social care for this severely affected patient group and contribute to improved practices for clinical care.

Abbreviations
ANCOVA: Analysis of covariance; ANOVA: Analysis of variance; CLaSP: Care of Late-Stage Parkinsonism; GDS: Geriatric Depression Scale; HY: Hoehn and Yahr stage; MDS : Movement Disorder Society; NPI: Neuropsychiatric Inventory; PD: Parkinson's disease; UPDRS-ADL: Unified Parkinson's Disease Rating Scale – part II, Activities of daily living

Acknowledgements
The authors wish to thank all patients and their families participating in the study and all staff members in the recruiting centres who are contributing to the study.

Funding
The CLaSP study is being funded by the European Commission (Joint Programme – Neurodegenerative Disease Research "European research projects for the evaluation of health care policies, strategies and interventions for Neurodegenerative Diseases") through national funding bodies in all six countries (Economic and Social Research Council ES/L009250/1; BMBF, Marburg, Germany 01ED1403A, Munich, Germany 01ED1403B, Bordeaux, France: ANR-13-JPHC-0001-07, Lisbon, Portugal: HC/0002/2012, Lund, Sweden: HC-559-002, Nijmegen, Holland, 733051003). AS was supported by the National Institute for Health Research UCL/UCLH Biomedical Research Centre.

Authors' contributions
AS and RD conceived the program and wrote the protocol, and WM, BB, PO, MW, JF, SL provided critical review. MBG drafted the manuscript and all authors reviewed and approved the final version of the manuscript.

Ethics approval and consent to participate
All study sites received approval of their local ethics committee before study start; all patients gave their written informed consent before study participation. The CLaSP study is being conducted in compliance with the Helsinki Declaration [35], i.e. detailed oral and written information is given to the patients and their informant to ensure that the patient fully understands potential risks and benefits of the study. The study protocol was approved by the local ethics committees of all participating study sites (London:Camden and Islington NRES Committee 14/LO/0612, Bordeaux: South West and Overseas Protection Committee III (South West and Overseas Protection Committee). 2014-A01501–46, Lisbon:Centro Hospitalar Lisboa Norte, DIRCLN-19SET2014–275, Lund: EPN Regionala etikprovningsnamnden: Lund (EPN Regional Ethics Name: Lund). *JPND NC 559–002*, Marburg: Ethik-Kommission bei der Landesarztekammer Hessen (Ethics Commission at the State Medical Association Hesse). MC 309/2014, Munich: Ethikkommission bei der LMU Munchen (Ethics committee at the LMU Munchen). 193–14, Nijmegen: Radboud universitair medisch centrum,

Concernstaf Kwaliteit en Veiligheid, Commissie Mensgebonden Onderzoek Regio Arnhem-Nijmegen (Radboud university medical center,Group staff Quality and Safety Human Research Committee, Arnhem-Nijmegen region). DJ/CMO300).

Informed consent

Participants (patients and their caregivers) are included in the study after giving their written informed consent. In case the patient lacks capacity to give consent to the study due to severe cognitive impairment, the decision on study participation is made by a legal guardian or consultee, depending on the ethical and legal requirements at each site. All participants (patients and caregivers) can withdraw from the study at any point in time without any negative implications.

Competing interests

The authors declare that they have no competing interests.

Author details

[1]Department of Neurology, Philipps-University Marburg, Marburg, Germany. [2]Instituto de Medicina Molecular Universidad di Lisboa, Lisboa, Portugal. [3]Department of Neurology, Lund University Hospital, Lund, Sweden. [4]Donders Institute for Brain, Cognition and Behaviour, Department of Neurology, Radboud University Medical Center, Nijmegen, The Netherlands. [5]Service de Neurologie, CHU de Bordeaux, 33000 Bordeaux, France. [6]Institut des Maladies Neurodégénératives, University de Bordeaux, UMR 5293, 33000 Bordeaux, France. [7]Interdisziplinäres Zentrum für Palliativmedizin und Klinik für Neurologie Universität München - Klinikum Großhadern, Munich, Germany. [8]Institute of Nursing Science and –Practice, Salzburg, Austria. [9]Coordinating Centre for Clinical Trials (KKS), Philipps-University Marburg, Marburg, Germany. [10]Department of Geriatric Medicine, University Hospital Essen, Essen, Germany. [11]UCL Institute of Neurology, University College London, Royal Free Campus, Rowland Hill street, NW3 2PF, London, UK.

References

1. Gustavsson A, Svensson M, Jacobi F, Allgulander C, Alonso J, Beghi E, et al. Cost of disorders of the brain in Europe 2010. Eur Neuropsychopharmacol. 2011;21:718–79. https://doi.org/10.1016/j.euroneuro.2011.08.008.
2. Barone P, Antonini A, Colosimo C, Marconi R, Morgante L, Avarello TP, et al. The PRIAMO study: a multicenter assessment of nonmotor symptoms and their impact on quality of life in Parkinson's disease. Mov Disord. 2009;24: 1641–9. https://doi.org/10.1002/mds.22643.
3. Aarsland D, Larsen JP, Karlsen K, Lim NG, Tandberg E. Mental symptoms in Parkinson's disease are important contributors to caregiver distress. Int J Geriatr Psychiatry. 1999;14:866–74.
4. Goetz CG, Stebbins GT. Risk factors for nursing home placement in advanced Parkinson's disease. Neurology. 1993;43:2227–9.
5. Vossius C, Nilsen OB, Larsen JP. Parkinson's disease and nursing home placement: the economic impact of the need for care. Eur J Neurol. 2009; 16:194–200. https://doi.org/10.1111/j.1468-1331.2008.02380.x.
6. Beiske AG, Loge JH, Ronningen A, Svensson E. Pain in Parkinson's disease: prevalence and characteristics. Pain. 2009;141:173–7. https://doi.org/10.1016/ j.pain.2008.12.004.
7. Ghoche R. The conceptual framework of palliative care applied to advanced Parkinson's disease. Parkinsonism Relat Disord. 2012;18(Suppl 3):S2–5. https://doi.org/10.1016/j.parkreldis.2012.06.012.
8. Hoehn MM, Yahr MD. Parkinsonism: onset, progression and mortality. Neurology. 1967;17:427–42.
9. Coelho M., Destri, K. Fabbri M., Schrag A., Ferreira J., b.C. Consortium. Efficacy and safety of therapeutic interventions to treat motor symptoms in late stage Parkinson's disease: a systematic review. Mov Disord 2017.
10. Weerkamp NJ, Zuidema SU, Tissingh G, Poels PJE, Munneke M, Koopmans RTCM, Bloem BR. Motor profile and drug treatment of nursing home

11. Findley LJ, Wood E, Lowin J, Roeder C, Bergman A, Schifflers M. The economic burden of advanced Parkinson's disease: an analysis of a UK patient dataset. J Med Econ. 2011;14:130–9. https://doi.org/10.3111/ 13696998.2010.551164.
12. Reese JP, Dams J, Winter Y, Balzer-Geldsetzer M, Oertel WH, Dodel R. Pharmacoeconomic considerations of treating patients with advanced Parkinson's disease. Expert Opin Pharmacother. 2012;13:939–58. https://doi. org/10.1517/14656566.2012.677435.
13. Valldeoriola F, Coronell C, Pont C, Buongiorno MT, Cámara A, Gaig C, Compta Y. Socio-demographic and clinical factors influencing the adherence to treatment in Parkinson's disease: the ADHESON study. Eur J Neurol. 2011;18:980–7. https://doi.org/10.1111/j.1468-1331.2010.03320.x.
14. Bach J-P, Riedel O, Klotsche J, Spottke A, Dodel R, Wittchen H-U. Impact of complications and comorbidities on treatment costs and health-related quality of life of patients with Parkinson's disease. J Neurol Sci. 2012;314:41–7. https://doi.org/10.1016/j.jns.2011.11.002.
15. Coelho M, Balzer-Geldsetzer M, Ferreira JJ, Odin P, Bloem BR, Meissner W, Lorenzl S, Wittenberg M, Dodel R, Schrag AE, Care of Late-Stage Parkinsonism (CLASP). A longitudinal cohort study. Eur J Neurol. 2018; 25(Suppl. 2):277–573.
16. Schwab RS, England AC Jr, editors. Projection technique for evaluating surgery in Parkinson's disease. Edinburgh: E & S Livingstone; 1969.
17. Hughes AJ, Daniel SE, Kilford L, Lees AJ, Accuracy of clinical diagnosis of idiopathic Parkinson's disease. A clinico-pathological study of 100 cases. J Neurol Neurosurg Psychiatry. 1992;55:181–4.
18. Dubois B, Burn D, Goetz C, Aarsland D, Brown RG, Broe GA, et al. Diagnostic procedures for Parkinson's disease dementia: recommendations from the movement disorder society task force. Mov Disord. 2007;22:2314–24. https://doi.org/10.1002/mds.21844.
19. von Campenhausen S, Winter Y, Rodrigues e Silva A, Sampaio C, Ruzicka E, Barone P, et al. Costs of illness and care in Parkinson's disease: an evaluation in six countries. Eur Neuropsychopharmacol. 2011;21:180–91. https://doi.org/ 10.1016/j.euroneuro.2010.08.002.
20. Brooks R, EuroQol. The current state of play. Health Policy. 1996;37:53–72.
21. Peto V, Jenkinson C, Fitzpatrick R, PDQ-39. A review of the development, validation and application of a Parkinson's disease quality of life questionnaire and its associated measures. J Neurol. 1998;245(Suppl 1):S10–4.
22. Fegg MJ, Kramer M, L'hoste S, Borasio GD. The schedule for meaning in life evaluation (SMiLE): validation of a new instrument for meaning-in-life research. J Pain Symptom Manag. 2008;35:356–64. https://doi.org/10.1016/j. jpainsymman.2007.05.007.
23. Smith SC, Lamping DL, Banerjee S, Harwood RH, Foley B, Smith P, et al. Development of a new measure of health-related quality of life for people with dementia: DEMQOL. Psychol Med. 2007;37:737–46. https://doi.org/10. 1017/S0033291706009469.
24. Zarit SH, Reever KE, Bach-Peterson J. Relatives of the impaired elderly: correlates of feelings of burden. Gerontologist. 1980;20:649–55.
25. Fahn S, Elton R. Members of the updrs development committee. Florham Park: Recent Developments in Parkinson's Disease; 1987.
26. Guy W. ECDEU Assessment Manual for psychopharmacology. Rockville: U.S. Department of Health, education, and welfare; 1976.
27. Folstein MF, Folstein SE, McHugh PR. "Mini-mental state". A practical method for grading the cognitive state of patients for the clinician. J Psychiatr Res. 1975;12:189–98.
28. Agrell B, Dehlin O. The clock-drawing test. Age and ageing. 1998;27:399–403.
29. Holtzer R, Goldin Y, Zimmerman M, Katz M, Buschke H, Lipton RB. Robust norms for selected neuropsychological tests in older adults. Arch Clin Neuropsychol. 2008;23:531–41. https://doi.org/10.1016/j.acn. 2008.05.004.
30. Cummings JL, Mega M, Gray K, Rosenberg-Thompson S, Carusi DA, Gornbein J. The neuropsychiatric inventory: comprehensive assessment of psychopathology in dementia. Neurology. 1994;44:2308–14.
31. Chaudhuri KR, Martinez-Martin P, Brown RG, Sethi K, Stocchi F, Odin P, et al. The metric properties of a novel non-motor symptoms scale for Parkinson's disease: results from an international pilot study. Mov Disord. 2007;22:1901– 11. https://doi.org/10.1002/mds.21596.
32. Yesavage JA, Brink TL, Rose TL, Lum O, Huang V, Adey M, Leirer VO. Development and validation of a geriatric depression screening scale: a preliminary report. J Psychiatr Res. 1982-1983;17:37–49.

residents with Parkinson's disease. J Am Geriatr Soc. 2012;60:2277–82. https://doi.org/10.1111/jgs.12027.

33. Miyasaki JM, Okun MS. The emerging field of palliative care for Parkinson's disease. Letter from the guest. Parkinsonism Relat Disord. 2012;18(Suppl 3): S1. https://doi.org/10.1016/j.parkreldis.2012.10.012.

34. Charlson ME, Pompei P, Ales KL, MacKenzie CR. A new method of classifying prognostic comorbidity in longitudinal studies: development and validation. J Chronic Dis. 1987;40:373–83.

35. World Medical Association Declaration of Helsinki. JAMA. 1997;277:925. https://doi.org/10.1001/jama.1997.03540350075038.

36. Makoutonina M, Iansek R, Simpson P. Optimizing care of residents with parkinsonism in supervised facilities. Parkinsonism Relat Disord. 2010;16:351–5. https://doi.org/10.1016/j.parkreldis.2010.02.010.

37. Dorsey ER, Bloem BR. The Parkinson pandemic: a call to action. JAMA Neurology. 2018;75(1):9–10.

Comparative effectiveness of beta-interferons and glatiramer acetate for relapsing-remitting multiple sclerosis

G. J. Melendez-Torres[1]*(iD), Xavier Armoiry[1], Rachel Court[1], Jacoby Patterson[2], Alan Kan[1], Peter Auguste[1], Jason Madan[1], Carl Counsell[3], Olga Ciccarelli[4,5] and Aileen Clarke[1]

Abstract

Background: We systematically reviewed the comparative effectiveness of injectable beta-interferons (IFN-β) and glatiramer acetate (GA) on annualised relapse rate (ARR), progression and discontinuation due to adverse events (AEs) in RRMS, using evidence from within the drugs' recommended dosages.

Methods: We updated prior comprehensive reviews, checked references of included studies, contacted experts in the field, and screened websites for relevant publications to locate randomised trials of IFN-β and GA with recommended dosages in RRMS populations, compared against placebo or other recommended dosages. Abstracts were screened and assessed for inclusion in duplicate and independently. Studies were appraised using the Cochrane risk of bias tool. Rate ratios for ARR, hazard ratios for time to progression, and risk ratios for discontinuation due to AEs were synthesised in separate models using random effects network meta-analysis.

Results: We identified 24 studies reported in 42 publications. Most studies were at high risk of bias in at least one domain. All drugs had a beneficial effect on ARR as compared to placebo, but not compared to each other, and findings were robust to sensitivity analysis. We considered time to progression confirmed at 3 months and confirmed at 6 months in separate models; while both models suggested that the included drugs were effective, findings were not consistent between models. Discontinuation due to AEs did not appear to be different between drugs.

Conclusions: Meta-analyses confirmed that IFN-β and GA reduce ARR and generally delay progression as defined in these trials, though there was no clear 'winner' across outcomes. Findings are additionally tempered by the high risk of bias across studies, and the use of an impairment/mobility scale to measure disease progression. Future research should consider more relevant measures of disability and, given that most trials have been short-term, consider a longitudinal approach to comparative effectiveness.

Review registration: PROSPERO CRD42016043278.

Keywords: Multiple sclerosis, Clinically isolated syndrome, Beta-interferon, Glatiramer acetate, Systematic review, Economic evaluation

* Correspondence: g.melendez-torres@warwick.ac.uk
[1]Warwick Evidence, Warwick Medical School, University of Warwick, Coventry CV4 7AL, UK
Full list of author information is available at the end of the article

Background

Injectable beta-interferons (IFN-β) and glatiramer acetate (GA) are mainstays of first-line treatment for relapsing-remitting multiple sclerosis (RRMS), with the primary goals of reducing the rate of relapses and delaying disease progression. Newer therapies such as alemtuzumab yield greater effects in reducing relapse rate and slowing disease progression, and patients may prefer therapies such as dimethyl fumarate or teriflunomide because of their oral mode of administration. However, amongst other disease-modifying therapies (DMTs), IFN-β and GA both have well-established long-term safety profiles without the severe side effects presented by other drugs. While IFN-β and GA are not appropriate for aggressive forms of RRMS (i.e. highly active RRMS or rapidly evolving-severe RRMS), the Association of British Neurologists (ABN) classifies these as 'drugs of moderate efficacy' [1]. Beginning in 2017, an appraisal committee of the UK National Institute for Health and Care Excellence received evidence as part of its reconsideration of the clinical and cost effectiveness of IFN-β and GA for use in the UK National Health Service. The work presented here, the full record of which can be found at [2], draws from our report to this appraisal committee.

There are currently five licensed IFN-β drugs indicated for RRMS. These include: two IFN β-1a (Avonex® (Biogen, Cambridge, Massachusetts, USA), administered via intramuscular injection once weekly at a dose of 30 μg; and Rebif® (Merck, Darmstadt, Germany), administered via subcutaneous injection three times weekly at a dose of either 44 or 22 μg); one pegylated IFN β-1a (Plegridy® (Biogen, Cambridge, Massachusetts, USA), administered via subcutaneous injection every 2 weeks at a dose of 125 μg); and two equivalent IFN β-1b (Betaferon® (Bayer, Leverkusen, Germany) and Extavia® (Novartis, Bale, Switzerland), both administered via subcutaneous injection every other day at a dose of 250 μg). Moreover, there are two licensed formulations of GA (Copaxone® (Teva, Petah Tikva, Israel)), both administered via subcutaneous injection: one at a dose of 20 mg daily, and another at a dose of 40 mg three times weekly. The mechanisms by which either type of drug exerts its effects in patients with MS are not fully understood, but it is now thought that these drugs induce a broad immunomodulatory effect that modifies the immune processes responsible for the pathogenesis of MS.

Though several systematic reviews incorporating network meta-analyses (NMAs) have considered the comparative effectiveness of treatments for RRMS, these have considered doses that do not correspond to the marketing authorisation and thus are not relevant to clinical practice (Tramacere et al. [3], Filippini et al. [4]), excluded relevant doses within drugs' marketing authorisations (Tolley et al. [5]), or included trials across differing severities of MS (Hadjigeorgiou et al. [6]). Our goal in this systematic review and NMA is to provide an up-to-date and consistent summary of the comparative effectiveness of IFN-β and GA on annualised relapse rate (ARR), disability progression and discontinuation due to adverse events (AEs) in RRMS, using evidence from within the drugs' recommended dosages.

Methods

This systematic review was part of a larger evidence synthesis project considering the effectiveness of treatments for several types of MS. Our protocol is registered on PROSPERO as CRD42016043278. The methods and results described here draw on our closely related work for the UK National Institute for Health and Care Excellence, the full report of which was provided to the National Institute for Health Research [2]. In the original protocol, we described that we would stratify comparisons by type of MS. Here, we report clinical effectiveness findings relating to RRMS specifically.

Searches

We identified and examined past relevant systematic reviews, conducted update searches in multiple databases, checked references of included studies, contacted experts in the field, and screened websites for relevant publications. We undertook the main database searches in January and February 2016. These update searches were limited by date to the beginning of 2012 (the year the searches were undertaken for the last comprehensive systematic review and NMA by Filippini et al. [4]) onwards, although we included trials without regard to publication date. This review was chosen because of the breadth of its scope, search strategy and eligibility criteria. A full record of searches is provided in Additional file 1.

We included: a) randomised controlled trials published as full-text reports in English (as well as systematic reviews, or meta-analyses to enable reference checking), b) in people diagnosed with RRMS, c) where the intervention was one of the drugs used within indication at the recommended dosage according to the summary of product characteristics as authorised by the European Medicines Agency (EMA), and d) where the comparator was placebo or best supportive care without DMTs, or another of the interventions when used within indication. Included trials had patient populations primarily comprised of RRMS patients. Our primary outcomes were relapse frequency, disease progression, and discontinuation due to adverse events. Outcomes assessed were relapse rate, time to progression, or discontinuation due to adverse events as outcomes. Full exclusion criteria can be found in the review protocol.

Study selection

First, two authors (XA and GJMT) independently examined relevant past systematic reviews (including Tramacere et al. [3], Filippini et al. [4], and Clerico et al. [7]) for studies meeting the inclusion criteria. We verified inclusion of these studies by examining their full text. For updated and new searches, we collected all retrieved records in a specialised database and removed duplicate records. We pilot-tested a screening form based on the predefined study inclusion and exclusion criteria. Subsequently, two reviewers (XA and GJMT) applied the inclusion/exclusion criteria and screened all identified bibliographic records on title/abstract and then using full texts. Any disagreements over eligibility were resolved through consensus or by a third party reviewer (AC). Reasons for exclusion of full text papers were documented.

Appraisal and extraction

All primary studies were appraised using the Cochrane risk of bias assessment tool [8]. For all included studies, the relevant data were extracted independently by two reviewers using a data extraction form informed by the Centre for Reviews and Dissemination [9]. Extracted data were entered into summary evidence Tables. A sample data extraction form is available in Additional file 1. Uncertainty and/or any disagreements were cross-checked with recourse to a third reviewer where necessary and resolved by discussion.

Meta-analysis

We undertook separate meta-analyses corresponding to each of our review outcomes. Data preparation methods to generate summary effect sizes for each study are detailed in Additional file 1.

First, for relapse frequency, we elected to meta-analyse rate ratios (RR) of relapses as an overall measure. This was the most commonly reported measure for relapse frequency. Where necessary, we converted arm-level data into rate ratios. Where studies presented different estimates for relapse frequency, we preferred estimates of protocol-defined, clinician-confirmed relapses over non-protocol-defined relapses or self-reported relapses.

Second, disease progression is frequently defined in clinical trials of DMTs in MS using the Expanded Disability Status Scale (EDSS), a scale which ranges from 0 to 10. While the EDSS is described as a disability scale (and thus, trials present this as disability progression), it is perhaps better understood as a scale measuring impairment and mobility. We used hazard ratios (HR) to examine differences between study arms in time to progression, where progression was confirmed at either 3 or 6 months after an initial signal (generally an increase in EDSS of 0.5 or 1.0 points). We separated estimates for progression confirmed at 3 months and confirmed at 6 months, as we could not establish whether measures were commensurate.

Third, we estimated models for discontinuation due to AEs, using risk ratios as a summary measure. We also estimated one model with studies closest to 24 months of follow-up. This was because risk ratios are time dependent and we could not reliably estimate person-years of follow-up in each arm across all studies to convert study-level estimates to rate ratios.

We pooled outcomes for each intervention-comparator contrast using random effects meta-analysis in Stata v14 and examined these pairwise meta-analyses for heterogeneity, measured as Cochran's Q and I^2. Subsequently, we used the package -network- [10] in Stata v14 to estimate network meta-analyses. We used a common heterogeneity model, where the between-studies variance is assumed equal across comparisons. After estimating a consistency model (i.e. where direct evidence for a contrast between two treatments is assumed to agree with indirect evidence for that contrast), we checked for inconsistency using an omnibus Wald test from a design-by-treatment interaction model and the side-splitting method to test for differences in the effectiveness estimates between direct and indirect evidence. Where evidence of inconsistency existed, we considered the direction of inconsistency. We also assessed transitivity conceptually by examining networks of evidence for imbalance of trial-level effect modifiers (e.g. sex, age and duration of MS diagnosis; date of trial publication), though we did not have enough studies on each comparison to undertake network meta-regression.

Lastly, we used a bootstrapping method to resample from our estimates of intervention effectiveness and develop probabilities of each treatment's relative position to the others. We then used the surface under the cumulative ranking curve (SUCRA) to produce a unified ranking of treatments.

Publication bias

We aimed to use funnel plots to examine studies for the presence of asymmetry, possibly due to publication bias, other reporting biases, heterogeneity or methodological inadequacies in included studies, in pairwise comparisons where there were more than 10 studies for an intervention-comparator contrast.

Results

Search results

We identified 6420 potentially relevant records. We removed 6146 records which did not meet our inclusion criteria at title/abstract stage, leaving 274 records to be examined at full-text. Among these, we excluded 232, leading to 42 publications meeting our inclusion criteria and corresponding to 24 primary studies. Study selection is summarised in Fig. 1. Additional studies related to other MS phenotypes and are described in the full report of our work for the National Institute for Health and Care Excellence [2].

Excluded studies

We excluded two trials in relevant populations and interventions because they did not present relevant outcomes (Schwartz 1997 [11]) or did not present outcomes in a form suitable for meta-analysis (Mokhber 2014 [12]). We also excluded one small trial with a mixed RRMS/SPMS population (REMAIN 2012 [13], RRMS $n = 13$) as treatment switching was explicitly allowed and data were not stratified by type of MS. Breakdown of studies by exclusion criterion is summarised in Additional file 2.

Included studies

We included 24 trials published between 1987 and 2015. Included studies are detailed in Table 1. In total, 14 trials were placebo-controlled, of which three (BRAVO 2014 [14], CONFIRM 2012 [15] and Kappos 2011 [16]) principally aimed to test the effectiveness of a new agent against either IFN-β or GA alongside a placebo control. The remaining 10 trials only compared active drugs against each other. One trial (AVANTAGE 2014 [17]) reported only adverse events data. The modal follow-up was 24 months.

Risk of bias

Risk of bias assessments are detailed in Table 2. All studies that adequately detailed their method of randomisation ($n = 15$, 63%) were appraised as being at low risk of

bias in this domain. A similar number of studies ($n = 15$) were judged to be at low risk of bias from allocation concealment, though one study (Bornstein 1987 [18]) was classed as at high risk of bias in this domain. We judged that most studies were at high risk of bias in blinding of participants and personnel ($n = 24$, 83%) and blinding of outcome assessment ($n = 18$, 75%) due to a combination of injection site reactions in placebo-controlled trials and an open label design. Five studies (21%) were at high risk of bias from incomplete outcome data due to differential attrition between arms, and we believed that four studies (17%) were at high risk of bias from selective reporting. Finally, most studies ($n = 17$, 71%) were at high risk of bias from other sources, generally stemming from industry sponsorship.

Annualised relapse rates

Direct evidence from comparisons is shown in Fig. 2. All drugs had a beneficial effect on ARR as compared to placebo. None of the pooled comparisons showed evidence of a statistically significant effect favouring one drug over another drug. Heterogeneity quantified by I^2 ranged from 0% (IFN β-1b 250 μg SC every other day, IFN β-1a 30 μg IM once a week) to 43% (IFN β-1a 44 μg SC thrice weekly) and 73% (GA 20 mg SC once daily). However, there were too few studies in each comparison to enable exploration of heterogeneity.

Findings derived from the NMA for comparisons between each drug and placebo substantially mirrored those of the pairwise comparisons, and reflected statistically significant reductions in ARR in patients receiving active drugs (see Table 3). There was little evidence of superiority of one drug over another. However, GA 20 mg SC once daily (RR = 0.82, 95% CI [0.73, 0.93]),

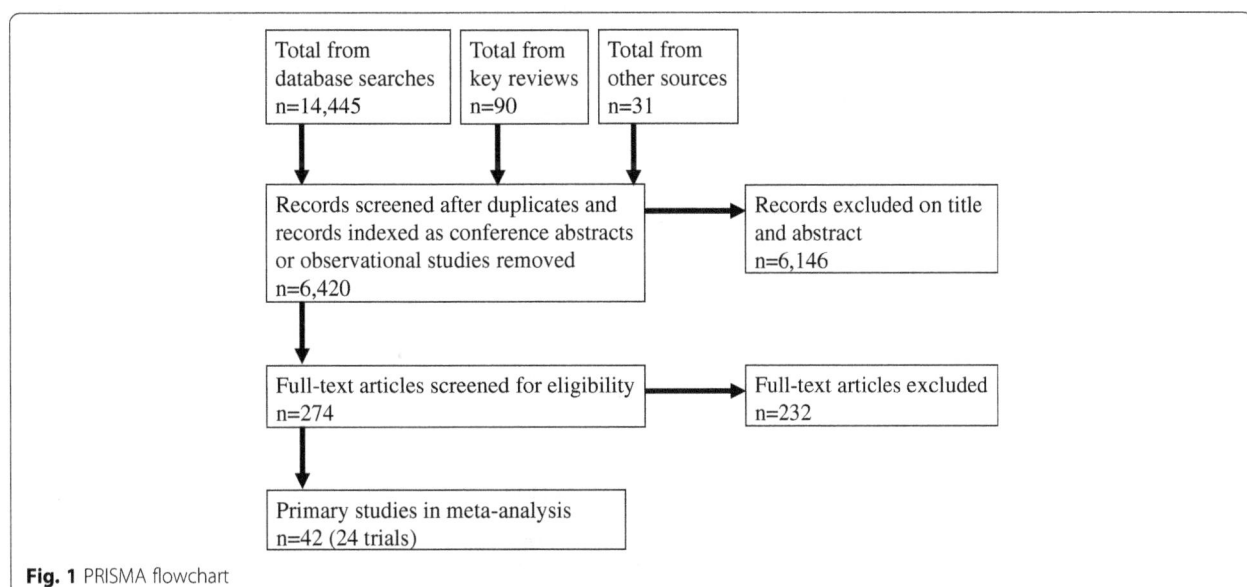

Total from database searches n=14,445

Total from key reviews n=90

Total from other sources n=31

Records screened after duplicates and records indexed as conference abstracts or observational studies removed n=6,420

Records excluded on title and abstract n=6,146

Full-text articles screened for eligibility n=274

Full-text articles excluded n=232

Primary studies in meta-analysis n=42 (24 trials)

Fig. 1 PRISMA flowchart

Table 1 Characteristics of included studies

Study ID MS type (diagnostic criteria)	Study details	Characteristics of participants at baseline	Intervention	Participants
ADVANCE 2014 RRMS (2005 McDonald criteria)	Country: USA, Belgium, Bulgaria, Canada, Chile, Colombia, Croatia, Czech Republic, Estonia, France, Georgia, Germany, Greece, India, Latvia, Mexico, Netherlands, New Zealand, Peru, Poland, Romania, Russian Federation, Serbia, Spain, Ukraine, United Kingdom. No. of countries: 26 Centres: 183 Study period: June 2009 and November 2011. Sponsor: Biogen Idec	Mean age: 36.5 (9.9) Mean sex: 71% female Race: 82% white EDSS Score: 2.5 Relapse rate: 1.6 within the previous 12 months, 2.6 within the previous 36 months Time from diagnosis of MS: 3.6 years Other clinical features of MS: Time from first MS symptoms: 6.6 years	Arm 1: pegylated IFN β-1a 125 µg SC every 2 weeks (Plegridy) Arm 2: Placebo	Randomised 512 arm 1 500 arm 2
AVANTAGE 2014 RRMS/CIS, diagnostic criteria unclear	Country: France No. of countries: 1 Centres: 61 Study period: March 2006–April 2008, 3 months follow up Sponsor: Bayer	Mean age: 38.7 Mean sex: 75% female Race: NA EDSS Score: 1.8 ± 1.3 Mean number of relapse rate: 2.1 ± 1.1 Time from diagnosis of MS: 3.3 (6.4) years Other clinical features of MS: NA	Arm 1: IFN β-1b 250 µg SC every other day (Betaferon) via Betaject Arm 2: IFN β-1b 250 µg SC every other day (Betaferon) via Betaject light Arm 3: IFN β-1a 44 SC three times weekly (Rebif) via Rebiject II	Included: 73 arm 1 79 arm 2 68 arm 3
BECOME 2009 RRMS/CIS (likely McDonald 2001 or 2005)	Country: USA No. of countries: 1 Centres: 2 Study period: Not specified, follow up over 2 years Sponsor: Bayer Schering pharma	Mean age: 36 Mean sex: 69% females Race: 52% white Median EDSS Score: 2 Relapse rate: 1.8 and 1.9 ARR Time from diagnosis of MS: between 0.9 and 1.2 Other clinical features of MS: 81% RRMS, 19% CIS; MSFC median 0.13	Arm 1: IFN β-1b 250 µg SC every other day (Betaferon) Arm 2: GA 20 mg SC daily (Copaxone)	Randomised 36 arm 1 39 arm 2
BEYOND 2009 RRMS (McDonald 2005)	Country: Not specified No. of countries: 26 Centres: 198 Study period: November, 2003, and June, 2005. Follow up between 2 and 3.5 years Sponsor: Bayer	Mean age 35.6 Mean sex: 69.4% female Race: 91.9% white EDSS Score: 2.33 Relapse rate: 1.6 relapses in last year Time from diagnosis of MS: 5.2 years Other clinical features of MS: 3.6 relapses previously; 70.6% had two or more relapses in past 2 years	Arm 1: IFN β-1b 250 µg SC every other day (Betaferon) Arm 2: GA 20 mg SC daily (Copaxone)	Randomised 897 arm 1 448 arm 2
Bornstein 1987 RRMS (Poser)	Country: USA No. of countries: 1 Centres: Not specified Study period: Not specified, follow up over 2 years Sponsor: public (grant from the National Institute of Neurological and Communicative Disorders and Stroke and grant from the National Institutes of Health)	Mean age: 30.5 Mean sex: 42% male/58% female Race: 96% white EDSS Score: 3.11 Relapse rate: 3.85 over 2 years Time from diagnosis of MS: 5.5 years duration of disease Other clinical features of MS: NA	Arm 1: GA 20 mg SC daily (Copaxone) Arm 2: Placebo	Randomised 25 arm 1 25 arm 2
BRAVO 2014 RRMS (McDonald 2005)	Country: US, Bulgaria, Croatia, Czech Republic, Estonia, Georgia, Germany, Israel, Italy, Lithuania, Macedonia, Poland, Romania, Russia, Slovakia, South Africa, Spain, Ukraine and others not specified No. of countries: 18 Centres: 140 Study period: April 2008 to June 2011. 24 months follow up Sponsor: Teva Pharmaceutical	Mean age: Median: 37.5 placebo, 38.5 IFN Mean sex: 71.3% females in placebo arm, 68.7% females in IFN arm Race: N/A EDSS Score: Median: 2.5 placebo, 2.5 IFN Median Relapse rate: previous year: 1.0 placebo, 1.0 IFN; previous 2 years: 2.0 placebo, 2.0 IFN Median Time from diagnosis of MS: 1.2 placebo, 1.4 IFN	Arm 1: IFN β-1a 30 µg IM once weekly (Avonex) Arm 2: Oral placebo once-daily with neur-ologist monitoring	Randomised 447 arm 1 450 arm 2

Table 1 Characteristics of included studies *(Continued)*

Study ID MS type (diagnostic criteria)	Study details	Characteristics of participants at baseline	Intervention	Participants
	Industries	Other clinical features of MS: NA		
Calabrese 2012 RRMS (McDonald 2005)	Country: Italy No. of countries: 1 Centres: 1 Study period: 1 Jan 2007–30 June 2008 Follow up over 2 years Sponsor: grant from Merck Serono S.A	Mean age: 36.5 (9.9) Mean sex: 70.2% of female/20.8% of male Race: NA EDSS Score: 2.1 (1.1) Relapse rate: 1.2 (0.7) Time from diagnosis of MS: 5.6 years (2.4) Other clinical features of MS: None	Arm 1: IFN β-1a 44 SC three times weekly (Rebif) Arm 2: IFN β-1a 30 μg IM once weekly (Avonex) Arm 3: GA 20 mg SC daily (Copaxone)	Randomised 55 arm 1 55 arm 2 55 arm 3
CombiRx 2013 RRMS (McDonald 2001, Poser)	Country: United States, Canada No. of countries: 2 Centres: 68 Study period: January 2005–April 2012. Minimally 36 months follow up Sponsor: NIH, with materials provided by Biogen and Teva	Mean age 38.3 Mean sex: 70.3% female Race: 87.6% white EDSS Score: 2.0 Relapse rate: 1.7 relapses in last year, on average Time from diagnosis of MS: 1.2 Other clinical features of MS: NA	Arm 1: IFN β-1a 30 μg IM once weekly (Avonex) Arm 2: GA 20 mg SC daily (Copaxone)	Randomised 250 arm 1 259 arm 2
CONFIRM 2012 RRMS (McDonald 2005)	Country: USA, Belarus, Belgium, Bosnia and Herzegovina, Bulgaria, Canada, Costa Rica, Croatia, Czech Republic, Estonia, France, Germany, Greece, India, Ireland, Israel, Latvia, Macedonia, Mexico, Republic of Moldova, New Zealand, Poland, Puerto Rico, Romania, Serbia, Slovakia, Spain, Ukraine No. of countries: 28 Centres: 200 Study period: 2 year follow up Sponsor: Biogen idec	Mean age 36.8 Mean sex: 70% female Race: 84% white EDSS Score: 2.6 Relapse rate: 1.4 in prior 12 months Time from diagnosis of MS: 4.6 years Other clinical features of MS: any prior DMTs (%) = 29%	Arm 1: GA 20 mg SC daily (Copaxone) Arm 2: 2 placebo capsules orally thrice daily	Randomised 360 arm 1 363 arm 2
Cop1 MSSG 1995 RRMS (Poser)	Country: USA No. of countries: 1 Centres: 11 Study period: October, 1991, and May, 1992. 2 year follow up. Sponsor: the FDA orphan drug program, the National multiple sclerosis society, and TEVA pharmaceutical	Mean age 34.4. Mean sex: 73% female Race: 94% white EDSS Score: 2.6 Relapse rate: 2.9 prior 2-year rate MS duration:6.9 years Other clinical features of MS: ambulation index = 1.1	Arm 1: GA 20 mg SC daily (Copaxone) Arm 2: Placebo	Randomised 125 arm 1 126 arm 2
ECGASG 2001 RRMS (Poser)	Country: Canada No. of countries: 7 Centres: 29 Study period: Enrollment started in February 1997 and concluded in November 1997. 9 month follow up Sponsor: Teva Pharmaceutical Industries	Mean age 34 Mean sex: NA Race: NA EDSS Score: 2.4 Relapse rate: 2.65 Disease duration (years): 8.1 Other clinical features of MS: ambulation index = 1.15	Arm 1: GA 20 mg SC daily (Copaxone) Arm 2: Placebo SC injections	Randomised 119 arm 1 120 arm 2
Etemadifar 2006 RRMS (Poser)	Country: Iran No. of countries: 1 Centres: 1 Study period: September 2002 and September 2004. 24 month follow up Sponsor: Not specified	Mean age 28.5 Mean sex: 76% female Race: NA EDSS Score: 2.0 Relapse rate 1 year prior: 2.2 Time from diagnosis of MS: 3.2 years Other clinical features of MS: None	Arm 1: IFN β-1b 250 μg SC every other day (Betaferon) Arm 2: IFN β-1a 30 μg IM once weekly (Avonex) Arm 3: IFN β-1a 44 SC three times weekly (Rebif)	Randomised 30 arm 1 30 arm 2 30 arm 3
EVIDENCE 2007 RRMS (Poser)	Country: USA, France, UK, Norway, Austria, Germany, France, Finland, Sweden, Canada	Mean age 37.9 Mean sex: 74.8% female Race: 91.0% Caucasian	Arm 1: IFN β-1a 44 SC three times weekly (Rebif)	Randomised 339 arm 1 338 arm 2

Table 1 Characteristics of included studies *(Continued)*

Study ID MS type (diagnostic criteria)	Study details	Characteristics of participants at baseline	Intervention	Participants
	No. of countries: 10 Centres: 56 Study period: Unclear. Minimally 48 weeks follow up, average 64.2 Sponsor: Serono	EDSS Score: 2.3 Median: 2.0 Relapse rate: 2.6 Median 2.0 relapses in last 2 years Duration of MS: 6.6. Median: 4.0–4.1 years Other clinical features of MS: Time since last relapse (months): Median 3.9 to 4.4; mean 5.1	Arm 2: IFN β-1a 30 μg IM once weekly (Avonex)	
GALA 2013 RRMS (McDonald 2005)	Country: United States, Bulgaria, Croatia, Germany, Poland, Romania, and Ukraine and others No. of countries: 17 Centres: 142 Study period: Not specified. 12 months follow up. Sponsor: TEVA pharmaceutical industries	Mean age 37.6 Mean sex: 68% female Race: 98% Caucasian EDSS Score: 2.7 Relapse rate: 1.3 in the prior 12 months, 1.9 in the prior 24 months Time from diagnosis of MS: NA Other clinical features of MS: Time from onset of first symptoms of MS = 7.7 years	Arm 1: GA 40 mg SC three times weekly (Copaxone) Arm 2: SC placebo injections	Randomised 943 arm 1 461 arm 2
GATE 2015 RRMS (McDonald 2010)	Country: USA, Belarus, Bosnia and Herzegovina, Bulgaria, Croatia, Czech Republic, Estonia, Georgia, Germany, Italy, Mexico, Republic of Moldova, Poland, Romania, Russian Federation, Serbia, South Africa, Ukraine, United Kingdom No. of countries: 20 Centres: 118 Study period: Recruited between December 7, 2011, and March 21, 2013; last follow-up December 2, 2013. Follow up 9 months (double-blind follow-up) + additional 15 months (open-label) Sponsor: Synthon BV	Mean age 33.1 Mean sex: 66.4% female Race: NA EDSS Score: 2.7 Relapse rate: 1.9 in prior 2 years Time from diagnosis of MS: NA Other clinical features of MS: • Time to onset of first symptoms to randomisation (years): 5.9 • No history of prior disease treatment: 16.1%	Arm 1: GA 20 mg SC daily (Copaxone) Arm 2: Placebo	Randomised 357 arm 1 84 arm 2
IFNB MSSG 1995 RRMS (Poser)	Country: USA and Canada No. of countries: 2 Centres: 11 Study period: after 2 years of follow-up, all subjects were given the option of continuing treatment in a double-blind fashion, extending the total treatment period to 5.5 years for some patients Sponsor: Triton Biosciences, Berlex Laboratories	Mean age 35.6 Mean sex: 70% female Race: 94% white EDSS Score: 2.9 Relapse rate: 3.5 in prior 2 years Time from diagnosis of MS:4.3 years Other clinical features of MS: Baseline Scripps neurological rating scale: 80.8	Arm 1: IFN β-1b 250 μg SC every other day (Betaferon) Arm 2: SC injections placebo	Randomised 124 arm 1 123 arm 2
IMPROVE 2012 RRMS (McDonald 2005)	Country: Italy, Germany, Serbia, Canada, Bulgaria, Estonia, Lithuania, Romania, Russia, Spain No. of countries: 10 Centres: 5 Study period: December 2006 to February 2009. Follow up 16 weeks for the double-blind phase, then 24 weeks where all patients received interferon beta 1-a, at last 4 weeks of safety period observation Sponsor: Merck Serono S.A.	Mean age NA Mean sex: NA Race: NA EDSS Score: NA Relapse rate: NA Time from diagnosis of MS: NA Other clinical features of MS: NA	Arm 1: IFN β-1a 44 SC three times weekly (Rebif) Arm 2: SC injections of placebo	Randomised 120 arm 1 60 arm 2
INCOMIN 2002 RRMS (Poser)	Country: Italy No. of countries: 1	Mean age 36.9 Mean sex: 65% female	Arm 1: IFN β-1b 250 μg SC every other	Randomised 92 arm 1

Table 1 Characteristics of included studies *(Continued)*

Study ID MS type (diagnostic criteria)	Study details	Characteristics of participants at baseline	Intervention	Participants
	Centres: 15 Study period: October, 1997, and June, 1999. 2 year follow up Sponsor: Istituto Superiore di Sanita' of the Italian Ministry of Health and the Italian MS Society	Race: NA EDSS Score: 1.97 Relapse rate 2 years prior: 1.45 Time from diagnosis of MS: 6.3 years Other clinical features of MS: None	day (Betaferon) Arm 2: IFN β-1a 30 μg IM once weekly (Avonex)	96 arm 2
Kappos 2011 RRMS (McDonald 2001)	Country: Belgium, Bulgaria, Canada, Czech Republic, Denmark, France, Germany, Italy, Mexico, Romania, Russian Federation, Serbia, Slovakia, Spain, Switzerland, Ukraine, United Kingdom, USA and others No. of countries: 20 Centres: 79 Study period: Not specified. Up to 96 weeks follow up. Sponsor: F Hoffmann-La Roche Ltd., Biogen Idec Inc	Mean age 37.5 Mean sex: 65% female Race: 96% white EDSS Score: 3.3 Relapse rate: NA Time from diagnosis of MS: median only Other clinical features of MS: NA	Arm 1: IFN β-1a 30 μg IM once weekly (Avonex) Arm 2: placebo injection every other week	Randomised 55 arm 1 54 arm 2
Knobler 1993 RRMS (Poser)	Country: USA No. of countries: 1 Centres: 3 Study period: June and October 1986. Follow up 3 years (24 weeks of initial follow-up for the 5 groups then all the patients that had received 0.8 mU, 4MU and 16MU for 24 weeks received a dose of 8MU from week 24 to 3 years) Sponsor: Triton Biosciences, Inc. and Berlex Laboratories, Inc	Mean age 35.6 Mean sex: 48% female Race: NA EDSS Score: 3.1 Mean exacerbation in prior 2 years: 2.84 Time from diagnosis of MS: 6.6 years Other clinical features of MS: mean Scripps Neurological Rating Scale (NRS): 76.6	Arm 1: IFN β-1b 250 μg SC every other day (Betaferon) Arm 2: Subcutaneous injection of placebo (1 mL like Betaseron 8 MU)	Randomised 6 arm 1 7 arm 2
MSCRG 1996 RRMS (Poser)	Country: USA No. of countries: 1 Centres: 4 Study period: November, 1990 to early 1993 2 years follow up for all-patients + 2 additional years for patients completing dosing before the end of the first period of follow-up. Sponsor: National Institutes of Health, National Institute of Neurological Disorders and Stroke (NINDS) grant R01–26321 and Biogen, Inc.	Mean age 36.8 Mean sex: 73.7% female Race: 93% white EDSS Score: 2.4 Relapse rate: 1.2 MS duration (years): 6.5 Other clinical features of MS: None	Arm 1: IFN β-1a 30 μg IM once weekly (Avonex) Arm 2: Placebo	Randomised 158 arm 1 143 arm 2
PRISMS 1998 RRMS (Poser)	Country: Australia, Belgium, Canada, Finland, Germany, Netherlands, Sweden, Switzerland, UK No. of countries: 9 Centres: 22 Study period: May 1994 to February 1995 with 2 years follow up. Sponsor: Ares- Serono	Mean age Median: 34.9 Mean sex: 69% female Race: NA EDSS Score: 2.5 (SD 1.2) Relapse rate: 3.0 (SD 1.2) Time from diagnosis of MS: Median: 5.3 years) Other clinical features of MS: NA	Arm 1: IFN β-1a 22 μg SC three times weekly (Rebif) Arm 2: IFN β-1a 44 SC three times weekly (Rebif) Arm 3: Placebo	Randomised 189 arm 1 184 arm 2 187 arm 3
REFORMS 2012 RRMS (McDonald 2005, Poser)	Country: USA No. of countries: 1 Centres: 27 Study period: December 2006–November 2007. 12 weeks follow up Sponsor: EMD Serono, Pfizer	Mean age 40.52 (SD 9.65) Mean sex: 70% female Race: 87.6% white EDSS Score: NA Relapse rate: 1.33 (SD 0.49) (of those with relapses) Time from diagnosis of MS: 1.47 yrs.	Arm 1: IFN β-1a 44 SC three times weekly (Rebif) Arm 2: IFN β-1b 250 μg SC every other day (Betaferon)	Randomised 65 arm 1 64 arm 2

Table 1 Characteristics of included studies *(Continued)*

Study ID MS type (diagnostic criteria)	Study details	Characteristics of participants at baseline	Intervention	Participants
		(3.31) Other clinical features of MS: Percentage with no relapse in last 12 months: 24 (18.6%) Time since onset: 5.12 yrs. (6.68) Percentage diagnosed with Poser criteria: 36 (27.9%) Time since last relapse, of those with last-year relapses: 3.76 mos (2.93) Steroid treatment episodes: 0.50 (0.55) Percentage needing more than one course of steroids: 49 (38.0%)		
REGARD 2008 RRMS (McDonald 2001)	Country: Argentina, Austria, Brazil, Canada, France, Germany, Ireland, Italy, Netherlands, Russia, Spain, Switzerland, UK, and USA No. of countries: 14 Centres: 80 Study period: February and December 2004, with 96 weeks follow up Sponsor: EMD Serono, Pfizer	Mean age 36.8 Mean sex: 29.5% male Race: 93.6% white EDSS Score: 2.34 Relapse rate: Presented as distribution of relapses; months since last relapse about 5 on average Time from diagnosis of MS: Years since first relapse: 6.2 Other clinical features of MS: Receiving steroid treatment in last 6 months: 43.7%	Arm 1: IFN β-1a 44 SC three times weekly (Rebif) Arm 2: GA 20 mg SC daily (Copaxone)	Randomised 386 arm 1 378 arm 2

RRMS relapsing remitting MS, *SPMS* secondary progressive MS, *CIS* clinically isolated syndrome, *IFN* interferon, *GA* glatiramer acetate, *IM* intramuscular, *SC* subcutaneous, *NA* not available, *EDSS* Expanded Disability Status Score

IFN β-1a 44 μg SC thrice weekly (0.85, [0.76, 0.95]) and IFN β-1b 250 μg SC every other day (0.86, [0.76, 0.97]) all produced significant reductions in ARR as compared to IFN β-1a 30 μg IM once a week. Ranking of the drugs suggested that the drug with the highest cumulative probability of superiority was GA 20 mg SC once daily. We found no evidence of inconsistency.

Sensitivity analyses

Several characteristics of the trials included in this network suggested that additional analyses would confirm the robustness of our findings. All of these analyses were post hoc. First, after exclusion of the REFORMS 2012 [19] trial from the analysis (where relapses were self-reported by subjects instead of being documented by an examining neurologist), effect estimates remained essentially unchanged for all pairwise comparisons. Second, we compared findings for studies with 'true', blinded placebos against studies that did not have blinded placebos. That is, several studies did not deliver placebos via the same route of administration [14–16]. We found that effects for these drugs against placebo were robust to inclusion of a covariate in the model for trials without a blinded placebo. Third, after exclusion of the Bornstein 1987 [18] trial that was an outlier in the comparison between GA 20 mg SC once daily and placebo, the pooled rate ratio for relapses still suggested a reduction in ARR as compared to placebo (RR = 0.71, 95% CI [0.62, 0.82]), with I^2 of 0% (see Additional file 2). Re-estimation of the NMA yielded a change in the SUCRA-based rankings,

with GA 20 mg SC once daily now ranked third, but point estimates and confidence intervals were not substantially different in the new model.

Time to progression confirmed at three months

Direct evidence from comparisons is shown in Fig. 3. GA 40 mg thrice weekly was not represented in this analysis. Comparison of drugs against placebo showed a mixed pattern of results. None of the three direct comparisons between active drugs suggested a benefit of one over another. Most comparisons were informed by only one study.

Comparisons for active drugs vs. placebo were similar between the NMA and the pairwise meta-analyses (see Table 4). Notably, additional information from indirect comparisons yielded a more precise estimate of effectiveness for both IFN β-1a 30 μg IM once a week vs placebo (HR = 0.73, 95% CI [0.53, 1.00], $p = 0.0499$) and GA 20 mg SC once daily (0.76, [0.60, 0.97]). Comparisons between active drugs estimated from the NMA did not indicate that any one drug was statistically better than the others, but ranking of the drugs suggested that the drug with the highest cumulative probability of superiority was IFN β-1a 44 μg SC thrice weekly. We found no evidence of inconsistency.

Time to progression confirmed at six months

Direct evidence from comparisons is shown in Fig. 3. All comparisons drew from a single study, except for IFN β-1a 30 μg IM once a week as compared to placebo.

Table 2 Risk of bias judgments for included studies

Reference	Random sequence generation	Allocation concealment	Blinding of participants and personnel	Blinding of outcome assessment	Incomplete outcome data	Selective reporting	Other sources of bias
ADVANCE 2014	Low risk	Low risk	High risk	High risk	High risk	Low risk	High risk
AVANTAGE 2014	Unclear risk	Unclear risk	High risk	High risk	Unclear risk	Low risk	Low risk
BECOME 2009	Unclear risk	Unclear risk	High risk	High risk	Low risk	Low risk	High risk
BEYOND 2009	Low risk	Low risk	High risk	High risk	Unclear risk	Low risk	High risk
Bornstein 1987	Unclear risk	High risk	High risk	High risk	Low risk	Low risk	Low risk
BRAVO 2014	Low risk	Low risk	High risk	Low risk	Low risk	High risk	High risk
Calabrese 2012	Low risk	Low risk	High risk	High risk	Low risk	High risk	Low risk
CombiRx 2013	Low risk	Low risk	Low risk	Low risk	High risk	Low risk	Low risk
CONFIRM 2012	Low risk	Low risk	High risk	High risk	High risk	Low risk	High risk
Cop1 MSSG 1995	Unclear risk	Low risk	High risk	High risk	Low risk	Low risk	Low risk
ECGASG 2001	Low risk	Low risk	High risk	High risk	Low risk	Unclear risk	High risk
Etemadifar 2006	Unclear risk	Unclear risk	High risk	High risk	Low risk	Unclear risk	Unclear risk
EVIDENCE 2007	Low risk	Low risk	High risk	High risk	Low risk	Low risk	High risk
GALA 2013	Unclear risk	Low risk	High risk	High risk	Unclear risk	Low risk	High risk
GATE 2015	Low risk	Low risk	High risk	High risk	Low risk	Low risk	High risk
IFNB MSSG 1995	Unclear risk	Unclear risk	High risk	High risk	High risk	Low risk	High risk
IMPROVE 2012	Unclear risk	Low risk	Unclear risk	Unclear risk	Unclear risk	High risk	High risk
INCOMIN 2002	Low risk	Low risk	High risk	High risk	Low risk	Low risk	Low risk
Kappos 2011	Low risk	Low risk	High risk	High risk	Low risk	High risk	High risk
Knobler 1993	Unclear risk	Unclear risk	High risk	High risk	Unclear risk	Unclear risk	High risk
MSCRG 1996	Low risk	Unclear risk	Low risk	Low risk	High risk	Unclear risk	High risk
PRISMS 1998	Low risk	Low risk	Unclear risk	Low risk	Low risk	Low risk	High risk
REFORMS 2012	Low risk	Unclear risk	High risk	High risk	Unclear risk	Low risk	High risk
REGARD 2008	Low risk	Unclear risk	High risk	Low risk	Low risk	Low risk	High risk

Only three drugs, GA 20 mg SC one daily, IFN β-1a 30 μg SC once weekly and IFN β-1a pegylated 125 μg every 2 weeks, were compared against placebo.

In the NMA, estimates for GA 20 mg SC once daily (HR = 0.82, 95% CI [0.53, 1.26]), IFN β-1a 30 μg IM once a week (0.68, [0.49, 0.94]) and IFN β-1a pegylated 125 μg every 2 weeks (0.46, [0.26, 0.81]) compared to placebo mirrored the direct evidence (see Table 4). Indirect comparisons suggested that both IFN β-1a 44 μg SC thrice weekly (0.47, [0.24, 0.93]) and IFN β-1b 250 μg

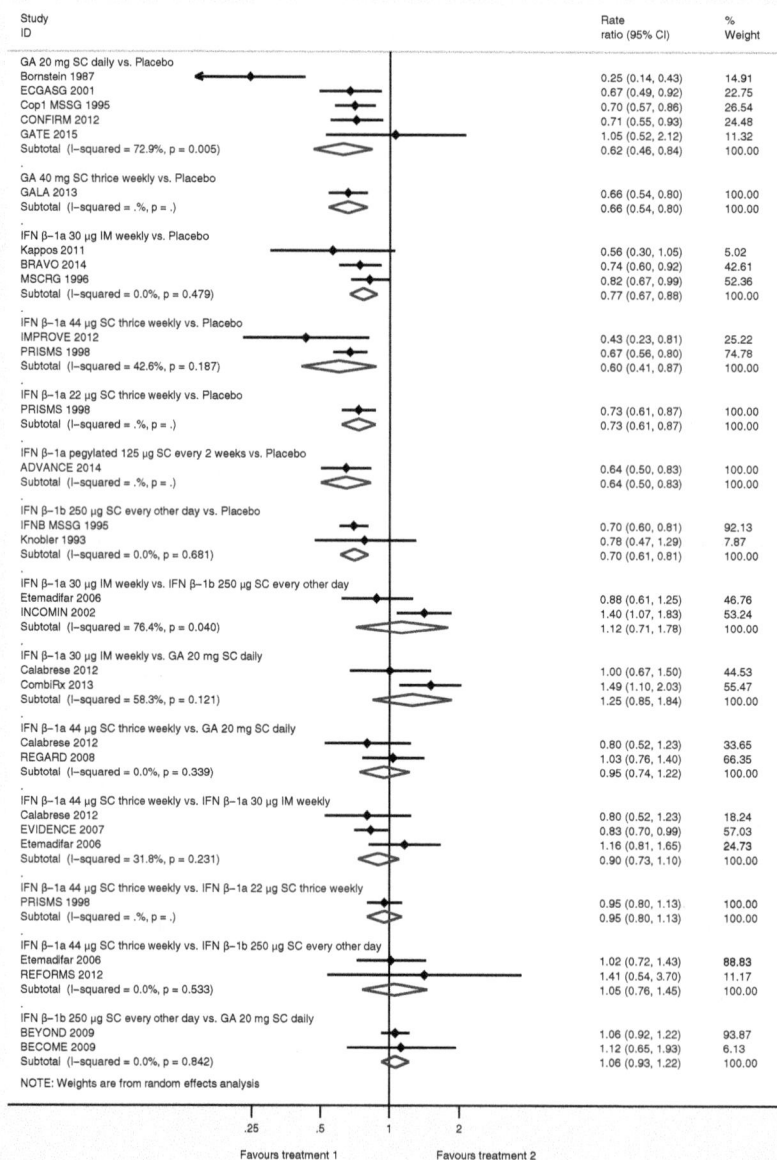

Fig. 2 Pairwise meta-analyses for annualised relapse rate. IFN: interferon, GA: glatiramer acetate, IM: intramuscular, SC: subcutaneous

SC every other day (0.34, [0.18, 0.63]) showed evidence of delaying disability progression as compared to placebo. The NMA suggested that IFN β-1b 250 μg SC every other day was superior both to IFN β-1a 30 μg IM once a week (HR = 0.50, 95% CI [0.29, 0.87]) and to GA 20 mg SC once daily (0.41, [0.21, 0.83]), but these findings were driven by the INCOMIN 2002 trial [20] and relied on a hazard ratio estimated from summary statistics. Ranking of the drugs suggested that the drug with the highest cumulative probability of superiority was IFN β-1b 250 μg SC every other day. Tests of inconsistency in the network did not suggest that direct and

indirect evidence were in disagreement; however, the network was sparse and only one comparison included more than one study.

Discontinuation due to AEs

Two NMA models were estimated: one for studies with 24-month follow-up and one including all studies with the follow-up of greatest maturity. Neither NMA found evidence that one drug was more likely to lead to discontinuation than another. However, confidence intervals were wide and NMA-based estimates were often numerically different to estimates from the direct

Table 3 Network meta-analysis results for annualised relapse rate[a]

Drug	SUCRA	GA 20 mg daily	PegIFN β-1a 125 µg every 2 weeks	GA 40 mg thrice weekly	IFN β-1a 44 µg SC thrice weekly	IFN β-1b 250 µg SC every other day	IFN β-1a 22 µg SC thrice weekly	IFN β-1a 30 µg IM weekly	Placebo
GA 20 mg daily	0.77		1.01 (0.77, 1.33)	1.00 (0.80, 1.24)	0.97 (0.85, 1.10)	0.95 (0.86, 1.05)	0.91 (0.76, 1.08)	0.82 (0.73, 0.92)	0.65 (0.59, 0.72)
PegIFN β-1a 125 µg every 2 weeks	0.73			0.98 (0.71, 1.35)	0.95 (0.72, 1.26)	0.94 (0.71, 1.23)	0.89 (0.66, 1.21)	0.81 (0.62, 1.06)	0.64 (0.50, 0.83)
GA 40 mg thrice weekly	0.70				0.97 (0.77, 1.22)	0.96 (0.77, 1.19)	0.91 (0.71, 1.17)	0.82 (0.66, 1.03)	0.66 (0.54, 0.80)
IFN β-1a 44 µg SC thrice weekly	0.64					0.99 (0.86, 1.13)	0.94 (0.80, 1.10)	0.85 (0.76, 0.95)	0.68 (0.60, 0.76)
IFN β-1b 250 µg SC every other day	0.56						0.95 (0.79, 1.14)	0.86 (0.76, 0.97)	0.69 (0.62, 0.76)
IFN β-1a 22 µg SC thrice weekly	0.43							0.91 (0.76, 1.08)	0.72 (0.61, 0.85)
IFN β-1a 30 µg IM weekly	0.18								0.80 (0.72, 0.88)
Placebo	0								
Test for inconsistency (χ^2, df, p)		11.71, 11, 0.38							

[a]Findings are expressed as rate ratio (RR) with 95% CI

IFN interferon, *GA* glatiramer acetate, *IM* intramuscular, *SC* subcutaneous, *SUCRA* surface under the cumulative ranking curve

evidence alone. Moreover, both networks of evidence included some indication of inconsistency. In the 24-month follow-up model, the sidesplitting test suggested that direct and indirect evidence were in conflict for the comparison between GA 20 mg SC once daily and placebo, with indirect evidence suggesting that risk of discontinuation due to AEs was higher than presented in the direct evidence ($p = 0.037$). In the all-studies model, the overall Wald test suggested some signal of inconsistency ($p = 0.09$), though sidesplitting tests did not indicate an obvious source of inconsistency. Full results are in Additional file 2.

Discussion

Meta-analyses confirmed that the different formulations of IFN-β and GA reduce ARR and generally delay progression as defined in these trials. There was little evidence that any one drug was superior to others, except for progression confirmed at 6 months, but networks were especially sparse. Findings for discontinuations due to AEs, which are intended to be indicative, did not suggest that one drug was more likely to result in discontinuation than another, but these findings relied on networks with some limited evidence of inconsistency.

Challenges with the clinical evidence

These conclusions are tempered by several considerations. Analyses did not show a clear 'winner' across outcomes, and, again, comparisons between drugs estimated as part of NMA models were in the main inconclusive. Though the main model for ARR was relatively well populated, analyses for time to progression confirmed at six months were especially sparse. In particular, several comparisons of drugs vs. placebo estimated as part of this last model relied exclusively on indirect evidence. Moreover, analyses for time to progression confirmed at three and at six months did not show a consistent pattern, except that all drugs were beneficial in delaying progression where progression was defined using the EDSS. This is particularly concerning, as progression confirmed at six months is considered to be a 'stronger' outcome than progression confirmed at three months.

Measurement of disease progression also relied on the EDSS, a measure that, while broadly accepted in clinical trials, may be of dubious value in measuring disability per se. The EDSS is heavily weighted towards mobility over other important aspects of disability affected by disease progression in MS, such as cognitive function. Additionally, progression outcomes based on confirmed

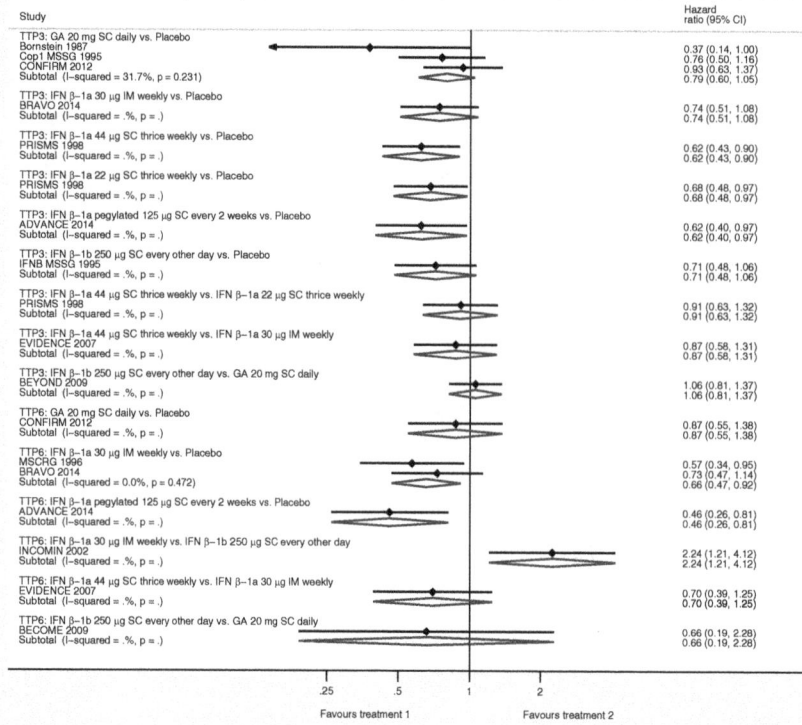

Fig. 3 Pairwise meta-analyses for time to progression. IFN: interferon, GA: glatiramer acetate, IM: intramuscular, SC: subcutaneous; TTP3: time to progression confirmed at 3 months; TTP6: time to progression confirmed at 6 months

progression at 3 or 6 months overestimate the accumulation of permanent disability by up to 30% [21]. This is in part because recovery from relapses may take longer than several months, and thus 'confirmed' progression may reflect residual relapse-related symptoms. Consequently, while time to progression confirmed at 3 or 6 months may be standard within the relatively short timeframe of clinical trials, these outcomes may not capture the true accumulation of MS-related disability over the lifecourse, and thus true differences between DMTs in delaying disease progression.

NMA models also had imbalanced risk of bias across the networks of studies. For example, most trials comparing two active treatments were open-label, whereas most trials comparing active treatments against placebos were blinded. Many trials relied on short follow-up, generally less than two years in duration, which increases the risk of spurious results [21]. Thus, participants were aware of the drugs they were receiving. This might have posed a greater risk for unblinding of outcome assessors than in ostensibly double-blinded trials. In addition, the majority of studies were judged as high risk of bias under the 'other' category of the Cochrane tool given that most of these were funded by drug companies. Although no research has specifically been undertaken

in the field of MS trials, empirical examination of trials suggests that industry-sponsored RCTs are more likely to have favourable results than non-industry sponsored RCTs [2]. A final issue is that patient populations recruited into trials may not be the same over time, given the nearly 20-year span of the trials included in our models. These differences may well extend to diagnostic definitions of MS, and detection and diagnosis of relapses and disease progression. Again, insufficient studies on each pairwise comparison prevented exploration of this problem, but it is conceivable that this might have affected transitivity of our networks of evidence.

Review-level strengths and limitations
We used a rigorous and exhaustive search to locate primary studies, which included updating existing high-quality systematic reviews. Additionally we used auditable and transparent methods to include and synthesise studies. Where appropriate, we undertook post hoc sensitivity analyses in our clinical effectiveness assessments to check the robustness of our findings. However, a limitation of our work, inherent to all systematic reviews, is publication bias. Methods for detecting publication bias in NMAs are still in development, and we did not have enough studies in any one

Table 4 Network meta-analysis results for time to progression[a]

Time to progression confirmed at 3 months

Drug	SUCRA	IFN β-1a 44 µg SC thrice weekly	PegIFN β-1a 125 µg every 2 weeks	IFN β-1a 22 µg SC thrice weekly	IFN β-1a 30 µg IM weekly	GA 20 mg daily	IFN β-1b 250 µg SC every other day	Placebo	GA 40 mg SC thrice weekly
IFN β-1a 44 µg SC thrice weekly	0.77		1.01 (0.59, 1.74)	0.92 (0.65, 1.30)	0.86 (0.62, 1.19)	0.82 (0.56, 1.22)	0.81 (0.53, 1.22)	0.63 (0.46, 0.86)	Not included in this analysis
PegIFN β-1a 125 µg every 2 weeks	0.75			0.91 (0.52, 1.59)	0.85 (0.49, 1.46)	0.81 (0.49, 1.34)	0.80 (0.47, 1.34)	0.62 (0.40, 0.97)	
IFN β-1a 22 µg SC thrice weekly	0.62				0.94 (0.62, 1.42)	0.90 (0.59, 1.36)	0.88 (0.57, 1.36)	0.68 (0.49, 0.96)	
IFN β-1a 30 µg IM weekly	0.5					0.96 (0.65, 1.42)	0.94 (0.62, 1.43)	0.73 (0.53, 1.00)*	
GA 20 mg daily	0.44						0.98 (0.78, 1.24)	0.76 (0.60, 0.97)	
IFN β-1b 250 µg SC every other day	0.39							0.78 (0.59, 1.02)	
Placebo	0.02								
Test for inconsistency (χ2, df, p)	0.35, 2, 0.84								

Time to progression confirmed at 6 months

Drug	SUCRA	IFN β-1b 250 µg SC every other day	PegIFN β-1a 125 µg every 2 weeks	IFN β-1a 44 µg SC thrice weekly	IFN β-1a 30 µg IM weekly	GA 20 mg daily	Placebo	PegIFN β-1a 125 µg every 2 weeks	GA 40 mg thrice weekly
IFN β-1b 250 µg SC every other day	0.9		0.74 (0.32, 1.71)	0.71 (0.32, 1.60)	0.50 (0.29, 0.87)	0.42 (0.21, 0.83)	0.34 (0.18, 0.63)	Not included in this analysis	
PegIFN β-1a 125 µg every 2 weeks	0.71			0.97 (0.40, 2.33)	0.68 (0.35, 1.31)	0.56 (0.28, 1.15)	0.46 (0.26, 0.81)		
IFN β-1a 44 µg SC thrice weekly	0.7				0.70 (0.39, 1.25)	0.58 (0.27, 1.27)	0.47 (0.24, 0.93)		
IFN β-1a 30 µg IM weekly	0.4					0.83 (0.49, 1.41)	0.68 (0.49, 0.94)		
GA 20 mg daily	0.25						0.82 (0.53, 1.26)		
Placebo	0.05								
Test for inconsistency (χ2, df, p)	0.77, 1, 0.38								

[a]Findings are presented as HR (95% CI)

IFN interferon, *GA* glatiramer acetate, *IM* intramuscular, *SC* subcutaneous, *SUCRA* surface under the cumulative ranking curve

comparison to test for small-study bias. This may be especially relevant since many of the early trials of IFN and GA for MS were small trials. Another important limitation was the selective and inconsistent reporting of outcomes. For example, one of the reasons we did not undertake a meta-analysis of time to first relapse is that there was inconsistent and often poor reporting, especially across multiple reports of the same study, which prevented imputation of hazard ratios. We were also unable to obtain meta-analysable data for one study [12],

due to the tight timeline within which the original work was undertaken.

Our analysis methods had a number of statistical advantages as well as some limitations. In examining the effect of IFN and GA on progression, we used time to event outcomes and hazard ratios instead of calculating risk ratios or odds ratios at different follow-up points. Thus, trial findings were reported at their fullest 'maturity' [22] and all relevant data were included. We were unable to verify empirically whether hazard ratios and rate ratios were time-varying due to few comparisons on every node of the study networks. On the other hand, we judged that stratifying analyses by time to follow-up would have resulted in excessively sparse networks that would have been difficult to interpret collectively. Thus, our decision to pool study estimates across follow-up times for analyses of clinical outcomes was both a strength and a potential limitation. Notably, we stratified analyses by time to follow-up in NMAs of discontinuations due to AEs, because we judged that the only feasible estimator in these analyses was the risk ratio.

Deviations from protocol

In our protocol, we specified that the comparator of interest was best supportive care without DMTs. In practice, this includes both best supportive care and also placebo, as reported in included trials. Though we sought to examine 10 outcomes relevant to RRMS in our original protocol, we report here findings for relapse rate, disability and discontinuation due to adverse events, as synthesis for other outcomes was limited and in many parts meta-analysable. Detailed findings for each of these outcomes are available in the main report [2]. Moreover, disability was ultimately measured and included in these meta-analyses as 'time to progression', as this was the most common outcome across trials. Finally, we implemented network meta-analyses in a frequentist paradigm rather than using WinBUGS as specified in the protocol.

In relation to research and practice

Our findings updated prior reviews, though comparability of findings is limited. We included trials examining IFN and GA against each other and against a no-treatment comparator, and restricted inclusion to doses and formulations within their marketing authorisation as compared to Tramacere et al. [3] who broadly examined immunomodulators and immunosuppressants for RRMS. Because they included studies across drugs and because they used risk ratios as the sole outcome estimator, our analyses and theirs are largely incommensurate. Our systematic review and NMA may however offer more clinically relevant evidence because of our focus on doses used in clinical practice. However, our analyses for discontinuation due to AEs agreed with theirs. Neither review suggested that any one drug had a significant effect on discontinuation due to AEs relative to placebo.

Our findings agree with the ABN guidelines [1] in that the guidelines classify IFN-β and GA as drugs of 'moderate efficacy', and observe that there is not much data to support differences in effectiveness between them. Our analysis does suggest that these drugs are effective in reducing relapse rate, which may have an effect on progression.

Longer-term observational cohorts have also examined DMT effectiveness over time and shed some doubt on the findings from randomised trials. In the year 8 analyses from the UK Risk Sharing Scheme, DMTs were not found to be cost-effective and the drugs assessed were not substantially different in terms of delays in disease progression (personal communication with UK Department of Health, 2016). An analysis from the MSBase study, an international registry with 'real-world' data from MS patients, has suggested that GA or subcutaneous IFN-β-1a are more effective in controlling relapse rate than other IFN-β, though drugs were not different on disease progression [23]. While this analysis relied on matching to overcome lack of randomisation, a strength is that it used disability progression confirmed at 12 months instead of at 3 or 6 months.

Future research

First, findings from this review will require updating as generic versions of the DMTs considered here are authorised. For example, the GATE trial also tested a generic version of glatiramer acetate against the branded version and placebo [24]. Key flaws in the assembled clinical effectiveness evidence included the lack of long-term follow-up and the absence of a measure for disease progression adequately capturing worsening of disability. A large-scale, longitudinal randomised trial comparing active first-line agents and using clinically meaningful and robust measures of disability progression would contribute towards resolving uncertainty about the relative benefits of different IFN or GA formulations (and other first line agents). While other, newer first line agents were beyond the remit of our systematic review, few randomised comparisons exist and thus a large trial could resolve remaining questions of comparative effectiveness. It may also be that using standardised definitions for relapses and disease progression together with blinded adjudicator panels could attenuate the risk of bias accruing to an open-label trial. Because of this lack of long-term follow-up, DMT trials are not informative on whether drugs delay progression to SPMS. Understanding long-term effectiveness of DMTs as described above would will also provide better information for informing cost-effectiveness evaluations, the effectiveness estimates for which currently rely on extrapolation from short-term trials. Use of a more relevant measure for disability and disease progression, especially as regards the development of secondary progressive MS, will also lead to better and more robust valuation of benefits accruing from DMTs.

Finally, above and beyond the broad interpretation that DMTs reduce ARR, there is a need to understand who responds best to DMTs; especially who does not respond to IFN or GA early on, to enable more targeted therapeutic decisions. Though several trials included in our clinical effectiveness review used subgroup analyses, based for example, on presenting lesions or demographic characteristics, a more fine-grained understanding can help patients and clinicians make better-informed decisions.

Conclusions

Our meta-analyses confirmed that IFN-β and GA reduce ARR and generally delay progression as defined in these trials. We found, however, that there was no clear 'winner' across outcomes, and our findings were qualified by the high risk of bias across studies, and the use of an impairment/mobility scale to measure disease progression. Future research should consider more relevant measures of disability and, given that most trials have been short-term, consider a longitudinal approach to comparative effectiveness.

Additional files

Additional file 1: Detailed search and data preparation methods. This file includes search strings, grey literature search sources, a sample data extraction form, and additional details on the statistical procedures undertaken to prepare study data for meta-analysis. (DOCX 47 kb)

Additional file 2: Additional results. This file includes detailed reasons for exclusion, tables of included publications, and sensitivity analyses for ARR, and detailed findings for discontinuation due to adverse events. (DOCX 265 kb)

Abbreviations

ABN: Association of British Neurologists; AEs: Adverse events; ARR: Annualised relapse rate; DMT: Disease-modifying therapy; EDSS: Expanded Disability Status Scale; EMA: European Medicines Agency; GA: Glatiramer acetate; HR: Hazard ratio; IFN-β: Beta-interferon; NMA: Network meta-analysis; RR: Rate ratio; RRMS: Relapsing-remitting multiple sclerosis; SPMS: Secondary progressive multiple sclerosis; SUCRA: Surface under the cumulative ranking curve

Funding

This work is part of a larger report commissioned by the NIHR HTA Programme as project number ID809. Aileen Clarke and G.J. Melendez-Torres are partly supported by the National Institute for Health Research (NIHR) Collaboration for Leadership in Applied Health Research and Care West Midlands at the University Hospitals Birmingham NHS Foundation Trust. The views expressed are those of the authors and not necessarily those of the NHS, NIHR, NICE or the Department of Health and Social Care.

Authors' contributions

GJMT led the review, participated in all parts of the review process and led the meta-analyses and drafting of the article. XA and JVP participated in all parts of the review process and contributed to drafting of the article. JVP participated in all parts of the review process and contributed to drafting of the article. RC led the information retrieval strategy and contributed to drafting of the article. AK participated in all parts of the review process and contributed to drafting of the article. PA contributed to the review process and to drafting of the article. JJM provided methodological advice and contributed to drafting of the article. CC and OC provided clinical advice and contributed to drafting of the article. AC provided methodological advice and contributed to drafting of the article. All authors read and approved the final manuscript.

Competing interests

Prof. Olga Ciccarelli received consultancy fees from Teva, Roche, Novartis, Biogen Idec, and Genzyme. She also received funds for research from the UK MS Society, National MS Society, EPSRC, Rosetree Trust; her research is supported by the National Institute for Health Research (NIHR) University College London Hospitals (UCLH) Biomedical Research Centre (BRC). She is an Associate Editor of *Neurology* for which she receives an honorarium. Dr. Carl Counsell received funding through Biogen Idec, who previously provided some funding for a departmental MS nurse. Dr. Carl Counsell has also authored a paper that was critical of the UK Risk Sharing Scheme for disease modifying therapies in MS (Sudlow, CLM, Counsell, CE. Problems with UK government's risk sharing scheme for assessing drugs for multiple sclerosis. BMJ 2003; 326:388–392). The remaining authors have no competing interests to declare.

Author details

[1]Warwick Evidence, Warwick Medical School, University of Warwick, Coventry CV4 7AL, UK. [2]Independent research consultant, Windsor, UK. [3]Institute of Applied Health Sciences, University of Aberdeen, Aberdeen, UK. [4]Queen Square Multiple Sclerosis Centre, University College London Institute of Neurology, London, UK. [5]National Institute for Health Research University College London Hospitals Biomedical Research Centre, London, UK.

References

1. Scolding N, Barnes D, Cader S, Chataway J, Chaudhuri A, Coles A, Giovannoni G, Miller D, Rashid W, Schmierer K, et al. Association of British Neurologists: revised (2015) guidelines for prescribing disease-modifying treatments in multiple sclerosis. Pract Neurol. 2015;15(4):273–9.
2. Melendez-Torres GJ, Auguste P, Armoiry X, Maheswaran H, Court R, Madan J, Kan A, Lin S, Counsell C, Patterson J, et al. Clinical and cost-effectiveness of beta interferon and glatiramer acetate for treating multiple sclerosis: systematic review and economic evaluation. Health Technol Assess. 2017; 21(52):1–352.
3. Tramacere I, Del Giovane C, Salanti G, D'Amico R, Filippini G. Immunomodulators and immunosuppressants for relapsing-remitting multiple sclerosis: a network meta-analysis. Cochrane Database Syst Rev. 2015;9:CD011381.
4. Filippini G, Del Giovane C, Vacchi L, D'Amico R, Di Pietrantonj C, Beecher D, Salanti G. Immunomodulators and immunosuppressants for multiple sclerosis: a network meta-analysis. Cochrane Database Syst Rev. 2013;6:CD008933.
5. Tolley K, Hutchinson M, You X, Wang P, Sperling B, Taneja A, Siddiqui MK, Kinter E. A network meta-analysis of efficacy and evaluation of safety of subcutaneous Pegylated interferon Beta-1a versus other injectable therapies for the treatment of relapsing-remitting multiple sclerosis. PLoS One. 2015; 10(6):e0127960.
6. Hadjigeorgiou GM, Doxani C, Miligkos M, Ziakas P, Bakalos G, Papadimitriou D, Mprotsis T, Grigoriadis N, Zintzaras E. A network meta-analysis of randomized controlled trials for comparing the effectiveness and safety profile of treatments with marketing authorization for relapsing multiple sclerosis. J Clin Pharm Ther. 2013;38(6):433–9.
7. Clerico M, Faggiano F, Palace J, Rice G, Tintore M, Durelli L. Recombinant interferon beta or glatiramer acetate for delaying conversion of the first demyelinating event to multiple sclerosis. Cochrane Database Syst Rev. 2008;2:Cd005278.
8. Higgins JP, Altman DG, Gotzsche PC, Juni P, Moher D, Oxman AD, Savovic J, Schulz KF, Weeks L, Sterne JA. The Cochrane Collaboration's tool for assessing risk of bias in randomised trials. BMJ (Clinical research ed). 2011; d5928:343.

9.   Systematic Reviews: CRD's guidance for undertaking reviews in health care [http://www.york.ac.uk/media/crd/Systematic_Reviews.pdf].

10. Higgins JP, Jackson D, Barrett JK, Lu G, Ades AE, White IR. Consistency and inconsistency in network meta-analysis: concepts and models for multi-arm studies. Res Synth Methods. 2012;3(2):98–110.

11. Schwartz CE, Coulthard-Morris L, Cole B, Vollmer T. The quality-of-life effects of interferon beta-1b in multiple sclerosis. An extended Q-TWiST analysis. Arch Neurol. 1997;54(12):1475–80.

12. Mokhber N, Azarpazhooh A, Orouji E, Rao SM, Khorram B, Sahraian MA, Foroghipoor M, Gharavi MM, Kakhi S, Nikkhah K, et al. Cognitive dysfunction in patients with multiple sclerosis treated with different types of interferon beta: a randomized clinical trial. J Neurol Sci. 2014;342(1–2):16–20.

13. Rieckmann P, Heidenreich F, Sailer M, Zettl UK, Zessack N, Hartung HP, Gold R. Treatment de-escalation after mitoxantrone therapy: results of a phase IV, multicentre, open-label, randomized study of subcutaneous interferon beta-1a in patients with relapsing multiple sclerosis. Ther. 2012;5(1):3–12.

14. Vollmer TL, Sorensen PS, Selmaj K, Zipp F, Havrdova E, Cohen JA, Sasson N, Gilgun-Sherki Y, Arnold DL, Group BS. A randomized placebo-controlled phase III trial of oral laquinimod for multiple sclerosis. J Neurol. 2014;261(4): 773–83.

15. Fox RJ, Miller DH, Phillips JT, Hutchinson M, Havrdova E, Kita M, Yang M, Raghupathi K, Novas M, Sweetser MT, et al. Placebo-controlled phase 3 study of oral BG-12 or glatiramer in multiple sclerosis. [erratum appears in N Engl J med. 2012 Oct 25;367(17):1673]. N Engl J Med. 2012;367(12):1087–97.

16. Kappos L, Li D, Calabresi PA, O'Connor P, Bar-Or A, Barkhof F, Yin M, Leppert D, Glanzman R, Tinbergen J, et al. Ocrelizumab in relapsing-remitting multiple sclerosis: a phase 2, randomised, placebo-controlled, multicentre trial. Lancet. 2011;378(9805):1779–87.

17. Bayer HealthCare AG. Clinical Study Synopsis: The AVANTAGE study - A randomized, multicenter, phase IV, open-label prospective study comparing injection site reaction and injection site pain in patients with relapsing remitting multiple sclerosis (RRMS) or after a first demyelinating event suggestive of MS newly started on interferon beta-1b (Betaferon®) or interferon beta-1a (Rebif®). 2013. http://trialfinder.pharma.bayer.com/omr/online/91489_Study_Synopsis_CTP.pdf. Accessed 10 May 2013.

18. Bornstein MB, Miller A, Slagle S, Weitzman M, Crystal H, Drexler E, Keilson M, Merriam A, Wassertheil-Smoller S, Spada V, et al. A pilot trial of cop 1 in exacerbating-remitting multiple sclerosis. N Engl J Med. 1987;317(7):408–14.

19. Singer B, Bandari D, Cascione M, LaGanke C, Huddlestone J, Bennett R, Dangond F, Group RS. Comparative injection-site pain and tolerability of subcutaneous serum-free formulation of interferonbeta-1a versus subcutaneous interferonbeta-1b: results of the randomized, multicenter, phase IIIb REFORMS study. BMC Neurol. 2012;12:154.

20. Durelli L, Verdun E, Barbero P, Bergui M, Versino E, Ghezzi A, Montanari E, Zaffaroni M. Every-other-day interferon beta-1b versus once-weekly interferon beta-1a for multiple sclerosis: results of a 2-year prospective randomised multicentre study (INCOMIN). Lancet. 2002;359(9316):1453–60.

21. Kalincik T, Cutter G, Spelman T, Jokubaitis V, Havrdova E, Horakova D, Trojano M, Izquierdo G, Girard M, Duquette P, et al. Defining reliable disability outcomes in multiple sclerosis. Brain. 2015;138(Pt 11):3287–98.

22. Flacco ME, Manzoli L, Boccia S, Capasso L, Aleksovska K, Rosso A, Scaioli G, De Vito C, Siliquini R, Villari P, et al. Head-to-head randomized trials are mostly industry sponsored and almost always favor the industry sponsor. J Clin Epidemiol. 2015;68(7):811–20.

23. Kalincik T, Jokubaitis V, Izquierdo G, Duquette P, Girard M, Grammond P, Lugaresi A, Oreja-Guevara C, Bergamaschi R, Hupperts R, et al. Comparative effectiveness of glatiramer acetate and interferon beta formulations in relapsing-remitting multiple sclerosis. Mult Scler. 2015;21(9):1159–71.

24. Cohen J, Belova A, Selmaj K, Wolf C, Sormani MP, Oberye J, van den Tweel E, Mulder R, Koper N, Voortman G, et al. Equivalence of generic Glatiramer acetate in multiple sclerosis: a randomized clinical trial. JAMA Neurol. 2015; 72(12):1433–41.

Association between medication-related adverse events and non-elective readmission in acute ischemic stroke

James A. G. Crispo[1*], Dylan P. Thibault[1,2], Yannick Fortin[3], Daniel Krewski[3] and Allison W. Willis[1,2]

Abstract

Background: There is limited data on the effects of medication-related adverse events occurring during inpatient stays for stroke. The objectives of our study were to characterize reasons for acute readmission after acute ischemic stroke (AIS) and determine if medication-related adverse events occuring during AIS hospitalization were associated with 30-day readmission. Secondary objectives examined whether demographic, clinical, and hospital characterisitcs were associated with post-AIS readmission.

Methods: We used the Nationwide Readmission Database to identify index AIS hospitalizations in the United States between January and November 2014. Inpatient records were screened for diagnostic and external causes of injury codes indicative of medication-related adverse events, including adverse effects of prescribed drugs, unintentional overdosing, and medication errors. Nationally representative estimates of AIS hospitalizations, medication-related adverse events, and acute non-elective readmissions were computed using survey weighting methods. Adjusted odds of readmission for medication-related adverse events and select characteristics were estimated using unconditional logistic regression.

Results: We identified 439,682 individuals who were hospitalized with AIS, 4.7% of whom experienced a medication-related adverse event. Overall, 10.7% of hospitalized individuals with AIS were readmitted within 30 days of discharge. Reasons for readmission were consistent with those observed among older adults. Inpatients who experienced medication-related adverse events had significantly greater odds of being readmitted within 30 days (adjusted odds ratio (AOR): 1.22; 95% CI: 1.14–1.30). Medication-related adverse events were associated with readmission for non-AIS conditions (AOR, 1.26; 95% CI: 1.17–1.35), but not with readmission for AIS (AOR, 0.91; 95% CI: 0.75–1.10). Several factors, including but not limited to being younger than 40 years (AOR, 1.12; 95% CI: 1.00–1.26), Medicare insurance coverage (AOR, 1.33; 95% CI: 1.26–1.40), length of stay greater than 1 week (AOR, 1.38; 95% CI: 1.33–1.42), having 7 or more comorbidites (AOR, 2.20; 95% CI: 2.08–2.34), and receiving care at a for-profit hospital (AOR, 1.20; 95% CI: 1.12–1.29), were identified as being associated with all-cause 30-day readmission.

Conclusions: In this nationally representative sample of AIS hospitalizations, medication-related adverse events were positively associated with 30-day readmission for non-AIS causes. Future studies are necessary to determine whether medication-related adverse events and readmissions in AIS are avoidable.

Keywords: Acute ischemic stroke, Readmission, Medication-related adverse events, Nationwide readmission database

---

* Correspondence: jcris021@uottawa.ca
[1]Department of Neurology, University of Pennsylvania Perelman School of Medicine, Blockley Hall, 423 Guardian Drive, Office 811, Philadelphia, PA 19104, USA
Full list of author information is available at the end of the article

Background

Despite improvements in population health contributing to decreasing stroke incidence, mortality, and age-adjusted hospitalization rates in the United States (US) over the last decade [1–3], stroke remains a leading cause of death, hospitalization, and healthcare expenditure [1, 4]. Estimates suggest that approximately 795,000 individuals experience a new or recurrent stroke each year in the US [1], and that readmissions following hospitalizations for stroke are relatively common and often occur for potentially avoidable causes, including urinary tract infections, uncontrolled diabetes, and pneumonia [4–6].

Hospital readmission is considered to be a useful indicator of quality of healthcare services [7–9], which has prompted some governments and insurers to implement hospital reimbursement schedules that are dependent on short-term hospital readmission rates [10, 11]. In effort to better understand factors contributing to readmission after stroke and identify populations at greatest risk of re-hospitalization, a number of studies have examined whether patient and care setting factors are associated with post-stroke readmission [5, 12–15]. Differences in study design, exposure and outcome definitions, and statistical analyses across studies have led to inconsistencies in reported results [8]. Nonetheless, length of index admission [6, 16, 17], discharge disposition [5], and stroke severity [13, 18] have been identified as consistent predictors of post-stroke readmission and may be essential measures in the development of risk-standardized readmission models for stroke.

Previously, a large multi-center study of stroke readmission in Australia found that experiencing an adverse event or severe complication, such as recurrent stroke, penumonia, urinary tract infection, or fall, during hospitalization was significantly associated with readmission within 28 days (adjusted odds ratio (AOR), 2.81; 95% confidence interval (CI): 1.55–5.12) [19]. Based on these findings, it is important to examine whether a similar relationship exists in the US, and whether the reported association between inpatient adverse events and acute readmission extends to medication-related adverse events. To enhance our understanding of medication-related adverse events among stroke inpatients, we examined acute ischemic stroke (AIS) hospitalizations and readmissions using the US Healthcare Cost and Utilization Project's (HCUP) 2014 Nationwide Readmissions Database (NRD). Our primary objectives were to characterize reasons for readmission within 30 days of discharge and determine if medication-related adverse events occuring during AIS hospitalization were associated with acute readmission. Our secondary objectives were to examine whether demographic, clinical, and hospital characteristics were associated with post-AIS readmission.

Methods

Data source

Using the 2014 NRD, we performed a cross-sectional analysis of hospitalizations for AIS and associated readmissions. Sponsored by the Agency for Healthcare Research and Quality, the NRD is a family of databases developed as part of the HCUP to support national readmission analyses for all payer classes in the US, including the uninsured. The NRD contains detailed demographic (including age, sex, and health insurance status), clinical (such as diagnoses, procedures, and length of stay), and hospital data (size, location, and teaching status) for approximately 35 million annual discharges. Persons admitted to NRD contributing hospitals may be longitudinally followed within calendar years, but not across years.

Study Population

A validated algorithm for stroke classification was employed to identify all 2014 discharges where a diagnosis of AIS was recorded [20], hereinafter referred to as index AIS hospitalizations. The utilized algorithm was specifically developed for the detection and classification of stroke (AIS, intracerebral hemorrhage, and subarachnoid hemorrhage) using administrative claims data from the US, with a reported sensitivity of 86% and specificity of 95% for AIS discrimination [20]. We identified index AIS hospitalizations by querying all diagnostic fields for documentation of any of the following International Classification of Diseases, Ninth Revision (ICD-9) codes: 433.x 1, 434.x 1, and 436. Index AIS hospitalizations with documented diagnoses of traumatic brain injury (ICD-9 codes: 800.xx-804.xx, 850–854.xx) or primary procedure indicative of rehabilitation care (ICD-9 code: V57) were excluded from the study population. Hospitalizations with undocumented length of stay and encounters where the patient died in-hospital were also excluded. Since source state data for the NRD database employ different patient identifiers, it is not possible to track encounters for the same individual across state boundaries. Therefore, index AIS hospitalizations were restricted to discharges where individuals were a resident of the same state as the hospital where they received care. To ensure the availability of 30-day readmissions data, December discharges of index AIS hospitalizations were also excluded.

Demographics, comorbidities, and care settings

Personal data extracted from index AIS hospitalizations included age, sex, health insurance status, length of stay, and discharge disposition. Comorbidities documented during the inpatient stay were assessed according to enhanced ICD-9 coding algorithms for Elixhauser comorbidities [21]. A single comorbidity score per encounter was computed as the sum of distinct comorbidities recorded during the hospitalization. Care setting characterisitcs of interest from index AIS hospitalizations included hospital size, geographic location, and teaching status.

Medication-related adverse events

Medication-related adverse events occurring during the index AIS hospitalization were identified using ICD-9 and External Causes of Injury codes (E codes) indicative of adverse drug events and medication errors [22]. Documentation of one or more of the following ICD-9 or E codes within index AIS hospitalization records served to indicate the occurrence of a medication-related adverse event: 357.6 (neuropathy due to drugs); 692.3 (contact dermatitis due to drugs and medicines in contact with skin); 693.0 (dermatitis due to drugs or medicines taken internally); 960.0–964.9, or 965.02–969.5, or 969.8–979.9 (poisoning by drugs, medicinal and biological substances); E850.1–E858.9 (accidental poisoning by drugs, medicinal substances, and biological substances); and E930.0–E934.9, or E935.1–E949.9 (drugs, medicinal, and biological substances causing adverse effects in therapeutic use). Index AIS hospitalizations with adverse drug events associated with illicit drug use, intentional harm, or poisonings unknown to be accidental were excluded from our analyses: 965.00 (opium poisoning); 965.01 (heroin poisoning); 969.6 (psychodysleptic poisoning); E850.0 (accidental poisoning by heroin); E854.1 (accidental poisoning by hallucinogens); E854.2 (accidental poisoning by psychostimulants); E935.0 (adverse effects of heroin); E939.6 (adverse effects of hallucinogens); E939.7 (adverse effects of psychostimulants); E950.0–E950.9 (suicide and self-inflicted poisoning); E962.0–E962.9 (assault by poisoning); and E980.0–E980.9 (poisoning undetermined to be accidental).

Readmissions

Same state readmissions within 30 days of index AIS hospitalization discharge were coded as the first readmission within 30 days. In instances where individuals were readmitted on multiple occasions within 30 days, only the encounter with the earliest time to readmission was retained for our analyses. Of these readmissions, elective readmissions were excluded. Time to readmission was calculated as the number of days between index AIS hospitalization discharge date and the date of first readmission. Readmissions where AIS was diagnosed according to the validated algorithm for stroke classifications were deemed to be for AIS. We summarized the principal causes of readmission (first diagnostic position) using HCUP's single-level Clinical Classifications Software [23], which aggregates ICD-9 diagnosed illnesses and conditions into 285 mutually exclusive and clinically meaningful categories.

Statistical analyses

Survey weighting methods that accounted for the NRD's sampling design were used to generate nationally representative estimates of all reported values, including the number of index AIS hospitalizations, the characteristics of these hospitalizations, and subsequent readmissions [24, 25]. Descriptive statistics were used to report individual, cormorbidity, and care setting characteristics for index AIS hospitalizations as a whole and by 30-day readmission status.

The chi-square test was used to make statistical comparisons between populations readmitted and not readmitted within 30 days of index AIS hospitalization discharge.

We examined differences in time to readmission by medication-related adverse event status within quartiles. We created population quartiles for each category of readmission. Applying the survey weights, we then compared proportions across medication-related adverse event status and population quartiles for time to readmission using the Wald chi-square test, which is based on the difference between observed and expected weighted cell frequencies. This approach allowed us to test for independence of medication-related adverse event status and time to readmission quartiles, while taking into account the NRD's complex survey design.

To examine the association between medication-related adverse events and readmission within 30 days of index AIS hospitalization discharge, we constructed weighted unconditional logistic regression models to estimate adjusted odds of readmission for those experiencing an adverse drug event during their hospitalization (compared to no adverse drug event). All models accounted for the survey design of the NRD and utilized the stratums and clustering of patients and hospitals to generate accurate variance estimates. Secondary analyses used similar models to assess associations between sociodemogaphic factors and readmission within 30 days of index AIS hospitalization discharge. Adjusted models included characterisitics that were hypothesized a priori to potentially confound modelled relationships. All analyses were completed using SAS v9.4 (SAS Institute Inc., Cary, NC, US).

Results
Cohort characteristics

We identified 439,682 unique individuals from the 2014 NRD who were hospitalized with acute ischemic stroke between January 1, 2014 and November 30, 2014. Cohort sociodemogaphic, clinical, and care setting characteristics are provided in Table 1. Nearly all (95.1%) index AIS hospitalizations were emergency admissions, with AIS documented 82.7% of the time as the primary reason for hospitalization. Overall, 4.7% of AIS inpatients were identifed as having experienced one or more medication-related adverse events during their index

Table 1 Characteristics of index AIS hospitalizations

Characteristic	Index Events n (%) n = 439,682
Age	
< 40	12,878 (2.9)
40–49	25,172 (5.7)
50–59	64,364 (14.6)
60–69	95,136 (21.6)
70–79	103,821 (23.6)
80–89	101,941 (23.2)
90+	36,371 (8.3)
Sex	
Female	225,570 (51.3)
Male	214,111 (48.7)
Primary payer[a]	
Private insurance	75,983 (17.3)
Medicare	295,655 (67.2)
Medicaid	39,091 (8.9)
Self-pay	16,303 (3.7)
No charge	2308 (0.5)
Median household income	
$66,000+	88,803 (20.2)
$51,000 - $65,999	99,932 (22.7)
$40,000 - $50,999	118,495 (27.0)
$1 - $39,999	126,668 (28.8)
Missing	5783 (1.3)
Length of stay	
0–7 days	306,786 (69.8)
> 7 days	132,896 (30.2)
Discharge disposition	
Routine	174,933 (39.8)
Transfer: short-term hospital	8551 (1.9)
Transfer: other type of facility	164,884 (37.5)
Home health care	86,989 (19.8)
Against medical advice	3531 (0.8)
Discharged alive, destination unknown	794 (0.2)
Comorbidities	
0–2	110,756 (25.2)
3–4	166,434 (37.9)
5–6	107,199 (24.4)
7+	55,292 (12.6)
Bed size of hospital	
Small	64,949 (14.8)
Medium	120,363 (27.4)
Large	254,370 (57.9)
Control/ownership of hospital	

Table 1 Characteristics of index AIS hospitalizations *(Continued)*

Characteristic	Index Events n (%) n = 439,682
Government, non-federal (public)	53,708 (12.2)
Private, not-for-profit (voluntary)	326,024 (74.1)
Private, investor-owned (proprietary)	59,950 (13.6)
Teaching status of hospital	
Metropolitan teaching	278,770 (63.4)
Metropolitan non-teaching	118,548 (27.0)
Non-metropolitan	42,364 (9.6)

[a]Some categories excluded due to small sample sizes

hospitalization, with 98.0% of medication-related adverse events being recorded as secondary diagnoses (conditions unlikely responsible for occasioning the admission).

Readmissions

In total, 47,170 (10.7%) of hospitalized individuals with AIS were readmitted within 30 days of discharge. The rate of all-cause 30-day readmission for inpatients hospitalized with AIS who experienced medication-related adverse events (15.4%) was greater than that of AIS inpatients who did not experience such events (10.5%) (Table 2). Primary documented reasons for re-hospitalization were consistent with those observed among older adult populations and included cerebrovascular disease, septicemia, congestive heart failure, renal failure, and urinary tract infections.

Of AIS inpatients readmitted within 30 days, 6205 (13.2%) were readmitted for AIS, with 40,965 (86.8%) readmitted for other reasons. Among individuals readmitted for AIS, those with a medication-related adverse event documented during their index hospitalization were more likely than those without to be readmitted between 2.4 and 15.0 days of discharge ($p = 0.003$) (Table 3). Time to readmission by medication-related event status during index hospitalization did not significantly differ for other examined reasons of readmission.

Factors associated with readmission

Compared to AIS inpatients who did not experience medication-related adverse events, inpatients who experienced medication-related adverse events had significantly greater odds of being readmitted within 30 days (AOR, 1.22; 95% CI: 1.14–1.30) (Table 4). Medication-related adverse events were found to be significantly associated with acute readmission for non-AIS conditions (AOR, 1.26; 95% CI: 1.17–1.35); however, were not associated with readmission for AIS (AOR, 0.91; 95% CI: 0.75–1.10).

Several other factors were associated with all-cause 30-day readmission (Table 5), including but not limited to: being younger than 40 years (AOR, 1.12; 95% CI: 1.00–1.26), Medicare (AOR, 1.33; 95% CI: 1.26–1.40) or Medicaid insurance (AOR, 1.41; 95% CI: 1.32–1.51) coverage, lowest

Table 2 Primary reasons for readmission within 30 days of hospital discharge

All Index Encounters n = 47,170 / 439,682; Readmission Rate = 10.7%	n (%)	Index Encounters With Medication-Related Adverse Event n = 3200 / 20,822; Readmission Rate = 15.4%	n (%)	Index Encounters Without Medication-Related Adverse Event n = 43,970 / 418,860; Readmission Rate = 10.5%	n (%)
Acute cerebrovascular disease	5833 (12.4)	Septicemia	464 (14.5)	Acute cerebrovascular disease	5591 (12.7)
Septicemia	5197 (11.0)	Acute cerebrovascular disease	241 (7.5)	Septicemia	4733 (10.8)
Congestive heart failure; nonhypertensive	1974 (4.2)	Congestive heart failure; nonhypertensive	165 (5.1)	Congestive heart failure; nonhypertensive	1809 (4.1)
Acute and unspecified renal failure	1852 (3.9)	Acute and unspecified renal failure	131 (4.1)	Acute and unspecified renal failure	1720 (3.9)
Urinary tract infections	1462 (3.1)	Pneumonia	118 (3.7)	Urinary tract infections	1356 (3.1)
Cardiac dysrhythmias	1412 (3.0)	Urinary tract infections	106 (3.3)	Cardiac dysrhythmias	1321 (3.0)
Gastrointestinal hemorrhage	1329 (2.8)	Cardiac dysrhythmias	91 (2.8)	Gastrointestinal hemorrhage	1252 (2.8)
Pneumonia	1272 (2.7)	Respiratory failure; insufficiency; arrest	88 (2.7)	Late effects of cerebrovascular disease	1158 (2.6)
Aspiration pneumonitis; food/vomitus	1223 (2.6)	Complications of surgical procedures or medical care	86 (2.7)	Pneumonia	1154 (2.6)
Late effects of cerebrovascular disease	1193 (2.5)	Aspiration pneumonitis; food/vomitus	80 (2.5)	Aspiration pneumonitis; food/vomitus	1143 (2.6)

income quartile (AOR, 1.08; 95% CI: 1.03–1.14), length of stay greater than 1 week (AOR, 1.38; 95% CI: 1.33–1.42), leaving hospital against medical advice (AOR, 2.41; 95% CI: 2.08–2.79), having 7 or more distinct comorbidites (AOR, 2.20; 95% CI: 2.08–2.34), and admission to a large hospital (AOR, 1.08; 95% CI: 1.02–1.15) or for-profit hospital (AOR, 1.20; 95% CI: 1.12–1.29) (Table 5). Individuals who were 90 or more years of age (AOR, 0.82; 95% CI: 0.74–0.91) and those who received care at non-metropolitan hospitals (AOR, 0.79; 95% CI: 0.73–0.85) were less likely to be readmitted following AIS hospitalization. Similar associations were observed for non-AIS readmissions (Table 5).

Having Medicaid insurance (AOR, 1.20; 95% CI: 1.02–1.42), leaving the hospital against medical advice (AOR, 3.12; 95% CI: 2.29–4.23), and having 7 or more distinct comorbidites (AOR, 1.34; 95% CI: 1.15–1.55) were identified as some

of the factors associated with readmission for AIS. Conversely, individuals who were 90 or more years of age (AOR, 0.72; 95% CI: 0.56–0.93) and those who were hospitalized for more than 1 week (AOR, 0.75; 95% CI: 0.68–0.83) were less likely to be readmitted for AIS following their initial AIS hospitalization.

Discussion

We analyzed nationally representative administrative claims from 439,682 individuals hospitalized with AIS between January and November 2014 in the US in order to characterize reasons for acute readmission and determine whether inpatient medication-related adverse events and select characteristics independently predicted readmission. Primary findings indicated that 10.7% of individuals were readmitted within 30 days of AIS

Table 3 Time to readmission by medication-related adverse event status during index hospitalization

Medication-related adverse event	Time to Readmission Median (IQR)	Time to Readmission Quartiles				p value[a]
		Quartile 1 n (%)	Quartile 2 n (%)	Quartile 3 n (%)	Quartile 4 n (%)	
	Any Readmission	1.0–4.0 days	4.1–10.0 days	10.1–18.6 days	18.7–30.0 days	
No	10.0 (4.0–18.5)	10,961 (24.9)	11,050 (25.1)	10,364 (23.6)	11,595 (26.4)	0.492
Yes	10.4 (4.5–18.8)	734 (22.9)	815 (25.5)	767 (24.0)	883 (27.6)	
	AIS Readmission	1.0–2.3 days	2.4–6.8 days	6.9–15.0 days	15.1–30.0 days	
No	6.9 (2.2–15.1)	1396 (23.5)	1329 (22.4)	1720 (28.9)	1499 (25.2)	0.003
Yes	6.7 (3.4–13.5)	31 (11.8)	83 (31.8)	89 (34.1)	58 (22.3)	
	Non-AIS Readmission	1.0–4.4 days	4.5–10.5 days	10.6–18.9 days	19.0–30.0 days	
No	10.5 (4.4–18.9)	8805 (23.2)	9547 (25.1)	9238 (24.3)	10,436 (27.4)	0.819
Yes	10.7 (4.7–19.0)	651 (22.1)	731 (24.9)	718 (24.5)	837 (28.5)	

Abbreviations: AIS Acute ischemic stroke, IQR Interquartile range
[a]Chi-square test

Table 4 Association between medication-related adverse events and 30-day readmission in AIS

Medication-related adverse event	30-Day Readmission		p value[a]	AOR[b] (95% CI)
	Yes n (%)	No n (%)		
	Any Readmission			
No	43,970 (93.2)	374,890 (95.5)	<.001	Reference
Yes	3200 (6.8)	17,622 (4.5)		1.22 (1.14–1.30)***
	AIS Readmission			
No	5944 (95.8)	412,916 (95.3)	0.172	Reference
Yes	261 (4.2)	20,561 (4.7)		0.91 (0.75–1.10)
	Non-AIS Readmission			
No	38,026 (92.8)	380,834 (95.5)	<.001	Reference
Yes	2939 (7.2)	17,883 (4.5)		1.26 (1.17–1.35)***

Abbreviations: *AIS* Acute ischemic stroke, *AOR* Adjusted odds ratio, *CI* Confidence interval

***$p < 0.001$

[a]Chi-square test

[b]Adjusted for age, sex, primary payer, number of Elixhauser comorbidities, median household income, length of stay, discharge disposition, bed size of hospital, hospital control/ownership, and hospital teaching status

discharge, that readmissions were primarily for reasons frequently observed in older adult populations, and that experiencing a medication-related adverse event greatly increased the likelihood of being readmitted within 30 days for reasons other than AIS. Our secondary findings showed that: (1) several factors, including, but not limited to, younger age, public health insurance, leaving the hospital against medical advice, and multimorbidity, were associated with an increased odds of all-cause acute readmission, and (2) that the eldest individuals and those receiving care at non-metropolitan hospitals were less likely to be readmitted following inpatient care for AIS.

Dramatic reductions in stroke incidence and related mortality have been observed in the US during the last decade and the age-adjusted AIS hospitalization rate decreased by 18.4% between 2000 and 2010 [2], with improvements being similar across sex and race [3]. Nevertheless, stroke remains a leading national cause of hospitalization and patient disability. Readmission following AIS hospitalization is common, with a large study of Medicare beneficiaries hospitalized for AIS in 2005–2006 reporting that 14.4% of patients were readmitted within 30 days of discharge and that nearly 12% of all readmission were for preventable causes [4]. During the year following AIS discharge, rates of readmission are estimated to be as high as 27% [14]. Our finding that 10.7% of patients with AIS were readmitted within 30 days of discharge suggests that there has been little overall improvement to the national rate of post-stroke acute readmission in recent years. Acute readmissions following AIS hospitalization in

the US are almost always (~ 90%) unplanned, are associated with more than $17 billion of annual healthcare spending, and in some circumstances may serve as an indicator of the quality of healthcare services received [5]. Although not all unplanned readmissions are preventable, knowledge of modifiable and non-modifiable risk factors associated with readmission provides the opportunity to develop validated readmission risk prediction tools to identify patients at greatest risk of acute readmission. Ideally, such tools could help target the delivery of health services, including enhanced discharge planning, to those found to be at great risk of readmission. In turn, this may improve individual health outcomes and lead to more efficient healthcare spending [26].

Medication-related adverse events may include side effects to medications taken as prescribed, accidental overdosing by patients, and medication errors [22]. Such events contribute to acute readmission and up to 50% of medication-related adverse events occurring post-discharge are considered preventable [27, 28]. Recently, a study of more than 500 readmissions to a large academic hospital in the US found that approximately 13% of all 30-day preventable readmissions were attributable to medication-related adverse events [27]. Of readmissions classified as preventable, one half were the result of prescribing errors, while the other half resulted from insufficient patient monitoring or education [27]. These findings highlight potential population and health system benefits that may result from interventions aimed at mitigating the risk of experiencing medication-related adverse events.

To date, studies of risk factors for readmission following inpatient stroke care have largely focused on patient or stroke-related factors, including, but not limited to, age, sex, socioeconomic status, place of residence, medical history, and the National Institutes of Health Stroke Scale/ Score [4–6, 17]. Similar to our findings, prior investigations have consistently identified recurrent stroke, infections, and cardiac conditions as primary causes of acute readmission in AIS, and longer length of index AIS hospitalization and increasing morbidity to be independently associated with readmission [4, 17, 29]. Other reported patient and stroke-related risk factors for short- and long-term readmission after stroke include prior coronary heart disease, heart failure, and diabetes, as well as having a feeding tube or urinary catheter [17]. Although we have confirmed prior reports that patient and geographic disparities in AIS exist and contribute to observed undesirable health outcomes such as acute readmission, characteristics such as individual age, sex, socioeconomic status, and place of residence are unlikely to be modified. At best, knowledge of these particular disparities may provide baseline data for future population-based research into other patient-level risk factors for readmission after AIS.

The path from patient and geographic disparity to timely, effective, and sustainable intervention is presumed

Table 5 Odds of readmission in AIS according to demographic, clinical, and care setting characteristics

Characteristic	Any Readmission		p value[a]	AOR[b] (95% CI)	AIS Readmission		p value[a]	AOR[b] (95% CI)	Non-AIS Readmission		p value[a]	AOR[b] (95% CI)
	Yes n (%) n = 47,170	No n (%) n = 392,512			Yes n (%) n = 6205	No n (%) n = 433,477			Yes n (%) n = 40,965	No n (%) n = 398,717		
Age												
< 40	1311 (2.8)	11,567 (2.9)	<.001	1.12 (1.00–1.26)*	135 (2.2)	12,743 (2.9)	<.001	0.76 (0.55–1.04)	1176 (2.9)	11,702 (2.9)	<.001	1.20 (1.06–1.36)**
40–49	2379 (5.0)	22,793 (5.8)		Reference	365 (5.9)	24,807 (5.7)		Reference	2014 (4.9)	23,158 (5.8)		Reference
50–59	6212 (13.2)	58,151 (14.8)		0.97 (0.88–1.05)	929 (15.0)	63,434 (14.6)		1.01 (0.83–1.21)	5283 (12.9)	59,080 (14.8)		0.96 (0.87–1.05)
60–69	9649 (20.5)	85,487 (21.8)		0.93 (0.85–1.01)	1431 (23.1)	93,705 (21.6)		1.08 (0.90–1.30)	8218 (20.1)	86,918 (21.8)		0.90 (0.83–0.99)*
70–79	11,992 (25.4)	91,829 (23.4)		0.97 (0.88–1.06)	1590 (25.6)	102,231 (23.6)		1.12 (0.91–1.37)	10,402 (25.4)	93,419 (23.4)		0.95 (0.86–1.05)
80–89	11,861 (25.1)	90,080 (22.9)		0.93 (0.85–1.02)	1389 (22.4)	100,551 (23.2)		0.99 (0.81–1.22)	10,472 (25.6)	91,469 (22.9)		0.93 (0.84–1.02)
90+	3766 (8.0)	32,605 (8.3)		0.82 (0.74–0.91)***	366 (5.9)	36,005 (8.3)		0.72 (0.56–0.93)*	3400 (8.3)	32,971 (8.3)		0.84 (0.75–0.94)**
Sex												
Female	24,509 (52.0)	201,061 (51.2)	0.087	Reference	3024 (48.7)	222,546 (51.3)	0.013	Reference	21,485 (52.4)	204,085 (51.2)	0.005	Reference
Male	22,661 (48.0)	191,450 (48.8)		1.03 (1.00–1.07)	3181 (51.3)	210,930 (48.7)		1.07 (0.99–1.17)	19,480 (47.6)	194,631 (48.8)		1.02 (0.99–1.06)
Primary payer[c]												
Private insurance	5834 (12.4)	70,149 (17.9)	<.001	Reference	1002 (16.1)	74,981 (17.3)	0.159	Reference	4832 (11.8)	71,151 (17.8)	<.001	Reference
Medicare	34,216 (72.5)	261,439 (66.6)		1.33 (1.26–1.40)***	4160 (67.0)	291,495 (67.2)		1.02 (0.90–1.16)	30,057 (73.4)	265,598 (66.6)		1.39 (1.30–1.47)***
Medicaid	4794 (10.2)	34,297 (8.7)		1.41 (1.32–1.51)***	636 (10.2)	38,455 (8.9)		1.20 (1.02–1.42)*	4158 (10.2)	34,933 (8.8)		1.44 (1.34–1.55)***
Self-pay	1264 (2.7)	15,040 (3.8)		1.04 (0.93–1.16)	231 (3.7)	16,072 (3.7)		1.05 (0.81–1.37)	1033 (2.5)	15,270 (3.8)		1.03 (0.92–1.16)
No charge	169 (0.4)	2139 (0.5)		1.01 (0.72–1.41)	42 (0.7)	2266 (0.5)		1.38 (0.85–2.25)	127 (0.3)	2181 (0.5)		0.92 (0.64–1.34)
Median household income												
$66,000+	9260 (19.6)	79,543 (20.3)	<.001	Reference	1312 (21.1)	87,492 (20.2)	0.014	Reference	7948 (19.4)	80,855 (20.3)	<.001	Reference
$51,000 - $65,999	10,175 (21.6)	89,756 (22.9)		0.97 (0.92–1.02)	1327 (21.4)	98,605 (22.7)		0.90 (0.79–1.03)	8848 (21.6)	91,083 (22.8)		0.99 (0.94–1.04)
$40,000 - $50,999	12,546 (26.6)	105,950 (27.0)		1.01 (0.96–1.06)	1544 (24.9)	116,952 (27.0)		0.88 (0.78–1.01)	11,002 (26.9)	107,493 (27.0)		1.04 (0.98–1.09)
$1 - $39,999	14,620 (31.0)	112,048 (28.5)		1.08 (1.03–1.14)**	1952 (31.5)	124,717 (28.8)		1.03 (0.91–1.17)	12,668 (30.9)	114,000 (28.6)		1.09 (1.03–1.15)**
Missing	569 (1.2)	5214 (1.3)		n/a	71 (1.1)	5712 (1.3)		n/a	498 (1.2)	5285 (1.3)		n/a
Length of stay												
0–7 days	27,070 (57.4)	279,716 (71.3)	<.001	Reference	4557 (73.4)	302,229 (69.7)	<.001	Reference	22,513 (55.0)	284,273 (71.3)	<.001	Reference
> 7 days	20,100 (42.6)	112,796 (28.7)		1.38 (1.33–1.43)***	1648 (26.6)	131,248 (30.3)		0.75 (0.68–0.83)***	18,452 (45.0)	114,444 (28.7)		1.50 (1.44–1.55)***
Discharge disposition												
Routine	13,069 (27.7)	161,864 (41.2)	<.001	Reference	2265 (36.5)	172,667 (39.8)	<.001	Reference	10,803 (26.4)	164,129 (41.2)	<.001	Reference
Transfer: short-term hospital	1306 (2.8)	7245 (1.8)		1.91 (1.70–2.14)***	327 (5.3)	8224 (1.9)		3.08 (2.44–3.90)***	979 (2.4)	7571 (1.9)		1.63 (1.44–1.84)***
Transfer: other type of facility	22,491 (47.7)	142,394 (36.3)		1.52 (1.45–1.59)***	2168 (34.9)	162,716 (37.5)		1.06 (0.95–1.19)	20,322 (49.6)	144,562 (36.3)		1.59 (1.51–1.67)***

Table 5 Odds of readmission in AIS according to demographic, clinical, and care setting characteristics *(Continued)*

Characteristic	Any Readmission		p value[a]	AOR[b] (95% CI)	AIS Readmission		p value[a]	AOR[b] (95% CI)	Non-AIS Readmission		p value[a]	AOR[b] (95% CI)
	Yes n (%) n = 47,170	No n (%) n = 392,512			Yes n (%) n = 6205	No n (%) n = 433,477			Yes n (%) n = 40,965	No n (%) n = 398,717		
Home health care	9693 (20.5)	77,296 (19.7)		1.26 (1.20–1.32)***	1298 (20.9)	85,691 (19.8)		1.19 (1.07–1.33)**	8395 (20.5)	78,594 (19.7)		1.27 (1.20–1.34)***
Against medical advice	595 (1.3)	2936 (0.7)		2.41 (2.08–2.79)***	##	##		3.12 (2.29–4.23)***	450 (1.1)	3081 (0.8)		2.13 (1.83–2.47)***
Discharged alive, destination unknown	16 (0.0)	777 (0.2)		0.20 (0.11–0.38)***	##	##		0.16 (0.02–1.08)	15 (0.0)	779 (0.2)		0.21 (0.11–0.42)***
Comorbidities												
0–2	7125 (15.1)	103,632 (26.4)	<.001	Reference	1364 (22.0)	109,392 (25.2)	0.001	Reference	5761 (14.1)	104,995 (26.3)	<.001	Reference
3–4	16,020 (34.0)	150,414 (38.3)		1.36 (1.30–1.43)***	2400 (38.7)	164,034 (37.8)		1.20 (1.07–1.34)**	13,620 (33.2)	152,814 (38.3)		1.40 (1.32–1.47)***
5–6	14,413 (30.6)	92,786 (23.6)		1.78 (1.68–1.87)***	1629 (26.2)	105,571 (24.4)		1.31 (1.16–1.47)***	12,784 (31.2)	94,415 (23.7)		1.86 (1.75–1.97)***
7+	9612 (20.4)	45,680 (11.6)		2.20 (2.08–2.34)***	812 (13.1)	54,479 (12.6)		1.34 (1.15–1.55)***	8800 (21.5)	46,492 (11.7)		2.34 (2.19–2.49)***
Bed size of hospital												
Small	6334 (13.4)	58,615 (14.9)	<.001	Reference	920 (14.8)	64,028 (14.8)	0.533	Reference	5414 (13.2)	59,535 (14.9)	<.001	Reference
Medium	12,747 (27.0)	107,616 (27.4)		1.04 (0.98–1.11)	1762 (28.4)	118,601 (27.4)		1.02 (0.88–1.17)	10,985 (26.8)	109,379 (27.4)		1.05 (0.97–1.12)
Large	28,089 (59.5)	226,281 (57.6)		1.08 (1.02–1.15)*	3523 (56.8)	250,847 (57.9)		1.00 (0.88–1.13)	24,566 (60.0)	229,803 (57.6)		1.10 (1.02–1.18)*
Control/ownership of hospital												
Government, non-federal (public)	5348 (11.3)	48,360 (12.3)	<.001	Reference	732 (11.8)	52,976 (12.2)	0.081	Reference	4616 (11.3)	49,093 (12.3)	<.001	Reference
Private, not-for-profit (voluntary)	34,592 (73.3)	291,432 (74.2)		1.04 (0.97–1.11)	4529 (73.0)	321,495 (74.2)		1.00 (0.86–1.16)	30,063 (73.4)	295,961 (74.2)		1.04 (0.97–1.12)
Private, investor-owned (proprietary)	7229 (15.3)	52,720 (13.4)		1.20 (1.12–1.29)***	944 (15.2)	59,006 (13.6)		1.09 (0.91–1.30)	6286 (15.3)	53,664 (13.5)		1.21 (1.13–1.30)***
Teaching status of hospital												
Metropolitan teaching	30,821 (65.3)	247,949 (63.2)	<.001	Reference	3856 (62.1)	274,914 (63.4)	0.161	Reference	26,965 (65.8)	251,806 (63.2)	<.001	Reference
Metropolitan non-teaching	12,662 (26.8)	105,886 (27.0)		0.97 (0.93–1.01)	1786 (28.8)	116,762 (26.9)		1.08 (0.97–1.19)	10,876 (26.5)	107,671 (27.0)		0.95 (0.91–1.00)*
Non-metropolitan	3687 (7.8)	38,677 (9.9)		0.79 (0.73–0.85)***	563 (9.1)	41,801 (9.6)		0.92 (0.77–1.11)	3124 (7.6)	39,240 (9.8)		0.77 (0.71–0.84)***

##Data suppressed - 10 or fewer observations in some cells
Abbreviations: *AIS* Acute ischemic stroke, *AOR* Adjusted odds ratio, *CI* Confidence interval
***p < 0.001; **p < 0.01; *p < 0.05
[a]Chi-square test
[b]Adjusted for all factors listed in table
[c]Some categories excluded due to small sample sizes

to be very long and uncertain. In consideration of these challenges, our study focused on the association between medication-related adverse events in the inpatient setting and acute readmission after AIS discharge, since medication-related adverse events are potentially modifiable events that may affect all patients. Our research adds to the growing body of literature pertaining to the role of hospital environments, both physical and social, in contributing to

readmission after hospitalization for AIS [14, 17, 30, 31]. Specifically, our finding that medication-related adverse events during hospitalization for AIS are associated with acute readmission may in part explain readmission risks observed among patients with AIS treated by hospitalists (compared to non-hospitalists; hazard ratio, 1.30; 95% CI: 1.11–1.52) [14] and those receiving care at hospitals with higher use of hospice (compared to non-use; OR, 5.86;

95% CI: 1.13–30.3) [30]. Moreover, our findings provide a clinically important contribution to knowledge of potentially avoidable outcomes related to modifiable events occurring within the hospital environment, and inspire new questions pertaining to inpatient medication monitoring and drug safety, areas that are often understudied in neurology.

Our study has a number of strengths. We used nationally representative and longitudinal health claims data and a US-validated algorithm to identify inpatients with AIS [20]. As such, it is unlikely that individuals included in our study were admitted primarily for hemorrhagic stroke, transient ischemic attack, traumatic brain injury, or other cerebrovascular conditions. Inpatient medication-related adverse events were coded using a method reported by the Agency for Healthcare Research and Quality to be efficient at classifying drug-related events in HCUP data [22]. In-depth demographic, clinical, and hospital NRD data enabled us to examine the association between various potential risk factors and acute readmission, and to control for several likely sources of confounding in our analyses. Collectively, our study methods permitted an assessment of the national inpatient burden of AIS with high external validity.

Despite these strengths, our study has certain limitations. Individuals receiving AIS care at hospitals outside of their home state were excluded from our study since it is not possible to track longitudinal follow-up across state boundaries. Therefore, the reported number of individuals admitted to hospital during our study period likely underestimates the true burden of AIS. It is also possible that not all medication-related adverse events experienced by inpatients were adequately documented within the source administrative claims data for this study. Notwithstanding this potential bias, misclassification of medication-related adverse event status is presumed to be non-differential and would therefore bias our reported associations towards the null. In addition, it remains possible that extraneous variables that could not be controlled for within our study (such as stroke severity, outpatient medication use, and comorbidities diagnosed prior to index hospitalization) may confound reported associations between examined risk factors and readmission.

Conclusions

In conclusion, using nationally representative health claims data from the US, we found that readmission within 30 days of inpatient care for AIS is common and associated with medication-related adverse events occurring during the index hospitalization. Although study replication is warranted, our initial findings provide compelling evidence that acute readmissions in AIS may be avoidable through implementation of interventions focused on modifiable risk factors within the hospital environment. Future studies are needed to fully elucidate how potentially modifiable factors within the hospital environment (such as medication

monitoring activities, pharmacist involvement in patient management, available nursing expertise, and communication methods) influence patient risk of medication-related adverse events and acute readmission. Population-based studies are also required to characterize inpatient medication-related adverse events in AIS by medication class and determine whether such adverse events and associated readmissions are avoidable. Lastly, future studies should examine whether the odds of acute readmission after AIS hospitalization vary by type of medication-related adverse event experienced during the index admission.

Abbreviations

AIS: Acute ischemic stroke; AOR: Adjusted odds ratio; CI: Confidence interval; HCUP: Healthcare Cost and Utilization Project; ICD-9: International Classification of Diseases, Ninth Revision; IQR: Interquartile range; NRD: Nationwide Readmissions Database; US: United States

Acknowledgements

We thank Mr. Derrick Tam and Dr. Dominique Ansell for proofreading the final version of our manuscript and recommending editorial changes.

Funding

This study was supported by the Department of Neurology Translational Center of Excellence for Neuroepidemiology and Neurology Outcomes.

Authors' contributions

JAGC designed the study, performed analyses, interpreted results, and wrote the manuscript. DPT assisted with study design and guided statistical analyses. YF assisted with study design, provided input on statistical analyses, and interpreted results. DK provided input on statistical analyses, and interpreted results. AWW assisted with study design, provided input on statistical analyses, and interpreted results. All authors read and approved the final manuscript.

Competing interests

JAGC, DPT, YF, and AWW declare that they have no competing interests. DK serves as Chief Risk Scientist of Risk Sciences International, a Canadian company formed in partnership with the University of Ottawa in 2006 (www.risksciences.com) that conducts risk assessment work for public and private sector clients in Canada and internationally. To date, RSI has not conducted work on the subject of the present research paper. DK holds a Natural Sciences and Engineering Council of Canada (NSERC) Industrial Research Chair in Risk Science, through a peer-reviewed university-industry partnerships program administered by NSERC. None of the industrial partners in this program are from the pharmaceutical industry.

Author details

[1]Department of Neurology, University of Pennsylvania Perelman School of Medicine, Blockley Hall, 423 Guardian Drive, Office 811, Philadelphia, PA 19104, USA. [2]Department of Biostatistics, Epidemiology and Informatics, University of Pennsylvania Perelman School of Medicine, Blockley Hall, 423 Guardian Drive, Office 811, Philadelphia, PA 19104, USA. [3]McLaughlin Centre for Population Health Risk Assessment, University of Ottawa, 600 Peter Morand Crescent, Room 216A, Ottawa, ON K1G 5Z3, Canada.

References

1. Mozaffarian D, Benjamin EJ, Go AS, Arnett DK, Blaha MJ, Cushman M, Das SR, de Ferranti S, Despres JP, Fullerton HJ, et al. Executive summary: heart disease and stroke statistics--2016 update: a report from the American Heart Association. Circulation. 2016;133(4):447–54.
2. Ramirez L, Kim-Tenser MA, Sanossian N, Cen S, Wen G, He S, Mack WJ, Towfighi A. Trends in acute ischemic stroke hospitalizations in the United States. J Am Heart Assoc. 2016;5(5):e003233.

3. Koton S, Schneider AL, Rosamond WD, Shahar E, Sang Y, Gottesman RF, Coresh J. Stroke incidence and mortality trends in US communities, 1987 to 2011. JAMA. 2014;312(3):259–68.

4. Lichtman JH, Leifheit-Limson EC, Jones SB, Wang Y, Goldstein LB. Preventable readmissions within 30 days of ischemic stroke among Medicare beneficiaries. Stroke. 2013;44(12):3429–35.

5. Bhattacharya P, Khanal D, Madhavan R, Chaturvedi S. Why do ischemic stroke and transient ischemic attack patients get readmitted? J Neurol Sci. 2011;307(1–2):50–4.

6. Nahab F, Takesaka J, Mailyan E, Judd L, Culler S, Webb A, Frankel M, Choi D, Helmers S. Avoidable 30-day readmissions among patients with stroke and other cerebrovascular disease. Neurohospitalist. 2012;2(1):7–11.

7. Chin DL, Bang H, Manickam RN, Romano PS. Rethinking thirty-day hospital readmissions: shorter intervals might be better indicators of quality of care. Health Aff (Millwood). 2016;35(10):1867–75.

8. Lichtman JH, Leifheit-Limson EC, Jones SB, Watanabe E, Bernheim SM, Phipps MS, Bhat KR, Savage SV, Goldstein LB. Predictors of hospital readmission after stroke: a systematic review. Stroke. 2010;41(11):2525–33.

9. Hansen LO, Young RS, Hinami K, Leung A, Williams MV. Interventions to reduce 30-day rehospitalization: a systematic review. Ann Intern Med. 2011; 155(8):520–8.

10. Centers for Medicare & Medicaid Services (CMS) Readmissions Reduction Program. https://www.cms.gov/Medicare/Medicare-Fee-for-Service-Payment/ AcuteInpatientPPS/Readmissions-Reduction-Program.html. Accessed 10 Dec 2017.

11. Chen C, Scheffler G, Chandra A. Readmission penalties and health insurance expansions: a dispatch from Massachusetts. J Hosp Med. 2014;9(11):681–7.

12. Fonarow GC, Smith EE, Reeves MJ, Pan W, Olson D, Hernandez AF, Peterson ED, Schwamm LH. Hospital-level variation in mortality and rehospitalization for medicare beneficiaries with acute ischemic stroke. Stroke. 2011;42(1):159–66.

13. Hsieh CY, Lin HJ, Hu YH, Sung SF. Stroke severity may predict causes of readmission within one year in patients with first ischemic stroke event. J Neurol Sci. 2017;372:21–7.

14. Howrey BT, Kuo YF, Goodwin JS. Association of care by hospitalists on discharge destination and 30-day outcomes after acute ischemic stroke. Med Care. 2011;49(8):701–7.

15. Lichtman JH, Leifheit-Limson EC, Jones SB, Wang Y, Goldstein LB. 30-day risk-standardized mortality and readmission rates after ischemic stroke in critical access hospitals. Stroke. 2012;43(10):2741–7.

16. Bjerkreim AT, Thomassen L, Brogger J, Waje-Andreassen U, Naess H. Causes and predictors for hospital readmission after ischemic stroke. J Stroke Cerebrovasc Dis. 2015;24(9):2095–101.

17. Rao A, Barrow E, Vuik S, Darzi A, Aylin P. Systematic review of hospital readmissions in stroke patients. Stroke Res Treat. 2016;2016:9325368.

18. Leitao A, Brito A, Pinho J, Alves JN, Costa R, Amorim JM, Ribeiro M, Pinho I, Ferreira C. Predictors of hospital readmission 1 year after ischemic stroke. Intern Emerg Med. 2017;12(1):63–8.

19. Kilkenny MF, Longworth M, Pollack M, Levi C, Cadilhac DA. Factors associated with 28-day hospital readmission after stroke in Australia. Stroke. 2013;44(8):2260–8.

20. Tirschwell DL, Longstreth WT Jr. Validating administrative data in stroke research. Stroke. 2002;33(10):2465–70.

21. Quan H, Sundararajan V, Halfon P, Fong A, Burnand B, Luthi JC, Saunders LD, Beck CA, Feasby TE, Ghali WA. Coding algorithms for defining comorbidities in ICD-9-CM and ICD-10 administrative data. Med Care. 2005; 43(11):1130–9.

22. Lucado J, Paez K, Elixhauser A. Medication-related adverse outcomes in U.S. hospitals and emergency departments, 2008: statistical brief #109. In: Healthcare cost and utilization project (HCUP) statistical briefs. Rockville: Agency for Healthcare Research and Quality (US); 2011.

23. U.S. Agency for Healthcare Research and Quality. HCUP Clinical Classifications Software (CCS). Healthcare Cost and Utilization Project (HCUP). Updated March 2017. http://www.hcup-us.ahrq.gov/toolssoftware/ ccs/ccs.jsp. Accessed 10 Dec 2017.

24. U.S. Agency for Healthcare Research and Quality. 2014 Introduction to the NRD. Healthcare Cost and Utilization Project (HCUP). www.hcup-us.ahrq. gov/db/nation/nrd/NRD_Introduction_2014.jsp. Accessed 10 Dec 2017.

25. U.S. Agency for Healthcare Research and Quality. HCUP Methods Series: Calculation Nationwide Readmissions Database (NRD) Variances. Report # 2017–01. https://www.hcup-us.ahrq.gov/reports/methods/2017-01.pdf. Accessed 18 Dec 2017.

26. Kansagara D, Englander H, Salanitro A, Kagen D, Theobald C, Freeman M, Kripalani S. Risk prediction models for hospital readmission: a systematic review. JAMA. 2011;306(15):1688–98.

27. Dalleur O, Beeler PE, Schnipper JL, Donze J. 30-day potentially avoidable readmissions due to adverse drug events. J Patient Saf. 2017. https://doi. org/10.1097/PTS.0000000000000346.

28. Davies EC, Green CF, Mottram DR, Rowe PH, Pirmohamed M. Emergency re-admissions to hospital due to adverse drug reactions within 1 year of the index admission. Br J Clin Pharmacol. 2010;70(5):749–55.

29. Fehnel CR, Lee Y, Wendell LC, Thompson BB, Potter NS, Mor V. Post–acute care data for predicting readmission after ischemic stroke: a Nationwide cohort analysis using the minimum data set. J Am Heart Assoc. 2015;4(9): e002145.

30. Burke JF, Skolarus LE, Adelman EE, Reeves MJ, Brown DL. Influence of hospital-level practices on readmission after ischemic stroke. Neurology. 2014;82(24):2196–204.

31. Smith MA, Frytak JR, Liou JI, Finch MD. Rehospitalization and survival for stroke patients in managed care and traditional Medicare plans. Med Care. 2005;43(9):902–10.

The psychometric properties of the Childhood Health Assessment Questionnaire (CHAQ) in children with cerebral palsy

Soojung Chae[1], Eun-Young Park[1] and Yoo-Im Choi[2*]

Abstract

Background: The evaluation of children with cerebral palsy (CP) focuses on activity level measurement to examine the effect of health-care interventions on their physical functioning in the home, school, and community settings. This study aimed to identify the psychometric properties of the Korean version of the Childhood Health Assessment Questionnaire (CHAQ) by applying the Rasch model. The use of the Rasch model has an advantage in that item characteristic curve estimation is not affected by the characteristics of subject groups.

Methods: Data were collected from 65 children with CP aged 75–190 months using the Korean version of the CHAQ. Response data were analyzed according to the Rasch model, and item fitness and difficulty and the appropriateness and reliability of the rating scale were evaluated.

Results: Among the 30 items of the Korean version of the CHAQ, two items (nail-cutting and opening a bottle cap that was already opened) were shown to be misfit items with low fitness. The analysis results for item difficulty indicated the requirement for modification of item difficulty, pointing out the need for the addition of question items with both higher and lower difficulty. The use of 4-point rating scale in the evaluation questionnaire was shown to be appropriate. With respect to analysis outcomes, the subjects' separation reliability value and separation index were 0.97 and 5.92, respectively. In contrast, the separation reliability value and separation index for the question items were 0.95 and 4.51, respectively.

Conclusions: The results of this study suggest the need for the modification of item fitness and difficulty. The psychometric properties of the Korean version of the CHAQ were identified using the item response theory-based Rasch analysis.

Keywords: Children with cerebral palsy, Childhood health assessment questionnaire, Health-related quality of life, Rasch analysis

Background

Cerebral palsy (CP) is a permanent and nonprogressive developmental disability. Despite medical treatment and rehabilitation, various motor limitations associated with CP may reduce functionality and affect skills required for the performance of activities of daily living (ADLs) [1]. Premature mortality in children with CP is rapidly decreasing, and most of them survive until adulthood [2, 3]. The acquisition of high-level information about the functional status of children with CP has progressively become imperative [4, 5]. However, information on health-related quality of life (HRQL) in children with CP, which could provide critical perspectives in preparation for the future of these children, remains lacking [6].

Unlike in the past, the evaluation of children with CP focuses on activity level measurement to examine the effect of health-care interventions on their physical functioning in the home, school, and community settings [7, 8]. The

* Correspondence: tiffaniey@wku.ac.kr
[2]Department of Occupational Therapy, School of Medicine and Institute for Health Improvement, Wonkwang University, Iksan, South Korea
Full list of author information is available at the end of the article

International Classification of Functioning (ICF) has provided a framework for the collection of data on aspects of activity limitation and impairment, urging the exploration of the correlation between activity limitation and impairment. The ICF defines activity as the execution of any specific task by an individual [9]. When assessing disability, all relevant circumstances must be taken into account, and the extent to which individuals with disabilities can perform essential functions or major life activities should be measured.

Recently, evaluation has included the role of childhood or how children with disabilities feel in the course of solving obstacles that they face [10–12]. HRQL, a concept pertaining to aspects of life quality that are directly associated with health status, has been assessed [13, 14]. A HRQL assessment inventory had been developed for the past 10 years, with some general scales of HRQL having already been applied to children with disabilities and used for the evaluation of physical and psychological damage [15–18]. Various assessment inventories have been adapted in Korea, including the Korean version of EuroQol-5 Dimensions, which is designed to assess health status with respect to five areas of HRQL, namely mobility, self-care, usual activities, pain/discomfort, and anxiety/depression. The indices for each area are substituted with the assessment index equation to calculate the subjective HRQL indices [19, 20]. The Korean version of the 12-item Short Form Health Survey developed for the Medical Outcomes Study is also a tool used to measure HRQL and comprises physical and mental component summaries (12 items in total), with a higher score indicating a higher HRQL level. Moreover, the entire inventory was reported to be reliable (Cronbach's α = 0.810) [21]. The Korean version of the World Health Organization (WHO) Quality of Life Scale, an abbreviated modified version of the WHO Quality of Life Assessment Instrument-100 translated into Korean [22], is a 5-point scale inventory consisting of four domains (physical health, psychological, social, and environmental) for each of 24 facets related to quality of life. A response of "never" and "always" corresponds to a score of 1 point (lowest score) and 5 points (highest score), respectively.

These assessment tools have been used to evaluate HRQL in children with different types of disabilities. Based on the results, various plans have been proposed, and assistance has been recommended and provided. However, general scales for HRQL do not directly address functionality or ADL-related concepts, with only few tools among several scales being suitable for children with CP [23–25]. In particular, there remains a lack of information about HRQL in children with CP in Korea, possibly owing to the absence of feasible tools for HRQL measurement.

Recently, the Childhood Health Assessment Questionnaire (CHAQ), a tool specially developed for the assessment of functional capacity and independence in everyday life, has been utilized in children with CP. The CHAQ is a validated questionnaire comprising specific items used to evaluate juvenile idiopathic arthritis in children and adolescents [26] and has been considerably applied to patients with current mobility restrictions due to other chronic diseases such as pediatric spondyloarthropathies, spina bifida, joint hypermobility syndrome, and systemic lupus erythematosus [27–31]. The CHAQ has already been translated into several languages and used in many countries [32]. In Korea, the CHAQ was adapted by Park [33]; since then, its usefulness for the health-related assessment of children with CP has been reported.

The rapidly growing development of comprehensive question items to measure functional health status and quality of life in children has left a task of whether measurement of general aspects or specific conditions should be considered in selecting a tool [34–36]. The tool should provide appropriate information, and its psychometric properties could be measured to check its validity. Further, the tool can be selected only when it is practical, reliable, and appropriate and is able to measure change or sensitive to the change [37].

The classical method of scale verification is to confirm construct validity using factor analysis. However, determining the construct validity of the scale by factor analysis is limited because it is not a confirmation at the level of question [38]. The scale verified by factor analysis is occasionally adapted in other cultural regions in the course of its utilization and is applied to other groups with different characteristics from the respondent group participating in scale development. As scales are diversely utilized, an argument emerges from a study on scale development that factor analysis itself cannot accurately evince validity [39]. Therefore, in order to accurately estimate the fitness and difficulty of items derived from factor analysis, attempts to verify them using various statistical methods are required.

Among these attempts, the Rasch model is one of the item response theory models increasingly used as an appropriate research method for the assessment of the appropriateness of item fitness and difficulty [40]. When measuring the ability of a subject using traditional methods, the same subject will attain a higher and lower score if administered with a lower and higher level of test, respectively. In other words, in traditional methods, the characteristics of children with CP could affect ability measurement, possibly influencing the validity analysis of measurement tools. As the psychometric properties of an instrument can vary among different population groups and can be particularly affected by the cultural context, a systematic assessment of psychometric properties is imperative before an instrument can become extensively used within a specific patient population [41].

Therefore, in order to evaluate the psychometric properties of the CHAQ for assessing HRQL in children with CP in Korea, it is necessary to use data obtained from Korean children with CP. An item response theory-based analysis could be utilized to scrutinize question items using the item characteristic curve unique for each item, examine the difficulty and discrimination power of each item, and estimate the real ability of the subject based on analysis results. In addition, the use of the Rasch model has an advantage in that item characteristic curve estimation is not affected by the characteristics of subject groups [42]. Although the suitability of the Korean version of the CHAQ as a tool based on the classical test theory has already been confirmed in a validity testing study [33], attempting to verify the nature of question items by applying the Rasch model based on the item response theory remains essential to accurately evaluate item fitness and difficulty.

Therefore, this study aimed to identify the psychometric properties of the Korean version of the CHAQ in children with CP by applying the Rasch model. In view of the objective of this study, the following specific research questions were raised: First, is the item fitness of the Korean version of the CHAQ appropriate for children with CP? Second, is the item difficulty of the Korean version of the CHAQ appropriate for children with CP? Third, are the response categories of the Korean version of the CHAQ appropriate for children with CP? Fourth, is the Korean version of the CHAQ reliable when used in children with CP?

Methods

Subjects

For subject recruitment, the researchers sent letters to professionals at a hospital or community welfare center, asking for referrals of eligible subjects. Initially, 73 children with CP desired to participate in this study. Subsequently, the researchers sent letters describing the details of this study and received 65 informed consent forms for participation from the parent(s) of children with CP. As incentive, gift cards equivalent to approximately 20,000 won each were provided to the subjects' parent(s) and therapists. School-age children diagnosed with spastic CP who provided parent consent for their participation in the study were included, whereas those who underwent elective dorsal rhizotomy and had spina bifida and associated musculoskeletal disorders such as muscular dystrophy and myopathy were excluded from the study. Evaluation was performed by one physiotherapist and one caregiver per one child with CP for over 6 months of treatment. The general characteristics of children with CP are summarized in Table 1. The mean age of subjects in this study was 113.14 months (standard deviation = 30.03; range, 75–190 months) (Table 1).

Table 1 General characteristics of the study subjects

Classification		Number	%
Gender	Male	45	69.2
	Female	20	30.8
Site of Palsy	Quadriplegia	15	23.1
	Triplegia	4	6.2
	Paraplegia	28	43.1
	Hemiplegi	15	23.1
	Missing Data	3	4.6
Type	Spastic	53	81.5
	Athetoid	9	13.8
	Hypotensive	1	1.5
	Combined Type	2	3.1
Gross Motor Function Classification System	Level 1	16	24.6
	Level 2	14	21.5
	Level 3	10	15.4
	Level 4	6	9.2
	Level 5	19	29.2
Total		65	100

Tools

Childhood health assessment questionnaire

The CHAQ is a tool developed to assess health status and HRQL in children and adolescents with juvenile idiopathic arthritis. It has already been applied to children with various types of disabilities to measure their functional capacity and independence in performing ADLs during the previous week at evaluation time point. The CHAQ covers the following eight domains: dressing and grooming, standing, eating, walking, hygiene, hand stretch, catching, and activities. Items in these respective areas are rated on a 4-point rating scale, with score ranging from 0 to 3 points. A score of 0, 1, or 2 points denotes the performance of certain tasks without difficulty, with some difficulty, and with much difficulty, respectively, whereas a score of 3 points suggests inability to execute tasks. Because some questions are not applicable to young children, such item is marked as "not applicable." A higher score means low functional capacity. The CHAQ includes two visual analogue scales for the evaluation of overall well-being and pain severity. The eight domains are evaluated with the highest score for the detailed items being recorded, and the overall average is interpreted using the CHAQ Disability Index, with 0 point and 3 points indicating the absence of disability and presence of serious physical disability, respectively [32]. In calculating the CHAQ Disability Index, the highest score for the subquestions under each area is selected. A score of at least 2 points is indicated when a child requires some help in performing certain activities, and the average score for each area is considered the value for the CHAQ Disability Index. In this study, we used the CHAQ adapted to the Korean population [33].

Gross motor function classification system

The Gross Motor Function Classification System (GMFCS) was used for the evaluation of gross motor function in children with CP. The GMFCS, a tool designed to evaluate motor disorders in children with CP, categorizes these children into the following five levels: level 1 children, or those who can walk without restrictions; level 2 children, or those who walk with some limitations in most settings; level 3 children, or those who may walk without physical assistance but are using handheld crutches, canes, or walkers; level 4 children, or those who can move around with some limitations by themselves using electric-powered wheelchair or other means of transportation in most settings; and level 5 children, or those who have seriously limited ability to move around by themselves even with the use of assistive devices [43].

Procedures

Measured data from a total of 65 children with CP who provided informed consent for their participation in this study were collected to determine the psychometric properties of the CHAQ. In this study, a secondary analysis of data collected from a structural equation modeling study on factors affecting the participation of children with CP in daily life activities was performed [44]. The GMFCS was used by a physiotherapist with experience in treating children over 6 years, whereas the CHAQ was used by a caregiver.

Data processing

An infit mean square statistic (MNSQ) value < 0.5 or > 1.7 for each item denoted unacceptable item fitness [42]. The relation between individual attribute scores and item difficulty was analyzed using the distributions of items and subjects, which were included in a graph according to respective individual attribute scores to enable a direct comparison. Because the individual attribute scores and item difficulty were correspondingly converted into a logit scale for a direct comparison, it was possible to evaluate whether the item difficulty was appropriate for the analyzed group. When the ranges of two different distributions were consistent (i.e., similar distribution ranges for item difficulty such that item difficulty measurement could estimate all ranges of individual attribute scores), the distribution was considered sufficient [45].

The rating scale was analyzed using changes in threshold and the fit index of each subject for each rating score. In general, the higher the rating scores, the higher

the proficiency estimates and threshold were for subjects who responded to the questionnaire.

In Rasch analysis, the standard error of measurement is calculated based on all proficiency estimates apart from that of the sample group. This is shown as two concepts, namely the subject separation index and the item separation index. A larger value for these two separation indices indicates an accurate functional measurement level [42]. Based on these concepts, changes in separation reliability were drawn through removal of misfit items and subjects who inadequately responded. A total of 14 subjects inadequately responded in this study.

We used WINSTEPS version 3.6 [46] as statistical software to adapt the Korean version of the CHAQ and apply the Rasch model.

Results
Item fitness

The estimation results for the fitness of the 30 items of the CHAQ are summarized in Table 2. As shown in Table 2, the infit MNSQ value for items 4 and 23 following estimation of fitness among all items of the CHAQ was > 1.7 and < 0.5, respectively. After estimating the fitness of all items, the result for the fitness of four items among the 30 items of CHAQ indicated an infit MNSQ value of > 1.7, whereas the infit MNSQ value for item 23 was < 0.5 (Table 2).

Item difficulty

In the comparison of individual attribute scores and item difficulty, items 20 and 1 appeared to have the highest and lowest difficulty, respectively. Moreover, proficiency estimates were higher and lower than item difficulty in 22 and 24 subjects, respectively (Fig. 1).

Rating scale analysis

The estimation results for the 4-point rating scale of the CHAQ are shown in Table 3 and Fig. 2. The analysis results indicated that, for the CHAQ adapted to the Korean population, the increase in scale scores corresponded to an increase in the average proficiency estimate in subjects. Furthermore, the fit index for each scale score provided information on whether the rating scale was properly functioning. The fit index for the individual scale scores showed values ≥1.3 with respect to a value of 1.0, implying that the applicable scale was not properly functioning. The results of the analysis performed showed that there was no misfit scale in the CHAQ. With an increase in each estimate, similar to that in the average proficiency estimate in subjects, the threshold must show an increasing tendency as well. The analysis of the scale threshold showed that the threshold was proportional to the increase in scale scores in all subscales.

Table 2 Item fit statistics: entry order

Item	Measure	S.E.	Infit MNSQ	Infit Z-value	Outfit MNSQ	Outfit Z-value
1	29.93	2.42	1.03	0.20	0.88	0.00
2	33.73	2.40	0.58	−2.20	0.54	−0.70
3	58.70	2.76	0.84	−0.60	1.00	0.10
4	27.59	2.43	2.28	4.30	1.93	1.40
5	57.20	2.73	1.20	0.80	0.88	−0.20
6	61.83	2.84	1.27	1.10	0.73	−0.60
7	36.62	2.41	1.54	2.20	1.24	0.60
8	64.29	2.90	0.69	−1.20	0.81	−0.30
9	48.85	2.56	1.54	2.10	1.70	1.80
10	48.20	2.55	1.39	1.60	1.05	0.30
11	42.55	2.47	1.70	2.70	1.35	0.90
12	41.94	2.46	0.64	−1.80	0.66	−0.80
13	48.20	2.55	0.64	−1.70	0.50	−1.60
14	57.20	2.73	0.56	−2.10	0.44	−1.90
15	55.73	2.69	0.67	−1.50	0.57	−1.30
16	50.17	2.58	0.61	−1.90	0.54	−1.50
17	58.70	2.76	1.22	0.90	1.49	1.30
18	58.70	2.76	0.80	−0.80	0.61	−1.10
19	56.46	2.71	0.62	−1.70	0.58	−1.30
20	73.40	3.16	0.98	0.00	2.12	1.50
21	64.29	2.90	0.72	−1.10	0.87	−0.10
22	59.47	2.78	0.82	−0.70	0.79	−0.50
23	65.99	2.94	0.47	−2.40	0.79	−0.30
24	62.64	2.85	0.68	−1.30	0.76	−0.50
25	62.64	2.85	0.58	−1.80	0.78	−0.40
26	36.04	2.41	0.93	−0.30	0.78	−0.20
27	36.04	2.41	0.87	−0.50	0.67	−0.50
28	36.62	2.41	0.47	1.90	1.14	0.40
29	32.02	2.39	1.08	0.40	0.98	0.20
30	34.31	2.40	1.43	1.80	1.11	0.40

MNSQ Mean Square, *SE* Standard Error

Separation reliability

The separation reliability of the CHAQ adapted to the Korean population is shown in Table 4.

The subjects attained a separation reliability value of 0.97 and separation index of 5.92, whereas the separation reliability value and separation index for the items were 0.95 and 4.51, respectively.

Discussion

This study aimed to identify the fitness and difficulty of the CHAQ items adapted to the Korean population and verify the appropriateness and reliability of the rating scale in children with CP. To address such objectives,

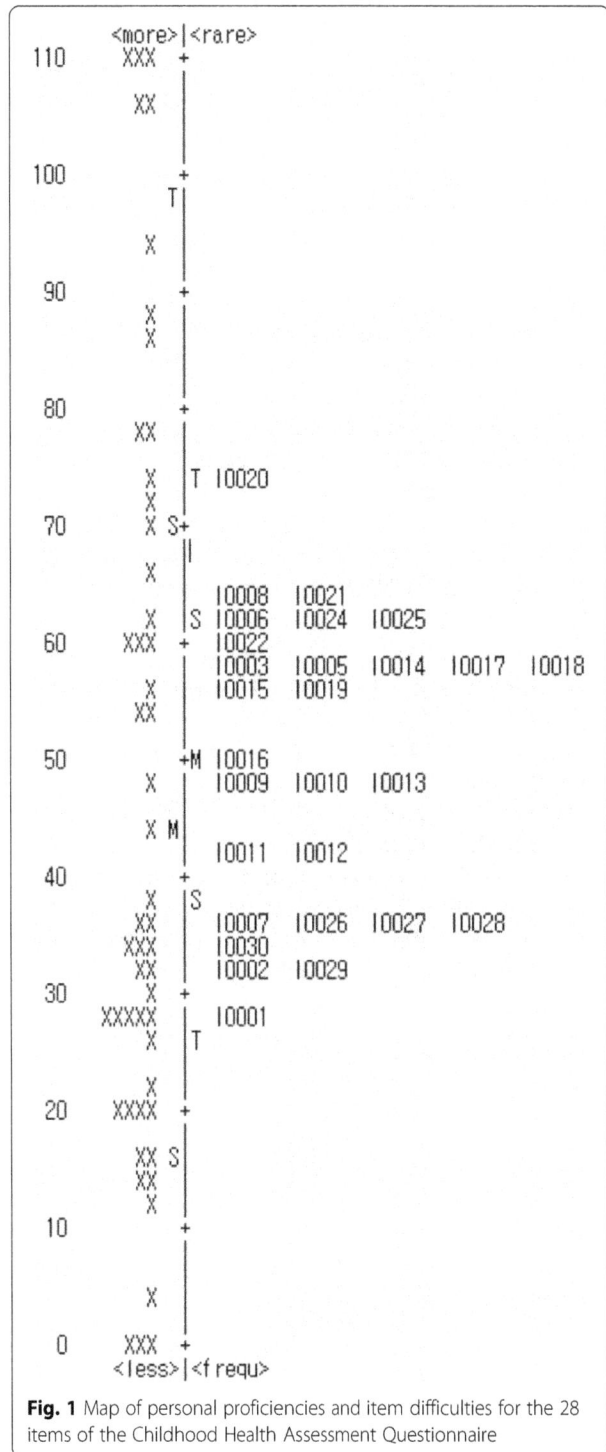

Fig. 1 Map of personal proficiencies and item difficulties for the 28 items of the Childhood Health Assessment Questionnaire

Rasch analysis of 65 subjects was performed using the CHAQ adapted to the Korean population.

When the fitness of the CHAQ items was determined, 2 of 30 items were shown to be misfit items. Item fitness is used to confirm the unidimensional nature of test items and is estimated using the MNSQ value via the utilization of the rating scale model, which could reveal

Table 3 Summary of the rating scale analysis of original 4 point scale

Category Level	Observed Average	Infit MNSQ	Outfit MNSQ	Structure Calibration
0	−33.19	0.92	0.95	None
1	−11.77	1.02	1.01	−17.48
2	8.18	0.87	0.70	1.50
3	33.06	1.31	1.26	15.95

how each item is adequately configured to confirm its unidimensional nature. A high MNSQ value indicates that the item does not have homogeneity with other items within the scale. In contrast, a low value means that the item is redundant with other items [45]. The MNSQ presents two values: the infit index and the outfit index. The infit and outfit indices are standardized, with the standardized value presented as Z value. In the Rasch model, an MNSQ value of 1 represents an ideal value. In this study, each item with an infit index < 0.5 or > 1.7 was regarded as a misfit item in order to determine item fitness [42]. Item 4, which pertained to nail-cutting, had an infit index ≥1.7, whereas item 23, which involved opening a bottle cap that was already opened, had an infit index ≤0.5.

Difficulties associated with the use of the CHAQ adapted to the Korean population were analyzed by comparing individual attribute scores and item difficulty. When the distribution ranges of the individual attribute scores and item difficulty were consistent (i.e., similar distribution ranges for item difficulty such that item difficulty

measurement could estimate all ranges of individual attribute scores), the distribution was considered sufficient [45]. The analysis results indicated that the difficulty for item 1 (tying shoe laces and buttoning) was the lowest among the 28 items with low fitness, whereas the difficulty for item 20 (turning the head to see behind the shoulder) was the highest. With respect to item difficulty for the CHAQ adapted to the Korean population, 23.5% and 13.7% of children showed a lower and higher capacity, respectively. A high percentage of floor effect for the measurement tool indicates that the item difficulty is higher than the proficiency estimate assessed using a tool in subjects. Conversely, a high percentage of ceiling effect for the measurement tool indicates that the item difficulty is lower than the proficiency estimate in subjects; hence, it is impossible to assess subjects exhibiting higher proficiency estimates as the item difficulty is too low. In the study of Park [33], the percentage of floor effect was reported to be 4.3–38.6%, with the rate for standing, walking, hand stretching, and catching exceeding 20%. In the case of ceiling effect, the percentage of floor effect was reported to be 1.4–25.7%, with the rate for walking and hygiene exceeding 20%. In the study of Morales et al. [32], the percentage of floor and ceiling effects was reported to be 2.1–26.0% and 30.2–68.8%, respectively. The high percentage of ceiling effect in the study of Morales et al. [32] should be considered, as the proportion of level 1 subjects according to the GMFCS was high (37.5%), and the results of Park's study [33] should had been affected by the fact that the proportion of level 1 children was 22.2%. Unlike in previous studies that identified item difficulty based on

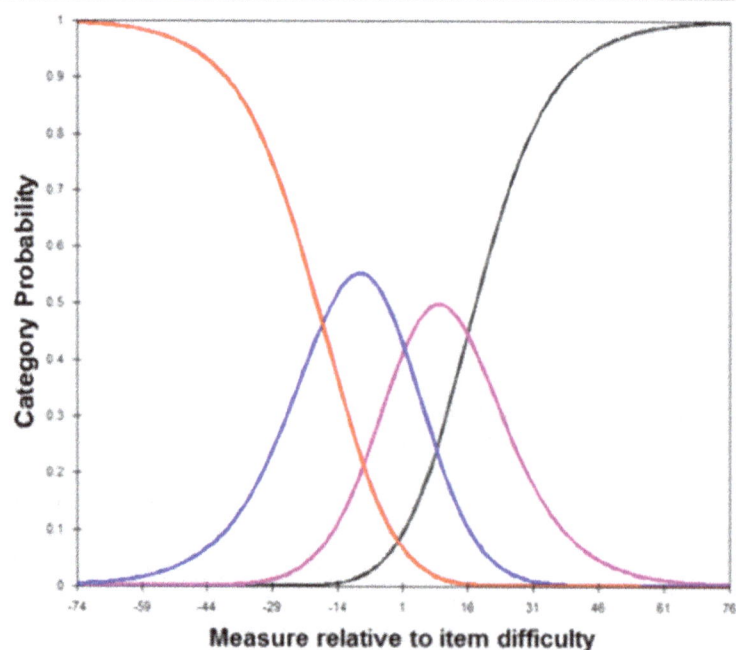

Fig. 2 Category probability curve for the Childhood Health Assessment Questionnaire

Table 4 Separation Reliability of the Study Subjects and the Items

	Mean	Standard Deviation	Separation Reliability	Separation Index
Subjects	34.0	26.8	.97	5.92
Items	67.3	18.0	.95	4.51

the classical test theory, the subjects' proficiency estimates and item difficulty in this study were converted into logit interval scales and analyzed, making it possible to overcome the limitations of subjects. Nevertheless, the results of this study showed that there was a need to add items characterized by both high and low difficulty to the CHAQ adapted to the Korean population.

The rating scale to be used for the development of a test should have a clear response level as same as potential variables to be measured and used to produce a test with a rating scale shall have a clear response level. Furthermore, fit indices for each scale score provide information on whether the rating scale is properly functioning. The fit index for the individual scale scores showed values ≥1.5 with respect to a value of 1.0, implying that the applicable scale was not properly functioning and providing possible information on whether the scale scores could be merged later [46, 47]. In the analysis, the 4-point rating scale of the CHAQ adapted to the Korean population was determined to be appropriate. The scale threshold estimate showed a tendency similar to that of the average proficiency estimate in which the scale threshold increased with an increase in scale scores. The scale threshold estimate differs from the average proficiency estimate in subjects in that the former is an estimate calculated by observation frequency based on the sample, whereas the latter is an estimate calculated using the Rasch model [42]. The analysis results showed that the rating scale of the Korean version of the CHAQ is proportional to the increase in scale score, indicating that the response range was appropriate.

The Rasch analysis estimates two types of separation reliability: subject separation reliability and item separation reliability. The Rasch model is able to estimate the concurrent validity through the subject separation reliability and estimate the construct validity through the item separation reliability [48]. The subject separation reliability is the same concept as the conventional reliability, Cronbach's α [46]. When the CHAQ separation reliability was estimated after excluding the misfit subjects and misfit topics, the subject separation reliability was 0.97, and the separation index was 5.92, whereas the item separation reliability was 0.95, and the separation index was 4.51. These results showed the CHAQ adapted to the Korean population had a high level of reliability.

This study has some limitations. First, it would have been preferable to have more than 65 children with CP as subjects. Further study with a larger sample size is required to increase the power and possibility for generalization of study results. Second, this study only included children with CP aged 75–190 months. This could potentially affect the feasibility to generalize the results to the entire pediatric population with CP. Future studies on infants (0–36 months) and/or young children (36–72 months) with CP should be performed. Lastly, this study did not examine differential item functioning. There may be items that function differently depending on the type of CP; hence, further analysis based on the types of CP is required.

Conclusions

In this study, the results of assessment performed using the CHAQ adapted to the Korean population were analyzed using the Rasch model to determine the psychometric properties of the CHAQ as a tool for HRQL measurement in children with CP. With the analysis, results for item fitness and difficulty, rating scale analysis, and reliability outcomes were derived. Based on the results, among the items of the CHAQ adapted to the Korean population, two items had low fitness, and modification of item difficulty was required. The rating scale was reliable and appropriate. Moreover, item development and modification were determined to be necessary to augment the usefulness of the CHAQ adapted to the Korean population in assessing HRQL in children with CP. Further studies clarifying the usefulness of tools in assessing quality of life in children with CP should be performed.

Abbreviations
ADLs: Activities of daily living; CHAQ: Childhood Health Assessment Questionnaire; GMFCS: Gross Motor Function Classification System; HRQL: Health-related quality of life; ICF: International Classification of Functioning; MNSQ: Mean square statistic; WHO: World Health Organization

Funding
This study was supported by Wonkwang University in 2017.

Authors' contributions
SC has made substantial contribution to the drafting of the manuscript. EY has made substantial contribution to data interpretation and analysis and drafting of the manuscript. YC has made substantial contribution to data collection and manuscript revision. All authors have read and approved the final version of the manuscript.

Competing interests
The authors declare that they have no competing interests.

Author details

[1]Department of Secondary Special Education, College of Education, Jeonju University, 1200 3-ga, Hyoja-dong, Wansan-gu, Jeonju 560-759, South Korea. [2]Department of Occupational Therapy, School of Medicine and Institute for Health Improvement, Wonkwang University, Iksan, South Korea.

References

1. Beckung E, Hagberg G. Neuroimpairments, activity limitations, and participation restrictions in children with cerebral palsy. Dev Med Child Neurol. 2002;44:309–16.
2. Hutton J, Pharoah PO. Life expectancy in severe cerebral palsy. Arch Dis Child. 2006;91:254–8.
3. Katz RT. Life expectancy for children with cerebral palsy and mental retardation: implications for life care planning. NeuroRehabilitation. 2003;18:261–70.
4. Bottos M, Feliciangeli A, Sciuto L, Gericke C, Vianello A. Functional status of adults with cerebral palsy and implications for treatment of children. Dev Med Child Neurol. 2001;43:516–28.
5. Donkervoort M, Roebroeck M, Wiegerink D, van der Heijden-Maessen H, Stam H. Transition research group south West Netherlands. Determinants of functioning of adolescents and young adults with cerebral palsy. Disabil Rehabil. 2007;29:453–63.
6. Young NL, Rochon TG, McCormick A, Law M, Wedge JH, Fehlings D. The health and quality of life outcomes among youth and young adults with cerebral palsy. Arch Phys Med Rehabil. 2010;91:143–8.
7. Palisano RJ, Copeland WP, Galuppi BE. Performance of physical activities by adolescents with cerebral palsy. Phys Ther. 2007;87:77–87.
8. Schenker R, Coster W, Parush S. Participation and activity performance of students with cerebral palsy within the school environment. Disabil Rehabil. 2005;27:539–52.
9. Wold Health Organization. International classification of functioning, disability and health. Geneva: World Health Organization; 2001.
10. Feldman BM, Grundland B, McCullough L, Wright V. Distinction of quality of life, health related quality of life, and health status in children referred for rheumatologic care. J Rheumatol. 2000;27:226–33.
11. Saigal S, Rosenbaum PL, Feeny D, Burrows E, Furlong W, Stoskopf BL, et al. Parental perspectives of the health status and health-related quality of life of teen-aged children who were extremely low birth weight and term controls. Pediatrics. 2000;105:569–74.
12. Sheridan RL, Hinson MI, Liang MH, Nackel AF, Schoenfeld DA, Ryan CM, et al. Long-term outcome of children surviving massive burns. JAMA. 2000; 283:69–73.
13. Bjornson KF, McLaughlin JF. The measurement of health-related quality of life (HRQL) in children with cerebral palsy. Eur J Neurol. 2001;8(Suppl 5): 183–93.
14. Guyatt GH, Naylor CD, Juniper E, Heyland DK, Jaeschke R, Cook DJ. Users' guides to the medical literature. XII How to use articles about health-related quality of life Evidence-Based Medicine Working Group. JAMA. 1997;277:1232–7.
15. Morales Nde M, Silva CH, Frontarolli AC, Araújo RR, Rangel VO, Pinto RM, et al. Psychometric properties of the initial Brazilian version of the CHQ-PF50 applied to the caregivers of children and adolescents with cerebral palsy. Qual Life Res. 2007;16:437–44.
16. Liptak GS, O'Donnell M, Conaway M, Chumlea WC, Worley G, Henderson RC, et al. Health status of children with moderate to severe cerebral palsy. Dev Med Child Neurol. 2001;43:364–70.
17. Vargus-Adams J. Health-related quality of life in childhood cerebral palsy. Arch Phys Med Rehabil. 2005;86:940–5.
18. Wake M, Salmon L, Reddihough D. Health status of Australian children with mild to severe cerebral palsy: cross-sectional survey using the child health questionnaire. Dev Med Child Neurol. 2003;45:194–9.
19. Kang IW, Cho WJ. The influence on mental health status and health-related quality of life in middle-aged women by the regular walking exercise by based on the Korea National Health and nutrition examination survey - KNHANES VI. J Korean Soc Wellness. 2016;11:207–15.
20. Kim SY, Yun JE, Kimm HJ, Jee SH. The relation of physical activity by the IPAQ to health-related quality of life - Korea National Health and nutrition examination survey (KNHANES) IV 2007-2008. Korean J Health Educ Promot. 2011;28:15–25.
21. Lee S. A study on employees' health status and quality of life by using SF-12: a case study of employees in large-scale workplaces in Daejeon and Chungcheong province. Seoul: Catholic University of Korea; 2010.
22. Min SK, Lee CI, Kim KI, Suh SY, Kim DK. Development of Korean version of WHO quality of life scale abbreviated version (WHOQOL-BREF). J Korean Neuropsychiatr Assoc. 2000;39:571–9.
23. Hammal D, Jarvis SN, Colver AF. Participation of children with cerebral palsy is influenced by where they live. Dev Med Child Neurol. 2004;46:292–8.
24. Nemer R, Blasco PA, Russman BS, O'Malley JP. Validation of a care and comfort hypertonicity questionnaire. Dev Med Child Neurol. 2006;48:181–7.
25. Schneider JW, Gurucharri LM, Gutierrez AL, Gaebler-Spira DJ. Health-related quality of life and functional outcome measures for children with cerebral palsy. Dev Med Child Neurol. 2001;43:601–8.
26. Machado CS, Ruperto N, Silva CH, Ferriani VP, Roscoe I, Campos LM, et al. The Brazilian version of the childhood health assessment questionnaire (CHAQ) and the child health questionnaire (CHQ). Clin Exp Rheumatol. 2001; 19:S25–9.
27. Brunner HI, Maker D, Grundland B, Young NL, Blanchette V, Stain AM, et al. Preference-based measurement of health-related quality of life (HRQL) in children with chronic musculoskeletal disorders (MSKDs). Med Decis Mak. 2003;23:314–22.
28. Lam C, Young N, Marwaha J, McLimont M, Feldman BM. Revised versions of the childhood health assessment questionnaire (CHAQ) are more sensitive and suffer less from a ceiling effect. Arthritis Rheum. 2004;51:881–9.
29. Moorthy LN, Harrison MJ, Peterson M, Onel KB, Lehman TJ. Relationship of quality of life and physical function measures with disease activity in children with systemic lupus erythematosus. Lupus. 2005;14:280–7.
30. Ruperto N, Malattia C, Bartoli M, Trail L, Pistorio A, Martini A, et al. Functional ability and physical and psychosocial well-being of hypermobile schoolchildren. Clin Exp Rheumatol. 2004;22:495–8.
31. Selvaag AM, Lien G, Sørskaar D, Vinje O, Førre Ø, Flatø B. Early disease course and predictors of disability in juvenile rheumatoid arthritis and juvenile spondyloarthropathy: a 3 year prospective study. J Rheumatol. 2005;32:1122–30.
32. Morales NM, Funayama CA, Rangel VO, Frontarolli AC, Araújo RR, Pinto RM, et al. Psychometric properties of the child health assessment questionnaire (CHAQ) applied to children and adolescents with cerebral palsy. Health Qual Life Outcomes. 2008;6:109.
33. Park EY. Exploration of utility for Korean translation of the childhood health assessment questionnaire in children with cerebral palsy. J Spec Child Educ. 2010;12:335–53.
34. Lindström B, Eriksson B. Quality of life among children in the Nordic countries. Qual Life Res. 1993;2:23–32.
35. Taylor RM, Wray J, Gibson F. Measuring quality of life in children and young people after transplantation: methodological considerations. Pediatr Transplant. 2010;14:445–58.
36. Vogels T, Verrips GH, Verloove-Vanhorick SP, Fekkes M, Kamphuis R, Koopman HM, et al. Measuring health-related quality of life in children: the development of the TACQOL parent form. Qual Life Res. 1998;7:457–65.
37. Waters E, Salmon L, Wake M. The parent-form child health questionnaire in Australia: comparison of reliability, validity, structure, and norms. J Pediatr Psychol. 2000;25:381–91.
38. Embretson SE, Hershberger SL. The new rules of measurement: what every psychologist and educator should know. London: Psychology Press; 1999.
39. Hammond SM. An IRT investigation of the validity of non-patient analogue research using the Beck depression inventory. Eur J Psychol Assess. 1995;11:14–20.
40. Rasch G. Probabilistic models for some intelligence and attainment tests. Chicago: Mesa Press; 1993.
41. Kim JH, Park EY. Rasch analysis of the Center for Epidemiologic Studies Depression scale used for the assessment of community-residing patients with stroke. Disabil Rehabil. 2011;33:2075–83.
42. Bond TG, Fox CM. Applying the Rasch model: fundamental measurement in the human sciences. 3rd ed. New York: Routledge; 2015.
43. Morris C, Bartlett D. Gross motor function classification system: impact and utility. Dev Med Child Neurol. 2004;46:60–5.
44. Park EY. Factors contributing on participation in everyday activities for children with cerebral palsy: structural equation modeling. J Phys Mult Health Disabil. 2013;56:1–19.
45. Hong S, Kim BS, Wolfe MM. A psychometric revision of the European American values scale for Asian Americans using the Rasch model. Meas Eval Couns Dev. 2005;37:194–207.
46. Linacre JM. WINSTEPS Rasch measurement computer program. Beaverton: Winsteps; 2006. http://www.winsteps.com/index.htm. Accessed 10 Aug 2018

Permissions

All chapters in this book were first published in NEUROLOGY, by BioMed Central; hereby published with permission under the Creative Commons Attribution License or equivalent. Every chapter published in this book has been scrutinized by our experts. Their significance has been extensively debated. The topics covered herein carry significant findings which will fuel the growth of the discipline. They may even be implemented as practical applications or may be referred to as a beginning point for another development.

The contributors of this book come from diverse backgrounds, making this book a truly international effort. This book will bring forth new frontiers with its revolutionizing research information and detailed analysis of the nascent developments around the world.

We would like to thank all the contributing authors for lending their expertise to make the book truly unique. They have played a crucial role in the development of this book. Without their invaluable contributions this book wouldn't have been possible. They have made vital efforts to compile up to date information on the varied aspects of this subject to make this book a valuable addition to the collection of many professionals and students.

This book was conceptualized with the vision of imparting up-to-date information and advanced data in this field. To ensure the same, a matchless editorial board was set up. Every individual on the board went through rigorous rounds of assessment to prove their worth. After which they invested a large part of their time researching and compiling the most relevant data for our readers.

The editorial board has been involved in producing this book since its inception. They have spent rigorous hours researching and exploring the diverse topics which have resulted in the successful publishing of this book. They have passed on their knowledge of decades through this book. To expedite this challenging task, the publisher supported the team at every step. A small team of assistant editors was also appointed to further simplify the editing procedure and attain best results for the readers.

Apart from the editorial board, the designing team has also invested a significant amount of their time in understanding the subject and creating the most relevant covers. They scrutinized every image to scout for the most suitable representation of the subject and create an appropriate cover for the book.

The publishing team has been an ardent support to the editorial, designing and production team. Their endless efforts to recruit the best for this project, has resulted in the accomplishment of this book. They are a veteran in the field of academics and their pool of knowledge is as vast as their experience in printing. Their expertise and guidance has proved useful at every step. Their uncompromising quality standards have made this book an exceptional effort. Their encouragement from time to time has been an inspiration for everyone.

The publisher and the editorial board hope that this book will prove to be a valuable piece of knowledge for researchers, students, practitioners and scholars across the globe.

List of Contributors

Biniyam Alemayehu Ayele and Yared Mamushet Yifru
Department of Neurology, College of Health Science, Addis Ababa Univeristy, Addis Ababa, Ethiopia

Diána Mühl
Department of Anaesthesiology and Intensive Therapy, Medical School, University of Pécs, Ifjúság Str. 13, Pécs HU-7624, Hungary

Ákos Mérei
Department of Anaesthesiology and Intensive Therapy, Medical School, University of Pécs, Ifjúság Str. 13, Pécs HU-7624, Hungary
Medical Skills Lab, Medical School, University of Pécs, Szigeti Str. 12, Pécs HU-7624, Hungary

Bálint Nagy and Gábor Woth
Department of Anaesthesiology and Intensive Therapy, Medical School, University of Pécs, Ifjúság Str. 13, Pécs HU-7624, Hungary
Medical Skills Lab, Medical School, University of Pécs, Szigeti Str. 12, Pécs HU-7624, Hungary
Department of Operational Medicine, Medical School, University of Pécs, Szigeti Str. 12, Pécs HU-7624, Hungary

Lajos Bogár
Department of Anaesthesiology and Intensive Therapy, Medical School, University of Pécs, Ifjúság Str. 13, Pécs HU-7624, Hungary
Department of Operational Medicine, Medical School, University of Pécs, Szigeti Str. 12, Pécs HU-7624, Hungary

János Lantos
Department of Surgical Research and Techniques, Medical School, University of Pécs, Szigeti Str. 12, Pécs HU-7624, Hungary

Ferenc Kövér
Department of Neurosurgery, Medical School, University of Pécs, Rét Str. 2, Pécs HU-7623, Hungary.

Emmanuel Bäckryd, Sofia Edström, Björn Gerdle and Bijar Ghafouri
Pain and Rehabilitation Center, and Department of Medical and Health Sciences, Linköping University, Linköping, Sweden

Ye-Ting Zhou, Song Ye, Ben-Wen Xu and Chen-Xi Yang
Department of Surgery, Affiliated Shuyang Hospital, Xuzhou Medical University, Xuzhou, Jiangsu, China

Dao-Ming Tong
Department of Neurology, Affiliated Shuyang Hospital, Xuzhou Medical University, Xuzhou, Jiangsu, China

Shao-Dan Wang
Department of Intensive Care Medicine, Affiliated Shuyang Hospital, Xuzhou Medical University, Xuzhou, Jiangsu, China

Ying Liu, Bing-Yun Wu and Juan-Juan Xu
Department of Electromyography, Shandong Provincial Qianfoshan Hospital, Shandong University, Jinan 250014, People's Republic of China

Zhen-Shen Ma
Department of radiology, Shandong Provincial Qianfoshan Hospital, Shandong University, Jinan 250014, People's Republic of China

Bing Yang, Heng Li and Rui-Sheng Duan
Department of Neurology, Shandong Provincial Qianfoshan Hospital, Shandong University, Jinan 250014, People's Republic of China

N. David Åberg, Daniel Åberg, Johan Svensson and Jörgen Isgaard
Department of Internal Medicine, Institute of Medicine, The Sahlgrenska Academy at University of Gothenburg, Gröna Stråket 8, SE-413 45 Gothenburg, Sweden

Katarina Jood and Christian Blomstrand
Department of Clinical Neuroscience, Institute of Neuroscience and Physiology, The Sahlgrenska Academy at University of Gothenburg, Gothenburg, Sweden.

Michael Nilsson
Department of Clinical Neuroscience, Institute of Neuroscience and Physiology, The Sahlgrenska Academy at University of Gothenburg, Gothenburg, Sweden
Hunter Medical Research Institute, University of Newcastle, Newcastle, Australia

H. Georg Kuhn
Department of Clinical Neuroscience, Institute of Neuroscience and Physiology, The Sahlgrenska Academy at University of Gothenburg, Gothenburg, Sweden
Center for Stroke Research Berlin, Charité – Universitätsmedizin Berlin, Berlin, Germany

Christina Jern
Institute of Biomedicine, The Sahlgrenska Academy at University of Gothenburg, Gothenburg, Sweden. Department of Clinical Genetics, The Sahlgrenska Academy at University of Gothenburg, Gothenburg, Sweden

Yiping Tang, Dengli Fu, Xinhai Gao, Zhengchao Lv and Xuetao Li
Department of Neurosurgery, The Second Affiliated Hospital of Kunming Medical University, Kunming 650101, Yunnan Province, China

Fengqiong Yin
Priority Ward, The Second Affiliated Hospital of Kunming Medical University, No. 374 Dianmian Avenue, Kunming 650101, Yunnan Province, China

Daniel O. Claassen
Department of Neurology, Vanderbilt University Medical Center, 1161 21st Avenue South A-0118, Nashville, TN 37232, USA

Charles H. Adler
Parkinson's Disease and Movement Disorders Center, Department of Neurology, Mayo Clinic College of Medicine, Mayo Clinic, 13400 East Shea Boulevard, Scottsdale, AZ 85259, USA

L. Arthur Hewitt
Medical Affairs, Lundbeck, 6 Parkway North, Deerfield, IL 60015, USA

Christopher Gibbons
Department of Neurology, Beth Israel Deaconess Medical Center, Harvard Medical School, 330 Brookline Avenue, Boston, MA 02215, USA

Jianlong Li
Department of Neurosurgery, The Second Affiliated Hospital of Harbin Medical University, 246 Xuefu Road, Nangang, 150086 Harbin, People's Republic of China
Department of Orthopaedic Surgery, Nanfang Hospital, Southern Medical University, Guangzhou 510515, China

Chuanlu Jiang, Ruiyan Li, Qingbin Li and Lin Lin
Department of Neurosurgery, The Second Affiliated Hospital of Harbin Medical University, 246 Xuefu Road, Nangang, 150086 Harbin, People's Republic of China
Neuroscience Institute, Heilongjiang Academy of Medical Sciences, Harbin 150086, China
Chinese Glioma Cooperative Group (CGCG), Beijing 100050, China

Rui Wang
Department of Neurology, The Second Affiliated Hospital of Harbin Medical University, Harbin 150086, China

Lingchao Chen
Department of Neurosurgery, Huashan Hospital, Fudan University, Shanghai 200040, China

Wenzhong Du
Department of Neurosurgery, The First Affiliated Hospital of Harbin Medical University, Harbin 150086, China

Yasuhiro Aso, Ryo Chikazawa, Yuki Kimura, Noriyuki Kimura and Etsuro Matsubara
Department of Neurology, Faculty of Medicine, Oita University, Yufu-city, Oita 879-5593, Japan

Weishuai Li, Si Wu, Qingping Meng, Xiaotian Zhang, Yang Guo, Lin Cong, Shuyan Cong and Dongming Zheng
Department of Neurology, Shengjing Hospital of China Medical University, Sanhao Street 36, Shenyang 110004, Liaoning, China

Thanh Thi Mai Pham, Hiroki Kato, Haruyoshi Yamaza, Keiji Masuda, Yuta Hirofuji, Hiroshi Sato, Huong Thi Nguyen Nguyen, Xu Han, Yu Zhang and Kazuaki Nonaka
Section of Oral Medicine for Child, Division of Oral Health, Growth and Development, Faculty of Dental Science, Kyushu University, Maidashi 3-1-1, Higashi-Ku, Fukuoka 812-8582, Japan

Tomoaki Taguchi
Department of Pediatric Surgery, Reproductive and Developmental Medicine, Graduate School of Medical Sciences, Kyushu University, Maidashi 3-1-1, Higashi-Ku, Fukuoka 812-8582, Japan

Wei Sun
Department of Neurology, Xuan Wu Hospital, Capital Medical University, No 45, Changchun Street, Xicheng District, Beijing 100053, China

Yanfeng Yang
Department of Neurology, Xuan Wu Hospital, Capital Medical University, No 45, Changchun Street, Xicheng District, Beijing 100053, China
Department of Neurosurgery, Xuan Wu Hospital, Capital Medical University, No 45, Changchun Street, Xicheng District, Beijing 100053, China

Guoguang Zhao
Department of Neurosurgery, Xuan Wu Hospital, Capital Medical University, No 45, Changchun Street, Xicheng District, Beijing 100053, China

Haixiang Wang and Wenjing Zhou
Epilepsy Center, Yuquan hospital, Tsinghua University, Beijing 100049, China

Tianyi Qian
Department of Radiology, Beijing Key Lab of magnetic resonance imaging (MRI) and Brain Informatics, Xuan Wu Hospital, Capital Medical University, Beijing 100053, China

Felix P. Bernhard, Jennifer Sartor, Kristina Bettecken and Carina Arnold
Department of Neurology and Neurodegenerative Diseases and Hertie Institute for Clinical Brain Research, University Tübingen, 72076 Tübingen, Germany
DZNE, German Center for Neurodegenerative Diseases, Tuebingen, Germany

Walter Maetzler and Markus A. Hobert
Department of Neurology and Neurodegenerative Diseases and Hertie Institute for Clinical Brain Research, University Tübingen, 72076 Tübingen, Germany
DZNE, German Center for Neurodegenerative Diseases, Tuebingen, Germany
Department of Neurology, University Hospital Schleswig-Holstein, Campus Kiel, Arnold-Heller-Str. 3, Haus 41, 24105 Kiel, Germany

Nils G. Margraf, Christian Schlenstedt and Clint Hansen
Department of Neurology, University Hospital Schleswig-Holstein, Campus Kiel, Arnold-Heller-Str. 3, Haus 41, 24105 Kiel, Germany

Yvonne G. Weber
Department of Neurology and Epileptology, University Tübingen, 72076 Tübingen, Germany

Sven Poli
Department of Neurology and Stroke, University Hospital Tübingen, Tübingen, Germany

Jian-Xin Zhou
Department of Critical Care Medicine, Beijing Tiantan Hospital, Capital Medical University, No 6, Tiantan Xili, Dongcheng District, Beijing, China

Han Chen
Department of Critical Care Medicine, Beijing Tiantan Hospital, Capital Medical University, No 6, Tiantan Xili, Dongcheng District, Beijing, China
Surgical Intensive Care Unit, Fujian Provincial Clinical College, Fujian Medical University, Fuzhou, Fujian, China

Kai Chen, Jing-Qing Xu, Ying-Rui Zhang and Rong-Guo Yu
Surgical Intensive Care Unit, Fujian Provincial Clinical College, Fujian Medical University, Fuzhou, Fujian, China

Gemma Clarke, Elizabeth Fistein, Sam Barclay and Stephen Barclay
Primary Care Unit, Department of Public Health and Primary Care, Cambridge Institute of Public Health, University of Cambridge School of Clinical Medicine, Box 113 Cambridge Biomedical Campus, Cambridge CB2 0SR, UK

Anthony Holland
The Health Foundation, Chair in Learning Disabilities, Cambridge Intellectual and Developmental Disabilities Research Group, Department of Psychiatry, University of Cambridge, Cambridge, UK

Jake Tobin
University of Cambridge, Cambridge, UK

Yangrui Zheng and Chen Wu
Department of Neurosurgery, Hainan Branch of Chinese People's Liberation Army General Hospital, Sanya, China

Craig Moore, David Sibbritt and Jon Adams
Faculty of Health, University of Technology Sydney, Level 8, Building 10, 235-253 Jones Street Ultimo, Sydney, NSW 2007, Australia

Andrew Leaver
Faculty of Health Science, University of Sydney, Sydney, Australia

Pernilla Vikström, Anders Björkman, Ingela K. Carlsson and Birgitta Rosén
Department of Translational Medicine – Hand Surgery, Skåne University Hospital and Lund University, Jan Waldenströms gata 5, SE-205 03 Malmö, Sweden

Anna-Karin Olsson
Department of Psychiatry, NU Health Care, Trollhättan and Department of Psychology, Karlstad University, Karlstad, Sweden

Joachim Ögren, Anna-Lotta Irewall and Thomas Mooe
Department of Public Health and Clinical Medicine, Umeå University, Östersund, Sweden

Lars Söderström
Unit of Research, Development and Education, Östersund, Sweden

Magdalena Naumovska, Rafi Sheikh, Malin Malmsjö and Björn Hammar
Department of Clinical Sciences Lund, Ophthalmology, Lund University, Skane University Hospital, Ögonklinik A Kioskgatan 1, SE-221 85 Lund, Sweden

Boel Bengtsson
Department of Clinical Sciences Malmo, Ophthalmology, Lund University, Lund, Sweden

Lisette Kogelman and Thilde Marie Haspang
Danish Headache Center, Department of Neurology, Rigshospitalet Glostrup, University Hospital of Copenhagen, Copenhagen, Denmark

Thomas Folkmann Hansen
Danish Headache Center, Department of Neurology, Rigshospitalet Glostrup, University Hospital of Copenhagen, Copenhagen, Denmark
Novo Nordisk Foundation Center for Protein Research, Faculty of Health and Medical Sciences, University of Copenhagen, Copenhagen, Denmark
Danish Headache Center, Neurological department, Copenhagen University Hospital, Nordre Ringevej 69, DK-2600 Glostrup, Denmark

Louise K. Hoeffding, Kristoffer Burgdorf, Henrik Ullum and Erik Sørensen
Department of Clinical Immunology, the Blood Bank, Rigshospitalet, University Hospital of Copenhagen, Copenhagen, Denmark

Christian Erikstrup
Department of Clinical Immunology, Aarhus University Hospital, Aarhus, Denmark

Ole Birger Pedersen
Department of Clinical Immunology, Naestved Hospital, Naestved, Denmark

Kaspar René Nielsen
Department of Clinical Immunology, Aalborg University Hospital, Aalborg, Denmark
Henrik Hjalgrim
Department of Epidemiology Research, Statens Serum Institut, Copenhagen, Denmark
Department of Hematology, Copenhagen University Hospital, Rigshospitalet, Copenhagen, Denmark

Helene M. Paarup
Department of Clinical Immunology, Odense University Hospital, Odense, Denmark

Thomas Werge
Institute of Biological Psychiatry, Mental Health Centre Sct. Hans, Copenhagen University Hospital, Roskilde, Denmark

Department of Clinical Medicine, University of Copenhagen, Copenhagen, Denmark
The Lundbeck Foundation Initiative for Integrative Psychiatric Research, iPSYCH, Copenhagen, Denmark

Monika Balzer-Geldsetzer and Richard Dodel
Department of Neurology, Philipps-University Marburg, Marburg, Germany
Department of Geriatric Medicine, University Hospital Essen, Essen, Germany

Joaquim Ferreira
Instituto de Medicina Molecular Universidad di Lisboa, Lisboa, Portugal

Per Odin
Department of Neurology, Lund University Hospital, Lund, Sweden

Bastiaan R. Bloem
Donders Institute for Brain, Cognition and Behaviour, Department of Neurology, Radboud University Medical Center, Nijmegen, The Netherlands

Wassilios G. Meissner
Service de Neurologie, CHU de Bordeaux, 33000 Bordeaux, France
Institut des Maladies Neurodégénératives, University de Bordeaux, UMR 5293, 33000 Bordeaux, France

Stefan Lorenzl
Interdisziplinäres Zentrum für Palliativmedizin und Klinik für Neurologie Universität München - Klinikum Großhadern, Munich, Germany
Institute of Nursing Science and –Practice, Salzburg, Austria

Michael Wittenberg
Coordinating Centre for Clinical Trials (KKS), Philipps-University Marburg, Marburg, Germany

Anette Schrag
UCL Institute of Neurology, University College London, Royal Free Campus, Rowland Hill street, NW3 2PF, London, UK

G. J. Melendez-Torres, Xavier Armoiry, Rachel Court, Alan Kan, Peter Auguste, Jason Madan and Aileen Clarke
Warwick Evidence, Warwick Medical School, University of Warwick, Coventry CV4 7AL, UK

Jacoby Patterson
Independent research consultant, Windsor, UK

Carl Counsell
Institute of Applied Health Sciences, University of Aberdeen, Aberdeen, UK

Olga Ciccarelli
Queen Square Multiple Sclerosis Centre, University College London Institute of Neurology, London, UK National Institute for Health Research University College London Hospitals Biomedical Research Centre, London, UK

James A. G. Crispo
Department of Neurology, University of Pennsylvania Perelman School of Medicine, Blockley Hall, 423 Guardian Drive, Office 811, Philadelphia, PA 19104, USA

Dylan P. Thibault and Allison W. Willis
Department of Neurology, University of Pennsylvania Perelman School of Medicine, Blockley Hall, 423 Guardian Drive, Office 811, Philadelphia, PA 19104, USA Department of Biostatistics, Epidemiology and Informatics, University of Pennsylvania Perelman School of Medicine, Blockley Hall, 423 Guardian Drive, Office 811, Philadelphia, PA 19104, USA

Yannick Fortin and Daniel Krewski
McLaughlin Centre for Population Health Risk Assessment, University of Ottawa, 600 Peter Morand Crescent, Room 216A, Ottawa, ON K1G 5Z3, Canada

Soojung Chae and Eun-Young Park
Department of Secondary Special Education, College of Education, Jeonju University, 1200 3-ga, Hyoja-dong, Wansan-gu, Jeonju 560-759, South Korea.

Yoo-Im Choi
Department of Occupational Therapy, School of Medicine and Institute for Health Improvement, Wonkwang University, Iksan, South Korea

Index

A

Acute Ischemic Stroke, 13, 54, 152, 217-219, 221-222, 224-226

Adenomyosis, 89-92

Adhd, 184-191

Alpha-1-antitrypsin, 14-15, 19-23, 25-26

Anticoagulation Therapy, 89, 91

Autoimmune Encephalitis, 93-94, 98-99

B

Beta-interferon, 200, 215

Brain Edema, 64, 66

C

Carotid Endarterectomy, 7, 10-13, 151-152

Carotid Stenting, 7, 12

Cerebral Palsy, 227, 234

Cerebrospinal Fluid, 14-15, 19, 21, 23-24, 26-27, 53, 93-94, 96, 99, 102, 109, 130, 134-135, 178

Cervicogenic Headache, 153, 155-161

Chiropractic, 153-161

Clinically Isolated Syndrome, 200, 208

Cognitive Function, 93, 97, 108, 196, 211

Conservative Method, 56, 58, 61-62, 64-65

Corticosteroids, 35, 37, 177-178, 180-183

Craniotomy, 56-66

Critical Illness, 28-33

D

Decision-making Capacity, 137-138, 140, 145

Decompressive Hemicraniectomy, 235, 241-242

Dementia, 15, 21, 26-27, 98, 127, 137-140, 142-145, 147, 193-198

Depression, 1-6, 16, 27, 98, 100, 121-122, 125-127, 159, 166, 191, 193-198, 228, 234

Dopamine Secretion, 101

Dopaminergic Neurons, 101-102, 108-109

Down Syndrome, 101, 108-109

Dysphagia, 74, 137-138, 143, 145, 147, 193

E

Electroclinical Characteristics, 110-111

Electromyography, 35-36, 42-43

Emt, 76-77, 79-81, 83-88

Epilepsy, 93, 97, 99-100, 110-111, 116-122

Esophageal Pressure, 129-131, 133-136

G

Glatiramer Acetate, 200, 208, 210-216

Glioma, 76-77, 79-88, 93-94, 96, 99-100

H

Head Injury, 28, 136

Health Assessment, 227-229, 231-234

Health-related Quality of Life, 122, 126-127, 167, 192, 194-195, 198, 227, 233-234

Herpes Zoster, 35, 42-43, 94

Human Exfoliated Deciduous Teeth, 101-102, 108-109

Huntington's Disease, 137-138, 146-147

Hypercoagulagulability, 89

Hypertensive Intracerebral Hemorrhage, 56-58, 60, 63-66

I

Inertial Sensor, 121

Infectious Neuropathy, 35

Insulin-like Growth Factor I, 44, 54-55

Intracerebral Hemorrhage, 28-30, 32-33, 56-58, 60, 63-66, 218

Intracranial Aneurysms, 148-152

Intracranial Pressure, 65, 129, 132, 135-136

Ischemic Cerebrovascular Diseases, 148-152

Ischemic Stroke, 13, 44-45, 47-48, 52, 54-55, 152, 169, 172, 175, 217-219, 221-222, 224-226

L

Large Hemispheric Infarction, 235, 241

Late Stage Parkinsonism, 192-193

M

Magnetic Resonance Imaging, 11, 41, 43, 89-90, 92-93, 97, 119, 151, 167, 236, 241

Manual Therapy, 153, 156, 161

Matrix Metalloproteinase, 7, 12-13

Median Nerve, 36, 40, 162, 167

Medication-related Adverse Events, 217, 219-220, 222, 224-225

Methylprednisolone, 94, 96, 177-178, 180-183

Midas, 1-2, 4-5, 154, 156, 159-161

Migraine, 1-6, 153-161, 184-191

Minimal Invasive Surgery, 56, 61-63, 65

Mir-139-5p, 76-79, 81, 83-88

Mmp-9, 7-13

Modifiable Risk Factors, 168, 172, 222

Mortality, 13, 28-29, 31-33, 56-58, 61-66, 99, 126, 136, 149, 169-171, 174-176, 192, 198, 218, 222, 226-227

Motor Neurone Disease, 137-139, 146-147

Multiple Cerebral Infarctions, 89, 92

Multiple Sclerosis, 121-122, 137-139, 147, 165-167, 177-179, 182-183, 200-201, 215-216

Multiple System Atrophy, 67-69, 74, 147

N

Nerve Conduction, 35-37, 39-40, 42

Nerve Mri, 35

Neurogenic Orthostatic Hypotension, 67, 69, 71, 73-75

Neurological Diseases, 121, 125, 137-138

Non-motor Complications, 192

Notch1, 76-88

O

Optic Neuritis, 177-178, 182-183

P

Parkinson's Disease, 27, 75, 121-122, 126-128, 137-139, 145-147, 192, 194-199

Perioperative Management, 148-149, 152

Phq-9, 1-6

Positive End-expiratory Pressure, 129, 132-133, 135-136

Postural Control, 121, 126

Precuneal Epilepsy, 110-111, 116, 118-119

Progressive Supranuclear Palsy, 137, 139, 146-147

Q

Quality of Care, 33, 66, 192, 226

R

Rasch Analysis, 227, 230-231, 233-234

S

Secondary Prevention, 152, 168, 174-176

Seeg, 110-120

Segmental Zoster Paresis, 35, 37-38, 40, 42-43

Sensory Profile, 162-167

Shed, 101-109, 214

Spinal Manipulation, 153, 158-159, 161

Stem Cells, 82, 88, 101-102, 106-109

Stroke, 6-13, 30-31, 33-34, 44-55, 66, 92, 121-122, 126, 136, 152, 163-164, 166-172, 174-176, 204, 207, 217-219, 221-222, 224-226, 234

Surgical Treatment, 57, 111-112, 120, 148-149, 151-152

T

Telemedicine, 168-169

Tension Headache, 6, 153, 155, 157-159

Tia, 149, 151-152, 168-172, 174-176

Timp-1, 7-12

U

Ulnar Nerve, 36, 162-163, 166-167